Handbook of MEMS for wireless and mobile applications

Related titles:

MEMS for automotive and aerospace applications
(ISBN 978-0-85709-118-5)

Smart sensors and MEMS
(ISBN 978-0-85709-502-2)

Semiconductor gas sensors
(ISBN 978-0-85709-236-6)

Details of these books and a complete list of titles from Woodhead Publishing can be obtained by:

- visiting our web site at www.woodheadpublishing.com
- contacting Customer Services (e-mail: sales@woodheadpublishing.com; fax: +44 (0) 1223 832819; tel.: +44 (0) 1223 499140 ext. 130; address: Woodhead Publishing Limited, 80 High Street, Sawston, Cambridge CB22 3HJ, UK)
- in North America, contacting our US office (e-mail: usmarketing@woodheadpublishing.com; tel.: (215) 928 9112; address: Woodhead Publishing, 1518 Walnut Street, Suite 1100, Philadelphia, PA 19102-3406, USA)

If you would like e-versions of our content, please visit our online platform: www.woodheadpublishingonline.com. Please recommend it to your librarian so that everyone in your institution can benefit from the wealth of content on the site.

We are always happy to receive suggestions for new books from potential editors. To enquire about contributing to our Electronic and Optical Materials series, please send us your name, contact address and details of the topic/s you are interested in to laura.pugh@woodheadpublishing.com. We look forward to hearing from you.

The team responsible for publishing this book:

Commissioning Editor: Laura Pugh
Publications Coordinator: Emily Cole
Project Editor: Elizabeth Moss
Editorial and Production Manager: Mary Campbell
Production Editor: Adam Hooper
Project Manager: Newgen Knowledge Works Pvt Ltd
Copyeditor: Newgen Knowledge Works Pvt Ltd
Proofreader: Newgen Knowledge Works Pvt Ltd
Cover Designer: Terry Callanan

Woodhead Publishing Series in Electronic and Optical Materials:
Number 45

Handbook of MEMS for wireless and mobile applications

Edited by
Deepak Uttamchandani

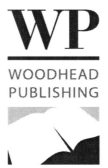

WOODHEAD
PUBLISHING

Oxford   Cambridge   Philadelphia   New Delhi

© Woodhead Publishing Limited, 2013

Published by Woodhead Publishing Limited,
80 High Street, Sawston, Cambridge CB22 3HJ, UK
www.woodheadpublishing.com
www.woodheadpublishingonline.com

Woodhead Publishing, 1518 Walnut Street, Suite 1100,
Philadelphia, PA 19102-3406, USA

Woodhead Publishing India Private Limited, 303 Vardaan House, 7/28 Ansari Road,
Daryaganj, New Delhi – 110002, India
www.woodheadpublishingindia.com

First published 2013, Woodhead Publishing Limited
© Woodhead Publishing Limited, 2013, except Chapter 12 © W. Ko and P. Feng, 2013.
The publisher has made every effort to ensure that permission for copyright material has been obtained by authors wishing to use such material. The authors and the publisher will be glad to hear from any copyright holder it has not been possible to contact. The authors have asserted their moral rights.

This book contains information obtained from authentic and highly regarded sources. Reprinted material is quoted with permission, and sources are indicated. Reasonable efforts have been made to publish reliable data and information, but the authors and the publishers cannot assume responsibility for the validity of all materials. Neither the authors nor the publishers, nor anyone else associated with this publication, shall be liable for any loss, damage or liability directly or indirectly caused or alleged to be caused by this book.

Neither this book nor any part may be reproduced or transmitted in any form or by any means, electronic or mechanical, including photocopying, microfilming and recording, or by any information storage or retrieval system, without permission in writing from Woodhead Publishing Limited.

The consent of Woodhead Publishing Limited does not extend to copying for general distribution, for promotion, for creating new works, or for resale. Specific permission must be obtained in writing from Woodhead Publishing Limited for such copying.

Trademark notice: Product or corporate names may be trademarks or registered trademarks, and are used only for identification and explanation, without intent to infringe.

British Library Cataloguing in Publication Data
A catalogue record for this book is available from the British Library.

Library of Congress Control Number: 2013942569

ISBN 978-0-85709-271-7 (print)
ISBN 978-0-85709-861-0 (online)
ISSN 2050-1501 Woodhead Publishing Series in Electronic and Optical Materials (print)
ISSN 2050-151X Woodhead Publishing Series in Electronic and Optical Materials (online)

The publisher's policy is to use permanent paper from mills that operate a sustainable forestry policy, and which has been manufactured from pulp which is processed using acid-free and elemental chlorine-free practices. Furthermore, the publisher ensures that the text paper and cover board used have met acceptable environmental accreditation standards.

Typeset by Newgen Knowledge Works Pvt Ltd
Printed by Lightning Source

Contents

Contributor contact details		*xiii*
Woodhead Publishing Series in Electronic and Optical Materials		*xvii*
Preface		*xxiii*

Part I	RF MEMS as an enabling technology for wireless applications	1
1	Overview of RF MEMS technology and applications T. PURTOVA and H. SCHUMACHER, Ulm University, Germany	3
1.1	Introduction	3
1.2	Radio frequency microelectromechanical systems (RF MEMS) operation principle and common realizations	4
1.3	RF MEMS design challenges	14
1.4	RF MEMS applications	16
1.5	Conclusion	24
1.6	Sources of further information and advice	25
1.7	Acknowledgements	25
1.8	References	25
2	Overview of wireless techniques for use with MEMS I. A. GLOVER, University of Huddersfield, UK and R. ATKINSON, University of Strathclyde, UK	30
2.1	Introduction	30
2.2	Transport layer issues	31
2.3	Network layer mobility issues	35
2.4	Data-link layer	38
2.5	Physical layer	43
2.6	The wireless link budget	59

2.7	Physical layer system design	63
2.8	Conclusion	65
2.9	References	65

3 RF MEMS fabrication technologies 67
K. GRENIER and D. DUBUC, LAAS-CNRS, University of Toulouse, France

3.1	Introduction	67
3.2	MEMS-based technologies for RF circuits with enhanced quality factor and minimized losses	68
3.3	Technologies for smart RF MEMS	79
3.4	Highlights on specific key steps in RF MEMS fabrication	81
3.5	Towards integrated technology for microsystem implementation	88
3.6	Emerging technologies in wireless applications	94
3.7	Conclusion	96
3.8	Acknowledgements	96
3.9	References	97

4 RF MEMS passive components for wireless applications 100
J. IANNACCI, Fondazione Bruno Kessler, Italy

4.1	Introduction	100
4.2	RF MEMS passive components and their applications	102
4.3	High-performance passive components enabled by RF MEMS technology	106
4.4	Complex networks based on RF MEMS passive components	126
4.5	Conclusion	131
4.6	References	131

5 RF MEMS phase shifters for wireless applications 136
V. PUYAL, CEA-LETI Laboratory, Minatec, France and LAAS-CNRS, Université de Toulouse, France and D. TITZ, Université Nice Sophia Antipolis, France

5.1	Introduction	136
5.2	Switched-line phase shifter	139
5.3	Loaded-line phase shifter	142
5.4	Reflection-type phase shifter	148
5.5	Distributed-line phase shifter	150

5.6	Mixed-architectures and exotic phase shifters	155
5.7	Towards global manufacturing	161
5.8	Applications	163
5.9	Conclusion	166
5.10	References	169

6 RF MEMS antennas for wireless applications — 176
D. RODRIGO, L. JOFRE and J. ROMEU, Universitat Politècnica de Catalunya, Spain

6.1	Introduction	176
6.2	RF MEMS antennas	177
6.3	Reconfigurable feeding networks	179
6.4	Reconfigurable antennas	185
6.5	Design considerations	197
6.6	Conclusion and future trends	201
6.7	Sources of further information and advice	202
6.8	References	202

7 RF MEMS-based wireless architectures and front-ends — 207
P. RÖJSEL, Lund University, Sweden

7.1	Introduction	207
7.2	Communication standards	209
7.3	Receivers, transmitters and transceivers: basic architectures	210
7.4	Conventional component technology	213
7.5	MEMS-based technology: filters, duplexers, switches, tunable devices and architecture	216
7.6	Diversity in receivers and transmitters	220
7.7	Multi-input multi-output (MIMO) systems	222
7.8	Systems-on-a-chip	223
7.9	Conclusion	223
7.10	Bibliography	224

8 RF MEMS technology for next-generation wireless communications — 225
F. GIACOMOZZI and J. IANNACCI, Fondazione Bruno Kessler, Italy

8.1	Introduction	225
8.2	RF MEMS technology	228
8.3	RF MEMS technology for high-performance passive components	231

8.4	Technology platform for the fabrication of RF MEMS complex circuits	244
8.5	Some examples of high-performance devices enabled by the RF MEMS technology	250
8.6	Conclusion	253
8.7	References	254

9 Wafer-level packaging technology for RF MEMS — 258
S. SEOK, IEMN CNRS, France

9.1	Introduction	258
9.2	Wafer-level zero-level packaging for RF MEMS	259
9.3	Electrical effects of the packaging material on the packaged devices	261
9.4	Packaging with hard cap materials	263
9.5	Packaging with a polymer cap	274
9.6	Conclusion	285
9.7	References	288

10 Reliability of RF MEMS — 291
I. DE WOLF, P. CZARNECKI, J. DE COSTER, O. V. PEDREIRA, X. ROTTENBERG and S. SANGAMESWARAN, imec, Belgium

10.1	Introduction	291
10.2	Overview of failure mechanisms in RF MEMS	292
10.3	Charging in RF MEMS	297
10.4	Analytical modelling	309
10.5	Electrostatic discharge	319
10.6	Reliability issues of MEMS packages	324
10.7	Conclusion	337
10.8	References	338

Part II Wireless techniques and applications of wireless MEMS — 343

11 Energy harvesters for powering wireless systems — 345
G. DE PASQUALE, Politecnico di Torino, Italy

11.1	Introduction	345
11.2	Kinetic energy harvesters	346
11.3	Design of kinetic energy harvesters	356
11.4	Other typologies of energy harvesters	384
11.5	Conclusion	392

| 11.6 | References | 392 |
| 11.7 | Appendix: list of symbols | 397 |

12 MEMS wireless implantable systems: historical review and perspectives — 401
W. Ko and P. X.-L. Feng, Case Western Reserve University, USA

12.1	Introduction	401
12.2	Basic considerations and characteristics of wireless MEMS implantable systems	403
12.3	Significant research on radio frequency implantable systems from 1955 to 1975	408
12.4	Progress of implantable systems from 1980 to 2010	416
12.5	Challenges of implantable/attached electronics	417
12.6	Conclusion and future trends	419
12.7	Acknowledgements	421
12.8	References	421

13 Wireless considerations in ocular implants based on microsystems — 424
W. Li, Michigan State University, USA

13.1	Introduction	424
13.2	Challenges of wireless ocular implants	425
13.3	Considerations of ocular microsystems	428
13.4	Applications of wireless microsystems in ocular implants	435
13.5	Necessary improvements in wireless ocular implants	449
13.6	Conclusion	450
13.7	References	451

14 MEMS-based wireless intraocular pressure sensors — 463
R. Blue and D. Uttamchandani, University of Strathclyde, UK

14.1	Introduction	463
14.2	Passive miniature implants for intraocular pressure (IOP) sensing	464
14.3	Introduction of active MEMS systems for IOP implants	467
14.4	Flexible parylene platforms for long-term MEMS implants	470
14.5	Design of custom ultra-low-power autonomous IOP sensors	474

14.6	Active and passive MEMS contact lenses for IOP monitoring	483
14.7	Conclusion	486
14.8	References	486

15	**Drug delivery using wireless MEMS**	**489**
	R. Sheybani, S. M. Schober and E. Meng, University of Southern California, USA	
15.1	Introduction	489
15.2	Wireless power and data for drug delivery applications	490
15.3	A MEMS approach to drug delivery	493
15.4	Biological constraints and requirements	502
15.5	Security concerns for wireless implants	503
15.6	Wireless inductive powering and uni-directional data system for a MEMS drug pump	505
15.7	Suggested improvements and future generation device	509
15.8	Conclusion	512
15.9	Acknowledgment	513
15.10	References	513

16	**RF MEMS for automotive radar**	**518**
	J. Oberhammer, N. Somjit, U. Shah and Z. Baghchehsaraei, KTH Royal Institute of Technology, Sweden	
16.1	Introduction	518
16.2	RF MEMS components for automotive radar	522
16.3	Example of RF MEMS-based automotive radar front-end technology	532
16.4	Unconventional MEMS radar beam-steering technologies	537
16.5	Conclusion	546
16.6	References	546

17	**Telecommunications reliability monitoring using wireless MEMS**	**550**
	M. Hautefeuille, Universidad Nacional Autónoma de México, Mexico	
17.1	Introduction	550
17.2	Typical reliability issues in telecommunication systems	551

17.3	Reliability monitoring with wireless MEMS	554
17.4	Case study: multi-MEMS platform	559
17.5	Conclusion	565
17.6	Acknowledgements	566
17.7	References	566
18	**Optical MEMS for displays in portable systems**	**569**
	W. O. DAVIS, MicroVision Inc., USA	
18.1	Introduction	569
18.2	MEMS-based direct-view displays	570
18.3	Handheld picoprojectors	576
18.4	Automobile head-up display	585
18.5	Eyewear displays	587
18.6	Conclusion	591
18.7	References	592
	Index	*595*

Contributor contact details

(* = main contact)

Editor

Professor Deepak Uttamchandani
University of Strathclyde
UK

E-mail: d.uttamchandani@strath.ac.uk

Chapter 1

Dr Tatyana Purtova and Professor Hermann Schumacher*
Institute of Electron Devices and Circuits
Ulm University
Albert-Einstein-Allee 45
89081 Ulm, Germany

E-mail: hermann.schumacher@uni-ulm.de

Chapter 2

Professor Ian A. Glover*
University of Huddersfield
Queensgate
Huddersfield
HD1 3DH, UK

E-mail: i.a.glover@hud.ac.uk

Robert Atkinson
University of Strathclyde
UK

E-mail: robert.atkinson@strath.ac.uk

Chapter 3

Dr Katia Grenier* and Dr David Dubuc
CNRS, LAAS, University of Toulouse
7 Avenue du Colonel Roche
F-31400 Toulouse, France

E-mail: grenier@laas.fr

Chapter 4

Dr Jacopo Iannacci
Center for Materials and Microsystems – CMM
Fondazione Bruno Kessler – FBK
Via Sommarive 18
38123, Povo
Trento, Italy

E-mail: iannacci@fbk.eu

Chapter 5

Dr Vincent Puyal*
CEA, LETI, DACLE/LAIR
MINATEC
17, rue des Martyrs
38054 Grenoble Cedex 9, France

E-mail: vincent.puyal@cea.fr

and

LAAS-CNRS
7, Avenue du Colonel Roche
  BP 54200
31031 Toulouse Cedex 4, France

Dr Diane Titz
EPIB, Université Nice-Sophia
  Antipolis
Lycée Jules Ferry
82, bd de la République
06400 Cannes, France

E-mail: diane.titz@unice.fr

Chapter 6

Daniel Rodrigo, Dr Lluis Jofre* and
  Jordi Romeu
Signal Theory and Communications
  Department
Universitat Politecnica de
  Catalunya
D3 Building
Jordi Girona, 1–3
Barcelona 08034, Spain

E-mail: rodrigo@tsc.upc.edu; jofre@
  tsc.upc.edu; romeu@tsc.upc.edu

Chapter 7

Dr Peter Röjsel
Lund University
Sweden

E-mail: peter.rojsel@gmail.com

Chapter 8

Flavio Giacomozzi* and Dr Jacopo
  Iannacci
Center for Materials and
  Microsystems – CMM
Fondazione Bruno Kessler – FBK
Via Sommarive 18
38123, Povo
Trento, Italy

E-mail: giaco@fbk.eu; iannacci@
  fbk.eu

Chapter 9

Dr Seonho Seok
IEMN UMR CNRS 8520
Laboratoire Central – Cité
  Scientifique – Avenue Poincaré –
  BP 60069 – 59652
Villeneuve d'ascq cedex, France

E-mail: seonho.seok@iemn.univ-
  lille1.fr

Chapter 10

Professor Ingrid De Wolf*, Dr Piotr
  Czarnecki, Dr Jeroen De Coster,
  Olalla Varela Pedreira, Dr Xavier
  Rottenberg and Dr Sandeep
  Sangameswaran
imec
Kapeldreef 75
B-3000 Leuven, Belgium

E-mail: ingrid.dewolf@imec.be

Chapter 11

Dr Giorgio De Pasquale
Department of Mechanical and
  Aerospace Engineering
Politecnico di Torino
Corso Duca degli Abruzzi 24
10129 Torino, Italy

E-mail: giorgio.depasquale@polito.it

Chapter 12

Dr W. Ko* and P. X.-L. Feng
Department of Electrical
  Engineering and Computer
  Science
Case School of Engineering
Case Western Reserve University
10900 Euclid Avenue
Cleveland
Ohio 44106, USA

E-mail: whk@cwru.edu; philip.
  feng@case.edu

Chapter 13

Dr Wen Li
Michigan State University
428 S. Shaw Lane
2120 Engineering Building
East Lansing
MI 48824, USA

E-mail: wenli@egr.msu.edu

Chapter 14

Dr Robert Blue and Professor
  Deepak Uttamchandani*
Centre for Microsystems and
  Photonics
Department of Electronic and
  Electrical Engineering
University of Strathclyde
204 George St
Glasgow G432YL, UK

E-mail: robert.blue@eee.strath.
  ac.uk; d.uttamchandani@strath.
  ac.uk

Chapter 15

R. Sheybani
Department of Biomedical
  Engineering 1042 Downey Way
University of Southern California
DRB-140 Los Angeles
CA 90089–1111 USA

E-mail: rsheyban@usc.edu

S. M. Schober
Ming Hsieh Department of
  Electrical Engineering
University of Southern California
3740 McClintock Avenue
EEB 100 Los Angeles
CA 90089–2560 USA

E-mail: schober@usc.edu

Dr Ellis Meng*
Department of Biomedical
  Engineering
1042 Downey Way
University of Southern California
DRB-140 Los Angeles
CA 90089–1111 USA

E-mail: ellis.meng@usc.edu

and

Ming Hsieh Department of
  Electrical Engineering
University of Southern California
3740 McClintock Avenue
EEB 100 Los Angeles
CA 90089–2560 USA

Chapter 16

Dr Joachim Oberhammer*,
Nutapong Somjit, Umer Shah
and Zargham Baghchehsaraei
KTH Royal Institute of Technology
School of Electrical Engineering
Microsystem Technology Lab
Osquldas väg 10
SE-100 44 Stockholm, Sweden

E-mail: joachim.oberhammer@ee.kth.se

Chapter 17

Dr Mathieu Hautefeuille
Universidad Nacional Autónoma de México
Facultad de Ciencias
Avenida Universidad 3000, Circuito Exterior S/N
Col. Universidad Nacional Autónoma de México C.U., CP 04510
Del. Coyoacán, Distrito Federal, Mexico

E-mail: mathieu_h@ciencias.unam.mx

Chapter 18

Dr Wyatt O. Davis
MicroVision, Inc.
6222 185th Ave NE, Redmond
Washington 98052, USA

E-mail: wyatt_davis@microvision.com

Woodhead Publishing Series in Electronic and Optical Materials

1 **Circuit analysis**
   J. E. Whitehouse
2 **Signal processing in electronic communications: For engineers and mathematicians**
   M. J. Chapman, D. P. Goodall and N. C. Steele
3 **Pattern recognition and image processing**
   D. Luo
4 **Digital filters and signal processing in electronic engineering: Theory, applications, architecture, code**
   S. M. Bozic and R. J. Chance
5 **Cable engineering for local area networks**
   B. J. Elliott
6 **Designing a structured cabling system to ISO 11801: Cross-referenced to European CENELEC and American Standards**
   Second edition
   B. J. Elliott
7 **Microscopy techniques for materials science**
   A. Clarke and C. Eberhardt
8 **Materials for energy conversion devices**
   Edited by C. C. Sorrell, J. Nowotny and S. Sugihara
9 **Digital image processing: Mathematical and computational methods**
   Second edition
   J. M. Blackledge
10 **Nanolithography and patterning techniques in microelectronics**
   Edited by D. Bucknall
11 **Digital signal processing: Mathematical and computational methods, software development and applications**
   Second edition
   J. M. Blackledge

12 **Handbook of advanced dielectric, piezoelectric and ferroelectric materials: Synthesis, properties and applications**
Edited by Z.-G. Ye
13 **Materials for fuel cells**
Edited by M. Gasik
14 **Solid-state hydrogen storage: Materials and chemistry**
Edited by G. Walker
15 **Laser cooling of solids**
S. V. Petrushkin and V. V. Samartsev
16 **Polymer electrolytes: Fundamentals and applications**
Edited by C. A. C. Sequeira and D. A. F. Santos
17 **Advanced piezoelectric materials: Science and technology**
Edited by K. Uchino
18 **Optical switches: Materials and design**
Edited by S. J. Chua and B. Li
19 **Advanced adhesives in electronics: Materials, properties and applications**
Edited by M. O. Alam and C. Bailey
20 **Thin film growth: Physics, materials science and applications**
Edited by Z. Cao
21 **Electromigration in thin films and electronic devices: Materials and reliability**
Edited by C.-U. Kim
22 ***In situ* characterization of thin film growth**
Edited by G. Koster and G. Rijnders
23 **Silicon-germanium (SiGe) nanostructures: Production, properties and applications in electronics**
Edited by Y. Shiraki and N. Usami
24 **High-temperature superconductors**
Edited by X. G. Qiu
25 **Introduction to the physics of nanoelectronics**
S. G. Tan and M. B. A. Jalil
26 **Printed films: Materials science and applications in sensors, electronics and photonics**
Edited by M. Prudenziati and J. Hormadaly
27 **Laser growth and processing of photonic devices**
Edited by N. A. Vainos
28 **Quantum optics with semiconductor nanostructures**
Edited by F. Jahnke
29 **Ultrasonic transducers: Materials and design for sensors, actuators and medical applications**
Edited by K. Nakamura

30 **Waste electrical and electronic equipment (WEEE) handbook**
  Edited by V. Goodship and A. Stevels
31 **Applications of ATILA FEM software to smart materials: Case studies in designing devices**
  Edited by K. Uchino and J.-C. Debus
32 **MEMS for automotive and aerospace applications**
  Edited by M. Kraft and N. M. White
33 **Semiconductor lasers: Fundamentals and applications**
  Edited by A. Baranov and E. Tournie
34 **Handbook of terahertz technology for imaging, sensing and communications**
  Edited by D. Saeedkia
35 **Handbook of solid-state lasers: Materials, systems and applications**
  Edited by B. Denker and E. Shklovsky
36 **Organic light-emitting diodes: Materials, devices and applications**
  Edited by A. Buckley
37 **Lasers for medical applications: Diagnostics, therapy and surgery**
  Edited by H. Jelínková
38 **Semiconductor gas sensors**
  Edited by R. Jaaniso and O. K. Tan
39 **Handbook of organic materials for optical and (opto)electronic devices: Properties and applications**
  Edited by O. Ostroverkhova
40 **Metallic films for electronic, optical and magnetic applications: Structure, processing and properties**
  Edited by K. Barmak and K. Coffey
41 **Handbook of laser welding technologies**
  Edited by S. Katayama
42 **Nanolithography: The art of fabricating nanoelectronic and nanophotonic devices and systems**
  Edited by M. Feldman
43 **Laser spectroscopy for sensing: Fundamentals, techniques and applications**
  Edited by M. Baudelet
44 **Chalcogenide glasses: Preparation, properties and applications**
  Edited by J.-L. Adam and X. Zhang
45 **Handbook of MEMS for wireless and mobile applications**
  Edited by D. Uttamchandani
46 **Subsea optics and imaging**
  Edited by J. Watson and O. Zielinski
47 **Carbon nanotubes and graphene for photonic applications**
  Edited by S. Yamashita, Y. Saito and J. H. Choi

48 **Optical biomimetics: Materials and applications**
   Edited by M. Large
49 **Optical thin films and coatings**
   Edited by A. Piegari and F. Flory
50 **Computer design of diffractive optics**
   Edited by V. A. Soifer
51 **Smart sensors and MEMS: Intelligent devices and microsystems for industrial applications**
   Edited by S. Nihtianov and A. Luque
52 **Fundamentals of femtosecond optics**
   S. A. Kozlov and V. V. Samartsev
53 **Nanostructured semiconductor oxides for the next generation of electronics and functional devices: Production, properties and applications**
   S. Zhuiykov

To Barbara for demonstrating strength and determination in adversity and Arun for perseverance with choir, golf, skiing, swimming, tae-kwon-do and violin.

Preface

The field of MEMS has made great advances over the last thirty years or so. The commercialization of MEMS from international research laboratories into everyday products has been impressive, and is an example of successful translational research originating from engineering science and technology. The incorporation of MEMS in radio-frequency (RF) devices and sub-systems is covered in a number of existing books and publications, and it is clear that there is yet more research to be undertaken and more innovation to be achieved in the field of radio-frequency microelectromechanical systems (RF MEMS). New processes, new materials and new device architectures remain to be discovered and implemented. There is, moreover, a high expectation that some of the initial research in this field is at the cusp of major commercialization.

In compiling this book, we have taken into consideration both the scope of those books and publications already available and the present status of RF MEMS technology. In order to add new knowledge to the field from a different perspective, we have followed the approach of addressing the advances that have been made in wireless systems and applications that incorporate microelectromechanical systems (MEMS) to achieve particular functions. This means that in this book we have looked at the latest trends in RF MEMS devices and components, and beyond that we have examined systems in which those other types of MEMS devices, such as MEMS microsensors, have been incorporated, and where portability and mobility using wireless technology are the key requirements. It is on this basis that the present volume differs from other books. The MEMS components and sub-systems that are covered herein do not all operate at RF frequencies; rather, we are looking at advanced systems and applications that use wireless protocols and technology to achieve mobility, and which incorporate various MEMS devices due to their advantages of size, weight, power consumption, cost and performance. For this reason we have included a chapter on energy harvesting, for instance, since this is an enabling technology for next generation wireless sensor nodes and networks.

This book is arranged in two parts. Part I, comprising ten chapters, deals with RF MEMS as an enabling technology. This part covers the latest trends in fabrication and technology: in RF MEMS components including RF antennas and RF front-ends, and wafer-level packaging and reliability. All the chapters are in the field that would traditionally be described as 'RF MEMS'. Also in this part of the book we have included an overview chapter on wireless techniques and protocols, so that the reader can gain a comprehensive systems overview and understanding of the protocols and issues associated with the flow of data in present day wireless nodes and networks.

Part II of the book, comprising eight chapters, focuses on applications addressing a diverse range of portable, wireless and mobile systems incorporating all types of MEMS. Chapters in this section cover energy harvesting for powering wireless systems, and implantable biomedical microsystems (for ocular and drug delivery applications), combining wireless technology and MEMS from a historical and present day perspective. MEMS in automotive radar, in telecommunication systems, and in portable display systems are also covered.

We believe that we have produced a unique volume which covers both 'basics' and 'applied'. I am very grateful to all of our very busy authors, who found the time to provide their valued contributions to what we all hope will be a significant and important book that will expand the knowledge in this field. I would also like to record my thanks to the staff at Woodhead Publishing for their professionalism and dedication in bringing this project to completion.

Deepak Uttamchandani

Part I
RF MEMS as an enabling technology for wireless applications

1
Overview of RF MEMS technology and applications

T. PURTOVA and H. SCHUMACHER,
Ulm University, Germany

DOI: 10.1533/9780857098610.1.3

Abstract: This chapter presents an introduction to radio frequency microelectromechanical systems (RF MEMS) technologies for wireless applications. It starts with reviewing the operation principle and common realizations of electrostatically actuated components. It is shown that RF MEMS advantages materialize especially at higher frequencies, and for applications requiring high linearity. The chapter then moves on to present exemplary RF MEMS applications. It is pointed out that while RF MEMS components have few opportunities as a one-on-one replacement for existing switch technologies, they are extremely attractive in RF MEMS-only subsystems. Besides, emerging monolithic BiCMOS-RF MEMS integration opens up new opportunities for millimeter-wave integrated circuits (ICs).

Key words: RF MEMS, millimetre-wave, switch, low-noise amplifier (LNA), voltage-controlled oscillator (VCO), impedance tuner.

1.1 Introduction

Switches and variable capacitors are important building blocks of radio frequency integrated circuits (RFICs). Due to the rapid advancement of RF complementary metal–oxide–semiconductor (CMOS) technologies, MOS switches are gaining in importance, but are still used typically below 6 GHz, and rarely up to 20 GHz (e.g. Talwalkar *et al.*, 2004; Pao *et al.*, 2006; Jin and Nguyen, 2007). For millimetre-wave applications III-V field effect transistors (FETs) or pin-diode switches can be used (e.g. Buber *et al.*, 2003; Kallfass *et al.*, 2008), but they suffer from increasing losses at high frequencies. Similar arguments apply to semiconductor varactors. Besides, the linearity of all semiconductor components is rather limited.

In contrast, radio frequency microelectromechanical systems (RF MEMS) can provide low loss even at elevated frequencies and inherently high linearity, since RF MEMS components do not contain non-linear elements, such as semiconductor junctions or ferroelectrics. The low loss originates mainly from the fact that RF MEMS can be fabricated at low temperatures and thus are often made of low-loss metals, such as gold, aluminium or copper. The insertion loss of a single-pole–single-throw switch can be as low as 0.3 dB up to 100 GHz, with the upper RF power limit of 15 dBm (hot switching) (Kaynak *et al.*, 2011, 2012). With proper techniques, RF MEMS components with several watts power handling have also been developed (e.g. Palego *et al.*, 2010).

The purpose of this chapter is to explain concisely the operational principles of the most common RF MEMS components, their electromagnetic and electromechanical modelling, and their fabrication procedure. Those aspects in which MEMS are better than their semiconductor counterparts are discussed, while associated challenges and bottle-necks are identified. Finally, several applications for which RF MEMS are significantly more advantageous than semiconductor-based components are presented.

1.2 Radio frequency microelectromechanical systems (RF MEMS) operation principle and common realizations

The main distinguishing feature of RF MEMS is that their electromagnetic properties are mechanically reconfigurable by moveable parts. It clearly differentiates them from just 'micromachined', or membrane-supported, components, where no moveable parts are present and the goal is to either improve quality factors of passive components (e.g. spiral inductors (Lin *et al.*, 2005) or transmission lines (Neculoiu *et al.*, 2001)) or to increase antenna bandwidth (Neculoiu *et al.*, 2004). The movement can be utilized for design of microelectromechanical switches with either capacitive or ohmic contacts. Besides, tuneable or switchable capacitors and, to a lesser extent, switchable inductors can be developed.

The moving force can be of electrostatic, thermal, electromagnetic or piezoelectric origin (a detailed description can be found, for example, in Pelesko and Bernstein (2003)). Electrostatic actuation is by far the most commonly used, due to its negligible DC power consumption, fast switching (as compared to other MEMS actuation mechanisms, for example thermal), the possibility of biasing with high-resistivity lines not interfering with the RF signal, as well as a fabrication process compatible with standard microelectronics techniques. Due to the practical importance of electrostatic actuation, its electromechanical and electromagnetic aspects are briefly reviewed below.

1.2.1 Electromechanical analysis of electrostatic MEMS

Despite the large number of possible RF MEMS realizations, all of them can be generally described by an equivalent mass-spring model (Pelesko and

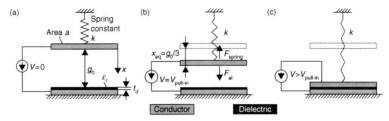

1.1 Parallel-plate model of an electrostatically actuated RF MEMS: (a) initial position, (b) at static pull-in, (c) after static pull-in. In practice, the spring displacement is much smaller than the not-to-scale figure shows.

Bernstein, 2003). Figure 1.1 shows such a model for the electrostatic case (Purtova, 2012). It consists of a pair of plates: one suspended in the air by a spring, and one fixed to a surface. Due to an applied potential difference, V, charges of opposite polarity arise on the two plates, generating an attractive electrostatic force, which moves the suspended plate towards the fixed plate. The model has one degree of freedom, allowing movement only along the x-axis. For simplicity, but without loss of physical insight, the following analysis neglects fringing electric fields and bending of the moveable plate, resulting in an ideal parallel-plate movement (Pelesko and Bernstein, 2003).

Static pull-in

Static analysis assumes that the applied voltage is increasing slowly enough that at any moment of time the system is in static equilibrium, that is, the total force is zero and the moveable plate is at rest. Thus, inertia and damping have no effect on the movement of the membrane. This somewhat artificial approach facilitates understanding of important physical processes, as shown in the following.

Initially, the two plates are at the same DC-potential (Fig. 1.1a, $V = 0$) and the spring is in equilibrium. As a small potential difference V is applied (Fig. 1.1b), an attractive electrostatic force F_{el} is created between the plates and the suspended plate moves towards the fixed plate. Simultaneously, the spring force F_{spring} increases to oppose this movement. For most RF MEMS, the displacement is small (typically below 1% of the spring's length), so that the spring remains linear and the spring force F_{spring} is defined by Hooke's law (Equation [1.1]):

$$F_{spring} = -kx \qquad [1.1]$$

The conductive plates in Fig. 1.1 have an area a, are separated from each other by a distance g_0, the dielectric thickness is t_d and the suspending spring has a spring constant k and the electrostatic force F_{el} is given by Equation [1.2]:

$$F_{el} = -\frac{1}{2}\frac{\varepsilon_0 a V^2}{\left(g_0 + \dfrac{t_d}{\varepsilon_r} - x\right)^2} \qquad [1.2]$$

For small V both forces balance each other at equilibrium position g_0-x_{eq}, obtained by equating force magnitudes: $|F_{el}| = |F_{spring}|$. However, above a certain voltage called 'static pull-in voltage', the electrostatic force exceeds the spring force for all displacements. Thus, no equilibrium position exists and the suspended plate moves all the way down onto the fixed plate, as illustrated in Fig. 1.1c. The application of this so-called 'pull-in' effect in microelectronics circuits was first reported by Nathanson et al. more than 40 years ago in their research on resonant gate transistors (Nathanson et al., 1967).

The pull-in effect can be easily explained using Fig. 1.2, where magnitudes of electrostatic and spring forces are qualitatively plotted against the displacement x (Purtova, 2012). Curve A corresponds to a small voltage, at which an equilibrium position does exist (despite the two possible equilibrium positions, only one of them is physical). Curve C corresponds to a high voltage, when $|F_{el}|$ is always larger than $|F_{spring}|$ and there is no stable point for the moving plate. Curve B illustrates the limiting case, corresponding to the 'pull-in' condition. The pull-in voltage $V_{pull-in}$, and the corresponding equilibrium position $x_{pull-in}$, are derived from the cross-sectional point of the curve B and the spring force in Fig. 1.2, where both magnitudes and their partial derivatives are equal:

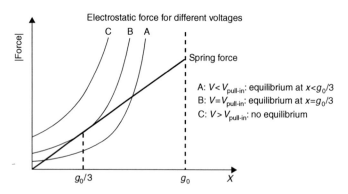

1.2 Magnitudes of electrostatic and spring forces acting on a suspended plate shown in Fig. 1.1 versus plate displacement x.

$$\begin{cases} |F_{el}| = |F_{spring}| \\ \dfrac{\partial |F_{el}|}{\partial x} = \dfrac{\partial |F_{spring}|}{\partial x} \end{cases}$$

Then the solutions for $x_{\text{pull-in}}$ and $V_{\text{pull-in}}$ are:

$$\begin{cases} x_{\text{stat.pull-in}} = \dfrac{\left(g_0 + (t_d/\varepsilon_r)\right)}{3} \\ V_{\text{stat.pull-in}} = \sqrt{\dfrac{8k\left(g_0 + (t_d/\varepsilon_r)\right)^3}{27\varepsilon_0 a}} \end{cases} \quad [1.3]$$

Thus, the static pull-in happens when the equilibrium position x_{eq} equals exactly one-third of the zero-voltage plates separation $g_0 + t_d/\varepsilon$ (Fig. 1.1b) and x_{eq} is independent of any other system parameter.

Dynamic pull-in

As mentioned earlier, static analysis assumes that the applied voltage is increased slowly. However, often electrostatic MEMS are actuated by a voltage step-function, causing fast movement of the membrane. Thus, inertia and damping must be taken into account. If damping is small and inertia is large, it is expected that the membrane will overshoot the static equilibrium position, at least for a short time. Besides, in the case of low damping, the pull-in voltage should be smaller as compared to the static case, since the inertial force is acting in the same direction as the electrostatic force.

These intuitive expectations can be confirmed analytically. A detailed analysis of the dynamic response for the case of a step-function actuation can be found in Elata and Bamberger (2004, 2006); Leus and Elata (2008). For convenience, final equations for the dynamic pull-in voltage and the corresponding deflection are repeated here:

$$\begin{cases} x_{\text{dyn.pull-in}} = \dfrac{\left(g_0 + (t_d/\varepsilon_r)\right)}{2} \\ V_{\text{dyn.pull-in}} = \sqrt{\dfrac{k\left(g_0 + (t_d/\varepsilon_r)\right)^3}{4\varepsilon_0 a}} \end{cases} \quad [1.4]$$

Comparing Equation [1.4] to Equation [1.3] reveals that the dynamic pull-in voltage is about 8% smaller than that derived from the static analysis. The maximum deflection corresponds to one-half of the initial plate separations, whereas for the static case it is only one-third. This confirms intuitive expectations that due to inertia the membrane can overshoot the static equilibrium position and the voltage required for the pull-in is smaller than that obtained from the static analysis.

Switching time

Switching time is determined as the time taken for the membrane to move from its initial position (unbiased) to the final state once the actuation voltage is applied. It is an important parameter, critical especially in such RF MEMS applications as transmit/receive (T/R) switches or phase shifters.

The equation for the switching time of the parallel-plate system shown in Fig. 1.1 has been derived numerically in (Leus and Elata, 2008), resulting in compact and accurate closed-form equations for the switching time. The solutions are repeated here for convenience:

$$t_s = \begin{cases} \dfrac{5.223 - \ln(\partial_1)}{2\omega_0}, & \text{for } V = V_{\text{dyn.pull-in}}(1-\partial_1) \\ \dfrac{2.068 - \ln(\partial_2)}{\omega_0}, & \text{for } V = V_{\text{dyn.pull-in}}(1+\partial_2) \end{cases} \quad [1.5]$$

Here, ∂_1 and ∂_2 determine V as a function of $V_{\text{dyn.pull-in}}$ with $0 < \partial_1 < 1$, and $0 < \partial_2 \ll 1$, and ω_0 is the mechanical resonance frequency of the system in the undamped case (m – spring mass):

$$\omega_0^2 = \frac{k}{m} \quad [1.6]$$

As follows from Equation [1.5], switching time is fully determined by the mechanical resonance frequency ω_0 and the applied voltage V.

Release time

When the actuation voltage is removed, the restoring spring force moves the plate upwards to its initial position. This process can be described by free oscillations of the mass-spring system shown in Fig. 1.1. The governing equation is given below, where η is the damping coefficient and ω_0 is given by Equation [1.6]:

$$\frac{dx^2}{dt^2} + \eta \frac{dx}{dt} + \omega_0^2 x = 0$$

The solution is a harmonic function given below:

$$\begin{cases} x(t) = e^{-\frac{\eta}{2}t}[c_1 \cos(\omega_d t) + c_2 \sin(\omega_d t)] \\ \omega_d = \sqrt{\omega_0^2 - \frac{\eta^2}{4}} \\ c_1 = x_{|t=0} \\ c_2 = \frac{1}{\omega_d}\left(\frac{\eta}{2} x_{|t=0} + \frac{dx}{dt_{|t=0}}\right) \end{cases} \quad [1.7]$$

Its angular frequency is ω_d and the amplitude is decaying with time according to $e^{-\eta/2 t}$ term. The parameters ω_d and η fully determine the release process of MEMS devices. The higher the frequency ω_d, the faster is the release of the RF MEMS component. The higher the damping coefficient η, the faster the oscillations following the release settle. The constants c_1 and c_2 are found by satisfying the initial conditions for position and velocity. Typically, at $t = 0$ the moveable plate is at the down position and is not moving, that is, $x_{|t=0} = g_0$ and $dx/dt_{|t=0} = 0$. However, Equation [1.7] assumes that the damping coefficient η does not vary with deflection. Generally, this is not true, since the damping force increases non-linearly with increasing deflection. Still, it is common to neglect such damping variations for simplicity (e.g. Gupta and Senturia, 1997).

1.2.2 Common RF MEMS components and their electromagnetic analysis

RF MEMS components can be realized in various ways, differing not only in actuation mechanism, but also in configuration (shunt or series), contact type (capacitive or ohmic) and mechanical design (bridge, cantilever, circular diaphragm). Quite frequently used combinations are electrostatically actuated shunt capacitive bridges and series ohmic cantilevers. These two types of RF MEMS are described later.

Shunt capacitive switches and switchable capacitors

Capacitive switches and switchable capacitors are often realized as moveable air-bridges placed in shunt to a transmission line, as schematically shown in Fig. 1.3. A coplanar configuration is used in most cases, since the air-bridge can be easily grounded. When no voltage is applied, the air-bridge is said to be in the up-state and it acts as a small shunt capacitor, mainly due to the overlap with the underlying signal line. If the applied voltage is above the pull-in value (Equation [1.4]), the bridge snaps down onto the underlying electrode covered with a dielectric layer, and the shunt capacitance greatly

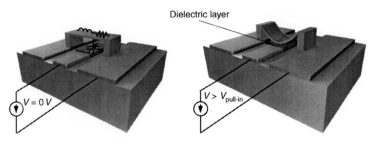

1.3 Schematic illustration of a MEMS bridge in shunt to a coplanar line in the up- (left) and down-states (right).

increases. Thus, a voltage-controlled capacitance is obtained, which can be utilized to construct shunt capacitive switches or switchable capacitors. The SEM image in Fig. 1.4 illustrates a typical example of a shunt capacitive switch, developed in Purtova (2012) using RF MEMS technology of the Fraunhofer Institute for Silicon Technology (ISiT) (Lisec *et al.*, 2004).

A simplified equivalent circuit of a shunt capacitive RF MEMS component is shown in Fig. 1.5. The impedance of the shunt bridge Z_{shunt} is generally formed by the MEMS capacitance, inductance and resistance as defined by Equation [1.8]:

$$Z_{shunt} = \frac{1}{j\omega C} + j\omega L + R \qquad [1.8]$$

The variation of the impedance with frequency is qualitatively described by Equation [1.9]:

$$Z_{shunt} = \begin{cases} \frac{1}{j\omega C} & f \ll f_{res} \\ R & f = f_{res} \\ j\omega L & f \gg f_{res} \end{cases} \qquad [1.9]$$

where f_{res} is the MEMS LC resonance frequency:

$$f_{res} = \frac{1}{2\pi\sqrt{LC}} \qquad [1.10]$$

The up-state capacitance C_{up} is typically small, resulting in a very low insertion loss (<0.5 dB). For a switchable capacitor operation, down-state capacitance C_{down} is only 3–6 times larger than the up-state capacitance. For a switch operation, the difference in capacitance should be maximized and C_{down} is typically 10–20 times larger than C_{up}. At the frequency f_{res},

Overview of RF MEMS technology and applications 11

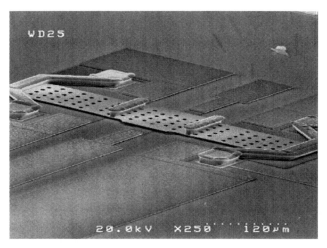

1.4 SEM image of a shunt RF MEMS switch.

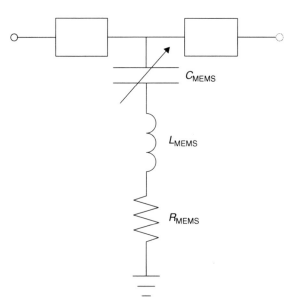

1.5 Equivalent circuit of a shunt capacitive MEMS switch or variable capacitor.

the down-state capacitance resonates with the MEMS inductance, leading almost to a short-circuit limited only by the resistance R_{MEMS}. Since this resistance is typically below 1 Ω, the isolation at f_{res} is often higher than 30 dB. Thus, the optimum operation point for such switches is around f_{res}, which is typically in the millimetre-wave frequency range.

Series switches with ohmic contact

Series switches with ohmic (metal-to-metal) contact are often constructed as a coplanar line with an interrupted centre conductor and a MEMS cantilever, as schematically illustrated in Fig. 1.6. The free end of the cantilever slightly overlaps the coplanar line centre conductor. The actuation electrode is DC-isolated from the coplanar line and is located below the cantilever. When a high enough voltage is applied, the cantilever snaps down and closes the gap in the coplanar line through a metal-to-metal contact. To prevent any short-circuit with the cantilever, the actuation electrode is covered with a dielectric. An SEM image shown in Fig. 1.7 illustrates such a component (Purtova, 2012) realized in ISiT RF MEMS technology (Lisec *et al.*, 2004).

A simplified equivalent circuit of a metal-to-metal contact MEMS cantilever is shown in Fig. 1.8. The impedance in the up-state state is dominated by the small capacitance C_{up}, resulting from the overlap of the cantilever's free end and the centre conductor and capacitance through substrate C_{coup}.

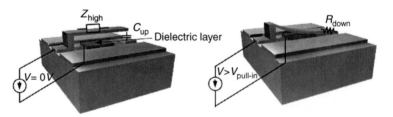

1.6 Schematic illustration a MEMS cantilever in series with a coplanar line in the up- (left) and down-states (right).

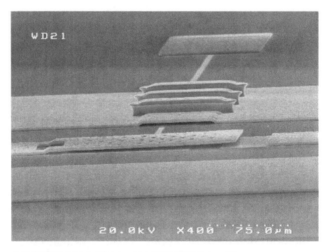

1.7 SEM image of a series RF MEMS cantilever.

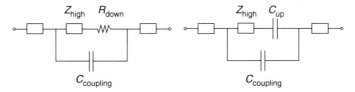

1.8 Equivalent circuit of a series MEMS switch with a metal-to-metal contact in the up- (left) and down-states (right).

The down-state impedance is mainly determined by the series resistance R_{down}, which includes contact resistance and the losses in the membrane. Such a switch works best up to microwave frequencies, since isolation considerably degrades as frequency increases to millimetre-waves.

1.2.3 RF MEMS fabrication

Up to now no standard RF MEMS manufacturing procedure has been developed. Practically each RF MEMS foundry or research lab has its own fabrication process, which may differ in substrate, metal, dielectric and sacrificial layers, micromachining techniques and release procedure. Still, some similarities can be defined, as briefly described in the following.

Most RF MEMS fabrication processes utilize surface micromachining, that is, deposition and structuring of diverse dielectric and metal layers on top of a substrate. Low-loss substrates, such as high-resistivity silicon, quartz, glass and GaAs, are usually chosen. Due to low fabrication temperatures, highly conductive metals such as gold, aluminium or copper can be used. Non-moveable electrodes (often called bottom electrodes or underpasses) are typically rather thin, about half a micron, and are often deposited via etching or lift-off. Such deposition techniques result in low surface roughness, important for high down-state capacitance in capacitive switches. However, over-smooth surfaces are undesirable, since they may lead to sticking of the moveable membrane in the down-state due to humidity or other effects. Moveable membranes are typically between half a micron to several microns in thickness and are deposited by electroplating or sputtering. The membrane thickness is an important parameter, since it influences both RF losses (thus, the thickness should be greater than several skin depths at the operation frequency) as well as the membrane's spring constant and mass (thus, the pull-in voltage and switching time) of the component.

As for dielectric layers, the most commonly used ones are plasma-enhanced chemical vapour deposition (PECVD) SiN, as well as low-temperature or PECVD SiO_2, since they are commonly available in many microelectronics processes. However, these materials, and especially SiN, are prone to accumulation of charges under high voltage conditions (so-called dielectric charging', see, e.g. Rebeiz, 2003) that degrade MEMS reliability. On the other hand, the less commonly available AlN has been shown to be much less prone to charging (Lisec *et al.*, 2004a; Ruan *et al.*, 2007) and is used for example in the Fraunhofer ISiT fabrication process (Lisec *et al.*, 2004).

An important step of RF MEMS fabrication is the release process, when the sacrificial layer is removed to obtain a free-standing structure. Most of the time photoresist is used as the sacrificial layer, but other materials (e.g. copper) can be used as well. Both wet and dry etching are possible. However, standard wet etching would lead to permanent adhesion of the membrane to the underlying layer during the drying stage. This problem can be avoided by subsequent critical point drying (as e.g. in Lisec *et al.*, 2004), or by using very thick membranes with high spring constant and resulting high restoring force (as e.g. in Majumder *et al.*, 2003).

1.3 RF MEMS design challenges

After initial proof-of-concept publications in the late 1990s (e.g. Goldsmith *et al.*, 1998), extensive work has been conducted worldwide to develop mature RF MEMS components with advanced performance. To mention but a few are the series ohmic switches of Radant (Majumder *et al.*, 2003) and Omron (Uno *et al.*, 2009), cantilever-type capacitive switches of EADS Innovation Works (Siegel *et al.*, 2005, 2006, 2007) and shunt capacitive RF MEMS switches monolithically integrated with the BiCMOS technology of IHP Microelectronics (Kaynak *et al.*, 2009).

Despite the potentially superior RF performance of RF MEMS components, their wide spread commercialization has been limited so far. The main reasons for that are reliability and yield, but also packaging, large size, high actuation voltage and large switching time. Currently, numerous RF MEMS research groups worldwide are working on new solutions to overcome these issues. The most promising strategies are briefly identified below. Only electrostatic RF MEMS are considered, since they became the de facto standard.

1.3.1 High actuation voltage

The pull-in voltage is one of the most important parameters of MEMS design. It was shown in Equation [1.4] that the pull-in voltage is inversely proportional to the actuation area. Thus, the actuation electrodes must be large enough, so that the actuation voltage is not unreasonably increased. As a result, footprints of many RF MEMS components are mainly determined by the actuation area and not by the 'useful' contact region. A typical compromise between small area and reasonable pull-in voltage is to choose actuation voltages in the range of tens of volts resulting in RF MEMS components of hundreds of micrometres in length and width.

Besides, if the required voltage is not available on-chip, a charge pump should be used. However, this requires high-breakdown voltage devices, at least as an option, as well as sufficiently robust on-chip capacitors. Additionally, charge pumps will consume power and chip area. Fortunately, high voltage is required only for a short time during switching. After that, the moveable membrane can be held in the down-state with a much smaller voltage, since the metal plates are now very close to each other and the electrostatic force is much larger. Thus, with some simple control circuitry, it is possible to switch off the charge pump immediately after switching, significantly reducing the overall power consumption.

Another issue following from the area/voltage compromise is a relatively large switching time. As Equation [1.5] shows, switching time is inversely proportional to the mechanical resonance frequency. Thus, it can be reduced by a higher spring constant, thus higher pull-in voltage, or smaller mass, hence smaller actuation area and again larger pull-in voltage. As a result, most present day RF MEMS components have switching times in the range of a few to tens of microseconds.

In principle, the pull-in voltage could be reduced by low spring constant designs. However, this is not used in practice, for the following reasons. Firstly, a low spring constant leads to a low restoring force, making the moveable membrane much more prone to sticking (e.g. due to moisture), significantly degrading its reliability. Besides, a low spring constant may greatly increase the switching time of MEMS devices, as follows from Equation [1.5]. In addition, low pull-in voltage makes the membrane susceptible to self-actuation at high RF power levels.

1.3.2 Reliability

Many RF MEMS components contain metal and/or dielectric surfaces, which come into direct contact with each other. This can lead to stiction. For ohmic contacts the main problem is contact welding when switching high RF power (hot switching). Thus, ohmic contact components should be operated under cold switching condition, that is, with RF power switched off during switching time. Alternatively, refractory contact materials can be used at the expense of an increased contact resistance. For capacitive contacts, main failure mechanisms are the remaining electric field in the dielectric layer originating from charging or capillary force, caused by a thin moisture film. In most cases stiction occurs between the actuation electrode and the moveable membrane, owing to the large contact area. These issues can be avoided by contact- and dielectric-less actuation, obtained by adding mechanical stoppers to the membrane, preventing a DC short with the electrode in the down-state. Alternatively, but less effectively, these problems can be mitigated by special dielectric layers less prone to charging (e.g. AlN; Lisec *et al.*, 2004a; Ruan *et al.*, 2007), and by reducing the contact surface area (the latter negatively affects the down-state capacitance).

1.3.3 Yield and temperature stability

A highly stable and reproducible fabrication process is required for high yield of MEMS structures. This is quite difficult to achieve in practice and has become one of the bottle-necks in MEMS commercialization. Owing to mismatch in temperature expansion, coefficients of MEMS structural materials and substrate, thin-film membrane may have residual stresses or stress gradients. Depending on the stress, it may lead to lateral bowing and/or buckling for bridge-type structures, or up- or downwards bending for cantilever-type MEMS. Such membrane deformations may be present already after fabrication, or develop with time as operational temperature conditions vary. For example, the SEM image in Fig. 1.4 shows a slight lateral bowing of the MEMS bridge, and the SEM image in Fig. 1.7 shows upwards bending of a cantilever. This may lead to a reduction or increase of the air-gap, as well as changes in the spring constant modifying the actuation voltage. Such problems can be prevented with stress-compensated and stress-decoupled mechanical MEMS designs, as has been demonstrated by several groups (e.g. Lisec *et al.*, 2004; Nieminen *et al.*, 2004; Schobel *et al.*, 2004; Kaynak *et al.*, 2011).

1.3.4 Packaging

To ensure long-term reliability, MEMS components should be packaged. This is necessary to prevent any contamination on the contact region, which may lead to reduction of the capacitance or increase of the contact resistance for capacitive and ohmic switches, respectively. Also, non-packaged MEMS may fail due to moisture films causing stiction of the membrane in the down-state. Some MEMS components must be hermetically packaged (e.g. if particular pressure is needed to reduce release oscillations), but some operate reliably with non-hermetic packages (Kaynak *et al.*, 2011).

1.4 RF MEMS applications

As was shown above, RF MEMS can outperform their semiconductor counterparts, but also have certain limitations. Thus, it should be carefully considered whether RF MEMS is indeed the best solution for a particular system. In the following, some sample applications where RF MEMS seems to be the right or the only choice are briefly presented.

1.4.1 Millimetre-wave switches and multi-band integrated circuits

As outlined earlier in this chapter, RF MEMS are particularly important for millimetre-wave applications, due to low loss and inherently high linearity even at elevated frequencies. However, RF MEMS components are often fabricated in non-standardized dedicated processes, not compatible with MMIC. Then, only a hybrid integration with active circuits is possible, resulting in high parasitics and increased size.

Thus, to extend millimetre-wave MMIC's portfolio with RF MEMS, a fully monolithic fabrication must be developed. It is an approach pursued by a few groups and IC foundries worldwide, as illustrated by the following examples. The French foundry OMMIC is working towards integration of MEMS into a high-frequency compound semiconductor MMIC technology. Here, the focus is on developing a series RF MEMS switch with a metal-to-metal contact for microwave frequencies. Suggestions for relevant RF MEMS circuits, such as tuneable matching networks, phase shifting elements and switching networks, have been presented in (Malmqvist *et al*., 2009; Simon *et al*., 2010; Rantakari *et al*., 2011). In Italy, Selex Systemi Integrati has developed MEMS components using its GaN MMIC technology (Crispoldi *et al*., 2009). The targeted frequency range is again below 50 GHz. IHP Microelectronics embedded an RF MEMS switch into the backend-of-line (BEOL) of its advanced Si/SiGe BiCMOS process (Kaynak *et al*., 2009, 2010). IHP Microelectronics aims at mm-wave frequency applications and the switch is optimized for W-band.

One of the most promising applications of monolithically integrated mm-wave RF MEMS technology is T/R switches and switchable multi-band circuits. This is particularly important for BiCMOS/CMOS technologies, due to the lack of high performance mm-wave switches (the performance of CMOS switches is typically not acceptable above 20 GHz).

Band-switchable 56/72 GHz LNA

Recently a 56/72 GHz RF MEMS-switchable LNA was developed (Ulusoy *et al*., 2012) using the IHP BiCMOS-RF MEMS technology (Kaynak *et al*., 2009). A micrograph of the LNA can be seen in Fig. 1.9 and its schematic is shown in Fig. 1.10. It is a two-stage cascade amplifier with inductors L_{1-8} realized as thin-film-microstrip lines. The IC consumes a total of 16 mA from a 2.5 V DC voltage source. RF MEMS shunt capacitive switches are integrated into the loads of the two stages L_2/L_3 and L_5/L_6, respectively. These transmission lines act as tapped inductors, where the tap can be shorted to the ground by the RF MEMS capacitance, if the switch is actuated. For the first stage, the total load inductance approximately equals L_4 in parallel with $(L_2 + L_3)$, if the RF MEMS bridge is in the up-state, and L_4 in parallel with L_2, if the bridge is

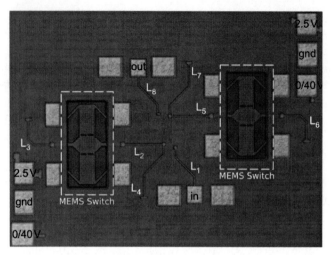

1.9 Micrograph of the RF MEMS band-switchable LNA. The total IC area is 0.75 × 1.05 mm² (© 2012 IEEE. Reprinted, with permission, from Ulusoy *et al.*, 2012).

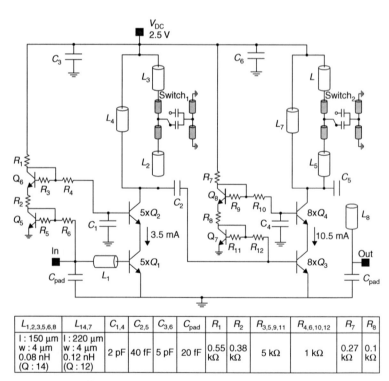

$L_{1,2,3,5,6,8}$	$L_{14,7}$	$C_{1,4}$	$C_{2,5}$	$C_{3,6}$	C_{pad}	R_1	R_2	$R_{3,5,9,11}$	$R_{4,6,10,12}$	R_7	R_8
l : 150 µm w : 4 µm 0.08 nH (Q : 14)	l : 220 µm w : 4 µm 0.12 nH (Q : 12)	2 pF	40 fF	5 pF	20 fF	0.55 kΩ	0.38 kΩ	5 kΩ	1 kΩ	0.27 kΩ	0.1 kΩ

1.10 Schematic of the RF MEMS band-switchable LNA (© 2012 IEEE. Reprinted, with permission, from Ulusoy *et al.*, 2012).

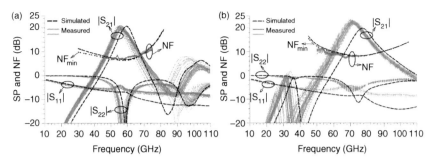

1.11 Measured and simulated performance of the RF MEMS band-switchable LNA (© 2012 IEEE. Reprinted, with permission, from Ulusoy *et al.*, 2012). (a) MEMS switch-up and (b) MEMS switch-down.

in the down-state. Consequently, the switchable 56/72 GHz dual-band LNA operation was achieved by properly adjusting the line lengths of L_{2-7}.

The measured S-parameters (for 46 out of 50 measured samples) and noise figure (for 27 out of 30 measured samples) are shown in Fig. 1.11. In the up-state of the MEMS switches, the gain reaches its maximum value of 20 dB at 56 GHz and the corresponding noise figure is around 7 dB. When the switches are actuated to the down-state by a 40 V signal, the peak gain shifts to 72 GHz and reaches 22 dB, and the resulting noise figure is about 8 dB. The designed switchable LNA achieves good performance in both bands, comparable to the state of the art in other BiCMOS technologies (Do *et al.*, 2007; Chen *et al.*, 2010). The switchable LNA outperforms conventional broadband designs, as in such designs more stages would be needed to maintain the high gain in both bands (Floyd *et al.*, 2005). These results verify the successful monolithic fabrication of the RF MEMS switches with the BiCMOS active devices, opening up many potential applications in the millimetre-wave frequency range.

Band-switchable 50/68 GHz VCO

Another interesting example of a band-switchable MMIC using the IHP BiCMOS-RF MEMS technology (Kaynak *et al.*, 2009) is a 50/68 GHz switchable VCO (Liu *et al.*, 2012). The circuit micrograph and schematic can be seen in Figs 1.12 and 1.13, respectively. This is a negative-resistance type VCO, and RF MEMS switches are used to modify the base inductance value to obtain the oscillation condition in two different frequency bands, depending on the switch state. The negative resistance is obtained by capacitive emitter degeneration indicated as C_{VAR} in the schematic. The RF MEMS switch, together with its feed line, forms a reconfigurable inductor, contributing to the resonance circuit. Switching the RF MEMS between up- and down-states results in a shift of the oscillation condition between the two bands of operation ('digital' tuning). In addition, 'analogue' frequency

20 Handbook of MEMS for wireless and mobile applications

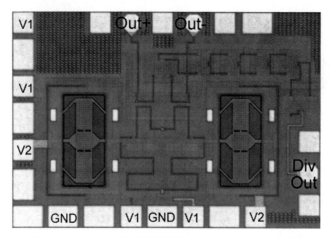

1.12 Micrograph of the RF MEMS band-switchable VCO (© 2012 IEEE. Reprinted, with permission, from Liu *et al.*, 2012).

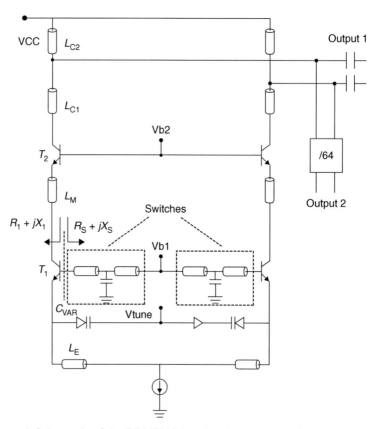

1.13 Schematic of the RF MEMS band-switchable VCO (© 2012 IEEE. Reprinted, with permission, from Liu *et al.*, 2012).

tuning within each band is done by changing the bias voltage of the variable capacitor (C_{VAR}). To improve the output power and isolate the VCO core from the load, a common base stage is cascaded with the VCO core. All inductors (except for the switch) are realized with thin-film-microstrip lines. To ease the characterization of the circuit and enable future use of the VCO in a phase-locked loop (PLL), a divide-by-64 frequency divider is designed and integrated with the VCO. The VCO and the frequency divider consume 17 mA and 40 mA from a 3.3 V supply, respectively. 28 V is applied to the switch for the down-state measurement and 0 V is applied for the up-state measurement. The complete circuit (including pads) occupies 0.68 mm².

Measured oscillation frequency and phase noise are shown in Figs 1.14 and 1.15, respectively. The RF MEMS switch frequency can be tuned from

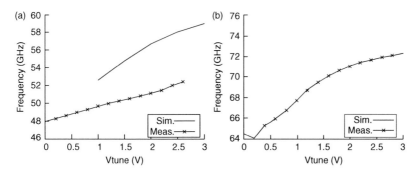

1.14 Measured and simulated oscillation frequency of the RF MEMS band-switchable VCO: (a) switch-up and (b) switch-down (© 2012 IEEE. Reprinted, with permission, from Liu *et al.*, 2012).

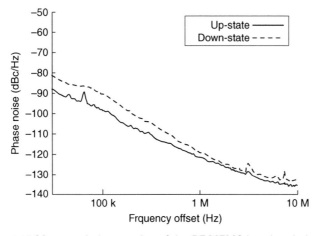

1.15 Measured phase noise of the RF MEMS band-switchable VCO (© 2012 IEEE. Reprinted, with permission, from Liu *et al.*, 2012).

48 to 52 GHz and from 64 to 72 GHz, for the up- and down-states of the RF MEMS switches respectively. The corresponding output power is 4 dBm and 5 dBm respectively, which is close to simulation. The phase noise is measured at the divided output. Due to the frequency division, the measured phase noise is improved by 36 dB (20log(64)), thus the estimated phase noise of the fundamental output is −86 dBc/Hz and −84 dBc/Hz at 1 MHz offset for the up- and down-state, which is close to simulation (−87 dBc/Hz).

1.4.2 Millimetre-wave impedance tuners

Impedance tuners are widely used in characterization of transistor noise parameters or load and source pulls. In most cases, the task is to move the 50 Ω impedance of measurement equipment to ideally any other point on the Smith Chart. To uniformly cover the entire area of the Smith Chart up to large voltage standing wave ratios (VSWRs), the tuners should have low loss. Besides, for load- and source-pull measurements, high linearity is especially important. Since low loss and high linearity are the key advantages of micromechanical components, RF MEMS impedance tuners are expected to outperform their semiconductor counterparts.

Despite inherent high linearity, there are limitations in RF MEMS power handling. In principle, MEMS membranes cannot follow RF and microwave signals, since their mechanical resonance frequencies are typically below 1 MHz. However, they do respond to the root mean square (rms) voltage of the RF signal. Thus, devices with an RF signal on the actuation electrodes may suffer from so-called hold-down (latching in the down-state) or unwanted self-actuation in the up-state. Still, capacitive RF MEMS components with several watts power handling have been developed (e.g. Palego et al., 2010). Another issue exclusively associated with ohmic contact switches is sticking due to contact welding during hot switching, i.e. with an applied RF signal (Majumder et al., 2003). However, with proper choice of contact geometry, ohmic contact components with up to 1 W power handling have been reported (Chow et al., 2007).

Impedance tuners can be realized in different ways. The most commonly used topologies are stub-based tuners (Vähä-Heikkilä et al., 2004) and distributed MEMS transmission lines (DMTLs) tuner (Vähä-Heikkilä and Rebeiz, 2004; Lu et al., 2005; Purtova, 2012). It has been shown (Vähä-Heikkilä, 2008) that DMTL circuits can withstand higher RF power levels and thus this topology is often preferred. It consists of a transmission line, periodically loaded with reconfigurable elements, typically with shunt switchable capacitors. Figure 1.16 shows an SEM image of such a W-band impedance tuner fabricated in the Fraunhofer ISiT MEMS technology. It consists of a coplanar transmission line loaded with eight tri-state RF MEMS capacitors

(Purtova, 2012). Thus, the circuit can generate $3^8 = 6561$ different impedance states. A simplified equivalent circuit of the tuner is shown in Fig. 1.17. A measured reflection coefficient constellation is shown in Fig. 1.18. Due to a large number of possible impedance states, to reduce the measurement setup complexity the MEMS capacitors were switched only between the low and intermediate capacitance states, and Fig. 1.18 shows only $2^8 = 256$ states of

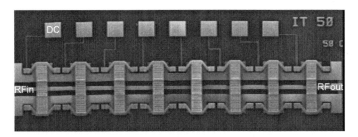

1.16 SEM image of the W-band DMTL impedance tuner.

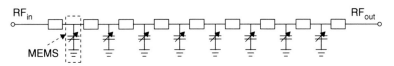

1.17 Equivalent circuit of the impedance tuner with capacitive tuning.

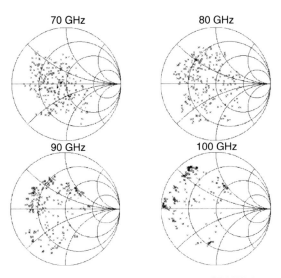

1.18 Measured impedance coverage of DMTL impedance tuner using RF MEMS capacitors.

the tuner. The optimum frequency band is 80–90 GHz, when the impedance tuner generates the largest VSWR and the achieved impedances cover all four quadrants of the Smith Chart.

1.4.3 Non-semiconducting 'all-MEMS' system

All-MEMS systems without any semiconductor devices are very promising and potentially disruptive as they do not face competition from semiconductor switches, as they commonly do in component-to-component replacements. The most typical realization of such system is a beam-steerable antenna array with either RF MEMS phase shifters or antenna elements, adjustable with MEMS components. This allows realization of large area components on inexpensive non-semiconducting substrates. Besides, since soft substrates can be used as well, this approach is applicable to conformal arrays and is especially attractive, for example, for aircrafts.

One example of such an 'all-MEMS' system has been presented in Gautier *et al.* (2009). It is a Ka-band (35 GHz) phased array with RF MEMS phase shifters. The 4 × 4 antenna array has been fabricated on a low-loss LTCC substrate at VIA Electronic GmbH. The 3-bit RF MEMS phase shifters are fabricated on a high-resistivity silicon substrate at EADS Innovation Works. The antenna and RF MEMS phase shifters are integrated with bond-wires. Depending on the states of the phase shifters, the beam angle has been steered to −15, 0 and +15 degrees (Gautier *et al.*, 2009).

1.4.4 Tuneable filters

Another application where RF MEMS can provide a significant advantage is tuneable filters. Often multi-band systems have to employ filter banks occupying large areas. Tuneable or switchable filters may provide the same functionality in a more compact and flexible way. RF MEMS switches and switchable capacitors are an attractive technology for adjusting the filter properties due to low loss and high linearity. Both planar as well as substrate-integrated RF MEMS tuneable filters have been reported. The former benefit from simple fabrication and potentially monolithic integration, but their quality factors are limited (see e.g. Pothier *et al.*, 2005; Malczewski *et al.*, 2011). On the other hand, substrate-integrated cavity-based filters, though they are more difficult to produce, offer much higher quality factors, as has been reported, for example, in (Schulte *et al.*, 2011; Sekar *et al.*, 2011). A detailed description of RF MEMS tuneable filters is given further down in a dedicated chapter.

1.5 Conclusion

It has been shown in this chapter that RF MEMS are particularly important for millimetre-wave applications, due to low loss and inherently high linearity even at elevated frequencies. Electromechanical aspects of the RF MEMS design were briefly reviewed, covering static and dynamic pull-in, as well as switching and release processes. Shunt capacitive and series ohmic components have been studied in more detail due to their practical importance. A general overview of the most commonly used fabrication steps of electrostatic components was given. The most critical issues hindering RF MEMS commercialization, such as high actuation voltage, yield and temperature stability and packaging have been identified and possible solutions discussed. Finally, several applications for which RF MEMS are significantly more advantageous than semiconductor-based components have been presented: mm-wave switches and multi-band circuits, mm-wave impedance tuners and non-semiconducting 'all-MEMS' systems.

1.6 Sources of further information and advice

For those who wish to read more about RF MEMS technology and applications, the book by Gabriel Rebeiz, RF MEMS – Theory, Design and Technology (Rebeiz, 2003) is recommended for anyone who approaches these components for the first time. A more recent compendium of RF MEMS knowledge is Advanced RF MEMS, edited by Stepan Lucyszyn (Lucyszyn, 2010). The work is largely an outcome of the European AMICOM project – the network of excellence for RF MEMS and RF Microsystems.

1.7 Acknowledgements

The authors thank Dr-Ing. Gang Liu and Dr-Ing. Ahmet Cagri Ulusoy for their contributions to the sections on millimetre-wave band-switchable circuits.

1.8 References

Buber, T., Kinayman, N., Yun, Y.-H. and Brogle, J. 'Low-loss high-isolation 60–80 GHz GaAs SPST PIN switch', in Proc. IEEE MTT-S Int. Microwave Symp. Digest, vol. **2**, (2003), pp. 1307–1310.

Chen, A. Y.-K., Baeyens, Y., Chen, Y.-K. and Lin, J. 'A low-power linear sige bicmos low-noise amplifier for millimetre-wave active imaging', *IEEE Microwave and Wireless Components Letters*, vol. **20**, no. 2, pp. 103–105 (2010).

Chow, L. L. W., Volakis, J. L., Saitou, K. and Kurabayashi, K. 'Lifetime extension of rf mems direct contact switches in hot switching operations by ball grid array dimple design', *IEEE Electron Device Letters*, vol. **28**, no. 6, pp. 479–481 (2007).

Crispoldi, F., Pantellini, A., Lavanga, S., Nanni, A., Romanini, P., Rizzi, L., Farinelli, P. and Lanzieri, C. 'New fabrication process to manufacture RF-MEMS and HEMT on GaN/Si substrate', in Proc. European Microwave Integrated Circuits Conf. EuMIC 2009 (2009), pp. 387–390.

Do, V.-H., Subramanian, V. and Boeck, G. '60 GHz SiGe LNA', in Proc. 14th IEEE Int. Conf. Electronics, Circuits and Systems ICECS 2007 (2007), pp. 1209–1212.

Elata, D. and Bamberger, H. 'A lower bound for the dynamic pull-in of electrostatic actuators', in Proc. Eur. Micro Nano Syst., Paris, France (2004), p. 8385.

Elata, D. and Bamberger, H. 'On the dynamic pull-in of electrostatic actuators with multiple degrees of freedom and multiple voltage sources', *Journal of Microelectromechanical Systems*, vol. **15**, no. 1, pp. 131–140 (2006).

Floyd, B. A., Reynolds, S. K., Pfeiffer, U. R., Zwick, T., Beukema, T. and Gaucher, B. 'SiGe bipolar transceiver circuits operating at 60 GHz', *IEEE Journal of Solid-State Circuits*, vol. **40**, no. 1, pp. 156–167 (2005).

Gautier, W., Ziegler, V., Stehle, A., Schoenlinner, B., Prechtel, U. and Menzel, W. 'RF-MEMS phased array antenna on low-loss LTCC substrate for Ka-band data link', in Proc. European Microwave Conf. EuMC 2009 (2009), pp. 914–917.

Goldsmith, C. L., Yao, Z., Eshelman, S. and Denniston, D. 'Performance of low-loss RF MEMS capacitive switches', *IEEE Microwave and Guided Wave Letters*, vol. **8**, no. 8, pp. 269–271 (1998).

Gupta, R. K. and Senturia, S. D. 'Pull-in time dynamics as a measure of absolute pressure', in Proc., IEEE. Workshop Tenth Annual Int Micro Electro Mechanical Systems MEMS '97 (1997), pp. 290–294.

Jin, Y. and Nguyen, C. 'Ultra-Compact High-Linearity High-Power Fully Integrated DC-20-GHz 0.18-µm CMOS T/R Switch', *IEEE Transactions on Microwave Theory and Techniques*, vol. **55**, no. 1, pp. 30–36 (2007).

Kallfass, I., Diebold, S., Massler, H., Koch, S., Seelmann-Eggebert, M. and Leuther, A. 'Multiple-throw millimetre-wave fet switches for frequencies from 60 up to 120 GHz', in Proc. 38th European Microwave Conf. EuMC 2008 (2008), pp. 1453–1456.

Kaynak, M., Ehwald, K. E., Drews, J., Scholz, R., Korndorfer, F., Knoll, D., Tillack, B., Barth, R., Birkholz, M., Schulz, K., Sun, Y. M., Wolansky, D., Leidich, S., Kurth, S. and Gurbuz, Y. 'BEOL embedded RF-MEMS switch for mm-wave applications', in Proc. IEEE Int. Electron Devices Meeting (IEDM) (2009), pp. 1–4.

Kaynak, M., Korndörfer, F., Wietstruck, M., Knoll, D., Scholz, R., Wipf, C., Krause, C. and Tillack, B. 'Robustness and reliability of BiCMOS embedded RF-MEMS switch', in Proc. IEEE 11th Topical Meeting Silicon Monolithic Integrated Circuits in RF Systems (SiRF) (2011), pp. 177–180.

Kaynak, M., Wietstruck, M., Scholz, R., Drews, J., Barth, R., Ehwald, K. E., Fox, A., Haak, U., Knoll, D., Korndorfer, F., Marschmeyer, S., Schulz, K., Wipf, C., Wolansky, D., Tillack, B., Zoschke, K., Fischer, T., Kim, Y. S., Kim, J. S., Lee, W.-G. and Kim, J. W. 'BiCMOS embedded RF-MEMS switch for above 90 GHz applications using backside integration technique', in Proc. IEEE Int. Electron Devices Meeting (IEDM) (2010).

Kaynak, M., Wietstruck, M., Zhang, W., Drews, J., Scholz, R., Knoll, D., Korndörfer, F., Wipf, C., Schulz, K., Elkhouly, M., Kaletta, K., Suchodoletz, M. V., Zoschke, K., Wilke, M., Ehrmann, O., Mühlhaus, V., Liu, G., Purtova, T., Ulusoy, A. C., Schumacher, H. and Tillack, B. 'RF-MEMS Switch Module in a 0.25 µm BiCMOS Technology', in Proc. IEEE 12th Topical Meeting on Silicon Monolithic Integrated Circuits in RF Systems (SiRF 2012), 16–18 Jan. (2012), Santa Clara, CA, USA, pp. 25–28.

Leus, V. and Elata, D. 'On the Dynamic Response of Electrostatic MEMS Switches', *Journal of Microelectromechanical Systems*, vol. **17**, no. 1, pp. 236–243 (2008).

Lin, J.-W., Chen, C. C. and Cheng, Y.-T. 'A robust high-Q micromachined RF inductor for RFIC applications', *IEEE Transactions on Electron Devices*, vol. **52**, no. 7, pp. 1489–1496 (2005).

Lisec, T., Huth, C., Shakhray, M. and Wagner, B. 'Surface-micromachined capacitive RF switches with high thermal stability and low drift using Ni as structural material', in Proc. MEMSWAVE 2004, Uppsala, June (2004), pp. C33–C36.

Lisec, T., Huth, C. and Wagner, B. 'Dielectric material impact on capacitive RF MEMS reliability', in Proc. 34th European Microwave Conf, vol. **1** (2004), pp. 73–76.

Liu, G., Kaynak, M., Purtova, T., Ulusoy, A. C., Tillack, B. and Schumacher, H. 'Dual-band millimetre-wave VCO with embedded RF-MEMS switch module in BiCMOS technology', in Proc. IEEE 12th Topical Meeting Silicon Monolithic Integrated Circuits in RF Systems (SiRF) (2012), pp. 175–178.

Lu, Y., Katehi, L. P. B. and Peroulis, D. 'A novel MEMS impedance tuner simultaneously optimized for maximum impedance range and power handling', in Proc. IEEE MTT-S Int. Microwave Symp. Digest, 12–17 June (2005), pp. 927–930.

Lucyszyn, S., Ed., *Advanced RF MEMS*. The Cambridge RF and Microwave Engineering Series (2010).

Majumder, S., Lampen, J., Morrison, R. and Maciel, J. 'A packaged, high-lifetime ohmic MEMS RF switch', in Proc. IEEE MTT-S Int. Microwave Symp. Digest, vol. **3** (2003), pp. 1935–1938.

Malczewski, A., Pillans, B., Morris, F. and Newstrom, R. 'A family of MEM tunable filters for advanced RF applications', in Proc. IEEE MTT-S International Microwave Symposium, (2011), pp. 1–4

Malmqvist, R., Samuelsson, C., Rantakari, P., Frijlink, P., Smith, D., Simon, W., Saijets, J., Vaha-Heikkila, T. and Baggen, R. 'RF MEMS-MMIC building blocks for emerging wireless systems and RF-sensing applications', in Proc. European Microwave Integrated Circuits Conf. EuMIC 2009, (2009), pp. 363–366.

Nathanson, H. C., Newell, W. E., Wickstrom, R. A. and Davis Jr, J., 'The resonant gate transistor', *IEEE Transactions on Electron Devices*, vol. **14**, no. 3, pp. 117–133 (1967).

Neculoiu, D., Plana, R., Pons, P., Muller, A., Vasilache, D., Petrini, I., Buiculescu, C. and Blondy, P. 'Microwave characterization of membrane supported coplanar waveguide transmission lines – electromagnetic simulation and experimental results', in Proc. Int. Semiconductor Conf. CAS 2001, vol. **1** (2001), pp. 151–154.

Neculoiu, D., Pons, P., Saadaoui, M., Bary, L., Vasilache, D., Grenier, K., Dubuc, D., Muller, A. and Plana, R. 'Membrane supported Yagi-Uda antennae for millimetre-wave applications', *IEE Proceedings-Microwaves, Antennas and Propagation*, vol. **151**, no. 4, pp. 311–314 (2004).

Nieminen, H., Ermolov, V., Silanto, S., Nybergh, K. and Ryhanen, T. 'Design of a temperature-stable RF MEM capacitor', *Journal of Microelectromechanical Systems*, vol. **13**, no. 5, pp. 705–714 (2004).

Palego, C., Solazzi, F., Halder, S., Hwang, J. C. M., Farinelli, P., Sorrentino, R., Faes, A., Mulloni, V. and Margesin, B. 'Effect of substrate on temperature range and power capacity of RF MEMS capacitive switches', in Proc. European Microwave Conf. (EuMC), Paris, France, 28–30 September (2010), pp. 505–508.

Pao, K.-H., Hsu, C.-Y., Chuang, H.-R., Lu, C.-L. and Chen, C.-Y. 'A 3–10 GHz Broadband CMOS T/R Switch for UWB Applications', in Proc. 1st European Microwave Integrated Circuits Conf, (2006), pp. 452–455.

Pelesko, J. A. and Bernstein, D. H. *Modeling MEMS and NEMS*. Chapman & Hall/CRC (2003).

Pothier, A., Orlianges, J.-C., Zheng, G., Champeaux, C., Catherinot, A., Cros, D., Blondy, P. and Papapolymerou, J. 'Low–loss 2–bit tunable bandpass filters using MEMS DC contact switches', *IEEE Transactions on Microwave Theory and Techniques* (2005), vol. **53**, no. 1, pp. 354–360.

Purtova, T. *RFMEMS Periodic Structures: Modelling, Components and Circuits*, PhD Thesis, Ulm University, Germany (2012).

Rantakari, P., Malmqvist, R., Samuelsson, C., Leblanc, R., Smith, D., Jonsson, R., Simon, W., Saijets, J., Baggen, R. and Vähä-Heikkilä, T. 'Wide-band radio frequency micro electro-mechanical systems switches and switching networks using a gallium arsenide monolithic microwave-integrated circuits foundry process technology', *IET Microwaves, Antennas & Propagation*, vol. **5**, no. 8, pp. 948–955 (2011).

Rebeiz, G. M. *RF MEMS: theory, design, and technology*. John Wiley and Sons, (2003).

Ruan, J., Nolhier, N., Barfleur, M., Bary, L., Mauran, N., Coccetti, F., Lisec, T. and Plana, R. 'Dielectric Material Charging and ESD Stress of AlN-based Capacitive RF MEMS', in 8th International Symposium on RFMEMS and RF Microsystems MEMSWAVE, Barcelona, Spain (2007), pp. 179–182.

Schobel, J., Buck, T., Reimann, M., Ulm, M. and Schneider, M. 'W-band RF-MEMS subsystems for smart antennas in automotive radar sensors', in Proc. 34th European Microwave Conf, vol. **3** (2004), pp. 1305–1308.

Schulte, B., Ziegler, V., Schoenlinner, B., Prechtel, U. and Schumacher, H. 'RF–MEMS tunable evanescent mode cavity filters in LTCC technology in Ku–band', in: Proc. IEEE European Microwave Conference (2011), pp. 514–517.

Sekar, V., Armendariz, M. and Entesari, K. 'A 1.2–1.6-GHz substrate-integrated-waveguide RF MEMS tunable filter', in *IEEE Transactions on Microwave Theory and Techniques* (2011), vol. **59**, no. 4, pp. 866–876.

Siegel, C., Ziegler, V., Prechtel, U., Schonlinner, B. and Schumacher, H. 'Very low complexity RF-MEMS technology for wide range tunable microwave filters', in Proc. European Microwave Conference, vol. **1**, Oct. 4–6 (2005), 4pp.

Siegel, C., Ziegler, V., Schönlinner, B., Prechtel, U. and Schumacher, H. 'RF-MEMS based 2-bit reflective phase shifter at X-Band for reconfigurable reflect-array antennas', in 8th International Symposium on RF MEMS and Microsystems MEMSWAVE, Barcelona, Spain, June (2007).

Siegel, C., Ziegler, V., Schonlinner, B., Prechtel, U. and Schumacher, H. 'Simplified RF-MEMS Switches Using Implanted Conductors and Thermal Oxide', in Proc. 36th European Microwave Conference, Sep. 10–15 (2006), pp. 1735–1738.

Simon, W., Baggen, L. and Smith, D. 'Innovative RF MEMS switches on GaAs', in Proc. 14th Int Antenna Technology and Applied Electromagnetics & the American Electromagnetics Conf. (ANTEM-AMEREM) Symp. (2010), pp. 1–4.

Talwalkar, N. A., Yue, C. P., Gan, H. and Wong, S. S. 'Integrated CMOS transmit-receive switch using LC-tuned substrate bias for 2.4-GHz and 5.2-GHz applications', *IEEE Journal of Solid-State Circuits*, vol. **39**, no. 6, pp. 863–870 (2004).

Ulusoy, A. C., Kaynak, M., Purtova, T., Tillack, B. and Schumacher, H. 'A 60 to 77GHz Switchable LNA in an RF-MEMS Embedded BiCMOS Technology', *Microwave and Wireless Components Letters, IEEE*, vol. **22**, pp. 430–432, Aug. (2012).

Uno, Y., Narise, K., Masuda, T., Inoue, K., Adachi, Y., Hosoya, K., Seki, T. and Sato, F. 'Development of SPDT-structured RF MEMS switch', in Proc. Int. Solid-State Sensors, Actuators and Microsystems Conf. Transducers (2009), pp. 541–544.

Vähä-Heikkilä, T. Design and Modeling Issues for High Power Handling RF MEMS, ser. RF MEMS Industrial Workshop. Fodele, Greece: Workshop, 1 July (2008).

Vähä-Heikkilä, T. and Rebeiz, G. M. 'A 20–50 GHz reconfigurable matching network for power amplifier applications', in Proc. IEEE MTT-S International Microwave Symposium Digest, vol. **2**, June 6–11 (2004), pp. 717–720.

Vähä-Heikkilä, T., Varis, J., Tuovinen, J. and Rebeiz, G. M. 'A reconfigurable 6–20 GHz RF MEMS impedance tuner', in Proc. IEEE MTT-S Int. Microwave Symp. Digest, vol. **2**, 6–11 June (2004), pp. 729–732.

2
Overview of wireless techniques for use with MEMS

I. A. GLOVER, University of Huddersfield, UK and
R. ATKINSON, University of Strathclyde, UK

DOI: 10.1533/9780857098610.1.30

Abstract: This chapter reviews wireless communication concepts, protocols and calculations that could be applied to microelectromechanical systems (MEMS). The impacts of the unreliable wireless channel on the transport, network, data-link and physical layers of the protocol stack are discussed and the ways that wireless network protocols can mitigate these impacts described. Particular attention is given to flow control, congestion control, error control, addressing for mobility, radio/logical link control, medium access control, digital modulation and link budgets. The chapter ends with a template for how a physical layer system design might proceed.

Key words: wireless network protocols, transport layer, network layer, data-link layer, physical layer design.

2.1 Introduction

Wireless communications systems have, as a virtue of their untethered nature, an inherent capability to support remote measurement and control in static, portable and mobile applications, including applications incorporating micro-electromechanical systems (MEMS). Both cellular radio and wireless sensor networks have proved, in this context, to be useful and reliable technologies.

Wireless systems introduce some unique challenges over and above their wired counterparts. These challenges must be overcome if reliable communication is to be established with actuators and/or sensors connected over wireless links. One major difference, for example, between wired and wireless networks is the highly error-prone nature of radio links. This hostile channel poses significant problems for the transmission control protocol (TCP) – the dominant transport layer protocol used on the Internet. Another important difference is that wireless networks permit endpoints (i.e. nodes) to be mobile, that is, to change their point of attachment to the Internet. This creates significant issues with regards to routing data between sensors, actuators, controllers, etc. It is not unrealistic, for example, to consider scenarios where the various components of sensor systems each have their own IP address; a notion central to an intense area of current research – the Internet of Things (IoT).

In order to make the complexity of an entire digital communication system tractable, its functionality is split between the various layers of a 'protocol stack'. Each layer in the stack takes responsibility for a well-defined set of functions, a lower layer effectively offering a communications service to the layer immediately above it. Each layer offers a more sophisticated communications service than the one below, effectively adding value to the lower-layer service. The interfaces between layers are sufficiently well defined to allow a particular layer to be designed without regard to the implementation details of the adjacent layers. There are exceptions to this, for example, in 'cross-layer design' where advantage is taken of the implementation details of one layer to make the operation of another layer more efficient. The structure of this chapter, however, reflects that of a classical protocol stack, starting at the higher layers of the stack and moving downwards towards the lower layers. The physical layer, at the bottom of the stack, is that which interfaces to the wireless channel.

2.2 Transport layer issues

The transport layer in communications systems is used to enable addressing of end applications through the use of port numbers but also to, optionally, enable reliable end-to-end connectivity. The two dominant transport layer protocols are the user datagram protocol (UDP) (Postel, 1980) and TCP (Anon., 1981). As will be discussed later, TCP, in particular, does not perform well over wireless networks.

UDP is a lightweight protocol that is used to transport short-lived sessions, such as Domain Name System requests or to support the carriage of real-time data over reliable links. UDP provides checksum functionality to verify the integrity of received data, plus source and destination port numbers. While other protocols (such as Internet protocol version 4 (IPv4) and IPv6) have addressing functionality to address a particular device (e.g. a wireless sensor node), an internal addressing scheme is required to deliver data to particular applications (processes) running within these devices. On Internet-enabled computers these applications include browsers and email clients, on Internet-enabled sensor platforms these applications include monitoring processes for each on-board sensor, or conceivably each agent in a multi-agent system.

TCP has considerably more functionality than UDP and is the dominant transport protocol on the Internet. It has a range of functionality to ensure that data packets are delivered to applications reliably. Specifically, it will:

- Re-order packets at the receiver to match the order in which they were sent. (This is particularly important for command and control applications, where a sequence of commands must be executed in a specific order.)
- Detect if packets have been lost/discarded en route.
- Control the transmission rate of data. (Many sensor applications will be implemented on platforms with limited processing capability that may be unable to process incoming data at the rate that a high-end server can support.)

TCP was devised before the mass deployment of wireless networks and some assumptions, therefore, concerning the underlying nature of the Internet, which were valid at the time of design, are no longer valid today. These assumptions have significant repercussions for its behaviour. A brief overview of TCP is therefore now provided, followed by a description of the challenges facing its operation in wireless environments.

Central to the operation of TCP is the use of a positive acknowledgement system which utilises sequence numbers. Successive TCP segments are assigned an incremental sequence number upon transmission, so that receivers can place those segments in the order in which they were transmitted before delivering them to the end processes running on the hardware. A gap in the sequence number chain can be used to detect if a segment has been lost (or discarded) in transit. When the loss of a data packet occurs, the intended receiver will not transmit the acknowledgement for the missing segment of data and hence induce the sender to retransmit that segment. These measures alone are not sufficient to achieve reliability.

TCP also controls the transmission rate of data using two intertwined mechanisms: flow control and congestion control. The former is used to ensure that senders do not overwhelm receivers by sending data at a faster rate than receivers can process it, since this would lead to packets being discarded at the receiver – an important consideration for many sensor applications. The latter is used to ensure that senders do not overwhelm intermediate nodes (e.g. Internet routers or intermediate nodes that constitute a mesh-like wireless sensor network) between source and destination. This is a preventative measure, aimed at reducing the probability of packets being discarded en route.

Flow control is a fairly simple mechanism. Incoming TCP segments are stored in a receiver buffer before being delivered to their associated processes. When the receiver issues an acknowledgement for a received segment, it includes the residual buffer capacity within a special field contained within that acknowledgement. In this way the sender can deduce if the receiver is able to process further segments, and hence avoid receiver-end packet loss.

Overview of wireless techniques for use with MEMS

Congestion control is considerably more complicated and has serious ramifications for wireless networks. It would be unfeasible for every intermediate network node to advertise its residual buffer capacity to senders. TCP therefore uses a timer to estimate the level of congestion on the path between the sender and receiver. The operation is as follows. Each TCP sender continually monitors the time delay between transmitting a data segment and receiving its associated acknowledgement, that is, it continually monitors the round trip time (RTT). The RTT will depend on a number of factors:

- The number of hops between source and destination.
- The bandwidth of each link in the path between source and destination.
- The queuing delay in each of the routers between source and destination.

Assuming for the time being that the sender and receiver are stationary, the RTT will then be dependent on the cumulative queuing delay of intermediate nodes. The queuing delay in a particular node will be a function of the volume of traffic passing through it (localised congestion). Consequently, the RTT will be a function of the aggregated congestion along the path between the sender and receiver. The objective of TCP's congestion control functionality is to transmit data at as fast a rate as possible, yet not so fast as to cause congestion at intermediate nodes.

A simplified description of its operation follows. TCP initially transmits a single data packet. If that is positively acknowledged then it will transmit a further two. If they are positively acknowledged then it will transmit a further four, and so on. Thus the number of packets permitted to be in flight per RTT grows exponentially (1, 2, 4, 8, ...), as illustrated in Fig. 2.1. This behaviour translates into an exponential growth in transmission rate.

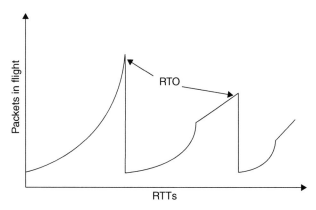

2.1 Packet loss detected.

As the transmission rate increases, so will the buffer occupancy levels (congestion) at nodes along the path between sender and receiver until packet loss occurs.

In actual fact detecting if packet loss has occurred is not quite as easy as it may seem. From an idealistic perspective, the absence of an acknowledgement for a data segment is indicative of packet loss. The possibility must be considered, however, that a packet may, instead, be indefinitely delayed. After all, how does the sender know that the acknowledgement will not arrive at some time in the future? A practical approach is to set an upper bound on the time that is permitted to elapse before an acknowledgement is received. If a segment of data has not been acknowledged upon expiry of this time period, known as the retransmission time-out (RTO), then it can be regarded as being lost for all practical purposes. The time-out value is based on a smoothed time-average of estimated RTTs, and on an estimate of the variation of RTTs (Paxson, 2011).

TCP can be regarded as a polite protocol, in that it will reduce its transmission rate when congestion is detected (as indicated by the time-out expiring before a particular acknowledgement is received). In doing so, congestion can be alleviated. Suppose one particular node is experiencing a high level of congestion. All TCP senders that transmit data on a path through that node will detect the congestion, and all will decrease their transmission rate. In doing so, they are not operating in a polite fashion for purely altruistic purposes. Rather they recognise that failure to reduce their transmission rates will perpetuate packet loss, and when loss occurs, retransmissions will be triggered with the effect of increasing still further the congestion level.

The salient point here is that TCP perceives packet loss to be caused by congestion. Within wired networks this inference is generally valid since the probability of noise-induced error is so small that data will generally only be lost in transit due to a buffer overflow at an intermediate node. As already stated, this is a historical assumption that did not consider the wide spread deployment of wireless networks.

Unfortunately, wireless channels are notoriously hostile to data transmission, giving rise to significant data corruption and loss due to noise, interference and distortion. When packet loss occurs during transmission over a wireless link, TCP will incorrectly interpret this as congestion-induced packet loss and reduce its transmission rate. TCP therefore takes a bad situation (external data loss) and makes it worse by reducing its transmission rate, that is, a lossy channel capable of high data rates becomes a lossy channel that supports only low data rates.

A number of variants of TCP have been proposed to cope with its undesirable behaviour over wireless links. These, however, have yet to be adopted en masse. Instead, most wireless communications systems attempt to implement a link-level automatic repeat request (ARQ) scheme to retransmit lost/corrupted segments before they are detected by upper layer protocols such as TCP. These solutions are discussed further in Section 2.4.1.

2.3 Network layer mobility issues

It is anticipated that in future most sensors, actuators and other devices will each have their own distinct, globally routable, IPv6 address (Deering, 1998). This is enabled by the vast address range of IPv6 (6.65×10^{23} addresses for each square metre on Earth). This capability presents new and exciting opportunities for measurement and control of mobile systems, including online engine diagnostics, etc.

The Internet addressing scheme has a logical structure: nodes are assigned an IP address, which is composed of a host identifier and network identifier (prefix) (Hinden, 2006). IP addresses are not assigned geographically, but rather contiguous blocks of addresses are awarded to organisations such as universities and Internet service providers (ISPs). The organisations can partition their portion of the address space as they see fit. A national ISP, for example, may assign sub-blocks of addresses on a city-by-city basis. Indeed, such a geographical partitioning may assist in routing packets to destinations while minimising the number of hops they take.

With the advent, and wide-scale deployment, of wireless technologies such as cellular systems and wireless local area networks (WLAN), a new problem presents itself: how to route a connection to a node that is mobile, and indeed mobile during a call/session? Mobility involves a change in geographical location, that is, a change in the point of attachment to the Internet, which in turn implies a change of IP address.

A naïve approach would assign a permanent IP address to a (sensor) node, and permit that node to advertise this address at each location it visits (at its point of attachment). Unfortunately, this approach would not be scalable: the advantage of having topologically similar IP addresses connected to the same network is that it permits traffic to be routed to them efficiently. In this context efficiency relates to the size of lookup (routing) tables within Internet routers or other intermediate nodes. Large routing tables imply large lookup times, that is, large processing delays. In order to avoid the necessity of holding a routing table entry per address, the grouping of topologically similar addresses permits the holding of a single entry per IP address block (i.e. a contiguous range of IP addresses). The naïve approach would lead to a fragmented address space that would substantially increase delays (and processing overhead) in routing packets; consequently, it is unworkable.

Another approach would be to allow the mobile node to change its IP address upon attachment to a new access point (i.e. a new subnet). However, this approach is flawed too, due to the historical context of the Internet's design. When the Internet architecture was designed, it was not anticipated that a node would change its IP address; consequently, an IP address has a secondary function.

Within the kernel of computer operating systems, sockets (communications interfaces) are used to allow applications to communicate with each other over the Internet. A socket represents one end of a connection. Applications communicate by reading and writing to/from an area of memory associated with the socket. Within the operating system, the socket is addressed using a 5-tuple:

- Destination IP address.
- Source IP address.
- Destination Port Number.
- Source Port Number.
- Protocol Type: generally either UDP or TCP.

The use of the protocol type and port numbers permit nodes to demultiplex streams of incoming data packets and deliver them to the appropriate applications. Port numbers effectively operate as part of an internal addressing system within the platform. A sensor node may have many sockets active simultaneously, and each will be addressed by a different combination of values of the 5-tuple.

It should be clear that if the IP address of an endpoint changes during a session then the associated applications using a socket addressed by the IP address will not be able to communicate, that is, the application would attempt to write to (or read from) a different area of memory based on the new IP address.

An IP address therefore acts not only as a locator (an address to deliver packets to across the Internet), but also as an identifier within operating systems. Any attempt to change the IP address of a host mid-session would result in data being written to the wrong place in memory, and consequently the connection would be severed.

The proposed solution offered by an extension to IPv6 (Mobile IPv6) (Johnson, 2004) is to assign two addresses to an Internet-enabled node: a permanent address (known as the home address) fulfils the function of an identifier, while a temporary address (known as the care-of address) fulfils the function of a locator. The operation of the protocol requires the assistance of an intelligent device (known as the home agent) that has a stable and well-known IP address. The operation is as follows.

Consider the scenario wherein a mobile node is attached to a wireless network, as shown in Fig. 2.2. The node will have a topologically correct temporary, care-of, address from that network. This address can be used to route packets to the node's true location on the Internet. However, this address may not be known to other entities (controllers, servers, etc.) which

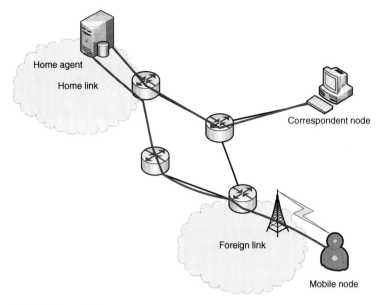

2.2 Node mobility.

wish to contact that node, and this represents a significant barrier to session establishment. Other entities (known as correspondent nodes) instead send packets to the (mobile) node's stable home address, where they are intercepted by the mobile node's home agent. The home agent will act as the mobile node's proxy by forwarding packets addressed to the home address on towards the care-of address. To achieve this, the home agent must first know that care-of address. Therefore, whenever a mobile node obtains a new temporary care-of address, it informs the home agent of this using a special message known as a binding update. The home agent maintains a special database (known as a binding cache) and processes the binding update by creating an entry in the binding cache associating the mobile node's home address with its care-of address. The forwarding is accomplished by IP-in-IP encapsulation (called tunneling), whereby the home agent puts an IP packet addressed to the mobile node's home address into the payload of a new packet which has its care-of address as the destination and the home agent's IP address as the source. Packets transmitted by the mobile node towards the correspondent node also travel via the home agent. The mobile node first constructs a packet with the source set to its home address and the destination set to that of the correspondent. This packet is then encapsulated within another packet, with the destination set to the address of the home agent and the source set to the care-of address. This packet within a packet is then sent to the home agent, which removes the outer packet (decapsulation) and forwards the inner packet towards the correspondent.

As the mobile node moves from access point to access point it will send a succession of binding updates to its home agent such that incoming data packets can be routed to its current location. Where the correspondent is also Mobile IPv6-enabled (i.e. not just IPv6-enabled), it can then also receive binding updates from the mobile node and hence route packets directly without the need to go through the home agent.

Another extension to the IPv6 protocol, network mobility (NEMO) (Devarpalli, 2005), proposes that the mobile node can be considered to be a mobile router. The router will have its own globally routable address block (in addition to its own home address) that can be assigned to various attached devices (sensors etc.), each device being given one of the addresses. As the mobile router changes its point of attachment to the Internet, its care-of address will change, and it will exchange binding updates with its home agent. All traffic for the nodes attached to the mobile router will be routed towards the router's care-of address before being forwarded to the end device. In this manner, the nodes attached to that router will be unaffected by any change in the router's care-of address; they will be able to keep a single, globally routable, IP address because they are effectively being shielded by the router. This technology may be particularly useful for mobile wireless sensor networks, perhaps employing a cluster-head for wide area communications.

2.4 Data-link layer

Within the open system interconnection (OSI) protocol framework, the data-link layer is composed of two sublayers. The higher sublayer is the logical link control (LLC) and is discussed in Section 2.4.1. The lower sublayer is the medium access control (MAC) and is discussed in Section 2.4.2.

2.4.1 Radio link control/logical link control

LLC operates on a link-by-link basis, in contrast to higher layer protocols that operate on an end-to-end basis. It can operate in acknowledged or unacknowledged mode. In acknowledged mode, frames of data that are received with errors are re-sent by the transmitter, that is, it provides a reliable service at link-level. In addition, it performs local flow control duties as well as segmenting and reassembling higher layer packets to suit the air-interface. In unacknowledged mode it operates transparently providing flow control and segmentation and reassembly, that is, erroneous frames are not retransmitted. The segmentation and reassembly function divides large data packets into a succession of smaller LLC frames for transmission over the local link where required. Wireless systems will generally support much smaller data packets than wired networks.

The reliability of acknowledged mode is achieved through the use of an ARQ scheme. ARQ is regarded as a backwards error correction scheme.

With this approach the receiver of a data packet determines whether it is erroneous and, if so, requests that it be retransmitted. Wireless systems employ robust error control coding schemes to make this determination. Redundant data in the form of parity bits, calculated from the information bits, are added to the original data to detect the erroneous bits/frames.

If sufficient redundancy is added, then the receiver can not only detect errors but can also correct them. This is called forward error correction coding (FECC). A significant advantage of FECC is reduced latency (delay) variation. FECC may also be used where the delay incurred by an ARQ system is unacceptable in absolute terms, for example, channels with large propagation delay.

The addition of redundancy for either error detection or error correction is referred to as channel coding and can be implemented using a variety of algorithms. Block coding (Lee, 2000) generates an output sequence of n bits from each block of k input (information) bits by adding $n-k$ parity check bits. Convolutional coding (Johnson, 2010) generates a sequence of output bits for each individual input bit. Convolutional codes are generally very effective at correcting errors that are randomly distributed within the bit sequence but poor at correcting bursts of error, that is, contiguous strings of erroneous bits. Block codes typically perform better than convolutional codes in the presence of burst errors.

Concatenated coding refers to the combined use of two different channel coding techniques to realise a very powerful error correction function. Typically outer block coding is followed by inner convolutional coding at the transmitter with corresponding inner convolutional decoding followed by outer block decoding at the receiver. A popular choice of outer code in such systems is Reed-Solomon (Lee, 2000).

The error correcting performance of many codes for a given raw (i.e. uncoded) error rate is better if the bit errors are randomly distributed than if bit errors occur in bursts. The signal fading that is characteristic of wireless channels means that these systems are particularly prone to error bursts. In order to obtain the best possible performance from the error correcting codes, the bits in each frame are reordered after Forward Error Control (FEC) coding at the transmitter and 're-reordered' at the receiver prior to FEC decoding – a process known as interleaving. Burst errors caused after coding at the transmitter by the channel then appear as random errors prior to decoding at the receiver.

Turbo coding (Johnson, 2010) is a recent innovation in channel coding in which a pair of codes is concatenated in parallel rather than in series, that is, each code operates directly on the uncoded information stream. This allows the information provided by one code about the location of errors to be used by the other code in the correction of errors. Turbo codes are very powerful and can result in almost errorless transmission of information at rates approaching the theoretical limit (as determined by the Shannon-Hartley

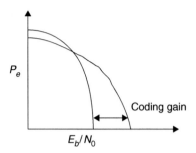

2.3 Probability of bit error versus E_b/N_0 with and without FECC.

capacity theorem). Such high-performance turbo codes can require large interleavers, however, resulting in high latency (i.e. long delay).

The performance of an error correcting code is summarised by its coding gain (measured in dB). This is the difference between the bit-energy to noise-power-spectral-density ratio, E_b/N_0 (or equivalently signal-to-noise ratio (SNR)), to achieve a specified probability of bit error, P_b, with and without coding. Coding gain is illustrated in Fig. 2.3. It is a function of error probability, although only weakly so in the low error probability regime.

Perhaps the most widely known LLC protocol is IEEE 802.2 (Anon, 1988), which was devised to operate in conjunction with Ethernet and other local area network technologies. This protocol provides three modes of operation:

1. Unacknowledged connectionless mode: no flow or error control.
2. Connection-oriented mode: connection established between peers a priori, flow and error control implemented.
3. Acknowledged connectionless mode: flow and error control utilised but no prior connection established.

The hostile nature of wireless links is such that both forward and backward error control are often utilised together. The various radio technologies implement customised ARQ mechanisms at various layers within their respective protocol stacks.

The well-known WLAN standard 802.11 implements a positive acknowledgement scheme as part of its MAC sublayer. Frames that are not acknowledged are retransmitted. Further robustness against data loss can be provided by utilising the functionality of IEEE 802.2.

Many cellular radio systems operate bespoke ARQ mechanisms over their radio interface. For example, the 2G system GSM/GPRS (i.e. Groupe Spécial Mobile/General Packet Radio Service) runs an LLC scheme between the mobile terminal and the serving GPRS support node (SGSN) – the entity within the core network that handles mobility management. An

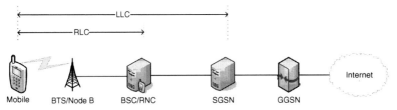

2.4 2G and 3G systems.

additional ARQ mechanism is implemented as part of its radio link control (RLC) protocol between the mobile terminal and base station controller (BSC) – the entity within the radio access network that controls a range of dumb base transceiver stations (BTS). Thus, the RLC operates as an inner loop to further segment LLC frames into RLC frames and retransmit lost data. If, after a number of unsuccessful attempts, it fails then the LLC outer loop will attempt retransmission of the entire LLC frame. If the LLC layer fails then the end-to-end ARQ scheme operated as part of TCP will invoke a retransmission of the entire segment.

The 3G Universal Mobile Telecommunication System (UMTS) operates on broadly similar principles; however, the entities involved have different names. The 3G equivalent of a BTS is a node B, and the equivalent of the BSC is the radio network controller (RNC). The operational scope of the RLC and LLC protocols for 2G and 3G systems is shown in Fig. 2.4.

The 4G long-term evolution (LTE) standard system employs a significantly different network architecture, in that the base station (known as the evolved node B) is not dumb and provides many of the functions of the node B and RNC combined. A single ARQ mechanism, therefore, operates between the mobile terminal and the evolved node B as part of its RLC protocol.

Radio systems are generally more bandwidth-constrained than wired systems. Several advanced techniques are therefore utilised to use the radio channel as efficiently as possible while still preserving the integrity of the transmitted data. More robust error control coding schemes can be used that permit errors to be not only detected but also corrected. Clearly, there is an overhead associated with the transmission of the greater number of parity bits that this requires but, depending on the characteristics of the radio channel, this may significantly reduce the number of retransmissions and, in doing so, result in a net decrease in bandwidth used. Modern cellular radio systems continuously monitor error rates and vary the ratio of parity bits to data bits to achieve optimum performance. Thus, mobile terminals in regions of favourable signal conditions will receive data with light error control coding, while those in adverse regions will receive data with heavy error control coding. The disadvantage of this approach is that terminals in areas of poor signal quality may receive poorer levels of throughput by virtue of the reduced number of data bits as a proportion of gross transmission rate. Designers of applications and services (including remote sensing and telemetry) must be aware, therefore, that the deliverable throughput may not be predictable in advance.

A simple way of combining ARQ with variable strength error correction codes is to transmit a frame with light protection. If that is erroneously received it is discarded and the ARQ mechanism requests a retransmission, however with stronger coding. This combination of error correction coding and ARQ is often referred to as (Type I) hybrid ARQ (HARQ).

Other approaches to bandwidth-efficient schemes are based on utilisation of as much information as possible to correct erroneous data. The idea is to reduce the number of retransmissions that are necessary to decode a transmitted frame. For example, whereas simple ARQ schemes will continually discard erroneous frames irrespective of the number of retransmission attempts, a more bandwidth-efficient approach would be to retain the erroneous frames. The original and subsequently retransmitted frames may be combined, say using a majority vote, to produce a corrected frame. In addition to being a more bandwidth-efficient approach, at the cost of little additional complexity, this approach has the potential to reduce average end-to-end latency since fewer retransmissions are required. The 3G high speed packet access (HSPA) service operates by transmitting the original block of data (including error correction code bits). If that is received in error then only additional error correction code bits are transmitted in response to an ARQ request, thus increasing the strength of the code on each retransmission using incremental redundancy (Type II HARQ).

2.4.2 Medium access control

The MAC protocol is the mechanism used by multiple terminals to coordinate communications over a shared medium. Most modern radio systems have their own bespoke MAC protocol. The space constraint here means, therefore, that it is not possible to describe all, or indeed any, of these in detail. Instead this section will focus on the key characteristic of MAC protocols for remote sensing and control applications: synchronous vs asynchronous systems.

The well-known local area network (LAN) technology Ethernet employs a technique known as carrier sense multiple access with collision detection (CSMA/CD) when deployed on a broadcast medium (bus topology). With this approach, terminals listen to the medium in an attempt to determine if another terminal is transmitting information. If not, they can commence transmission. Due to the fact that there is a finite propagation time for transmissions, it is possible for a terminal not to hear another terminal that has already commenced transmission. If the terminal in question were to attempt transmission then both transmissions would interfere with each other and cause corruption of data. When this happens, a collision is said to have occurred. Fortunately, both terminals can monitor the medium during transmission to detect collisions. When a collision is detected, both terminals wait a random time before sensing the medium again in an attempt to retransmit the corrupted data. The Wireless LAN technology 802.11 uses a similar approach, known as CSMA with collision avoidance (CSMA/CA). The principal difference between CSMA/CD and CSMA/CA is that unlike wired systems, wireless transceivers cannot monitor the medium (radio channel) while they transmit, and are therefore unable to implicitly determine if a collision has occurred. CSMA/CA systems rely on positive acknowledgements to indicate that data has been received uncorrupted. Both these schemes are examples of asynchronous MAC protocols.

Most cellular radio systems employ a synchronous MAC. For example, in the GPRS system terminals use a CSMA/CA-like procedure to contend for access to traffic channels (channels used for carrying user data) on a special random access channel. They use this channel to communicate their transmission requirements to a base station. Thereafter, the base station will reserve fixed resource blocks (time slots) on a particular radio frequency (RF) for the terminal to transmit user data. UMTS and LTE systems also use a synchronous MAC, although the definition of what constitutes a resource block varies from system to system.

The essential difference between a synchronous and an asynchronous system is that the former provides a dedicated logical channel for terminals, while the latter is based on random access, which can lead to some terminals dominating the transmission channel. The great advantage of being provided with dedicated resources is that the bandwidth and delay will be within fixed and predictable bounds. For real-time critical control applications, this may be an essential property. The disadvantage of this approach is that traffic channels may be under-utilised if the terminal transmits data only intermittently. Asynchronous systems have the potential to be more bandwidth-efficient (particularly at light load).

2.5 Physical layer

The physical layer of a communication system is the lowest layer in the protocol stack. It is concerned with the physical processes by which patterns of binary digits (which should strictly be referred to as 'binits' but are almost always referred to as bits) are conveyed from a transmitter to a receiver. The single most important function of the physical layer is to define the precise way that the bits are represented by (or mapped onto) a finite set of electrical waveforms or symbols. In the simplest case, two symbols are used, one symbol to represent binary zeros and one symbol to represent binary ones. (In this case the symbol is almost synonymous with the bit.) Groups of information bits (n-bit words) may be taken together, however, and mapped to $M = 2^n$ different symbols. The entire set of waveforms is often referred to as an alphabet.

In communication systems generally, the waveforms may be baseband (i.e. have a spectrum extending down, or almost down, to zero hertz) or they may be passband (i.e. be restricted to a band of frequencies starting well above zero hertz). In wireless systems, while baseband symbols may be used in the transmitter prior to modulation and in the receiver after demodulation, the symbols (i.e. signals or waveforms) transmitted across the channel are invariably passband, usually located in the RF part of the electromagnetic spectrum.

The simplest example of a baseband symbol alphabet is a positive rectangular voltage pulse to represent a binary one and a negative rectangular voltage pulse (of the same amplitude and duration) to represent a binary zero. The precise shapes of baseband pulses used to represent bits, or groups of bits, is called a line code. The example just given could be referred to as a polar binary line code. Another example of a popular binary line code is the use of a positive rectangular pulse for a binary one and no transmission at all (i.e. a zero amplitude, or null, pulse) for a binary zero. This could be referred to as a unipolar line code. It is also referred to as (baseband) on-off keying (OOK), since the digital ones in the binary data are used to turn (or 'key') the signal 'on'.

A disadvantage of both these line code examples is that their ($sinc^2$) power spectral densities are non-zero (in fact they are a maximum) at zero hertz. This means low frequencies have to be transferred faithfully from transmitter to receiver if the pulses are not to be distorted during transmission. This obviously precludes them from use in wireless transmission. (Even for wired communication systems which can utilise baseband transmission this is generally a problem, since it effectively excludes AC coupling of transmission lines.) A further disadvantage is that a long string of digital ones or zeros would result in an unchanging voltage – potentially resulting in loss of receiver synchronisation with the transmitted symbols. Many sophisticated line codes have been devised to address these problems, e.g. HDBn, making special provision to allow any arbitrary bit sequence to be successfully received (including long strings of ones and zeros). Such line codes are said to be 'transparent'.

Wireless communications systems must transmit symbols as signals or waveforms with a passband spectrum. This is required not only to allow the transmission to be located within the allocated radio channel but also to allow the use antennas with, simultaneously, reasonable radiation efficiency and reasonable size. This process of translating a set of baseband symbols to a set of bandpass symbols is called modulation (Glover and Grant, 2010).

2.5.1 Modulation

One method of translating the spectrum of a signal from baseband to passband is by multiplying the signal by a high frequency sinusoidal 'carrier' wave. If the carrier is a sinusoid of frequency f_c Hz then the (one-sided) power spectral density of the baseband signal $S(f)$ is shifted upwards in frequency by f_c Hz such that the (one-sided) passband signal has a spectrum $S(f - f_c)$. Figure 2.5 illustrates this schematically for the case of binary data with a unipolar baseband line code, and Fig. 2.6 illustrates the case for a binary data with a polar baseband line code. The carrier frequency is 900 MHz, and the bit rate is 40 Mbit/s in both figures.

The former modulation technique is usually referred to as OOK (for the same reasons as explained in the context of baseband OOK). More generically, however, it is referred to as binary amplitude shift keying (BASK), since the amplitude of the carrier is shifted between two levels by 'keying' with the baseband data.

The latter modulation technique is often referred to as phase reversal keying (PRK), since the effect of multiplying the carrier by a polar (±) bit stream is equivalent to shifting the phase of the carrier by π radians or 180°.

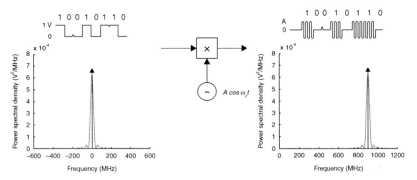

2.5 Schematic illustration of an OOK (BASK) modulation (Baseband spectrum two-sided, RF spectrum one-sided).

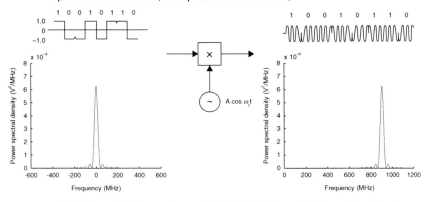

2.6 Schematic illustration of a PRK (BPSK) modulation (Baseband spectrum two-sided, RF spectrum one-sided).

The generic designation, however, is binary phase shift keying (BPSK), which allows the possibility of shifting between phase states separated by less than π radians. In this case the signal can be resolved into a PRK component and a constant (unmodulated) carrier. Such a BPSK system would sacrifice performance, in that the probability of bit error (P_b), also called the bit error ratio (BER), would be higher than for a PRK system. (BER and P_b are essentially synonymous and refer to the frequency with which digital ones are erroneously detected as digital zeros or vice versa.) The BER performance penalty arises because the power in the unmodulated component is 'wasted', in the sense that it carries no information, that is, it does not aid in distinguishing between digital ones and zeros. It does, however, provide a convenient signal which can be used to recover a carrier (typically via a phase locked loop) in the receiver. Such non-PRK BPSK systems can have some advantages, therefore, if the convenience provided by a 'pilot' carrier outweighs the BER performance penalty implied by the 'wasted' power.

The third (and final) generic binary modulation technique is binary frequency shift keying (BFSK). BFSK changes the frequency of a carrier (rather than its amplitude or phase angle) in sympathy with the baseband data. The resulting passband signal can be thought of as the sum (superposition) of two OOK signals: one signal in which the carrier is keyed on by the digital ones in the data, and one signal in which the carrier is keyed on by the digital zeros in the data. This is illustrated schematically in Fig. 2.7 for a carrier frequency of 900 MHz, a frequency deviation of 100 MHz, and a bit rate of 40 Mbit/s. Note that the tones have frequencies equal to the frequency of the suppressed carrier plus and minus the frequency deviation.

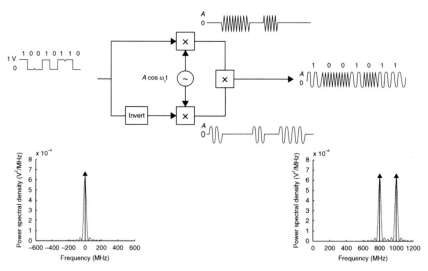

2.7 Schematic illustration of a BFSK modulation (Baseband spectrum two-sided, RF spectrum one-sided).

(The 'Invert' block, in Fig. 2.7, replaces 0 V with 1 V and 1 V with 0 V; it is not a linear gain of −1 but a gain of −1 plus a DC level of 1 V.)

Since the two OOK symbols represent bursts of carrier at different frequencies (tones) it is sometimes referred to as tone signalling. BFSK is a non-linear modulation technique, in that if two data streams are added at the modulator input the signal at the modulator output is not the sum of the two signals that arise if each input is applied separately.

There are two principal criteria against which modulation methods are benchmarked. These are power efficiency and bandwidth efficiency. (The word efficiency in both cases is a misnomer, in that it does not refer to a numerical value between 0 and 1 representing a ratio of output to input quantities. These terms are, however, widely used and accepted.)

Power efficiency refers to the SNR, or equivalently bit-energy to noise-power-spectral-density ratio (E_b/N_0), needed to realise a specified BER (e.g. 10^{-6}). A modulation scheme requiring lower SNR to realise the specified BER is said to be more power efficient. Modulation schemes with high power efficiency are preferred in applications where signal power is at a premium (e.g. where transmission loss and/or noise levels are high).

Bandwidth efficiency (measured in bit s^{-1} Hz^{-1}) refers to the bit rate (bit/s) offered by a modulation scheme divided by the bandwidth (Hz) of the modulated signal. The precise numerical value of bandwidth efficiency depends on the definition of bandwidth adopted (−3 dB, −10 dB, Gabor bandwidth, absolute bandwidth, etc.), but provided the same definition is adopted for all modulation schemes it does give a useful comparison of the relative 'efficiency' with which spectrum is being used. Modulation schemes with higher bandwidth efficiency are preferred in applications where the use of spectrum is especially costly.

The fundamental trade-off between power and bandwidth efficiency is reflected in the Shannon-Hartley channel capacity law, which is a statement of the maximum errorless information rate (channel capacity, C) that can be transmitted via a channel of bandwidth B that yields a received signal power S and a received noise power N, that is:

$$\frac{C}{B} = \log_{10}\left(1 + \frac{S}{N}\right) \text{ bit s}^{-1}\text{Hz}^{-1} \qquad [2.1]$$

The most power-efficient modulation scheme is PRK. This is because the two symbols are antipodal, that is, one binary symbol is precisely the opposite (i.e. the negative of) the other symbol. Their normalised correlation coefficient (the integral of the product of the symbols divided by the geometric mean of their energies) is therefore −1.0. There is no power wasted (e.g. in a pilot carrier) and the antipodal nature of the symbols means they are as different as it is possible for them to be. The two symbols are therefore most easily distinguished from each other in the presence of noise or interference and the required SNR for a specified BER is therefore a minimum.

OOK is an orthogonal modulation scheme. This means the correlation coefficient of the two symbols is zero and they are thus less dissimilar than the PRK symbols. Being less dissimilar they are less easily distinguished from one another in a noisy environment. The power efficiency of OOK is thus poorer than PRK. In the case of receivers using ideal detection (correlation or, equivalently, matched filter detection) the power efficiency penalty of OOK compared to PRK is 3 dB, that is twice the signal power (averaged over many bits) is required for OOK as is required for PRK to realise a specified BER. (An alternative, of course, to a requirement of twice the signal power would be half the noise power.)

The precise normalised correlation between the symbols of a BFSK system depends on the relationship between tone spacing and bit rate. The correlation is theoretically bounded by 1.0 (for the case of equal frequency symbols – useless, of course, for conveying information) and $-2/(3\pi)$ (for the case when the tone frequency difference is about 0.72 times the bit rate). In practical systems the tone frequencies and bit rate are typically chosen such that the correlation is close to zero, that is, the symbols are orthogonal, or at least nearly so. In this case the BFSK power efficiency is equal, or close, to that of OOK.

Equation [2.2] gives the probability of bit error, P_b, as a function of E_b/N_0 and the correlation coefficient (ρ) between symbols for an arbitrary binary modulation scheme – including the special cases of OOK, BFSK and PRK. (E_b/N_0 is the ratio of average bit-energy to one-sided noise-power-spectral-density.)

$$P_b = \frac{1}{2}\left[1 - erf\sqrt{\frac{1-\rho}{2}\left(\frac{E_b}{N_0}\right)^{\frac{1}{2}}}\right] \qquad [2.2]$$

Table 2.1 gives the value of ρ for the common binary modulation schemes.

For binary modulation schemes other than those listed in Table 2.1, the value of ρ can be calculated using:

$$\rho = \frac{1}{\sqrt{E_1 E_2}} \int_0^{T_0} v_1(t) v_2(t) dt \qquad [2.3]$$

where the subscripts distinguish the two symbols. The BER given by Equation [2.3] is for the case of ideal coherent detection (which means intersymbol-free signalling and either a correlation receiver or a matched filter receiver). For BPSK (including PRK), coherent detection is necessary since the information

Table 2.1 Correlation coefficient for common binary modulation methods

Modulation method	OOK	BFSK (orthogonal)	BPSK (optimum)	PRK ($\Delta\theta = \pi$)	BPSK ($\Delta\theta < \pi$)
ρ	0	0	$-2/(3\pi)$	-1	$\cos \Delta\theta$

resides in the phase angle of the symbols. Incoherent detection (e.g. an envelope detector followed by a low-pass filter) can always be used for OOK and can usually be used for BFSK (provided there is sufficient spacing between tones). Incoherent detection is simpler to implement than coherent detection but suffers a small penalty in power efficiency. The increase in BER can be compensated, however, by increasing the signal power (or reducing the noise power) by a small amount (typically about 1 dB for a BER around 10^{-4}). The modest increase in SNR necessary to compensate for the poorer BER offered by an incoherent receiver means that, in practice, incoherent detection is normally used in OOK and BFSK receivers.

Although BPSK (including PRK) systems require coherent detection, a technique exists that obviates the need for complex carrier recovery circuitry in the receiver. This is differential PSK (DPSK), in which the bit stream is differentially coded in the transmitter, a transition in the bit stream (0 to 1 or 1 to 0) being represented by one PRK symbol (e.g. phase 0) and no transition (0 to 0 or 1 to 1) being represented by the other symbol (e.g. phase π). In the receiver a simple one-bit delay can then be used to provide a coherent reference (the previous symbol) for the detection of the current symbol. This simplified receiver structure differentially decodes the received bit stream concurrently with detection. Since the coherent reference signal in such a receiver is now precisely as noisy as the symbol being detected it might be thought that DPSK suffers a 3 dB penalty in power efficiency compared to ideal detection in a correlation receiver of uncoded PRK. In practice, the penalty is less than this (around 1 dB), since the phase noise is not completely decorrelated between the adjacent bits, that is, there is some degree of 'noise cancellation' between the symbol being detected and the 'reference' signal. If differential coding of the bit stream is implemented at the transmitter, but conventional correlation or matched filter detection is used at the receiver followed by separate differential decoding, then the scheme is referred to as differentially encoded PSK (DEPSK). There is no simplification in receiver design in this case – indeed, there is the modest additional complexity of post-detection differential decoding. The performance penalty (for realistically small probabilities of error) is now simply a factor of 2 in BER, since both inputs to the differential decoder have the same probability of error. (For practical, that is, small, BERs the probability of both input bits being in error, and therefore the decoded bit being correct, can usually be neglected.)

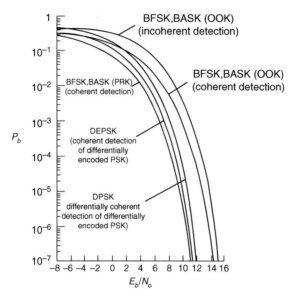

2.8 BER versus E_b/N_0 for common binary modulation techniques. (*Source*: Glover and Grant, 2010.)

Figure 2.8 shows a comparison of the BER vs E_b/N_0 curves for all the binary modulation schemes discussed above.

If bandwidth efficiency (also sometimes called spectral efficiency) is more important than power efficiency, then multiple bits can be mapped onto a single symbol, a bandwidth efficiency improvement arising since it is the symbol (or physical pulse) rate, rather than the bit rate, which determines bandwidth. The two most common 'higher order' modulation schemes used in practice are *M*-ary PSK (MPSK) and *M*-ary quadrature amplitude modulation (MQAM). In the former case the number of symbols (*M*) in the symbol alphabet is typically an integer power of two 2 (i.e. 4, 8, 16, 32, …) and the tips of the *M* symbol phasors form a constellation of points evenly distributed around a circle in the complex plane. In the latter case, *M* is typically an even integer power of 2 (i.e. 4, 16, 64, 256, …) and the symbol phasors form a square regular grid of constellation points. For *M* = 4, MPSK and MQAM are identical, and this modulation scheme is referred to as quadrature (or quaternary) phase shift keying (QPSK). Figure 2.9 shows the constellation diagrams for 16-PSK, 64-QAM and QPSK signalling systems.

The spectral efficiency of an *M*-ary modulation scheme, mapping $n = \log_2 M$ bits to each symbol, is given by:

$$\eta_s = \frac{\log_2 M}{T_0 B} \quad [\text{bit s}^{-1}\text{Hz}^{-1}] \qquad [2.4]$$

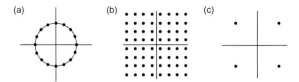

2.9 Constellations for (a) 16-PSK, (b) 64-QAM and (c) QPSK.

T_0 in Equation [2.4] is the reciprocal of the symbol, or baud, rate and B is the signal bandwidth. The T_0B product in the denominator of Equation [2.4] is a significant parameter in its own right. For a bandpass signal $T_0B \geq 1.0$ is a necessary (but not sufficient) condition if inter-symbol interference (ISI) is to be avoided. If $T_0B < 1.0$ then ISI cannot be avoided. ISI describes the smearing (time dispersion) of one received symbol into the adjacent symbol(s) due to the distorting effects of the channel such that decision instant samples no longer represent a single symbol. The channel frequency response that causes this distortion potentially includes contributions from the transmitter and receiver filters as well as the transmission medium. In a channel suffering ISI, each decision instant sample at the receiver represents the symbol that was intended to be sampled plus fractions of adjacent symbols. The result of ISI is a reduction in the robustness of the modulation scheme to noise, and thus an increase in BER. If the ISI is severe it may lead to bit errors, even in the absence of noise. The resulting BER is then referred to as 'irreducible', since it cannot be improved by increasing signal power. (It is of course reducible by more careful design of the transmitter and receiver filtering and/or equalisation of the channel distortion. The latter can be achieved by periodically measuring the channel frequency response and incorporating an adaptive filter in the receiver with a response that is, effectively, the reciprocal of that of the channel.) Transmit and receive filtering, which preserves ISI-free samples at the receiver decision circuit input, is called Nyquist filtering. One particular form of Nyquist filtering often used in practice is raised-cosine filtering. When this filter is split properly between transmitter and receiver, then ISI at the sampling instants is avoided while simultaneously preserving ideal (matched filter) detection.

The probability of bit error for ISI-free, Gray-coded, MPSK signalling is given approximately by:

$$P_b \approx \frac{1}{\log_2 M} \left\{ 1 - erf \left[\sin\left(\frac{\pi}{M}\right) \sqrt{\log_2 M} \left(\frac{E_b}{N_0}\right)^{\frac{1}{2}} \right] \right\} \qquad [2.5]$$

Gray coding (the mapping of bits to symbols such that the binary words represented by adjacent symbols differ by only one bit) is virtually always used in *M*-ary modulation schemes, since this minimises the BER for a given symbol error result (SER). (If symbol errors are dominated by those involving an adjacent symbol, as is the case for most types of noise when errors are relatively rare, then BER is approximately SER/*n* since each symbol error results in one bit error but *n*-1 bits remain correct.)

The probability of bit error for ISI-free Gray-coded MQAM signalling is given approximately by:

$$P_b \approx \frac{2}{\log_2 M} \left\{ \frac{M^{\frac{1}{2}} - 1}{M^{\frac{1}{2}}} \right\} \left[1 - erf \sqrt{\frac{3\log_2 M}{2(M-1)} \left(\frac{E_b}{N_0} \right)^{\frac{1}{2}}} \right] \quad [2.6]$$

Figure 2.10 compares the BER versus E_b/N_0 curves for a range of MPSK and MQAM systems.

Figure 2.11 locates MPSK and MQAM modulation schemes in the spectral efficiency/power efficiency plane. (The power efficiency here is represented by the SNR required for a BER of 10^{-6} assuming an ideal ISI-free matched filter receiver.) The Shannon channel capacity, rearranged to give maximum possible spectral efficiency versus SNR (Equation [2.1]) for error-free transmission, is also plotted in Fig. 2.11. This figure illustrates how closely a particular modulation scheme approaches the theoretical ideal. (Channel

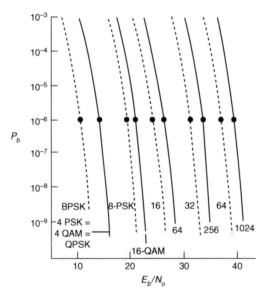

2.10 Comparison of BER versus E_b/N_0 for MPSK and MQAM systems. (*Source*: Glover and Grant, 2010.)

Overview of wireless techniques for use with MEMS

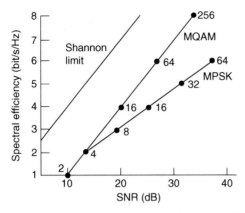

2.11 Comparison of spectral and power efficiencies of popular modulation schemes with the Shannon limit.

coding can be applied, of course, to move the combined modulation-coding scheme closer to the Shannon limit.)

2.5.2 Spread spectrum

Spread spectrum (Torrieri, 2011) refers to the technique in which an information signal with a (relatively) narrow bandwidth is spread over a wider band of frequencies by modulating it with a 'spreading' signal. (To qualify as a true spread spectrum technique the spreading signal must not be derived from the information signal.) Figure 2.12 illustrates the basic principle of direct sequence spread spectrum (DSSS), which is conceptually the simplest way of doing this.

The (voltage) spectrum of the spread signal is that of the pre-spread signal convolved with the (voltage) spectrum of the spreading waveform. If the bandwidth of the spreading waveform is much greater than the bandwidth of the pre-spread signal then the post-spread signal has, to a first approximation, the bandwidth of the spreading waveform.

The spreading waveform is deterministic and is therefore known at the receiver. It is usually a pseudo-random chip sequence (PRCS) – often generated using a shift register with feedback from its elements to its input via a modulo-2 adder. The terminology 'chip' is used to denote a single DSSS symbol to distinguish it from a 'bit', which relates to the longer, information-carrying symbol. The spread signal is usually then modulated onto an RF sinusoidal carrier at the transmitter in the normal way. At the receiver the spread signal is recovered from the RF signal by demodulation using a matched filter, correlation processor or incoherent detector as usual. De-spreading is achieved by multiplying by the same PRCS sequence as

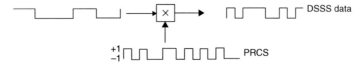

2.12 Basic DSSS.

used for spreading. (The reference PRCS sequence in this process is synchronised to that in the received signal.) That re-multiplication at the receiver of a DSSS signal with the same PRCS as applied at the transmitter de-spreads the signal is easy to see in the case of a polar binary chip sequence with values of ±1 since, after de-spreading, the information has been multiplied by the spreading sequence squared, that is, $(\pm 1)^2 = 1$.

There are several potential advantages to spreading the spectrum of a signal. These include:

- Security advantages – The spread signal has many properties in common with noise and, if the spectral density is low, it can be difficult to detect the presence of the signal unless the spreading sequence is known. (Spread spectrum is not a substitute, however, for proper data encryption if data privacy, authenticity and/or integrity are important.)
- Regulatory advantages – Radio regulatory authorities restrict the power spectral density of signals radiated in some frequency bands. Spread spectrum can be helpful in achieving low spectral density without compromising total radiated power.
- Interference suppression – Interference added after spreading will be spread by the PRCS sequence in the receiver at the same time as the wanted signal is de-spread. After filtering using the bandwidth of the de-spread information signal much of the interference is therefore removed.
- If mutually orthogonal (or nearly orthogonal) spreading sequences are applied to different information signals then each information signal can be recovered independently of the others by de-spreading with its own sequence. (All the other information signals spread by orthogonal sequences are thereby suppressed relative to the wanted signal.) This is the basis of the code division multiple access (CDMA) scheme used in third-generation mobile phone technology.

For white noise (or interference processes), de-spreading results in an SNR (or signal to interference ratio) processing gain, G_p, given by:

$$G_p = 10 \log_{10} \left(\frac{R_c}{R_b} \right) \text{ dB} \qquad [2.7]$$

where R_b and R_c are the bit rate and chip rate, respectively.

DSSS, as described above, is similar to an additional PRK modulation process, in that multiplying by chips with amplitude of ±1 results in (chip-by-chip) shifting of the carrier phase in the RF modulated signal by 0 or π radians. An alternative spectrum spreading technique, frequency hopping spread spectrum (FHSS), is similar to an additional FSK modulation process. In FHSS the frequency of the carrier is changed ('hopped') pseudo-randomly. If the frequency is hopped many times per symbol, then it is referred to as fast frequency hopping. If the frequency hopping rate is low compared to the symbol period, then it is referred to as slow frequency hopping. Measured on an appropriate time scale the spectrum of the RF signal in both cases is spread over a band between the highest and lowest frequencies in the hopping scheme.

At the receiver an FHSS signal is de-spread by hopping the local oscillator synchronously with frequency changes in the hopped data. FHSS offers similar advantages to DSSS.

DSSS is applied in third-generation cellular radio systems to realise CDMA and FHSS is applied in Bluetooth technology.

2.5.3 Orthogonal frequency division multiplexing

Orthogonal frequency division multiplexing (OFDM) takes a digital information signal with bit rate R_b, maps n-bit words on to $M = 2^n$ symbols (each symbol being a complex number representing the amplitude and phase of an M-ary modulation scheme), splits the resulting symbol stream (rate $R_s = R_b/n$) into N parallel streams (each of rate $R_{OFDM} = R_s/N$) and modulates each stream onto one of N different carriers (Li and Stubber, 2010). The N frequencies chosen for the carriers are such that the carriers are mutually orthogonal over one OFDM symbol period, $T_{OFDM} = 1/R_{OFDM}$, allowing independent recovery of each parallel information stream. Figure 2.13 shows the spectrum of a (small) number of adjacent (unmodulated) OFDM carriers.

The basic process of impressing the parallel symbol stream onto the orthogonal carriers is illustrated in Fig. 2.14.

The fundamental advantage of OFDM is that its symbol rate is a factor of N times lower than the original symbol stream (and Nn lower than the original bit stream). Time dispersion in the radio channel (caused by propagation of energy between transmitter and receiver along multiple propagation paths – some paths involving reflection from distant objects) results in echoes of earlier symbols overlapping with later symbols, that is, it causes ISI. Reducing the symbol rate on each orthogonal channel reduces the degree of overlap (as a proportion of the OFDM symbol duration), thereby greatly reducing the deleterious effects of ISI on BER.

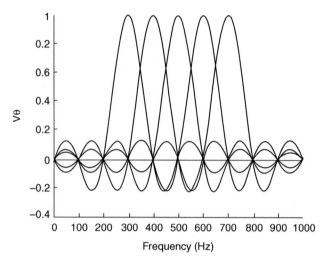

2.13 Five adjacent (unmodulated) OFDM carriers.

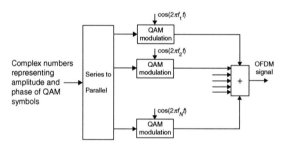

2.14 Conceptual representation of OFDM transmitter.

In practice the strict orthogonality of OFDM carriers is compromised by the multipath channel. Orthogonality can be re-established by extending the duration of each OFDM symbol using a 'cyclic prefix'. This prefix is a copy of the final part of an OFDM symbol added to the front of the OFDM symbol. To be entirely effective the prefix must be at least as long as the delay of the most delayed (significant) multipath echo.

OFDM has been adopted in the Terrestrial Digital Video Broadcast standard DVB-T and the 3GPP LTE. One of the developments that has made OFDM a popular recent solution for radio communications in severe multipath environments is the (very efficient) fast Fourier transform (FFT) algorithm. The impressing of symbols (complex numbers) on to a carrier determines the amplitude and phase of that carrier. N such symbols therefore determine (for one OFDM symbol period) the amplitude and phase (at the discrete carrier frequencies) of the OFDM signal spectrum. The inverse fast Fourier transform (IFFT) can therefore be used to realise the basic OFDM signal at the transmitter and the FFT can be used to recover (demultiplex) the symbols at the receiver.

2.5.4 Ultra-wideband

Ultra-wideband (UWB) refers to a signal that has a −10 dB bandwidth greater than 500 MHz or a fractional bandwidth (bandwidth divided by the band centre frequency) greater than 20%. There has been intense recent interest in the use of such signals for high data-rate, low power, short-range communications. Regulatory authorities around the world have agreed that unlicensed transmission of UWB signals can be allowed subject to certain restrictions. The most important of these restrictions is that the power spectral density (PSD) should not exceed limits determined by a PSD mask. The details of the mask differ depending on application and geography, but a common feature is that the PSD is always restricted to −41.3 dBm/MHz or less. Figure 2.15a shows the Federal Communications Commission (FCC) PSD mask for indoor applications in the USA and Fig. 2.15b shows the Ofcom mask adopted in the UK.

The spectral mask ensures that the power from a UWB system falling within the band of a co-located conventional communications system is sufficiently low to avoid significant interference. The PSD limit is lower than −41.3 dBm/MHz in some bands to give extra protection for some existing services, e.g. GPS. The low PSD of UWB systems typically restricts their range to around 10 m. The large bandwidth, however, results in potentially huge data rates.

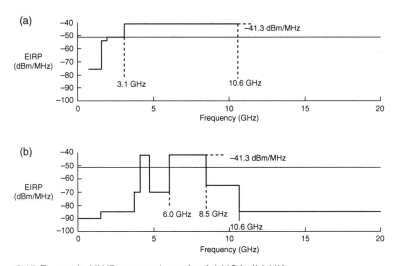

2.15 Example UWB spectral masks: (a) USA; (b) UK.

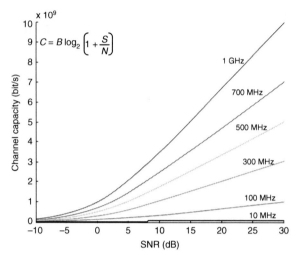

2.16 Channel capacity versus SNR and bandwidth.

Figure 2.16 illustrates the theoretical channel capacity (calculated using the Shannon-Hartley law) as a function of bandwidth and SNR.

UWB modulation schemes (Arslan *et al.*, 2006) can broadly divided into two categories: multi-carrier UWB (MC-UWB) and impulse radio (IR).

The most important MC-UWB variation is multi-band OFDM (MB-OFDM). A practical specification based on MC-UWB has been developed by the MB-OFDM Alliance – a group of organisations (including companies) that came together to champion this particular form of UWB technology.

Important variations of IR include Direct Sequence UWB (DS-UWB) and Pulse Position Modulation Time-Hopped UWB (PPM-TH-UWB). Both of these are included as part of the IEEE 802.15.3a standard.

DS-UWB is similar to DSSS except that each chip is transmitted as a short pulse with duration of the order of 1 ns. (The precise duration of the pulses, of course, depends on the desired UWB bandwidth.) The pulses are typically wavelet-like and are often modelled as a high-order time-derivative of a Gaussian pulse.

PPM-TH-UWB transmits narrow pulses but, rather than wavelets, they are typically monocycles or doublets, often modelled by the first and second time-derivative of a Gaussian pulse respectively. Information is coded onto the pulse stream using pulse position modulation (PPM). If the nominal pulse slot is divided into M sub-slots then $n = \log_2 M$ information bits determine the sub-slot to be used. To avoid particular bit patterns resulting in a transmitted pulse sequence with large amounts of power concentrated in discrete spectral lines, the position of the pulse slot is, itself, hopped in time within a larger symbol slot using a pseudo-random sequence. (The concentration of power in spectral lines is likely to result in a violation of the UWB spectral mask.)

2.5.5 Software radio and cognitive radio

The advent of cheap, fast, signal processing technologies (in particular fast analog-to-digital converters (ADCs) and digital-to-analog converters (DACs)) has allowed much of the communications signal processing that was formerly implemented in hardware to be implemented in software. This allows programmable transceivers to be realised in which carrier frequency bandwidth, modulation and coding can all be rapidly programmed for a specific application. This is what is commonly referred to as software radio (Rouphael, 2009). If the transceiver can be reconfigured sufficiently rapidly, and some element of environmental sensing is incorporated (e.g. sensing the occupancy or otherwise of the spectrum to which the transceiver has access), then these parameters may be dynamically optimised. This is an example of cognitive radio, that is, a radio system which is, at least to some extent, aware of its environment and adapts accordingly (Doyle, 2009). Spectrum that is notionally dedicated to a particular service, for example, but is unused in some bands at some times, is referred to (during the time, and within the bands, it is not used) as white spectrum. One (but not the only) application of cognitive radio is the detection and use of these white spaces. The spaces may be split into many non-contiguous fragments across a wide range of frequencies requiring the cognitive radio to divide data into parallel streams at the transmitter and reassemble these streams at the receiver. OFDM Access (OFDMA) techniques, in which OFDM carriers are assigned dynamically to the fragmented white spaces is a particularly attractive method of exploiting spectrum of this kind. The sensing and signal processing required to handle such dynamically changing fragmented spectrum opportunities is clearly challenging. The increasing cost of spectrum use, however, is a powerful driver of this type of technology.

2.6 The wireless link budget

The wireless link budget is fundamental to the physical layer of any wireless system. It is used to assess the required transmitter power and/or the required receiver noise figure to achieve acceptable link BER.

There are two distinct parts to the link budget: the signal-budget and the noise-budget. The basic signal-budget is represented by Equation [2.8].

$$P_R = P_T + G_T - L_P + G_R \qquad [2.8]$$

where P_R (dBW) is the received power, P_T (dBW) is the transmitted power, G_T (dBi) is the transmit antenna gain (defined with respect to an isotropic radiator), L_P (dB) is the path loss and G_R (dBi) is the receive antenna gain. There are often constraints on individual terms in Equation [2.8]. The transmitted power may be constrained, for example, by the energy capacity of the power supply and, if the power supply cannot be replaced, the required battery life of the system. Legal constraints imposed by radio regulatory bodies may limit the transmitted power, the effective isotropic radiated power (EIRP = $P_R + G_T$), the maximum power density (dB[W/m²]) at a specified range and/or the transmitted PSD (dB[W/Hz]). There are physical limitations on antenna gains that depend on the antenna's electrical size and there is the constraint that an isotropic antenna (i.e. one with a gain that is independent of direction) is not realisable. Despite such constraints transmitted power and antenna gains are, at least to some extent, under the control of the system designer. Path loss depends on link length and the environment, and is usually under the control of the designer only in so far as link length is a design variable. If link length is pre-determined by the application there is little, or no, control over this term.

The treatment of antennas here is restricted to the basic systems concept of antenna gain. For a transmitting antenna, gain is the ratio of the (far-field) radiation intensity (in W/sr) in a given direction (the direction of maximum gain unless otherwise specified) to the radiation intensity ($P_T/4\pi$) that would be delivered by an isotropic antenna. Alternatively (and equivalently), it is the ratio of the power density (in W/m²) in a given direction at a given (far-field) range, R, to the power density ($P_T/4\pi R^2$) that would be delivered at the same range by an isotropic antenna. For a receiving antenna, gain is the ratio of received power (available at the antenna terminals) due to a plane wave arriving from a particular direction to the power that would be available from an isotropic receiving antenna (i.e. an antenna whose sensitivity to a plane wave is independent of the wave's arrival direction).

Path loss, L_P, is the mean difference between transmitted and received power assuming isotropic transmit and receive antennas. (Taking the mean is necessary since path loss is usually subject to random fluctuations due interference between fields arising from multiple propagation paths. In some applications fading may also be caused due to shadowing by obstacles along the line-of-sight path.) Path loss can often be adequately modelled by a law of the form:

$$L_P = K + 10n \log_{10}\left(\frac{R}{R_0}\right) \text{ dB} \qquad [2.9]$$

where K and n are constants for a particular environment. n is sometimes referred to as the path loss index and is determined by the geometrical dilution of power density as energy propagates away from the transmitter. For free-space propagation $n = 2$ (corresponding to the inverse square law) and $K = 20 \log_{10}(4\pi/\lambda)$ where λ is wavelength. Free-space path loss increases at a rate of 6 dB/octave (i.e. received power in watts decreases by a factor of 4 for each factor of 2 increase in link length).

For propagation over a plane reflecting surface the path loss has a different character in two different range regions and must generally be modelled by a two-slope model of the form:

$$L_P = \begin{cases} K + 10n_1 \log_{10} R, & 0 \leq R \leq R_b \\ K + 10n_1 \log_{10} R_b + 10n_2 \log_{10}(R - R_b), & R_b \leq R \end{cases} \quad [2.10]$$

where R_b $(=4\pi h_T h_R/\lambda)$ is the break point between the two segments of the piece-wise linear law, n_1 and n_2 are the slopes of the law for ranges (from the transmitter) less than, and greater than, R_b, respectively, n_1 and K are the same as for free-space path loss, $n_2 = 4$ and h_T and h_R are the heights of the transmit and receive antennas above the reflecting surface. The path loss in region $R < R_b$ is subject to spatial fluctuations of power density or field strength due to the interference pattern formed by power arriving at the receive antenna directly from the transmitter along the line-of-site (LOS) path and power arriving at the receive antenna via reflection from the surface. The fluctuations in the simple model oscillate between +6 dB and $-\infty$ dB with respect to the free-space value. (The fluctuations are essentially sinusoidal, that is, the free-space value of received power in watts is multiplied by the factor $4\sin^2(2\pi h_T h_R/\lambda R)$.) The path loss in the region $R > R_b$ increases monotonically with a slope that is asymptotic to 12 dB/octave. The increased slope is composed of 6 dB/octave due to spreading loss (as in the free-space model) and 6 dB/octave due to increasingly complete cancellation between the LOS field and the reflected field.

Although the parameters in Equation [2.10] are defined above for the case of an ideal plane reflecting surface (sometimes referred to as planeearth propagation) it can be used to model path loss in more general environments in which case R_b, K, n_1 and n_2 may take on different values (often found by linear regression of experimentally measured path loss data). The same is true of the single-slope model, Equation [2.9]. In some environments, particularly those in which very short paths are of interest, a threeslope model may be required. The region closest to the transmitter may then model near-field coupling between antennas. (For electrically small antennas the near-field is confined to a region which extends to a distance of about one wavelength from the antenna.)

If a propagation medium is inherently lossy then the model for a nonlossy medium (often the free-space model) can be adapted by adding an attenuation term, A (dB), to the path loss. A is normally calculated from the specific attenuation A_s (dB/m) of the lossy medium (i.e. the attenuation per unit distance) using:

$$A = A_s L \qquad [2.11]$$

where L is the length of the path in the lossy medium (which may, of course, be the same as the link length R).

Local amplitude fluctuations (i.e. fluctuations in a region of space a few wavelengths in extent) due to the constructive and destructive interference between the fields arising from multiple propagation paths may be modelled, provided there is a sufficient number of paths and no path(s) dominates, by a random variable following a Rayleigh probability density function (pdf). Such fluctuations are normally referred to as fast fading (although they may result in signal enhancement as well as signal fades). If one path is much stronger than the others then the fading pdf is Rician and the ratio between the power carried by the strong path to the power carried by all other paths is referred to as the Rician K-factor. ($K = 0$ therefore corresponds to Rayleigh fading.) If the K-factor is known, then it is a relatively simple matter to calculate the fade level F (dB) exceeded in a given fraction of locations. If the transmitter, receiver or scattering objects are moving then F is also the fade level exceeded for a given fraction of time. F can therefore be interpreted as the fade level exceeded with a given probability.

In order to ensure a radio system, operating in a multipath environment, will have a specified availability (i.e. to ensure it will have received power that exceeds the minimum value required for acceptable system performance for a given fraction of locations or time) a fade margin (equal to F) can be added to the path loss.

In applications where signal fluctuation is due to shadowing by obstacles (rather than interference between multiple propagation paths) the fading is often referred to as slow fading and modelled by a log-normal process (i.e. a random fade expressed in dB that has a Gaussian pdf). In this case the median path loss is typically found from an empirical model (i.e. one based on measurements) such as Equation [2.9] or [2.10] and the severity of the fading is specified by the standard deviation of the scattered data. An appropriate fade margin is then given by the upper limit (M_F) in the integral from $-\infty$ to M_F of the (Gaussian) fade pdf that yields the required availability (i.e. the required fraction of locations, fraction of time or probability).

If multipath fading and (log-normal) shadowing are both present then they can usually be assumed to be statistically independent in which case the fading follows a Suzuki distribution (Suzuki, 1977).

The basic noise-budget is represented by Equation [2.12]:

$$N = k(T_a + T_e)B \quad \text{W} \qquad [2.12]$$

where N is the equivalent in-band noise power referred to the antenna terminals, k (=1.381×10^{-23} J/K) is Boltzmann's constant, T_a (K) is the antenna noise temperature, T_e (K) is the equivalent noise temperature of the receiver (representing the internal noise generated by the receiver electronics) and B (Hz) is the bandwidth of the receiver. (Strictly B is the noise bandwidth, which is the bandwidth of the filter with an ideal rectangular amplitude response that passes the same power as the cascaded filters in the receiver. For approximate calculations, however, the 3 dB bandwidth of the receiver can usually be substituted for the noise bandwidth.) The antenna noise temperature represents the noise arising from the antenna. This includes a contribution arising from noisy electromagnetic radiation received by the antenna and a contribution arising from the thermal motion of free charge in the material from which the antenna is made. For calculations of modest accuracy it is often sufficient to equate T_a to the mean physical temperature of the environment, for example, 290 K. This corresponds to a (conservative) assumption that the environment is made up of black body radiators. If a more accurate answer is required, or if the radiation efficiency of the antenna is low (as can be the case for electrically small antennas), then T_a may be calculated using:

$$T_a = T_A \eta_\Omega + T_{ph}(1 - \eta_\Omega) \text{ K} \qquad [2.13]$$

where T_A is antenna aperture temperature (representing the electromagnetic brightness of the material surrounding the antenna weighted by the antenna gain pattern), T_{ph} is the physical temperature of the antenna and η_Ω is the ohmic efficiency of the antenna (equal to the ratio of antenna radiation-resistance to antenna input-resistance).

The noise temperature of the receiver is related to its noise figure, f_n, by:

$$T_e = (f_n - 1)290 \text{ K} \qquad [2.14]$$

(f_n in Equation [2.14] is expressed as a linear ratio. It is more usually quoted, however, in decibels, that is, $F_n = 10 \log_{10} f_n$ dB.) The noise figure of a linear receiver can be calculated from the noise figure of its component subsystems using the Friis noise formula (Glover and Grant, 2010).

Equation [2.8] (supplemented with any necessary attenuation and fade margin terms) combined with Equation [2.12] will give the transmitter power needed if the required SNR is known or, alternatively, the SNR achievable if the maximum transmitter power is known.

2.7 Physical layer system design

The link budget is central to a communication system physical layer design. It normally involves several trade-offs and several iterations. Typically, however, such a design might proceed as follows:

1. Estimate the worst case antenna temperature (T_a) using either Equation [2.13] or the physical temperature of the environment. (This may depend on the chosen frequency band.)
2. Measure the receiver noise temperature (T_e) or calculate it from Equation [2.14] if its noise figure (or the noise figures of its component subsystems) is known.
3. Calculate the system noise-power-spectral-density $N_0 = k(T_a + T_e)$ W/Hz.
4. Establish the minimum bit rate (R_b) and maximum BER (P_b) required for the particular application.
5. Establish the maximum channel bandwidth (B) available for the particular application.
6. Assume a maximum (ISI-free) symbol rate $R_s = 1/B$. (The precise relationship between symbol rate and bandwidth will be determined by the pulse shaping.)
7. Calculate the minimum number of bits per symbol, $n \geq R_b/R_s$.
8. Calculate the minimum modulation order, $M \geq 2^n$, required to realise at least the minimum required bit rate.
9. Choose a modulation scheme of at least order M. (The choice of modulation scheme may depend on issues such as the relative importance of power efficiency and implementation cost.)
10. Calculate the required bit-energy E_b to achieve the required BER using the appropriate P_e versus E_b/N_0 formula (e.g. Equations [2.2], [2.5] or [2.6]).
11. Calculate the required received signal power using $P_R = E_b R_b$.
12. Estimate the mean path loss using an appropriate model (e.g. using Equation [2.9] or [2.10]).
13. If lossy attenuation is present add A (calculated using Equation [2.11]) to the path loss.
14. If fading is present add M_F (calculated using the appropriate fading statistics and the required availability) to the path loss.
15. Use Equation [2.8] to calculate the required transmit power.
16. If the required transmit power P_R (dBW) is greater than the maximum desirable transmit power $P_{R,max}$ (dBm) then chose a channel coding scheme with coding gain $G_c \geq P_R - P_{R,max}$ at the required BER.

The above design 'recipe' is only an example, of course, and the procedure will vary depending on which parameters are most tightly constrained. In reality the design is an iterative process with elements being repeated until a solution is found that satisfies all the important constraints. For complex systems several candidate designs, initially arrived at by a process similar to that described, may be investigated more thoroughly using simulation. Simulink (a MathWorks product) is an example of a popular simulation package that might be used for such simulations.

2.8 Conclusion

In this chapter the end-to-end transport of packets over a network has been reviewed. In particular, the traditional strategy for congestion control in TCP has been described and the difficulties this strategy presents for wireless networks has been pointed out. The importance of error control in wireless networks and its role in preventing packet loss on otherwise unreliable links has been emphasised. The various approaches to link-level error control including ARQ, forward error control coding and hybrid methods have been described.

The difficulty of routing data packets to mobile devices has been discussed and example solutions in the context of mobile IPv6 and NEMO have been outlined. MAC and the key choice between synchronous and asynchronous approaches for sensing and control applications have been discussed.

A range of modulation methods for wireless systems have been presented and their BER performance and spectral efficiencies compared. Spread spectrum, OFDM, ultra-wideband and cognitive radio techniques have been briefly reviewed and their particular advantages for wireless systems outlined. Link and noise budgets have been defined and their respective calculations presented. Finally, a typical step-by-step physical layer design process has been described.

2.9 References

Anon (1988), IEEE Standard For Information Technology, Telecommunications and information exchange between systems, Local and metropolitan area networks, Specific requirements, Part 2: Logical Link Control, ISO/IEC 8802-2:1998.

Anon (1981), *Transmission control protocol*, Internet Engineering Task Force, Request for comments 793, Sept. 1981.

Arslan H, Chen Z N and Di Benedetto M G (Eds) (2006), *Ultra wideband wireless communications*, New Jersey, Wiley, 2006.

Deering S (1998), *Internet protocol version 6 (IPv6) specification*, Internet Engineering Task Force, Request for comments 2460, Dec. 1998.

Devarpalli V (2005), *Network mobility (NEMO) basic support protocol*, Internet Engineering Task Force, request for comments 3963, Jan. 2005.

Doyle L E (2009), *Essentials of cognitive radio*, Cambridge, Cambridge University Press, 2009.

Glover I A and Grant P M (2010), *Digital communications*, 3rd edn., Harlow, Pearson Education, 2010.

Hinden R (2006), *IP version 6 addressing architecture*, Internet Engineering Task Force, Request for comments 4291, Feb. 2006.

Johnson D (2004), *Mobility support in IPv6*, Internet Engineering Task Force, Request for comments 3775, June 2004.

Johnson S J (2010), *Iterative error correction: Turbo, low-density parity-check and repeat-accumulate codes*, Cambridge University Press, Cambridge, 2010.

Lee L H C, *Error-control block codes for communications*, Norwood USA, Artech House, (2000).

Li G and Stubber G L (Eds), *Orthogonal frequency division multiplexing for wireless communications*, New York, Springer (2010).

Paxson V (2011), *Computing TCP's retransmission timer*, Internet Engineering Task Force, Request for comments 6298, June 2011.

Postel J (1980), *User datagram protocol*, Internet Engineering Task Force, Request for comments 768, Aug. 1980.

Rouphael T J (2009), *RF and digital signal processing for software defined radio*, Burlington, Elsevier, 2009.

Suzuki H (1977), A statistical model of mobile radio reception, *IEEE Trans. Communications*, vol. **25**, July 1977, pp. 673–680.

Torrieri D, *Principles of spread-spectrum communications* 2nd edn, New York, Springer (2011).

3
RF MEMS fabrication technologies

K. GRENIER and D. DUBUC,
LAAS-CNRS, University of Toulouse, France

DOI: 10.1533/9780857098610.1.67

Abstract: This chapter presents the developments enabled in wireless applications by microelectromechanical systems technologies. Based on surface and bulk micromachining techniques, the elaboration of passive components with improved performance in terms of losses and quality factor, as well as radio frequency (RF) tuneable and mechanical devices, is possible. Highlights of specific key steps in their fabrication are presented and discussed. Their implementation in complete microsystem integration is then considered. Finally, fabrication trends with new material combinations, such as carbon nanotubes, or openings to other disciplinary technologies, such as microfluidics, are given.

Key words: MEMS technology, sacrificial layer, micromachining, microwave.

3.1 Introduction

The constant race towards the performance enhancement, compactness, integrability and reconfigurability of communication systems has motivated the requirements of new technologies which could extend the traditional limits by providing a new dimensional level to circuits (De Los Santos, 1999). High linearity and isolation, as well as low losses and power consumption, indeed represent attractive characteristics, which translate into the performance enhancement and architectural evolution of communications systems. Adequate micro- and nano-technologies need consequently to be developed.

In the 1980s and 1990s, bulk and surface micromachining techniques had already proven their potential in high volume commercial applications, such as micro-mirrors in video projectors, so-called digital micro-mirror devices (DMDs), and inkjet printer heads. The step toward a natural migration and implementation of such traditional processes of the sensors and actuators into the 'community to the communications systems' was not so large, and led to the emergence of new radio-frequency (RF) components such as microelectromechanical systems (MEMS) based on bulk and surface micromachining. The 'RF MEMS' term normally refers to radio-frequency MEMS, which integrate movable parts to realize electronic tuneability through electromotive actuations. This denomination has nevertheless been enlarged and now includes all devices which integrate bulk or surface micromachining processes during their fabrication.

The goal of this chapter is therefore to describe the significance of MEMS technologies in the radio-frequency, microwave- and millimetre-wave ranges, and to provide a global vision of the different employments of MEMS-based technologies in wireless applications.

The examples given in this chapter are presented to illustrate the different breakthroughs brought by MEMS technologies to communications systems. There is no intention to make an exhaustive listing of all RF MEMS technologies, which have been developing for several decades. MEMS-based technologies have stimulated an enormous amount of research with the definition of many processes and continue to do so.

3.2 MEMS-based technologies for RF circuits with enhanced quality factor and minimized losses

One of the first integrations of MEMS technology with RF circuits concerned the bulk substrate micromachining of passive elements. It was in response to the requirements of satellite developments in the 1990s, which were associated with a drastic minimization of mass and volume, and enhanced performance, of high frequency electronics.

To achieve high-density integration, there were various technologies that constituted a strong challenge. Silicon substrates promised a completely unified electronic platform due to the emergence of SiGe-based transistors for high frequency circuits in complementarity to complementary metal-oxide-semiconductor (CMOS) technology for low frequency data treatment. Such a material, however, exhibits high losses in the microwave and millimetre-wave domains. For low price and technological process stability, the silicon substrates employed were indeed presenting low resistivity levels, in the order of few units to tens of Ω.cm. Such values induced very strong dielectric losses at high frequencies.

To overcome these substrate losses and deliver high quality factor (Q) devices for wireless applications, different MEMS-based technologies have consequently been developed. It was first initiated through the elaboration of **bulk micromachined waveguides**, which were intensively investigated in the 1990s, by Pr. Linda Katehi and Gabriel Rebeiz notably. These transmission lines consist of metallic conductive strips placed on a thin dielectric membrane which has previously been grown or spin-coated onto host wafer, then partly removed. Both microstrip and coplanar configurations of micromachined lines on GaAs and Si substrates (Herrick *et al.*, 1998b)

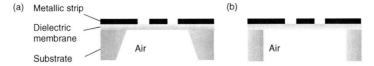

3.1 Illustration of bulk micromachined coplanar lines obtained with (a) wet and (b) dry etching techniques.

were investigated, as indicated in Fig. 3.1 in the case of coplanar lines. These waveguides could also integrate metallized shielding on the top or at the back.

From a technological point of view, the initially realized components utilized wet etching techniques. Potassium hydroxide (KOH)-based solutions were used for silicon attack. This imposed large surface area consumption, as the etching was stopping along specific crystalline substrate planes. Traditionally, <100> silicon substrate exhibits an edge angle of 54.74°, while the etching stops on <111> crystal planes. Due to the spreading of dry etching solutions with Deep Reactive Ion Etching (DRIE) equipment, a straight 90° attack angle was enabled, and this led to more compact micromachined circuits. This also eliminated the use of contaminating etchant solutions.

Moreover, the first devices were employing inorganic membranes based on the superposition of silicon oxide (SiO_2) and silicon nitrides (SiN) layers. To enable the correct reliability and standing of the membrane, a global tensile stress (around 100–200 MPa) was required. Quite large micromachined structures were then feasible. The fabrication of a device featuring a maximal length of approximately 1 cm was demonstrated on top of a SiO_2/SiN dielectric membrane of 1.4 µm thickness.

As far as thermal budget was concerned, the first Si-based membranes required extremely high fabrication temperatures. Thermal silicon oxidations imposed temperatures as high as 1000°C, whereas low pressure chemical vapour deposition (LPCVD) of nitrides employed temperatures close to 700°C. For compatibility with Integrated Circuits (ICs), dielectric layers obtained by plasma enhanced chemical vapour deposition (PECVD) should now be preferred, as good quality layers may be obtained even with a low thermal budget (from 200°C to 300°C approximately).

The latest developments have led to the use of organic membranes based on a single polymer layer of few micrometres thickness (Bouchriha *et al.*, 2006). Their technology is simple, involving a dielectric polymer deposition by spin-coating, followed by its curing for polymerisation at temperatures below 260°C. Finally, such membranes exhibit an inherent tensile stress with typical dielectric permittivities located in the range of 2–3, depending on the chosen polymer and the operating frequency. Additionally, organic layers are mostly photosensitive and consequently patternable, which favours the elaboration of interconnections during the post-processing of passive micromachined elements on top of ICs.

Such a micromachined technology permits reaching attenuation levels of 0.4–0.6 dB/cm at 20 GHz (Herrick *et al.*, 1998a) compared to a range of 15–20 dB/cm for transmission lines directly realized on top of 20 Ω.cm low resistivity silicon substrates (Peterson and Drayton, 2001). As illustrated in Fig. 3.2, the losses are proportional to the square root of the frequency, which translates into the predominance of ohmic losses in the metallic conductors. The suppression of the substrate indeed inhibits the impact of dielectric losses.

The evaluation of such a technology has also been extended to other types of passive elements, such as antennas, inductors (Chi and Rebeiz, 1995; Weller *et al.*, 1995) and filters (Bouchriha *et al.*, 2006; Drayton and Katehi, 1995; Katehi *et al.*, 1993) with both inorganic and organic membranes. An example of a micromachined antenna realized on organic membrane, with a 10 μm thick polymer layer of BenzoCycloButen from Dow Chemicals

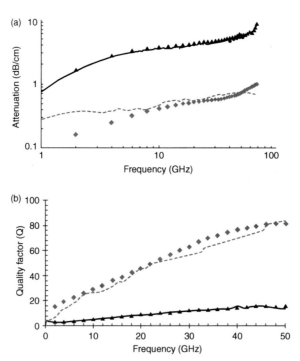

3.2 (a) Attenuation and (b) quality factors of bulk micromachined CPW (in grey) and CPW realized on top of a 10 μm thick polymer layer on low resistivity Si (in black).

RF MEMS fabrication technologies

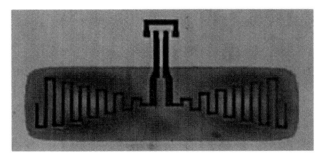

3.3 Image of bulk micromachined antenna realized on a 10 μm thick organic dielectric layer.

in that case, is given in Fig. 3.3. The surface of this differential coplanar antenna designed for a 24 GHz front-end was highly miniaturized with the use of meanders. The use of a 20 Ω.cm silicon substrate was overcome due to the silicon micromachining and led to an efficiency improvement of 70% in antenna performance.

An example of a bulk micromachined inductor is given in Fig. 3.4. The enhancement of its performance is shown in Fig. 3.5. The inductor value remains constant over a larger frequency range with the silicon substrate suppression, whereas the quality factor is increased.

The improvement of passive circuits with bulk micromachining has been consequently very impressive in terms of performance enhancements. However, this technique presents some limitations. The first is related to the low relative effective permittivity of the devices close to 1.4. The wavelength related to this technology is consequently very large, which leads to cumbersome surface area consumption of the circuits. The second is directly linked to the restrictions imposed by the DRIE technique. The etching efficiency is related to the size of the hole to be etched. As illustrated in Fig. 3.6, large holes are more quickly etched than smaller ones, which creates differences in terms of etched depth. Consequently, to ensure the correct etching of all targeted devices, the dry etching has to be prolonged, which leads to a local enlargement of the suppressed silicon at the bottom of the larger holes (called notching) (cf. Fig. 3.7). This effect may be avoided by using holes of similar size, but this is not practicable and may explain the poor use of bulk micromachining in wireless commercial components.

Despite these technological constraints, bulk micromachining remains an efficient means to overcome silicon dielectric losses and coupling in passive microwave circuits.

In a complementary approach, other **technologies based on surface micromachining** have also been investigated. Pr Linda Katehi and Dr George

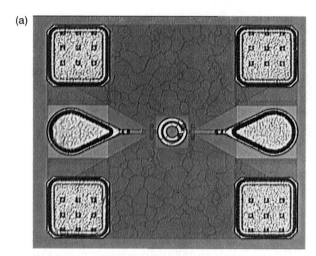
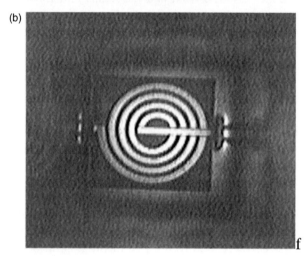

3.4 Photographs of bulk micromachined inductors from the (a) front side and (b) back side.

Ponchak initiated such technologies in the late 1990s (Herrick *et al.*, 1998a; Ponchak *et al.*, 2001). A few examples of surface-micromachined techniques are shown in Fig. 3.8. All involve the partial suppression of dielectrics or sacrificial layers on the front side of the wafers.

Globally, the investigated structures involve dielectric etchings into the coplanar apertures (cf. Fig. 3.8a, b and c) over a small, or even large, depth (up to 200 μm with SU-8 polymer in Newlin paper in 2002). Similar to bulk micromachined structures, both chemically wet and dry etching techniques

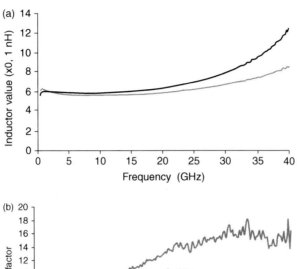
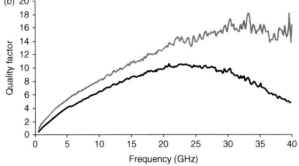

3.5 Performance of an inductor without (in black) and with bulk micromachining (in grey): (a) inductor value and (b) quality factor.

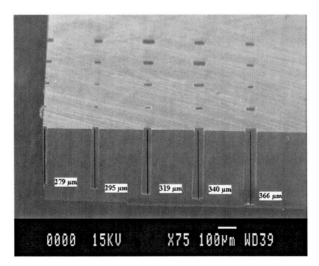

3.6 Efficiency of DRIE depending on the size of the holes.

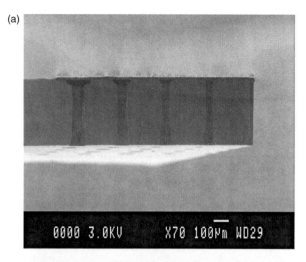

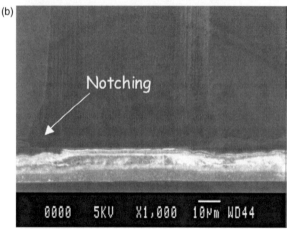

3.7 Observation of the notching effect on large etched holes in a silicon substrate: (a) view of several holes with different widths and (b) zoom on the notching effect.

have been employed. Other structures, such as that of Fig. 3.8d, include the use of a sacrificial layer, which is removed at the end of the process (Kim *et al.*, 2001; Lubecke *et al.*, 2001). For all these technologies, excellent performances have been achieved.

To have a better view of the different surface and bulk micromachining-based technologies and their associated performance, a summary is given in Table 3.1. The attenuation level obtained depends on the substrate resistivity, the dielectric material, and also the etched depth of the material. In the best case, the surface-micromachined technology may even compete

3.8 Illustration of various surface-micromachined configurations in planar passive elements: (a) surface dielectric isolation etching in the coplanar slots; (b) partial etching of the surface dielectric and the substrate; (c) partial substrate etching filled with the top dielectric isolation and (d) overlay CPW in air.

with the bulk micromachined one. In addition, it presents other attractive advantages: it necessitates only single-side wafer processing, very low cost development, ease in design and in fabrication, and it is also IC compatible.

Because of all these advantages, the surface micromachining technique has been applied to various microwave passive elements, such as filters (Herrick *et al.*, 1998a), inductors (Lubecke *et al.*, 2001; Rieh *et al.*, 1998; Yoon *et al.*, 2003), and even film bulk acoustic-wave resonators (FBAR) (Bi and Barber, 2008) and high Q resonators (Akgul *et al.*, 2011).

The technology presented in Fig 3.8c exhibits an additional advantage. As expected, its performance is directly related to the micromachining depth realized in the silicon substrate (as shown in Fig. 3.9). However, its topology is particularly adapted to three-dimensional integration. The lossy silicon substrate is replaced in the coplanar apertures by a low loss polymer material (Bouchriha *et al.*, 2003). This results in a planar technology, which allows the superposition of additional polymer and metallic layers, as illustrated in Fig. 3.10. The low attenuation level, associated with a wide range of characteristic impedance allowed by the technology, is suitable for the elaboration of enhanced passive circuits. The example of a three-dimensional (3-D) broadside coupler (Do *et al.*, 2007) is indicated in Fig. 3.11. It exhibits low insertion losses of 0.25 dB at 20 GHz, with an excellent compromise between strong coupling and wideband performance. Moreover, such a technology is compatible with IC integration.

To conclude this section, the implementation of MEMS technologies based on surface and bulk micromachining with high frequency electronics has led to the development of passive circuits enhanced in terms of minimized losses, improved quality factor and miniaturization. They also respond to the frequency increase of the communication systems and facilitate strong and various multi-chip integration.

These are not the only possibilities opened by MEMS technologies in wireless systems. Micromachining was initially developed to elaborate

Table 3.1 Summary of attenuation levels for bulk and surface-micromachined technologies on silicon substrates

Structure type	Substrate	Dielectric	Attenuation (dB/cm) at 20 GHz	Reference
	HRS	None	1–2	Gamble *et al.* (1999)
	LRS	None	15–20	Peterson (2001)
	LRS	SiO$_2$ 0.2 μm	20	Grenier *et al.* (2004)
	LRS	BCB 10–30 μm	3–5	Ponchak *et al.* (2002)
		Polyimide 20 μm	3–4	
	HRS	SiO$_2$/Si$_3$N$_4$/SiO$_2$ 1.5 μm	1–2	Herrick *et al.* (1998a)
	LRS	Si 60 μm (straight)	0.6–0.7	Strohm *et al.* (2002)
		Si 12 μm (triangular)	0.7	Herrick *et al.* (1998a)
		Polyimide 20 μm	1.9	Ponchak (2001)
		SU8 200 μm	0.18	Newlin *et al.* (2002)
		BCB 10 μm	4	Bouchriha *et al.* (2003)
	LRS	BCB 10 μm Si 30 μm	3	Bouchriha *et al.* (2003)
	HRS	SiO$_2$/Si$_3$N$_4$/SiO$_2$ 1.5 μm	0.45–0.6	Herrick *et al.* (1998a)
	LRS	BCB 10 μm	0.4–0.6	Bouchriha *et al.* (2006)

HRS: high resistivity silicon; LRS: low resistivity silicon.

RF MEMS fabrication technologies

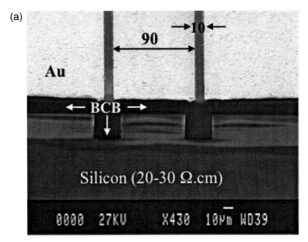

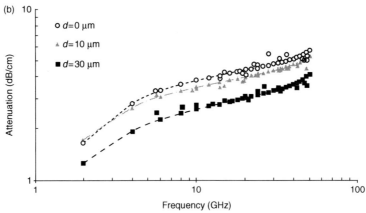

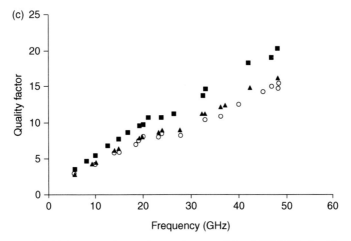

3.9 (a) SEM view of a surface-micromachined CPW filled with polymer, and its associated performance in terms of (b) attenuation and (c) quality factor for different etching depths.

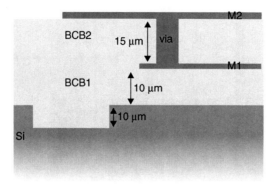

3.10 (a) 3-D integrated polymer technology with localized surface micromachining.

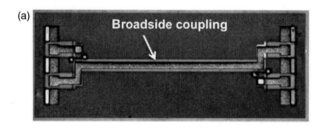

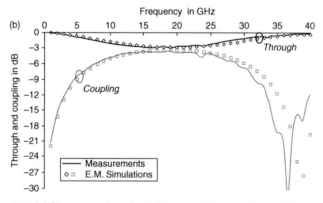

3.11 (a) Photography of a 3-D broadside coupler and (b) associated performances.

sensors, with famous commercial examples like accelerometers in air bag systems, inkjet printers, micro-mirrors in video projectors, and so on. Their common and major breakthrough resides in their tuning. This feature has also been envisaged to elaborate smart RF MEMS systems.

3.3 Technologies for smart RF MEMS

Contrary to the previous section dedicated to enhanced passives circuits with MEMS technologies, this section is dedicated to the fabrication of smart RF MEMS devices. This means that the technological process leads to the elaboration of movable parts which may be actuated with an electromotive force.

Historically, Dr Petersen from the IBM Research Division laboratory in California published the first movable RF MEMS device in 1979 (Petersen, 1979). An electrostatic force was applied between a bi-material membrane in SiO_2 and gold materials with a p-doped silicon layer in order to perform a switch function (cf. Fig. 3.12). An operation frequency of 200 kHz was assumed to be achievable. Larson et al. then demonstrated microwave performances in 1991 with a rotating transmission line switch (Larson et al., 1991). Measurements performed up to 45 GHz were already impressive with insertion losses lower than 0.5 dB and isolation greater than 35 dB. A few years later, in 1995, Goldsmith et al. introduced a bridge configuration for the RF MEMS switch, with a capacitive contact, as illustrated in Fig. 3.12c (Goldsmith et al., 1995, 1996). Rebeiz et al. followed these developments on a similar RF MEMS configuration (Barker and Rebeiz, 1998; Muldavin and Rebeiz, 1999).

These first RF MEMS switches clearly demonstrate the wide variety of possible RF MEMS topologies and consequently technologies. They may, however, be distinguished by their type of displacement. Most tuneable RF MEMS devices present bridge or cantilever configurations, respectively as shown in Fig. 3.13a and b. The movable membrane exhibits a vertical movement during actuation. The corresponding technologies are usually realized on top of the substrate, or even independently of it. On the other hand, RF MEMS with lateral movement, as illustrated in Fig. 3.13c, have also been investigated, and generally involve the etching of the substrate and

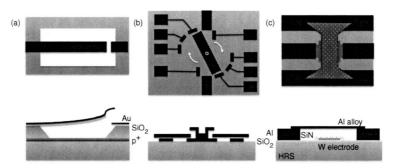

3.12 Schematics of RF MEMS switches from (a) Pertersen (1979) (b) Larson *et al.* (1991) and (c) Goldsmith *et al.* (1995, 1996) top views and cross sections.

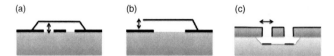

3.13 Vertical and lateral displacement configurations of RF MEMS: vertical movement for (a) a bridge or (b) a cantilever configurations; (c) lateral movement.

its participation in the movement. For instance, the switch developed by Oberhammer *et al.* (2006) involves the superposition of two bonded substrates, a silicon one placed on top of a glass wafer. The top silicon substrate is 60 μm thick and is dry-etched to realize the movable part, whereas the bottom glass wafer is wet-etched to allow free movement of the metallized silicon beam.

Different types of actuation have been studied. Most of the investigations worldwide have implemented RF MEMS with electrostatic forces, but electrothermal, piezoelectric and magnetostatic actuations may also be encountered (Rebeiz, 2003). Each of them presents specific advantages and drawbacks. The electrostatic one is the most common, because of its ease in fabrication and low power consumption.

3.3.1 Overview of a traditional movable RF MEMS process

In general, the process flow of movable RF MEMS with vertical displacement may be globally divided into six main steps, as illustrated in the case of a bridge configuration in Fig. 3.14. As a brief overview, the first step, depicted in Fig. 3.14a, consists in isolating the switch from the substrate in order to

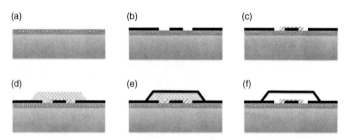

3.14 Traditional process flow of RF MEMS devices with a vertically deflected beam: (a) substrate isolation, (b) transmission line elaboration, (c) dielectric layer deposition and patterning, (d) sacrificial layer definition, (e) movable part fabrication and (f) MEMS release.

minimize the losses and also unwanted coupling effects. In the case of silicon substrates, various techniques exist, such as the use of a thick polymer interfacial layer or an oxide one. RF transmission lines are then defined in a second step, which is sketched with a coplanar waveguide in the Fig. 3.14b. In the case of capacitive switches, a dielectric layer is then deposited and patterned on the lines (see Fig. 3.14c). The next phase, described by the graph of Fig. 3.14d, consists in defining a sacrificial layer, to support the movable membrane during its fabrication, which is illustrated in the following sketch of Fig. 3.14e. Finally the sacrificial layer is removed to release the RF MEMS structure.

Schematically on paper, such a process does not present difficulties. However, it generated important complexities which required many years of research and development.

3.4 Highlights on specific key steps in RF MEMS fabrication

This section presents the basic building blocks of traditional RF MEMS switches, depending on the targeted use of the MEMS, with specific highlights on different key steps: sacrificial layers and MEMS release compared to stiction consideration, bias circuitry, dielectric considerations for capacitive switches, and metallic contact for ohmic MEMS.

3.4.1 Dielectric considerations in capacitive switches

For capacitive RF MEMS, various dielectric materials are possible. The required thickness is generally of the order of 0.25 µm, which allows the employment of both polymer and inorganic layers. Polymers may be possible candidates, but their non-conformal deposition and their low permittivity make the inorganic dielectrics better candidates. Dielectric layers such as SiO_2 or SiN obtained by PECVD are preferably used because of their low thermal budget, compatible with the metal of the transmission lines and also with possible ICs located underneath. Their process traditionally involves, after their deposition an RIE etching step with a photoresist mask. To simplify the understanding of the global process, the dielectric layer of Fig. 3.14 is realized on top of the transmission line, prior to the sacrificial layer step. As this layer is present to prevent any direct contact between the transmitted signal line and the movable membrane, it may also be elaborated during the formation of the tuneable part of the MEM element.

Other dielectric materials, as for example aluminium oxide, barium strontium titanate (BST) and zinc oxide, are also interesting because of their higher permittivity compared to SiO_2 or SiN. The use of such layers has,

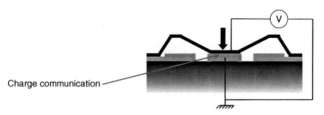

3.15 Dielectric charging in capacitive RF MEMS.

however, to be studied in terms of their reliability. Related to dielectrics, a main issue resides indeed in the RF MEMS operational reliability. When a voltage is applied to actuate the bridge or cantilever, charges accumulate in the dielectric, which lead to undesired stiction and operation of the membrane. This phenomenon is illustrated in Fig. 3.15.

To overcome this problem, several solutions have been investigated. One consists of replacing the dielectric layer with an air gap and by placing some dimples on the movable membrane in front of the slots in the bottom metallic layer, in order to avoid any contact between both membrane and transmission line during actuation. This solution is effective, but limits the performance of the switches in terms of capacitance ratio and consequently possible applications.

Another possibility resides in doping the dielectric layer, in order to better evacuate the charges during the application of the electrostatic force. This may be done through the doping of a SiN layer with Si, as patented by Goldsmith *et al.* (Ehmke *et al.*, 2002). It may also be performed through the incorporation of carbon nanotubes (CNT) in the dielectric layer (Bordas *et al.*, 2007). Figure 3.16 presents the technological process used to easily integrate the CNT into the SiN layer in two steps. After the definition of the metallic transmission line, a first SiN layer is deposited, exhibiting a thickness of 70 nm. The wafer is then immersed into a CNT and solvent-based mixture, which has been previously sonicated. Due to the capillary forces and the solvent evaporation, a layer of CNT is randomly dispersed on the first dielectric layer. The CNT are then encapsulated in a second SiN layer, which has a thickness of 180 nm. The delimitation of the global 2.5 µm thick dielectric layer is then traditionally done by an RIE step applied on top of a photoresist mask, which is afterwards removed. Such a technique using CNT doping translates into an improvement of the MEMS lifetime of several orders of magnitude.

3.4.2 Sacrificial layer considerations in movable RF MEMS

The sacrificial layer defines the height of the movable membrane. This dimension requires precision in the elaboration of capacitive MEMS to

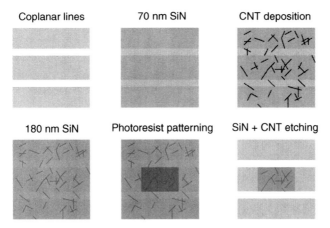

3.16 Elaboration of a CNT doped SiN layer for RF MEMS capacitive switches.

reach the expected capacitance ratio. Its value is often of the order of 3 μm in thickness. This layer should also respond to several requirements: able to sustain temperatures of at least 100–150°C necessary for the next technological steps and packaging, easy to remove without residue during the final release of the MEMS, and exhibiting a low intrinsic stress, in order not to add supplementary stress to the top membrane itself.

Various candidates appropriately fulfil these requirements: metallic layers, such as copper, aluminium; silicon, polysilicon; dielectric layers (different from the one used for the capacitive behaviour for chemical resistance during the final release of the MEMS); polymers and photoresists. The most frequent solution is photoresists, due to their ease of processing. They are simply spin-coated and the final thickness is well defined with the spin speed. The anchorages of the MEM membrane may be smoothed through the controlled reflow of the photoresists with temperature, as indicated in Fig. 3.17. Finally, they are simply removed with solvents. Holes in the MEM membrane are often designed to facilitate the sacrificial layer removal at the end of the process.

A common issue to all possible sacrificial materials resides in the flatness of the layer. As illustrated in Fig. 3.18, bottom relief of the substrate with RF transmission lines may induce important corrugation on the MEM membrane. A direct consequence is the incomplete contact of the MEM membrane on the bottom electrode, which leads to the degradation of the capacitance ratio limited to a value close to 10. To overcome this drawback, the transmission line is traditionally thinned below the MEM membrane. Capacitor ratios to the order of 30 are then achievable. On the other hand, to be compatible with low losses and high power handling requirements,

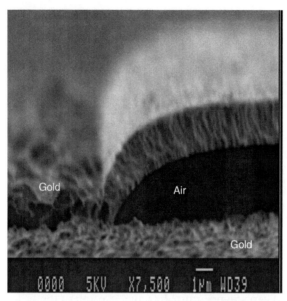

3.17 SEM view of the anchorage of a gold bridge obtained with a reflowing photoresist.

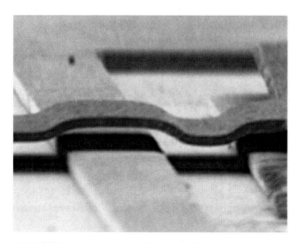

3.18 SEM view of a non-flat metallic membrane due to bottom relief.

capacitive MEMS switches have to present thick signal lines to decrease current density as much as possible. This creates important relief below the MEM membrane and constrains to planarize the bridge sacrificial layer to assure good contact quality and isolation in the down-state of the switches. One can then use the chemical mechanical polishing (CMP) technique (Chang *et al.*, 2003), which remains complex, or the stack of two sacrificial layers (Bordas *et al.*, 2006; Yu *et al.*, 2005). The principle is given in Fig. 3.19, with a first sacrificial layer patterned in the metallic slots and a second used to form the frame of the MEM membrane. This last solution is quite attractive, and satisfactory for both parallel and serial coplanar switches if some precautions are taken. Figure 3.20 presents a bridge which is not sufficiently flattened, due to an accentuated reflow of two similar photoresists in the serial gap. This phenomenon consequently degrades the switch capacitance ratio. To overcome this, two different sacrificial layer types presenting various viscosity and temperature properties (Hocheng *et al.*, 2002) have to be used. The bottom one, a polymer, is chosen with a low ability to reflow

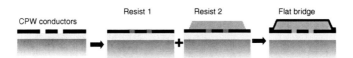

3.19 MEM planarization process flow.

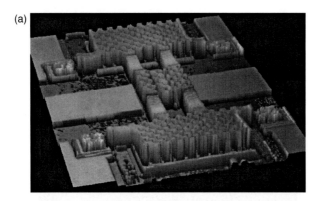

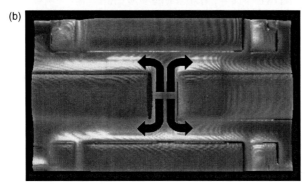

3.20 (a) Three-dimensional view of a shunt switch and (b) visualization of the accentuated photoresist reflow in the serial gap.

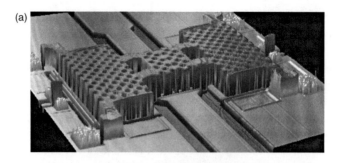

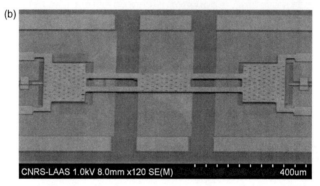

3.21 (a,b) SEM view of a flat metallic MEM bridge with a length of 900 μm.

below 200°C, whereas the second remains unchanged in order to retain the reflow benefit at the membrane anchorages. The composition of these two resists is so different that no intermixing appears during the bake procedure. The obtained MEM membranes are consequently flat, whatever the configuration: parallel or serial switches, as illustrated in Fig. 3.21 with the three-dimensional view of a serial capacitive switch and a scanning electron microscope (SEM) view of a parallel one 900 μm long.

3.4.3 Movable membrane

As far as the movable membrane is concerned, it must present a global low tensile stress (in the order of 100–200 MPa) to prevent any buckling at the final release and to minimize stiction. Various metals have been investigated, aluminium, gold, nickel, copper. Gold is most used in capacitive switches as it does not oxidize, and also for its compatibility with ICs in post-processing. Gold membranes are, however, subject to stress and modification with temperature increase or power application. This constitutes a major drawback, not only for their use but also for packaging issues. Curing steps before the final MEMS release, as well as relaxed spring anchorages permit extended temperature ability but these solutions remain limited. Nickel-based membranes better sustain temperatures up to 400°C, which is very attractive for packaging matter, but this material is not IC compatible.

In the case of piezostatic MEMS, the actuation material is integrated into the MEM membrane, which implies to take care specifically to the global stress of the membrane.

For ohmic switches, metallic considerations are mandatory to assure a good contact quality between the membrane and the RF transmission line. Because of rapid fatigue, gold–gold contacts were quickly skipped for the benefits of other materials. For instance, CEA-LETI in France has moved toward ruthenium-based contacts to enhance reliability and lower sensitivity to stiction, compared to gold-based contacts, for their ohmic RF MEMS switches in 2011.

Finally, the most crucial step in RF MEMS technologies corresponds to the final release, when the sacrificial layer is removed and the structure is dried. Stiction of the membrane on the substrate may appear easily. It is related to the metal and dielectric surfaces with regards to their roughness, the membrane stress, and thickness, all elements that favour capillary forces. The literature indicates two techniques to perform this release: dry and wet techniques.

Dry ones, such as oxygen plasma treatment for sacrificial layers realized with polymers or photoresists, are interesting as no liquid is used. It lowers the risk of stiction, but metallic membranes may suffer in terms of stress and buckle due to the temperature increase in the plasma chamber. The plasma etching should then be stopped periodically to allow the chamber temperature to decrease.

Wet etchings are also used with acid solutions to remove metals, or solvents in the case of photoresists. The critical step is then to dry the MEMS structures without any stiction effect. The solutions employed to dry RF MEMS devices is usually not clearly indicated in the literature, as this aspect is extremely critical and competitive. In silicon-based sensors with SiO_2 sacrificial layers, the efficiency of a CO_2-based supercritical dryer has been shown to avoid stiction. This technique may nevertheless not work appropriately with metallic RF MEMS, as it imposes low pressure and thus stress, and is totally material and shape dependent. One efficient solution consists in replacing the sacrificial layer remover by ethanol and drying it very quickly in a vacuum chamber.

3.4.4 Added elements such as bias circuitry with integrated resistors or metal/insulator/metal (MIM) or metal/air/metal (MAM) capacitors

Additional to RF MEMS devices, some other passive elements are required to build complete and complex circuits. Integrated resistors and MIM or

Table 3.2 Resistive materials

Materials	NiV	NiCr	TaN	SiCr	Ge
Resistivity (μΩ·cm)	60	100	150–200	20.10^3	46.10^6

MAM capacitors compatible with MEMS process have consequently been developed.

Integrated resistors are indeed required in RF MEMS switches to prevent any RF signal leakage through the bias circuitry. Traditional integrated resistors in microtechnologies are realized in NiV (Shen *et al.*, 2003), NiCr (Kola *et al.*, 1997; Shen *et al.*, 2003) and TaN (Shen *et al.*, 2003), which present limited resistivity values (as shown in Table 3.2). To be compatible with the rapid switching time of RF MEMS switches and MEMS capacitor values of few pF in the down-state and fF in the up-state, the resistors should exhibit kΩ to MΩ resistance. SiCr (Hayden and Rebeiz, 2003; Lakshminarayanan and Weller, 2006) and Ge (Grenier *et al.*, 2008) are appropriate materials to elaborate integrated resistors with RF MEMS devices. Resistors realized in SiCr suffer from quite long bias lines in order to reach adequate resistor values. The use of a germanium layer, which exhibits a larger resistive value compared to SiCr, permits realization of miniaturized resistors appropriate for RF MEMS components without any RF perturbations.

For circuits which requires low capacitive ratio, such as impedance matching networks, fixed capacitors placed close to the RF MEMS switches or capacitors are required. Both MIM and MAM capacitors have been added in RF MEMS processes. An example of MIM ones is given in the tuner configuration presented in Fig. 3.22.

3.5 Towards integrated technology for microsystem implementation

To enable the elaboration of highly integrated RF microsystems, the co-integration of RF MEMS with ICs has been investigated.

Before all possible combination of MEMS with ICs, one key element to be aware of is the tolerable thermal budget. The maximal allowed temperature during process with ICs has to be clearly defined, in order to maintain their correct operation. As far as CMOS technology is concerned, this limit is traditionally considered to be around 400°C. Above this temperature, the circuits start to present faults. As far as active components based on SiGe heterostructures are concerned, the maximal post-processing temperature is above 330°C. This temperature has been defined through the evaluation of test transistors submitted to different stress temperatures from 300°C up to 400°C. Noise measurements, which are presented

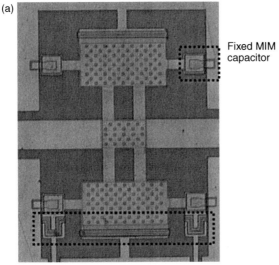
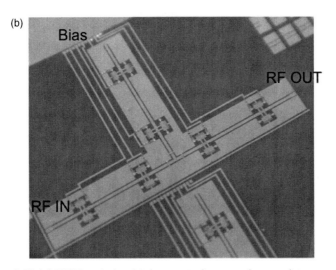

3.22 (a) MEM switch with integrated germanium resistors and MIM capacitors and (b) its implementation in a tuner.

in Fig. 3.23, have demonstrated a noticeable degradation for stress temperatures at or above 360°C.

The second key factor in the integration of RF MEMS passive components with ICs is cost. One may recall that IC substrate is particularly expensive because of the important masks number used for the process steps of transistors and integrated passives. Consequently, if the RF MEMS passive elements require a large surface area, their monolithic integration on the IC

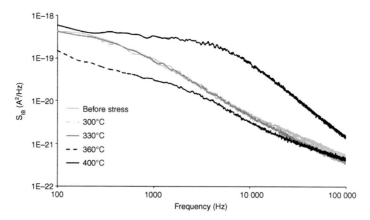

3.23 Low frequency noise spectral densities of the base current for different stress temperatures.

substrate would constitute a costly solution. The choice between monolithic and hybrid integrations is thus essentially driven by the surface consumption of the passive components. A trade-off has to be evaluated between the performance benefit and the global cost in order to decide between monolithic and hybrid integration.

3.5.1 Hybrid integration

In the case of hybrid integration, two different techniques exist to interconnect active circuits with MEMS technologies: wire bonding and flip chip implementations.

An example of a frequency-tuneable low-noise amplifier (LNA) connected to RF MEMS varactors using wire bonding is given in Fig. 3.24. The RF MEMS capacitors constitute matching networks located at the input and output of an SiGe-based LNA to enable the use of the circuit at two frequencies, 2.45 and 5.5 GHz. The length of the wire bondings had to be taken into account in the global RF design.

To lower the length of the wires, the IC circuit may also be inserted into a dedicated cavity in the host substrate. The corresponding hole and the IC report have to be performed before the RF MEMS fabrication. Special care with respect to the thermal expansion coefficient (CET) of host and IC substrates and the glue used to fix the IC substrate in the cavity has to be followed. This example clearly shows the important size of the passive elements compared to ICs and the justification, in this case, to use a hybrid configuration.

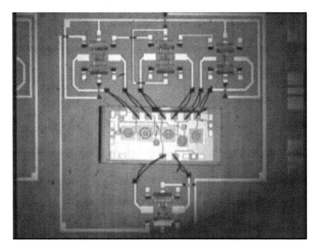

3.24 Image of a tuneable in frequency LNA with MEMS capacitors networks.

3.5.2 Monolithic integration

Traditionally, the monolithic integration of RF MEMS is realized through post-processing steps, after the realization of the ICs, as indicated in Fig. 3.25. For example C. Nguyen demonstrated vibrating disk mechanical resonators realized on a CMOS substrate to achieve integrated micromechanical radio front-ends (Nguyen, 2008). Metallization and dielectric layers were, until few years ago, still thin and some common MEMS metallizations, such as gold and copper, were prohibited for contamination reason. Wet chemical etching of silicon based on KOH was also avoided for the same reason. DRIE of silicon is on the other hand compatible with ICs if a simple design and fabrication rule is followed: the micromachined area should be kept at a minimum distance of 50 μm from the transistors in order to avoid any degradation of the ICs. This rule has been defined through low frequency noise measurements performed on SiGe-based test transistors. No deterioration of the active circuits has been observed except in the case of Si etching achieved below the IC, as described in Fig. 3.26 (Grenier *et al.*, 2004).

Based on this rule, a compact RF transceiver centred at 24 GHz has been achieved with a micromachined antenna for short-range radars and communication applications (Grenier *et al.*, 2005). Figure 3.27 presents the front and back sides pictures of the RF module, which monolithically integrates a micromachined antenna placed around the SiGe-based IC. The global size of the module corresponds to 9 mm^2. The antenna has been post-processed on top of the IC and includes a polymer membrane in

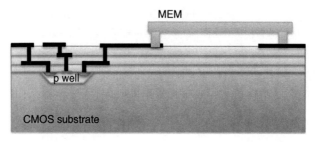

3.25 Post-processing of MEMS structures of CMOS or SiGe-based substrates.

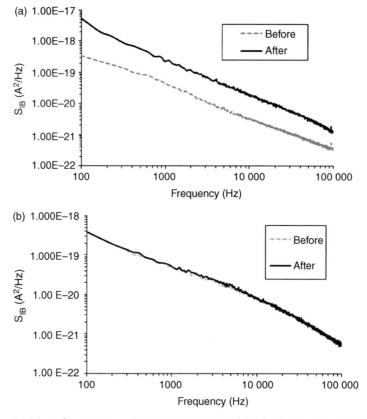

3.26 Low frequency noise measurement with a bulk micromachining localized (a) below or (b) at a minimal distance of 50 μm from the test transistor.

benzocyclobutene (BCB), which has been patterned to allow interconnections between the IC and the antenna. The antenna is obtained through a delimited metallization on top of the dielectric membrane and a final DRIE of the silicon substrate.

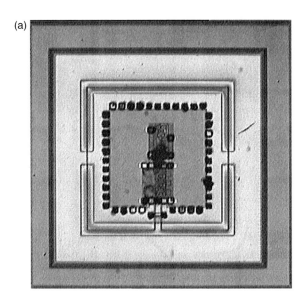

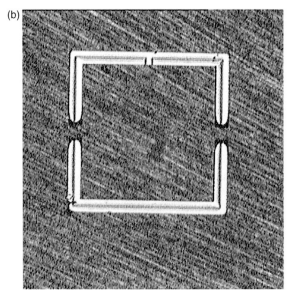

3.27 Photographs of an RF communication module centred at 24 GHz, which integrates a post-processed and bulk micromachined antenna: (a) top side and (b) back side.

More recently, new possibilities offered by thick dielectric and metallic layers with IC technologies open new horizons for integrated MEMS with ICs (Fedder *et al.*, 2008), as indicated with the schematic of Fig. 3.28. An excellent tuning ratio up to 60:1 of digital capacitors has been demonstrated

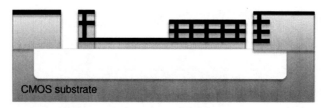

3.28 MEMS capacitor composed of top dielectric and metal layers of a CMOS substrate.

with the employment of the top dielectric and metallic layer available on ICs (Reinke *et al.*, 2011).

3.6 Emerging technologies in wireless applications

To conclude this chapter dedicated to RF MEMS technologies, this last part addresses new trends in wireless fabrication based on unconventional technologies. New materials, such as CNT or graphene, as well as microfluidic-based technologies for RF MicroElectroFluidic Systems, are emerging.

Among the recent investigations, CNT and graphene are being extensively tested as a new type of movable membrane in nanoelectromechanical systems (NEMS) structures. Such materials exhibit indeed very attractive mechanical, thermal and electrical properties, as well as a low mass. RF studies of NEMS using CNT or graphene are still at an early stage. However, NEMS functionalities with varactors or capacitive switches have been demonstrated with CNT-based membranes.

At LAAS-CNRS, a NEMS varactor in a cantilever configuration, which includes a beam of a CNT array, has been realized and actuated. As far as the technology is concerned, the CNT were randomly sprayed on a sacrificial layer and delimited through the patterning of a photoresist associated to a RIE step. Figure 3.29 presents the corresponding schematic of the CNT beam placed above a gold electrode and an image of the obtained device. The 3 μm thick expected gap was finally presenting a value of 0.5 μm certainly due to a lower membrane stress than the theoretical one. A tuning of 0.5 dB on the transmitted RF signal was however achieved on a large frequency range (1–30 GHz).

A clamped-clamped configuration of a high-density aligned CNT array has also been realized at the Ecole Polytechnique Fédérale de Lausanne (EPFL) (Acquaviva *et al.*, 2010) to perform a capacitive switch function. The CNTs are grown *in situ*, and a chemical treatment with isopropanol permits optimizing the density of the film. Combined to the bridge configuration of the switch, a low switching voltage of 6 V is reached. Figure 3.30 presents an image of such a device. The technological reproducibility, reliability, thermal

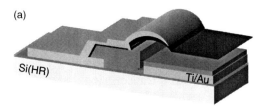

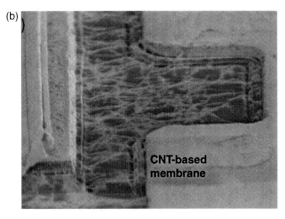

3.29 (a,b) NEMS varactor with a CNT-based membrane, in a cantilever configuration.

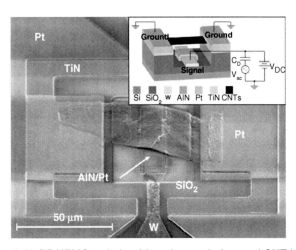

3.30 RF NEMS switch with a clamped-clamped CNT-based membrane (Acquaviva, 2010).

stability, power handling and other important features of these devices need now to be addressed and optimized, as was done previously with RF MEMS, but attractive performances of NEMS are already foreseen.

A new emerging field for RF MEMS is also related to the exploitation of microfluidic-based technologies. Tuneability may indeed be performed through the movement or the modification of fluids. A RF liquid-based switch has been, for instance, demonstrated at Purdue Univ. using the displacement of a microdroplet to shunt a transmission line with an applied electrostatic force (Chen and Peroulis, 2007). By modifying a liquid and notably colloidal concentration, RF components may also be tuned in terms of frequency for an antenna (Huff *et al.*, 2010) or delay in a transmission line (Dubuc and Grenier, 2010). Forecasted possibilities seem colossal. MEMS and NEMS technologies may provide unexplored areas and continue to participate in the development of future communications systems.

3.7 Conclusion

RF MEMS technologies for wireless applications have strongly benefited from all the developments performed for traditional sensors through various micromachining techniques and sacrificial layers implementation. These have enabled the enhancements of the passive circuits in terms of losses, quality factors and also tuneability through ohmic or capacitive RF MEMS switches, varactors and variable inductors.

Current investigations are currently more induced by material developments. CNT and graphene, due to their attractive properties, constitute good candidates for the elaboration of the future wireless circuits. Amazingly, metallic and dielectric fluids are of increasing interest. From employing liquids within microwave circuits, the step to then access and implement biological materials is not far. What about biological materials in the future wireless systems? Research to perform some elementary electrical behaviours have already been demonstrated, with DNA reaction circuits for instance.

3.8 Acknowledgements

The authors would like to thanks Fouad Bouchriha, Chloé Bordas, Nhut Do, Jean-Pierre Busquère and Sébastien Pacchini, Ph. D students under the supervision of David Dubuc and Katia Grenier from 2002 to 2008. Their work on RF MEMS design, fabrication and characterization contributed to increase the knowledge of the team.

Katia Grenier and David Dubuc also acknowledge the support of Thales Alenia Space, the French Defense Agency (DGA), ST-Microelectronics and the French Space Center CNES, as well as collaborations with Uppsala Univ., Ulm Univ, ATMEL and LPICM.

3.9 References

Acquaviva D, Arun A, Esconjauregui S, Bouvet D, Robertson J, Smajda R, Magrez A, Forro L, and Ionescu A M (2010), 'Capacitive nanoelectromechanical switch based on suspended carbon nanotube array', *APL*, **97**, 233508.

Akgul M, Schneider R, Ren Z, Chandler G, Yeh V, and Nguyen C T (2011), 'Hot filament CVD conductive microcrystalline diamond for high Q, high acoustic velocity micromechanical resonators', *IEEE Frequency Control Conference*, 1–6.

Barker N S and Rebeiz G M (1998), 'Distributed MEMS true-time delay phase shifters and wide-band switches', *IEEE T-MTT*, **46**, 11, 1881–1889.

Bi F Z and Barber B P (2008), 'Bulk acoustic wave RF technology', *IEEE Microwave Magazine*, 65–80.

Bordas C, Grenier K, Dubuc D, Flahaut E, Pacchini S, Paillard M, and Cazaux J L (2007), 'Carbon nanotube based dielectric for enhanced RF MEMS reliability', *IEEE International Microwave Symposium*, 375–378.

Bordas C, Grenier K, Dubuc D, Paillard M, Cazaux J-L, and Plana R (2006) 'Performances optimization of capacitive parallel MEMS switches', *IEEE Asian Pacific Microwave Conference*, 1365–1368.

Bouchriha F, Dubuc D, Grenier K, and Plana R (2006), 'IC-compatible low loss passive circuits for millimeter-wave applications', *36th European Microwave Conference (EuMC)*, Manchester, UK, 380–383.

Bouchriha F, Grenier K, Dubuc D, Pons P, and Plana R (2003), 'Minimization of passive circuits losses realized on low resistivity silicon using micro-machining techniques and thick polymer layers', *IEEE MTT-S International Microwave Symposium*, Philadelphia, USA, 959–962.

Chang H-P, Qian J, Cetiner B A, De Flaviis F, Bachman M, and Li G P (2003), 'RF MEMS switches fabricated on microwave-laminated printed circuit boards', *IEEE Electron Device Letters*, **24**, 4, 227–229.

Chen C H and Peroulis D (2007), 'Liquid RF MEMS Wideband Reflective and Absorptive Switches', *IEEE T-MTT*, **55**, 12, 2919–2929.

Chi C-Y and Rebeiz G M (1995), 'Planar microwave and millimeter-wave lumped elements and coupled-line filters using micro-machining techniques', *IEEE T-MTT*, **43**, 4, 730–738.

De Los Santos H J (1999), '*Introduction to Microelectromechanical (MEM) Microwave Systems,*' Boston – London, Hartech House.

Do M N, Dubuc D, Grenier K, and Plana R (2007), 'Low insertion losses broadside coupler in a multilayer above IC technology for K-band applications', *IEEE MTT-S*, 181–184.

Drayton R F and Katehi L P B (1995), 'Development of self-packaged high frequency circuits using micromachining techniques', *IEEE T-MTT*, **43**, 9, 2073–2080.

Dubuc D and Grenier K (2010), 'Microfluidic-based tunable RF true-time delay line', *IEEE European Microwave Week*, 1222–1224.

Ehmke J C, Goldsmith C L, Yao Z J, and Eshelman S M (2002), 'Method and apparatus for switching high frequency signals', *Patent No: US 6,391,675 B1*.

Fedder G K, Howe R T, King Liu T-J, and Quevy E P (2008), 'Technologies for cofabricating MEMS and electronics', *Proceedings of the IEEE*, **96**, 2, 306–322.

Gamble H S, Armstrong B M, Mitchell S J N, Wu Y, Fusco V F, and Stewart J A C (1999), 'Low-loss CPW lines on surface stabilized high-resistivity silicon', *IEEE Microwave and Guided Wave Letters*, **9**, 10, 395–397.

Goldsmith C, Lin T H, Powers B, Wu W R, and Norvell B (1995), 'Micromechanical membrane switches for microwave applications', *IEEE MTT-S Digest*, 91–94.

Goldsmith C, Randall J, Eshelman S, Lin T H, Denniston D, Chen S, and Norvell B (1996), 'Characteristics of micromachined switches at microwave frequencies', *IEEE MTT-S Digest*, 1141–1144.

Grenier K, Bordas C, Pinaud S, Salvagnac L, and Dubuc D (2008), 'Germanium resistors for RF MEMS based microsystems', *Microsystem Technologies Journal, Springer*, **14**, 4–5, 601–606.

Grenier K, Dubuc D, Mazenq L, Busquere J-P, Ducarouge B, Bouchriha F, Rennane A, Lubecke V, Pons P, Ancey P, and Plana R (2004), 'Polymer based technologies for microwave and millimeterwave applications', *50th IEEE International Electron Devices Meeting*, San Francisco, USA, 545–548.

Grenier K, Mazenq L, Dubuc D, Bouchriha F, Ojefors E, Lindberg P, Rydberg A, Berntgen J, Rabe W J, Sonmez E, Abele P, Schumacher H, and Plana R (2005), 'IC compatible MEMS technology', *IEEE European Microwave Conference*, 293–296.

Hayden J and Rebeiz G (2003), 'Very low-loss distributed X-band and Ka-band MEMS phase shifters using metal-air-metal capacitors', *IEEE T-MTT*, **51**, 1, 309–314.

Herrick K J, Yook J-G, and Katehi L P B (1998a), 'Microtechnology in the development of three-dimensional circuits', *IEEE T-MTT*, **46**, 11, 1832–1844.

Herrick K J, Schwarz T A, and Katehi L P B (1998b), 'Si-micromachined coplanar waveguides for use in high-frequency circuits', *IEEE T-MTT*, **46**, 6, 762–768.

Hocheng H, Pan C T, and Cheng C C (2002), 'Formation of micro-lens by reflow of dual photoresist', *Microprocesses and Nanotechnology Conference*, Nov. 6–8, 198–199.

Huff G H, Rolando D L, Walters P, and McDonald J (2010), 'A Frequency Reconfigurable Dielectric Resonator Antenna Using Colloidal Dispersions', *IEEE Antennas and Wireless Propagation Letters*, 9.

Katehi L P B, Rebeiz G M, Weller T M, Drayton R F, Cheng H-J, and Whitaker J F (1993), 'Micromachined circuits for millimeter and sub-millimeter-wave applications', *IEEE Ant. and Prop. Magazine*, **35**, 5, 9–17.

Kim H-T, Jung S, Park J-H, Baek C-W, Kim Y-K, and Kwon Y (2001), 'A new micromachined overlay CPW structure with low attenuation over wide impedance ranges and its application to low-pass filters', *IEEE T-MTT*, **49**, 9, 1634–1639.

Kola R, Lau M, Duenas S, Kumagai H, Smith P, Frye R, Tai K, and Sullivan P (1997), 'Thin film resistors and cpacitors for advanced packaging', *International Symposium on Advanced Packaging Materials*, 71–74.

Lakshminarayanan B and Weller T (2006), 'Design and modeling of 4-bit slow-wave MEMS phase shifters', *IEEE Trans. on MTT*, **54**, 1, 120–127.

Larson L E, Hackett R H, and Melendes M A (1991), 'Micromachined microwave actuator (MIMAC) technology – A new tuning approach for microwave integrated circuits', *IEEE Microwave and Millimeter-Wave Monolithic Circuits Symposium*, 27–30.

Lubecke V M, Barber B, Chan E, Lopez D, Gross M E, and Gammel P (2001), 'Self-assembling MEMS variable and fixed RF inductors', *IEEE T-MTT*, **49**, 11, 2093–2098.

Muldavin J B and Rebeiz G M (1999), '30 GHz tuned MEMS switches', *IEEE MTT-S Digest*, 1511–1514.

Newlin D P, Pham A-V, and Hariss J E (2002), 'Development of low loss organic-micromachined interconnects on silicon at microwave frequencies', *IEEE Trans. on Comp. and Pack. Tech.*, **25**, 3, 506–510.

Nguyen C T C (2008) 'Integrated micromechanical radio front-ends', *IEEE Int. Symposium on VLSI Technology, Systems and Applications*, 3–4.

Oberhammer J, Tang M, Liu A Q, and Stemme G (2006), 'Mechanically tri-stable in-line single-pole-double-throw all-metal switch', *IEEE MEMS conference*, 898–901

Petersen K E (1979), 'Micromechanical membrane switches on silicon', *IBM J Res Develop*, **23**, 4, 376–385.

Peterson R L and Drayton R F (2001), 'Dielectric properties of oxidized porous silicon in a low resistivity substrate', *IEEE MTT-S Digest*, 767–770.

Ponchak G E, Dalton E, Bacon A, Papapolymerou J, and Tentzeris E M (2002), 'Measured propagation characteristics of finite ground coplanar waveguide on silicon with a thick polyimide interface layer', *IEEE European Microwave Conference*.

Ponchak G E, Margomenos A, and Katehi L P B (2001), 'Low-loss CPW on low-resistivity Si substrates with a micromachined polyimide interface layer for RFIC interconnects', *IEEE T-MTT*, **49**, 5, 866–870.

Rebeiz G M (2003), *'RF MEMS theory, design, and technology'*, Hoboken, New Jersey, John Wiley & Sons.

Reinke J, Fedder G K, and Mukherjee T (2011) 'CMOS-MEMS 3-bit digital capacitors with tuning ratios greater than 60:1', *IEEE T-MTT*, **59**, 5, 1238–1248.

Rieh J-S, Lu L-H, Katehi L P B, Bhattacharya P, Croke E T, Ponchak G E, and Alterovitz S A (1998), 'X- and Ku-band amplifiers based on Si/SiGe HBT's and micromachined lumped components', *IEEE T-MTT*, **46**, 5, 685–694.

Shen H, Arreaga J, Ramanathan R, Knoedler H, Sawyer J, and Tiku S (2003), 'Fabrication and characterization of thin film resistors for GaAs-based power amplifiers', *International Conference on Compound Semiconductor Manufacturing Technology, CS ManTech*.

Strohm K M, Schmückle F J, Schauwecker B, Heinrich W, and Luy J-F (2002), 'Silicon micromachined CPW transmission lines', *IEEE European Microwave Conference*, 1–4.

Weller T M, Katehi L P B, and Rebeiz G M (1995), 'Single and double folded-slot antennas on semi-infinite substrates', *IEEE Trans. on Ant. and Prop.*, **43**, 12, 1423–1428

Yoon J-B, Kim B-I, Choi Y-S, and Yoon E (2003), '3-D construction of monolithic passive components for RF and microwave ICs using thick-metal surface micromachining technology', *IEEE T-MTT*, **51**, 1, 279–288.

Yu A B, Liu A Q, Zhang Q X, Alphones A, Zhu L, and Shacklock A P (2005), 'Improvement of isolation for MEMS capacitive switch via membrane planarization', *Sensors and Actuators A*, **119**, 206–213.

4
RF MEMS passive components for wireless applications

J. IANNACCI, Fondazione Bruno Kessler, Italy

DOI: 10.1533/9780857098610.1.100

Abstract: In this chapter an overview on the different classes of passive components that can be realized in radio frequency microelectromechanical systems (RF MEMS) technology is provided. A particular focus is oriented toward the performance description of RF passive components in MEMS technology, compared to their standard semiconductor counterparts. The crucial applications related aspects of RF MEMS passive components within transceivers and telecommunication platforms will also be stressed, drawing some considerations on the expected future trends in the diffusion of such a technology within large scale market applications.

Key words: RF MEMS, RF passive components, variable capacitors, inductors, micro-switches, complex networks, reconfigurability.

4.1 Introduction

Microelectromechanical systems (MEMS) technology has been exhibiting in the last 10–15 years a paramount potential with respect to the manufacturing and fabrication of passive components for radio frequency (RF) applications, such as variable capacitors (varactors), inductors, switches, and so on, commonly referred to as RF MEMS. The most relevant advantages of passive components in MEMS technology compared to their standard counterparts (e.g. in semiconductor technologies or based on discrete components) reside in their high-performance and low fabrication cost, as well as in the possibility of integrating RF MEMS devices to yield circuits and functional blocks entirely based on such a technology. For example, varactors and inductors in MEMS technology present good linearity and large tuning ranges, as wide as a ratio between the maximum and minimum capacitance values (C_{max}/C_{min}) better than 10:1 for capacitors, and a tuning range larger than 30–50% for inductors, respectively, with a quality factor (Q-factor) as good as 100–200, for both these reactive tunable elements.

On the other hand, MEMS switches are characterized by low insertion losses (in the range of 0.1–0.3 dB), very good isolation (better than

30–40 dB), and wide operability ranges in terms of frequency band, the last spanning between DC and 30–40 GHz, through which typical insertion loss and isolation are exhibited. Thereby, the typical features of RF MEMS components are significantly better than their counterparts implemented in standard semiconductor technology. For instance, varactors and switches realized with diodes and transistors exhibit smaller C_{max}/C_{min} ratios and are less linearly controllable. Moreover, with respect to standard switches, the insertion loss is often in the range of 3–6 dB, the isolation in the range of 20–30 dB, and more generally the frequency range operability is limited to 1–5 GHz. Another relevant advantage of MEMS-based tunable components is that the power consumption needed for their control and reconfiguration is virtually zero, as in the case of electrostatically controlled MEMS devices (discussed in the next pages). All these characteristics of MEMS passive components represent crucial issues, enabling better performance and wider usability and reconfigurability of transceivers and telecommunication systems employing such devices. Another significant advantage of RF MEMS technology abides in the typically low manufacturing costs. MEMS passive components, indeed, have dimensions ranging from a few tens to a few hundred of micrometres, so their typical footprint and geometrical features are a few orders of magnitude larger than semiconductor devices. Consequently, the tolerances and minimum features sizes in a MEMS fabrication process are significantly more relaxed as compared, for instance, to a complementary metal oxide semiconductor (CMOS) process, leading to reduced costs for all the fabrication steps from the lithography to the clean-room equipment required. On the other hand, relevant issues are still standing in the way of wider use of MEMS passive components in large scale market applications. Integration of MEMS components within circuits and systems in standard technology, their encapsulation (i.e. packaging) and protection, as well as the mechanical reliability, power handling and stability of performance, are issues that add to the cost of RF MEMS components. More simply, RF MEMS devices are cheap to fabricate and test as stand-alone devices, but expensive to be qualified and made suitable for a specific application. Despite these aspects, significant effort and resources are being invested in the development of high-performance RF MEMS passive components for very critical applications, such as space applications, where the demand on the components specifications and characteristics overwhelm the investment effort for the realization of just a small batch of RF MEMS passive components with outstanding characteristics. In conclusion, when the costs for the integration of RF MEMS passive components has become more standardized and, on the other hand, the demand for components with very high performance become the deciding point for a specific application, the diffusion of RF passives in MEMS technology will take significant steps forward.

4.2 RF MEMS passive components and their applications

As already mentioned, MEMS technology is particularly suitable for the fabrication of high-performance RF lumped components, such as variable capacitors (varactors), inductors and switches (also referred to as relays). In the following two subsections some basic information will be introduced concerning the technological process for the fabrication of RF MEMS passive components, and their applications.

4.2.1 Introduction to the technology platforms for the fabrication of RF MEMS

Concerning the technology platforms for the manufacturing of MEMS devices and components, they are typically constituted of a combination of process steps, most of which are in common with those for standard semiconductor devices, such as diodes and transistors. Indeed, the fabrication of micro-devices is always based on the selective deposition and removal of stacked conductive and insulating layers, by means of pattern transfer (i.e. lithography), and the subsequent execution of steps such as the electrodeposition or sputtering of metal layers (gold, silver, copper, aluminium, and so on), the growth of insulating layers (e.g. silicon oxide, silicon nitride), and the selective removal of the same layers (wet or dry etching, plasma oxygen, and so on) (Adams, 2009). A peculiar fabrication step of MEMS and RF MEMS devices is the exploitation of the so-called sacrificial layer, which is a film of material (typically photoresist or oxide) needed for defining the movable MEMS parts, and then removed in order to release the suspended structures (Zhang et al., 2009). The stacked deposition and selective removal of multiple conductive and insulating layers onto a substrate (typically a silicon wafer) is called surface micromachining (Liu et al., 2010), and it is commonly used for the fabrication of RF MEMS passive components. Differently from a typical surface micromachining process, another fabrication technique is frequently exploited for the realization of MEMS devices, although more in the field of sensors and actuators than for RF applications, that is the so-called bulk micromachining. In this, the (silicon) substrate is selectively removed (from the bottom side), forming suspended and deformable membranes made of the same material of the substrate, rather than layers deposited above it (Um et al., 2010). In general, the bulk micromachining process cannot be completely used for the fabrication of RF MEMS devices, as movable structures made of silicon (as constitutive material) would excessively attenuate the RF signal (i.e. large resistive losses) with respect to a surface micromachined metal layer, because of the resistivity of the first material being significantly larger than that of gold, for instance. A solution to circumvent this problem resides in coating the MEMS constitutive silicon parts with highly conductive material (e.g. evaporated metal layers), along the path where the RF signal is supposed to travel, reducing resistive losses. More interestingly, several examples of RF MEMS devices benefiting from a combination of surface and bulk micromachining processes are available in literature. For instance, the work reported in Zine-El-Abidine *et al.* (2004) discusses a metal RF MEMS tunable inductor below which the silicon was removed (bulk micromachining) in order to have a suspended (in air) micro-device, consequently achieving reduction of resistive losses and capacitive coupling toward the substrate. The inductor reported in this work shows a Q-factor larger than 9 at 5 GHz, and a self-resonance frequency above 15 GHz.

4.2.2 Applications of RF MEMS passive components

As already mentioned, MEMS technology is suitable for the realization of high-performance passive components to be employed within transceivers and telecommunication platforms. In this subsection, an overview of potential applications of MEMS basic passive components and complex networks within RF systems is provided. In terms of transceiver (i.e. transmitter/receiver) platforms for radio signals, one of the most widely diffused architectures is the super-heterodyne transmitter and receiver (Laskar *et al.*, 2004). Such an architecture operates a frequency up-conversion (transmitter) and down-conversion (receiver) of the baseband signal, to an intermediate frequency (IF) band lower than the RF band exploited for broadcasting the signal. The IF facilitates the manipulation and treatment of the signal to be transmitted/received (e.g. filtering, amplification, modulation/demodulation, and so on). Passive components in MEMS technology can replace traditional devices in several parts of a super-heterodyne transceiver, improving its performance and characteristics. The block diagram reported in Fig. 4.1 shows the typical configuration of a super-heterodyne receiver, as reported and discussed in Nguyen (2001). All the starred sub-blocks of the diagram can be replaced by implementations of passive components in RF MEMS technology. In particular, looking at the receiver from the antenna to the output of the demodulated received signal (In-phase – I and Quadrature – Q) a MEMS switching unit can be used to select the proper antenna (i.e. hardware selection). Moreover, MEMS varactors (i.e. variable capacitors) and inductors are suitable to realize high Q-factor filters (both RF and IF) and reconfigurable LC-tanks to tune the oscillation frequency of the voltage controlled oscillator (VCO). Finally, MEMS resonators can replace the typical quartz-based devices in the oscillators. Besides the realization of RF MEMS basic passive components, MEMS technology can be exploited for the fabrication of more complex

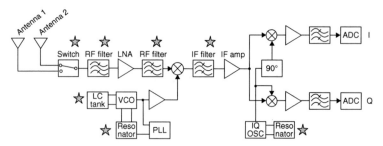

4.1 Block diagram of a super-heterodyne radio receiver, as reported in Nguyen (2001). The starred blocks can be realized with passive components based on RF MEMS technology, improving the performance and characteristics of the whole system.

blocks as well. Indeed, by merging several varactors, inductors and switches, it is possible to realize reconfigurable high-order switching matrices, phase shifters, impedance matching tuners, couplers, delay lines, and so on, as will be discussed later in this chapter. The availability of such networks leads to rethinking the architecture of a transceiver, rather than just replacing some of its base components with their MEMS counterparts, as discussed above. To this purpose, the architecture of the super-heterodyne receiver previously shown can be rearranged and simplified on the basis of MEMS complex networks (Nguyen, 2001), as shown in Fig. 4.2. In this architecture, the availability of a multi-channel selector (i.e. MEMS switches) with several filtering functions would simplify the hardware complexity of the whole platform. For instance, the typical low loss of MEMS-based devices and networks compared to standard technologies would reduce the number of power amplifiers needed for regenerating the signal. Moreover, the high-reconfigurability of MEMS can be exploited to realize a widely tunable oscillator, extending the range of possible received signals that can be mixed and demodulated by the receiver, through the integration of a mixer-filter IF block based on RF MEMS technology as well. It is easy to envisage that MEMS passive components could be employed in several RF systems and applications apart from transceivers. Although it is not the purpose of this chapter to discuss promising exploitations of MEMS technology in the RF field, another example is worth being briefly mentioned. In modern radar systems, the electronic steering of the antenna beam has replaced the old rotary mechanical antennae, leading to a significant reduction in complexity and space occupation, as well as to improved robustness of the system (Meikle, 2001). However, phase shifters in standard technology needed for antenna beam orientation are typically rather lossy, and consequently require additional power amplifiers duplicated for each of the antenna array delay lines. A block diagram of the radar system, close

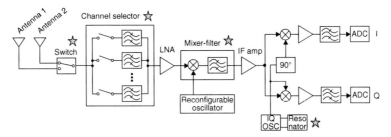

4.2 Block diagram of a super-heterodyne radio receiver, based on a modified architecture that features complex blocks entirely based on RF MEMS technology, namely, a multi-channel selector, a reconfigurable oscillator, and a mixer-filter, as reported in Nguyen (2001).

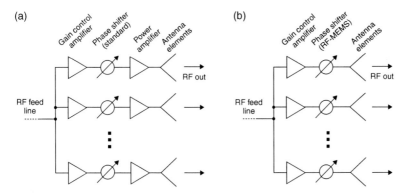

4.3 Block diagram of a radar system employing electronically steerable beam antennae (Haridas *et al.*, 2008). (a) Scheme employing phase shifters in standard technology, requiring power amplifiers on each branch to regenerate the signal attenuated by the lossy phase shifting elements. (b) Scheme employing phase shifters in RF MEMS technology. Due to the very low loss of such elements the power consumption and hardware complexity of the system can be significantly reduced.

to the transmitting antennae array and featuring standard phase shifters, is depicted in Fig. 4.3a and discussed in Haridas *et al.* (2008). As visible in the scheme, a power amplifier is necessary before and after the phase shifter element of each branch, in order to regenerate the attenuated RF signal. For mid-power radar systems, traditional phase shifters can be replaced by high-performance and low-loss realizations of such networks in RF MEMS technology. In the latter case, the power consumption and hardware complexity of the system can be considerably reduced, as an amplifying stage can be omitted on each branch (see Fig. 4.3b).

4.3 High-performance passive components enabled by RF MEMS technology

In this section more details concerning passive components realized in RF MEMS technology will be discussed. First of all, some critical basic concepts concerning the operation principles of such devices will be provided, both concerning their electromechanical and electromagnetic (RF) characteristics. Such features are common to all the different categories of RF MEMS passive components (such as varactors, inductors, and so on), and consequently will help in describing the specific characteristics of all the different device classes that will be presented in the following subsections.

4.3.1 Electromagnetic properties and mechanical actuation of RF MEMS passive components

Passive components in RF MEMS technology are always arranged as parts of waveguide (with a certain length). The RF signal, indeed, is driven from the input of the waveguide to the intrinsic MEMS device, such as a variable capacitor or a micro-relay, that is, the element that actually manipulates the signal, and then is driven to the output of the device. As is well known in microwave theory, several waveguide configurations are possible, depending on the number and placement of the conductive and ground planes, as well as of the insulating material/s (Mahmoud, 1991). Since MEMS structures are typically planar devices with movable parts built above silicon (surface micromachining) or made of silicon (bulk micromachining), they can be easily framed within planar waveguides, rather than coaxial or, in general, sandwiched configurations, where the metal conductive plane is embedded within multiple insulating layers. Given these considerations, the most diffused configurations of RF MEMS passive components are the coplanar waveguide (CPW) and the microstrip waveguide (Mahmoud, 1991), which, in general, are very widely used in RF and microwave circuits regardless of the presence of MEMS devices. A schematic three-dimensional (3D) view of a CPW is proposed in Fig. 4.4a, while that of a microstrip waveguide is reported in Fig. 4.4b. In a CPW, the metallizations are on the same side of a substrate made of insulating material (e.g. silicon, quartz, sapphire, and so on). Very often the CPW structure lies above a thin insulating layer (e.g. silicon oxide, aluminium oxide, etc.), in order to reduce losses to the substrate. In particular, the central signal line has two ground planes (ideally infinite) placed beside it, and separated by a suitable distance known as gap. As the RF signal propagates along the waveguide, the electromagnetic field is confined between the central line and the ground planes, partially through the dielectric material underneath the metal layers, and partially through the air above them. In a microstrip waveguide (see Fig. 4.4b), however, the

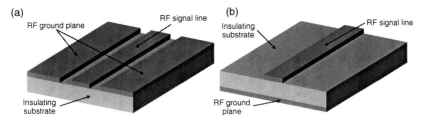

4.4 (a) 3D schematic of a CPW. It features three metallizations on the same side of an insulating substrate, namely, a central line for the RF signal and two lateral ground planes. (b) 3D schematic of a microstrip waveguide. It features two metallizations, namely, the RF signal line on top of the dielectric substrate, and the ground plane on its bottom face.

signal line metallization is placed on top of the insulating substrate, while a unique ground plane (ideally infinite) is patterned on the bottom face of the dielectric material. In this case, as the RF signal propagates along the waveguide, the electromagnetic field is mainly confined within the substrate, among the two metal layers (signal line and ground plane). The analytical modelling of CPWs and microstrip waveguides is well known, and discussed in detail in several scientific papers and books about microwave theory, as in Pozar (2005). Among the various features of CPWs and microstrip lines, the characteristic impedance and the losses are particularly critical. Indeed, the first one determines the impedance matching of the waveguide (and of the RF MEMS component) with the rest of the circuit, that is, before and after the waveguide section itself. The larger the impedance mismatch, the more critical is the RF signal reflection. On the other hand, the losses of a waveguide, determined by the characteristics of the metallization as well as of the insulating substrate, determine the attenuation of the RF signal, and consequently should be kept as small as possible. The analysis of the S-parameters (i.e. scattering parameters), for which a comprehensive theoretical explanation is given in Pozar (2005), helps understand the electromagnetic behaviour of waveguides. For example, the simulated reflection (S11 parameter) and transmission (S21 parameter) behaviour of an ideal 2 mm long CPW, designed to match the characteristic impedance of 50 Ω in the 10 GHz range, are shown in Fig. 4.5. The CPW material is gold, while the substrate is made of high resistivity silicon (HRS), presenting a resistivity of 4 kΩ.cm. The S11 parameter indicates the fraction of the RF signal reflected at the input port of the CPW, and as it is small on the whole frequency range (better than −12 dB), most of the RF signal flows into the waveguide. On the other hand, the S21 parameter indicates the amount of RF power reaching the output port of the CPW. Since its worst value (around −0.45 dB) is rather close to 0 dB (i.e. ideal zero losses), the attenuation of the RF signal

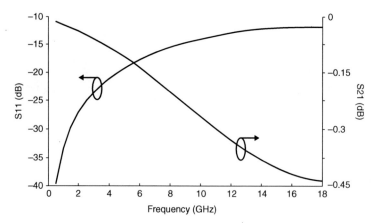

4.5 Simulated S-parameters behaviour (up to 18 GHz) of a standard CPW designed to match a characteristic impedance of 50 Ω. The S11 parameter (i.e. reflection) indicates a rather good impedance matching up to 8–10 GHz, while the S21 parameter (transmission) proves a rather low loss distributed along the transmission line (TL).

introduced by the waveguide is limited. A simple lumped element network suitable for describing the RF behaviour of CPWs and microstrip lines is proposed in Pozar (2005) and depicted in Fig. 4.6. Between the input and output ports of the waveguide (P_1 and P_2), a resistance and inductance are inserted, representing the series resistive (R_{cpw}) and inductive (L_{cpw}) contributions of the metal RF line, respectively. Moreover, the shunt-to-ground capacitance and resistance model the capacitive coupling (C_{gnd}) and the resistive losses (R_{gnd}) between the RF line and the ground plane/s, respectively, through the substrate material and through air. Frequently CPWs and microstrip lines are referred to as MEMS devices, although they do not encompass any movable or deformable part. This is because they are often fabricated using a combination of surface and bulk micromachining technology (see Subsection 4.2.1), that is, technology solutions that are very common in the manufacturing of RF MEMS components. For example, several CPWs are realized by patterning a metal layer above a silicon substrate (surface micromachining) and then removing the silicon underneath the waveguide, etching it from the bottom (bulk micromachining). This leads to the CPW lying above a very thin silicon membrane, and to a consequent significant reduction of losses, as reported and discussed in Shi *et al.* (2001) and Farrington and Iezekiel (2011). In the description of actual RF MEMS passive components, more focus will be given to examples in CPW configuration. This choice is based solely upon requirements of brevity, as RF MEMS in a microstrip waveguide configuration exhibit very good performance too, and all the considerations drawn in this book are applicable to

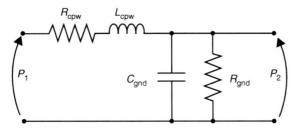

4.6 Typical lumped element network scheme describing the electromagnetic behaviour of a CPW or microstrip waveguide, as reported in Pozar (2005). The series elements account for the inductive and resistive characteristic of the metal RF line, while the shunt elements describe the capacitive coupling and resistive losses toward the RF ground plane/s through the substrate (and air in the case of the CPW).

both classes of devices. The second purpose of this subsection is to provide some fundamental information on the actuation mechanisms for RF MEMS devices and passive components. The multi-physical coupling through which the mechanical behaviour of the movable RF MEMS part is controlled (and its characteristics reconfigured) can take place basically according to four different actuation principles: electrostatic, electromagnetic, piezoelectric, and thermal/electro-thermal (Liu, 2005). A brief description of the four RF MEMS controlling mechanisms follows:

- *Electrostatic.* The floating RF MEMS membrane moves towards the underlying fixed electrode when a voltage drop is imposed between them, due to the force of electrostatic attraction. When the floating membrane collapses (i.e. pulls-in) onto the lower electrode/s the switch state changes. Figure 4.7a, b depicts a schematic view of an electrostatically actuated series ohmic micro-relay. In the rest position (i.e. when no bias is applied between the suspended and the fixed underlying electrode – i.e. between the Act_1 and Act_2 terminals of Fig. 4.7a) the switch is open (Lee *et al.*, 2004). On the other hand, when a voltage drop larger than the pull-in level is imposed between the movable and fixed electrode (Act_1 and Act_2 terminals), the first collapses onto the underlying contact pads, and a low-resistance path is established between the T_1 and T_2 terminals of Fig. 4.7b (closed switch). The same electrostatic control mechanism can be exploited for reconfiguring other characteristics of the RF MEMS component. In a variable capacitor (varactor), for instance, the capacitance between the movable suspended electrode and the fixed one in the rest position (see Fig. 4.7c) can be continuously tuned by applying a variable voltage between them (smaller than the pull-in level), as reported in Fig. 4.7d.

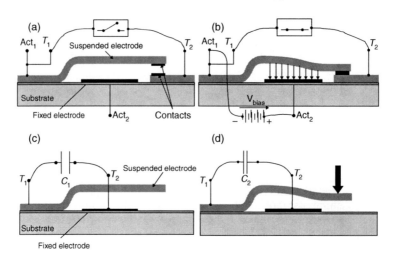

4.7 Schematic cross-section of an electrostatically controlled RF MEMS device. In (a) and (b) the device is a series ohmic switch in the rest position (open switch) and in the actuated (pulled-in) position (closed switch), respectively. In (c) and (d) the same RF MEMS component is exploited as a variable capacitor (varactor). In particular, in (c) the device is in the rest position and the capacitance realizes its minimum value (C_1), while, when the membrane moves towards the fixed electrode, as depicted in (d), the capacitance increases (C_2).

- *Electromagnetic.* The floating MEMS membrane is made of (or coated with) a ferromagnetic material and is surrounded by a variable magnetic field (i.e. current controlled). When a current is driven through the controlling coil the induced magnetic field causes the deformation of the MEMS membrane. When the MEMS movable part collapses onto the underlying electrodes (i.e. pulls-in) the device state changes (Cho *et al.*, 2005).
- *Piezoelectric.* The MEMS movable membrane is coated with a layer of piezoelectric material, which has the property of expanding when subjected to a voltage drop. As the piezoelectric material is coated onto the layer of structural material constituting the MEMS floating membrane (e.g. gold, copper, silver, and so on), the expansion of the first causes the downward bending and displacement of the whole MEMS structure (due to the induced momentum), until there is contact with the underlying electrodes, and the device commutation is achieved (Kawakubo *et al.*, 2005).
- *Thermal/electro-thermal.* In this case, the thermal expansion properties of the material realizing the RF MEMS device are exploited. When the floating metal (or constitutive material) is subjected to the imposition

of a voltage drop, the current flowing through it causes the thermal expansion of the suspended membrane and its buckling (downward direction) (Daneshmand et al., 2009). When the membrane collapses onto the underlying electrodes (i.e. pulls-in), the device state changes. Another option concerning the controlling principle here discussed is to employ two different materials (and/or geometries) for the MEMS movable part, so that the thermal expansion coefficient and/or electrical resistance are different. In this case, when a current flows through the device, the amount of heating is different for the two materials and/or geometries, inducing a momentum (torque) that causes deformation/actuation of the MEMS device (OZENINC.COM, 2011). MEMS actuator demonstrators, such as that just discussed, typically exhibit a resistance larger than 10–30 kΩ, and need a current in the range of a few mA to be operated, leading to a power consumption ranging from a few mW up to 100–200 mW.

To conclude this subsection, a few further considerations will be discussed with respect to the features of the electrostatic actuation of RF MEMS passive components. First of all, a typical measured vertical displacement vs applied bias characteristic (i.e. pull-in/pull-out characteristic) of an RF MEMS parallel-plate capacitor is shown in Fig. 4.8. Figure 4.8a shows the 3D schematic of the parallel-plate suspended electrode, while Fig. 4.8b reports the experimental pull-in/pull-out behaviour. The RF MEMS device is subjected to a ±20 V symmetric triangular waveform. The vertical displacement of the suspended structure presents two abrupt downward transitions at around ±16 V, corresponding to the pull-in (i.e. actuation) for positive and negative applied voltages, PI+ and PI−, respectively, and two abrupt upward transitions at ±9–10 V, being the pull-out (i.e. release) for the positive and negative bias, PO+ and PO−, respectively. Within an electrostatically actuated RF MEMS device, the electrostatic attraction force is balanced by the mechanical restoring force of the deformed flexible suspensions (Liu, 2005). When the applied voltage causes a vertical displacement larger than one-third of the air gap, there is instability in the balance of the electrostatic and mechanical force, and the movable suspended membrane collapses onto the underlying surface. By considering the RF MEMS movable membrane as a mass-spring system, the pull-in voltage (V_{PI}) can be expressed as:

$$V_{PI} = \sqrt{\frac{8kd_0^3}{27\varepsilon_0 A}} \qquad [4.1]$$

where k is the elastic constant of the deformable suspensions, d_0 the air gap (in the rest position), ε_0 the dielectric constant of air, and A is the area of the

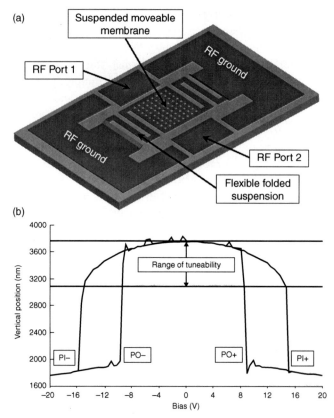

4.8 Typical measured pull-in/pull-out characteristic of an RF MEMS electrostatically controlled device, in response to an applied triangular symmetric bias. The schematic of the device is reported in (a) and refers to a parallel-plate capacitor (in-plane dimensions of 200 μm by 180 μm) kept suspended with two folded flexible suspensions. The pull-in (actuation) and pull-out (release) transitions for positive voltages are indicated in (b) as PI+ and PO+, while negative bias levels are labelled as PI– and PO–, respectively. The range of vertical displacement where it is possible to perform a continuous control of the RF MEMS position is one-third of the air gap, corresponding to an applied bias range from 0 V up to the pull-in voltage V_{PI}, at which the suspended membrane collapses abruptly on the underlying fixed electrode.

movable and fixed electrode. On the other hand, the pull-out voltage (V_{PO}) is expressed as follows:

$$V_{PO} = t_{ins}\sqrt{\frac{2kd_0}{\varepsilon_{ins}A}} \qquad [4.2]$$

where t_{ins} and ε_{ins} are the thickness and dielectric constant of the insulating material separating the actuated MEMS membrane from the underlying fixed electrode. Additional considerations on the physics and analytical description of all the actuation mechanisms of RF MEMS devices discussed in this subsection are reported in Liu (2005) and Busch-Vishniac (1999).

4.3.2 RF MEMS variable capacitors (varactors)

Capacitors are passive components that play an important role in the realization of bandpass or bandstop filters (Besser and Gilmore, 2003), matching networks and, more generally, in a large part of telecommunication systems (Haykin, 2001). The most important characteristics that lumped capacitors are requested to exhibit are the tuning range and the Q-factor, which should both be as large as possible. A wide tunability range for the capacitance enables a correspondingly large reconfigurability of the functional block that employs it (Chen *et al.*, 1979). On the other hand, a large Q-factor ensures a high selectivity with respect to passive filters and better performance in terms of low-losses (Martin and Downing, 1986). Variable capacitors (i.e. varactors) are widely realized in standard semiconductor technology by reverse biasing of diodes (Grajal *et al.*, 2000), with some limitations in terms of performance. A significant alternative solution to obtain varactors with better performance and characteristics is to fabricate them in MEMS technology, and this possibility has been widely researched in the past decade (Peroulis and Katehi, 2003). An example of RF MEMS varactor manufactured in a surface micromachining process (gold constitutive layers electroplated above a 5 kΩ.cm silicon substrate) is depicted in the microphotograph of Fig. 4.9, where all the critical device dimensions are reported. It is based on a gold floating electrode (electrostatically controlled) suspended by means of two meander-shaped flexible springs, and arranged in the CPW configuration. When the floating electrode is not biased (rest position) the capacitance presents the minimum value, as the air gap between the movable and the underlying fixed electrode is at maximum. However, when a DC bias (below the pull-in level) is applied, the capacitance increases due to the reduced gap, and it can be tuned continuously as a function of the bias level, while when the pull-in occurs the capacitance abruptly reaches the maximum value. The capacitance C between two parallel plates of area A is expressed as a function of the applied bias V_{bias} by the following well-known formula:

$$C(V_{bias}) = \frac{\varepsilon_{air} A}{d(V_{bias})} \qquad [4.3]$$

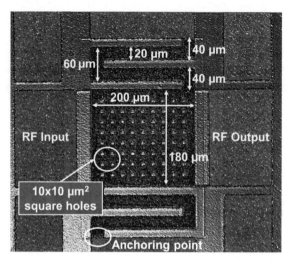

4.9 Micro-photograph of an RF MEMS varactor fabricated in a surface micromachining process. The movable electrode is suspended above the fixed one by means of two meander-shaped flexible beams. The device is realized in the CPW configuration.

The extent of the air gap as a function of V_{bias}, that is, $d(V_{bias})$, can be extracted by equating the electrostatic attraction force (F_{el}) and the restoring mechanical force (F_{me}), expressed as follows:

$$F_{el} = \frac{\varepsilon_{air} A V_{bias}^2}{2(d_0 - x)^2} \qquad [4.4]$$

$$F_{me} = kx \qquad [4.5]$$

where x is the spring elongation consequent to the imposition of V_{bias}. When the pull-in occurs, the maximum capacitance is expressed by:

$$C_{max} = \frac{\varepsilon_{ins} A}{t_{ins}} \qquad [4.6]$$

where ε_{ins} and t_{ins} are the dielectric constant and the thickness, respectively, of the insulating layer (e.g. silicon oxide) between the underlying fixed electrode and the collapsed movable plate. A typical C–V (capacitance versus applied voltage) characteristic of an RF MEMS varactor is reported in Fig. 4.10b (the 3D schematic of the RF MEMS device is reported in Fig. 4.10a). The capacitance can be continuously tuned within the range of 170 fF and 200 fF (see the sub-plot in Fig. 4.10b) before pull-in, while above 5 V it snaps to about 2.4 pF (collapsed movable plate). The tuning range of such a varactor, that is, the ratio between C_{max} and C_{min}, is 12. The pull-in

RF MEMS passive components for wireless applications

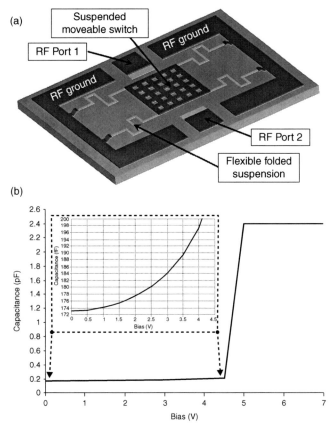

4.10 Typical C-V (capacitance vs applied voltage) characteristic of an RF MEMS varactor. The 3D schematic of the tunable device is shown in (a), and the in-plane dimensions of the suspended movable plate are 220 μm by 220 μm. The capacitance can be continuously tuned, as reported in (b), in the range of applied bias levels below the pull-in (see sub-plot), while it increases more than ten times when the movable electrode collapses onto the underlying one.

voltage is particularly low (about 5 V) because of the meander-like design of the flexible suspensions (see Fig. 4.10a), which drastically decreases their stiffness. A typical topology of a lumped element network describing the electromagnetic behaviour of an RF MEMS variable capacitor (in shunt configuration) is shown in Fig. 4.11. The variable capacitance (C_{mems}) realized by the movable and fixed electrodes is connected to the RF ground through a series resistance (R_{par}) and inductance (L_{par}), accounting for the losses through the air and metal structure and for the series inductance of the flexible suspensions (see Fig. 4.9), respectively. Finally, the transmission line (TL) blocks model the CPW (or microstrip) line branches connecting

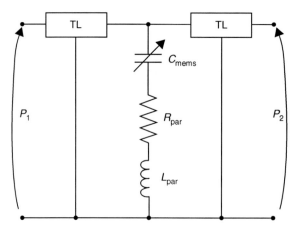

4.11 Lumped element network describing the electromagnetic behaviour of an RF MEMS varactor. The intrinsic variable capacitor (C_{mems}) is in series with a parasitic resistor (R_{par}) and inductor (L_{par}), accounting for the losses to RF ground and the inductance of the flexible suspensions, respectively. The input/output TL branches are described with the network of Fig. 4.6.

the intrinsic RF MEMS varactor to the input and output terminations. The scheme of the TL blocks is as shown in Fig. 4.6. As already mentioned, examples of MEMS-based varactors reported in the literature in recent years are numerous. Several design principles, actuation mechanisms, as well as solutions at fabrication and materials levels, have been investigated in order to increase the tuning range (Bakri-Kassem and Mansour, 2009), enhance the Q-factor (Bakri-Kassem *et al.*, 2008), reduce the actuation voltage (Zahirovic *et al.*, 2009), and to enlarge the power handling (Leidich *et al.*, 2008) of such reconfigurable passive components.

4.3.3 RF MEMS (variable) inductors

The second relevant class of passive reactive components that can be fabricated in RF MEMS technology is represented by inductors, being critical elements, together with capacitors and varactors, in the realization of filters, resonators, impedance matching networks, and so on (Besser and Gilmore, 2003). One of the most important features an inductor should present is a very high Q-factor, and MEMS technology enables improvement of this. The work reported in Fang *et al.* (2010) shows the realization of a metal spiral inductor framed within a CPW structure. The device concept is explained by the 3D schematic of Fig. 4.12. The centre of the spiral coil is connected with the output by means of an overpass, that is, a suspended metallization, which makes it possible to cross all the windings and

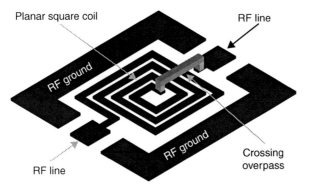

4.12 3D schematic of the RF MEMS inductor concept proposed in Fang *et al.* (2010). The planar (square) coil is framed within a CPW structure. The electrical interconnection from the centre of the coil to the output RF pad is realized by means of a suspended (in air) metal overpass which crosses the planar windings, indeed avoiding shorting the RF signal. The coil conductor width and spacing (between adjacent windings) are 40 μm and 30 μm, respectively, while the outer size of the inductive square coil is fabricated according to two variants, namely, 1000 μm and 1920 μm.

bring the RF signal to the output. The Q-factor of MEMS inductors can be increased by choosing a low-loss substrate, such as alumina, as reported by Blondy *et al.* (2007), as well as by reducing the coupling of the inductor windings with the substrate by depositing a good insulating layer in between them (van Beek *et al.*, 2003). By means of such solutions, improvements of the Q-factor from 5–10 up to 40–70 have been experimentally demonstrated. However, MEMS technology also enables other solutions at manufacturing level that significantly reduce the losses of inductors and, in turn, enhance the Q-factor. Such solutions consist of having the metal inductor coil suspended above an air layer (i.e. floating) rather than lying on silicon (Mizuochi *et al.*, 2009). A micro-photograph of an RF MEMS inductor with the coil suspended in air realized in a surface micromachining process is shown in Fig. 4.13. The thickness of the suspended gold wire and the gap between two adjacent windings is 10 μm, while the external edge of the square coil is 600 μm. The inductance of such a component can be approximated with the formula for a square loop inductor proposed in TECHNICK.NET (2011):

$$L \approx N^2 \frac{2W\mu_0\mu_{air}}{\pi}\left[\ln\left(\frac{W}{r}\right) - 0.77401\right] \qquad [4.7]$$

where N is the number of turns, W the width of the coil external square, $\mu_0\mu_{air}$ the magnetic permeability of air, and r the radius of the suspended

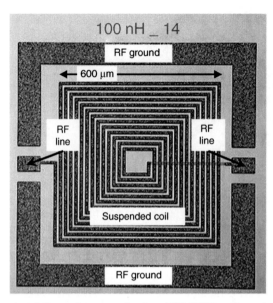

4.13 Micro-photograph of an RF MEMS suspended square loop inductor. The floating coil reduces drastically the substrate losses compared to a standard planar inductor, and consequently increases the Q-factor. The component is arranged in CPW configuration. The thickness of the suspended gold wire and the gap between two adjacent windings is 10 μm, while the external edge of the square coil is 600 μm.

coil metallization. Given the geometrical features of the inductor shown in Fig. 4.13, its inductance value is around 100 nH. As well as the inductor Q-factor improvement enabled by RF MEMS technology, other characteristics, such as self-resonant frequency and parasitic capacitance, benefit from the exploitation of Microsystems over standard semiconductor technology. Indeed, the fact of designing in RF MEMS technology offers additional degrees of freedom (DOF) with respect to standard solutions addressing, for example, an inductor's self-resonant frequency falling into a wider range. Moreover, the option of realizing a tunable inductor in RF MEMS technology (e.g. electrostatically or thermo-electro-mechanically controlled), yields devices with intrinsically reconfigurable properties without the need of any physical redundancy of hardware components (e.g. bank of switchable inductors of different values in standard technology). The typical S-parameter behaviour of an RF MEMS suspended coil inductor, similar to that just discussed, is depicted in the Smith chart (Pozar, 2005) shown in Fig. 4.14. The S11 parameter (simulated with a 3D electromagnetic simulator) is plotted in order to have an indication of the device characteristic impedance behaviour versus frequency. The simulation is performed from

RF MEMS passive components for wireless applications 119

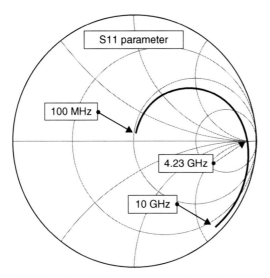

4.14 Simulated S11 parameter of a typical suspended RF MEMS inductor plotted on the Smith chart (from 100 MHz to 10 GHz) to highlight the characteristic impedance behaviour versus frequency. The device behaves as an inductor up to 4.23 GHz, while for higher frequencies the capacitive characteristic is dominating.

100 MHz up to 10 GHz, and the device presents an inductive behaviour up to 4.23 GHz (Smith chart region with positive impedance phase values). On the other hand, beyond such a frequency the trace moves in the negative phase region of the Smith chart (capacitive region). This means that the capacitive parasitic effects of the device dominate its inductive characteristics. Concerning the modelling of RF MEMS inductors, a typical scheme of a lumped element network is shown in Fig. 4.15. The intrinsic inductor (L_{mems} in the figure) is in series with a parasitic resistor (R_{par}), accounting for the losses due to the metal coil, and in parallel with a capacitor, which accounts for the input/output capacitive coupling through air (C_{air}). Finally, as in the case of the varactor lumped network, the input/output TL branches (CPW or microstrip line) are modelled with the same network of Fig. 4.6 and labelled TL. The reconfigurability typical of MEMS technology has been investigated also for lumped inductors, and the techniques enabling such a tuning capability are various. One of the most straightforward employs RF MEMS switches for varying the length of the metal line realizing the inductor (Choi *et al.*, 2009; Zhou *et al.*, 1997). Moreover, self-assembly techniques are also exploited in order to realize inductors with a Q-factor greater than 13 that can be tuned by thermally stressing the device (Lubecke *et al.*, 2000). Another solution consists of deploying a suspended movable metal plate on top of a spiral planar inductor. The metal membrane is electrostatically

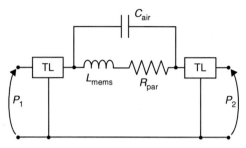

4.15 Lumped element network describing the electromagnetic behaviour of an RF MEMS inductor. The intrinsic inductor (L_{mems}) is in series with a parasitic resistor (R_{par}), accounting for the coil resistive losses, and in parallel with a capacitor (C_{air}) modelling the direct input/output capacitive coupling. The input/output TL branches are described with the network of Fig. 4.6.

actuated, and when it approaches the underlying coil the interaction of the plate with its magnetic field modifies the inductance (Okada *et al.*, 2006). More exotic approaches to reconfiguring the inductance of RF MEMS metal coils are also discussed in the literature. For instance, in Gmati *et al.* (2008) the inductance is modified by exploiting a micro-pump that injects a fluid between the spires, shortening the length of the electrical path and, in turn, the inductance.

4.3.4 RF MEMS ohmic and capacitive switches

The most common and well known class of RF MEMS devices is represented by micro-switches (ohmic and capacitive). The literature reports many valuable realizations of switches in MEMS technology for RF applications, as they represent the key-components capable, on the one hand, of enabling the reconfigurability of the network/platform comprising them, and also presenting, on the other hand, high performance and good characteristics as compared to the current implementations of relays in standard semiconductor technology. Concerning the mechanical working principles of RF MEMS micro-switches, two main classes can be identified, namely the clamped–clamped and the cantilever switches. A 3D image of an RF MEMS clamped–clamped switch, realized in a surface micromachining process, is reported in Fig. 4.16, and is acquired with a profiling system based on optical interferometry (the main geometrical features are mentioned in the figure caption). In a clamped-clamped (or fixed-fixed) RF MEMS switch a metal membrane is suspended and placed transversally above the signal line (Caekenberghe and Sarabandi, 2008). The membrane has two anchoring points (i.e. fixed at both ends), and typically is symmetric with respect to the

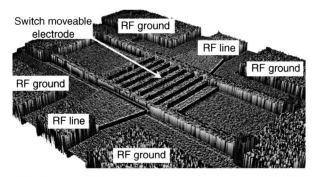

4.16 Measured 3D image of a clamped-clamped RF MEMS series ohmic switch fabricated in a surface micromachining technology platform, and designed in CPW configuration. The suspended membrane is electrostatically controlled. The distance between the two anchoring points is 450 µm, the in-plane dimensions of the central transducer are 150 µm by 150 µm, the suspending beams are long 150 µm and their width is 10 µm.

RF line (Thakur *et al.*, 2009), as Fig. 4.16 shows. On the other hand, cantilever-type RF MEMS switches are based on a membrane that is anchored just on one end. The free end realizes the contact with the electrodes underneath (when the RF MEMS switch is pulled-in) and the membrane can be placed both transversally (Iannacci *et al.*, 2009) on the RF line, or it can be aligned with it (Shen *et al.*, 2008). Besides the type of geometry chosen to realize an RF MEMS switch, the micro-relays can be divided into two categories depending on the switching function they realize, namely the series and shunt configurations. A series switch passes the RF signal between the input and output, while the shunt switch diverts the RF signal towards the RF ground. Both the series and shunt switches are characterized by two states, namely ON and OFF. The ON state corresponds to an activated switch (i.e. pulled-in or actuated), while the OFF state corresponds to a switch in the rest position (i.e. not biased). The schematic views reported in Fig. 4.17 help understand the function operated by the series and shunt switches in the ON and OFF states. The series and ohmic switches realize the functions described above when they are in the ON state, but they do not realize these functions when in the OFF state. This means that a series RF MEMS switch passes the RF signal from the input to the output port when it is in the ON state (i.e. actuated) as Fig. 4.17c reports, while it isolates the two ports when is in the OFF state (i.e. rest position) as shown in Fig. 4.17a. In other words, looking at the input/output transfer function of an RF MEMS series ohmic switch, it is CLOSED when the micro-relay is ON, and is OPEN when the MEMS switch is OFF. The plots in Figs 4.18 and 4.19 show the reflection (S11) and transmission (S21) parameters, respectively,

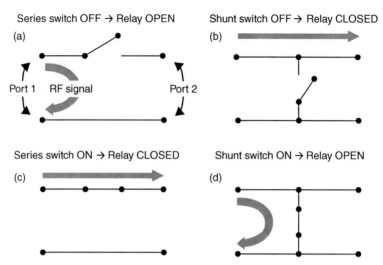

4.17 Schematic view of the transfer function that RF MEMS micro-switches operate on the RF signal (between the two terminals, namely, Port 1 and Port 2) depending on their configuration (series or shunt) and state (ON or OFF). In particular, a series switch reflects (i.e. blocks) the RF signal when it is OFF (a), while it passes (i.e. transmits) the RF signal when it is in the ON state (c). Concerning a shunt switch, it passes the RF signal when it is in the OFF state (b), and blocks the RF signal when the switch is in the ON state (d).

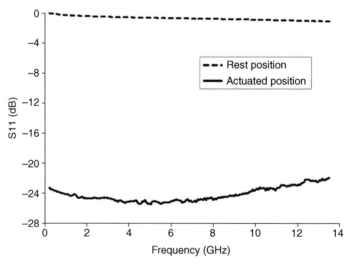

4.18 Measured reflection parameter (S11) characteristic (up to 13 GHz) typical of an RF MEMS series ohmic switch, both in the micro-relay rest (OFF) and actuated (ON) positions.

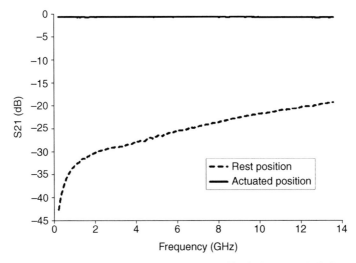

4.19 Measured transmission parameter (S21) characteristic (up to 13 GHz) typical of an RF MEMS series ohmic switch, both in the micro-relay rest (OFF) and actuated (ON) positions.

for an RF MEMS series ohmic switch measured up to 13 GHz, both for the rest and actuated positions of the micro-switch. The micro-switch has a topology similar to that of the device reported in Fig. 4.16 (i.e. a central metal plate kept suspended with four straight flexible suspensions), and is realized in gold above a HRS substrate (i.e. surface micromachining). In particular, in Fig. 4.18 the reflected RF signal has a large value (greater than about -1.5 dB on the whole frequency range) when the switch is OPEN as the power is reflected, while it shifts down to about -24 dB when the switch is CLOSED. Concerning the transmission (see Fig. 4.19), the S21 parameter in the OPEN state, also referred to as isolation, exhibits values better than –20 dB. On the other hand, in the CLOSED configuration, the S21 provides an indication of the attenuation introduced by the RF MEMS switch that is, as expected, rather limited, its value being better than -1 dB over the whole frequency span. The case of a shunt RF MEMS switch is dual with respect to that of a series micro-relay. A shunt switch diverts the RF signal towards the RF ground when it is in the ON state, while it passes the RF signal from the input to the output when it is in the OFF state. As done previously, looking at the input/output transfer function of an RF MEMS shunt switch, it is CLOSED when the micro-relay is OFF (see Fig. 4.17b), and it is OPEN when the MEMS switch is ON (see Fig. 4.17d). In the latter case, it is obvious that when the RF signal flows towards the RF ground it does not reach the device output. A further distinction that has to be made referring to RF MEMS switches (series and shunt) concerns the type of contact they realize with the pads underneath when are in the ON state. When the actuated MEMS metal membrane realizes a metal-to-metal contact with the underlying contact area, it is an ohmic-type micro-relay. On the other hand, if an insulating layer (deposited above the underlying fixed electrode/s) makes impossible a direct metal-to-metal contact, or if the MEMS switch is also meant not to touch the underlying electrode when it is in the ON state (i.e. contact-less switch), the RF MEMS micro-relay is capacitive. In the first case, when the RF MEMS switch is OFF the resistance between the suspended MEMS electrode and the one underneath is very large (in the range of several GΩ), virtually infinite, while a low-resistance ohmic contact (as low as 1–2 Ω) is established when the switch is ON. Concerning RF MEMS capacitive switches, a very small capacitance (typically in the range of 10–50 fF) is realized between the suspended and the underneath fixed parts, i.e. a very large impedance. However, that capacitance becomes significantly larger (e.g. from 1–5 pF up to 10–100 pF, depending on the design) when the RF MEMS switch is in the ON state, establishing a very low-impedance path between the movable (actuated) and the fixed parts. The measured S-parameter characteristic of an RF MEMS shunt capacitive switch is shown in Figs 4.20 and 4.21. Focusing on the reflection parameter (S11 reported in Fig. 4.20), its value is small (better than -10 dB) when the micro-relay is not actuated, but it increases to about -2 dB when the MEMS membrane pulls-in, as the capacitive switch commutes to the OPEN state, and the RF power at the input termination is shorted to RF ground. The steep variation of the

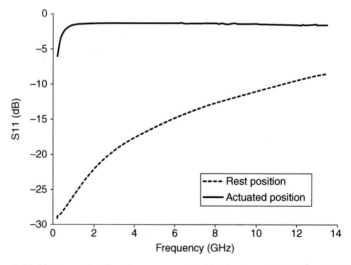

4.20 Measured reflection parameter (S11) characteristic (up to 13 GHz) typical of an RF MEMS shunt capacitive switch, both in the micro-relay rest (OFF) and actuated (ON) positions.

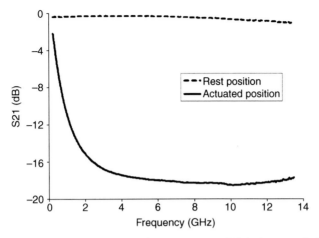

4.21 Measured transmission parameter (S21) characteristic (up to 13 GHz) typical of an RF MEMS shunt capacitive switch, both in the micro-relay rest (OFF) and actuated (ON) positions.

S11 for the OPEN configuration in the low-frequency range (below 2 GHz) is due to the fact that the capacitance behaves as an open circuit in the low-frequency range, so the impedance to ground seen by the RF signal, initially very large, tends to decrease as the frequency increases. All these characteristics and configurations can be combined in different fashions, obtaining several implementations of RF MEMS switches. For instance, it is possible to have cantilever-type series ohmic switches (Patel and Rebeiz, 2010; Shalaby *et al.*, 2009), as well as double-hinged shunt capacitive RF MEMS switches (Mahameed and Rebeiz, 2010; Thakur *et al.*, 2009) and so on (Martinez *et al.*, 2007), each of them with specific advantages and disadvantages in terms of their performance and characteristics, such as isolation, insertion loss (Mollah and Karmakar, 2001), power handling (Lahiri *et al.*, 2009), bandwidth, actuation and release voltages, performance stability (Hwang, 2007) versus time, and so on. The lumped element network describing the electromagnetic behaviour of a series ohmic RF MEMS switch is shown in Fig. 4.22. When the MEMS is actuated (i.e. CLOSED switch), the intrinsic micro-relay introduces a series resistance (R_{on}) due to the ohmic contacts, typically rather small (smaller than a few Ohms). On the other hand, when the switch is OPEN, the relay is modelled as the parallel of a resistance (R_{off}) and of a capacitor (C_{air}). The resistance models the losses through air and is typically very large (e.g. in the order of GΩ). On the other hand, C_{air} takes into account the small capacitive coupling between the input and output contact pads, typically in the range of 10–50 fF, depending on the design of the RF MEMS switch and on the dimensions of the ohmic contact pads. To complete the discussion on the lumped element networks

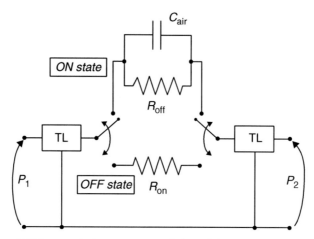

4.22 Lumped element network describing the electromagnetic behaviour of an RF MEMS series ohmic switch. In the ON state the micro-relay inserts a small resistance (R_{on}) between the input and output terminations (CLOSED switch). In the OFF state the RF MEMS switch introduces a parallel resistive (R_{off}) and capacitive (C_{air}) coupling isolating the input from the output.

describing the electromagnetic behaviour of RF MEMS micro-relays, the topology corresponding to a shunt capacitive switch (yielding the behaviour described in Figs 4.20 and 2.21) is as shown in Fig. 4.11 for an RF MEMS varactor. From the conceptual point of view, indeed, an RF MEMS varactor is basically equivalent to a capacitive switch. The difference resides in how the device is operated (e.g. reaching or avoiding the pull-in) and how the C_{max} is shaped. In conclusion, the lumped element network for an ohmic shunt switch, not reported here for the sake of brevity, is a combination of the schemes depicted in Figs 4.11, 4.22, presenting a topology similar to a shunt varactor, but with a variable ohmic resistance (like the one of Fig. 4.22) replacing the variable capacitor to ground.

4.4 Complex networks based on RF MEMS passive components

This section, which concludes the chapter, provides a short overview of complex networks and functional sub-blocks based on the basic RF MEMS passive components discussed in the previous pages. As already mentioned, RF MEMS components can be exploited in the replacement of standard passive elements within RF circuits and systems, indeed enhancing their performance. On the other hand, the availability of high-performance passive components has stimulated the scientific community into rethinking the architecture of functional RF sub-blocks and networks in RF MEMS technology, demonstrating a significant potential in the realization of high-performance and widely reconfigurable Microsystems-based RF circuits. In the following subsections some of the most relevant RF MEMS networks available in literature are listed and categorized.

4.4.1 Single pole double throws and switching matrices

Micro-relays based on RF MEMS technology represent the base elements to implement switching functions, and have been already discussed in detail in Subsection 4.3.4. When combined, RF MEMS switches enable the implementation of switching functions more complex than the simple opening/closing of a contact between two terminals. Following an incremental level of complexity, the combination of two RF MEMS switches enables the realization of Single Pole Double Throws (SPDT), i.e. switching elements with three terminals (one input and two outputs). Depending on the state of the two switches, the RF signal at the input can be directed to one of the two outputs, as well as to both of them (Rebeiz, 2003). A micro-photograph of a CPW-based RF MEMS SPDT realized in a surface micromachining process is shown in Fig. 4.23. The device is realized above a silicon substrate (5 kΩ. cm) and the RF MEMS main structural geometric features are indicated. The dimensions of the suspended micro-transducers are 200 µm by 200 µm. Several examples of RF MEMS-based SPDTs are available in literature. For instance, in Uno *et al.* (2009) RF MEMS SPDTs with insertion loss of -1 dB and isolation better than -40 dB up to 10 GHz are reported. The switching function order can be increased by adding more RF MEMS switching units. In this fashion, it is possible to realize Single Pole Four Throw (SP4T), Single Pole Six Throw (SP6T), as well as more in generality Single Pole Multiple Throw (SPMT), featuring four, six and multiple outputs, respectively, as reported in Gong *et al.* (2011) and Stehle *et al.* (2009). Finally, following the same incremental complexity approach, RF MEMS switches also enable the

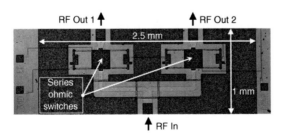

4.23 Micro-photograph of an SPDT fabricated in RF MEMS technology (surface micromachining). The two independently controlled electrostatic switches reconfiguring the switching function are highlighted.

realization of very compact high-order switching matrices, particularly interesting for space and satellite applications thanks to their reduced footprint and very limited weight. Some examples available in literature are reported in Fomani and Mansour (2009) and Yassini *et al.* (2004).

4.4.2 RF power attenuators and splitters/couplers

Another interesting class of networks in MEMS technology is represented by reconfigurable RF power attenuators and splitters/couplers. Such devices are commonly used in RF and microwave circuits for several purposes, such as the power level adjustment between cascaded blocks in a radio receiver, or the power redistribution between two or more branches of a microwave circuit implemented by splitters and couplers (Montgomery *et al.*, 1987). An example of a MEMS-based multi-state reconfigurable power attenuator is shown in the micro-photograph of Fig. 4.24, and discussed in Iannacci *et al.* (2010). The RF signal is attenuated by several resistors (in series on the RF line) that can be selectively shorted by controlling the RF MEMS cantilever-type ohmic switches highlighted in the figure, with in-plane dimensions of 70 μm by 130 μm. The attenuator experimental

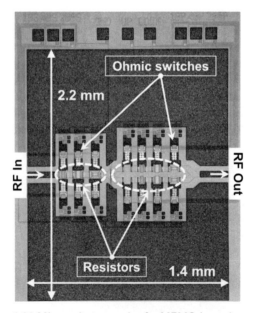

4.24 Micro-photograph of a MEMS-based reconfigurable RF power attenuator reported in Iannacci *et al.* (2010). The attenuation level is realized by several resistors and is tuned by controlling shorting MEMS ohmic switches (highlighted in figure).

testing has proved that it realizes several attenuation levels up to −19 dB, with a rather flat characteristic up to 30 GHz. For instance, the minimum attenuation level realized by the network ranges between −4 dB and −2 dB in the frequency span from 100 MHz up to 30 GHz, while the maximum attenuation level is confined to the range from −19 dB to −15 dB, referring to the same frequency span. On the other hand, several examples of microwave and RF couplers entirely realized in RF MEMS technology are also available in literature. Two significant prototypes are discussed in Nishino *et al.* (2009) and Ocera *et al.* (2007), concerning the CPW and microstrip configuration, respectively.

4.4.3 Impedance matching tuners

A diffused class of RF MEMS-based networks is represented by the reconfigurable impedance matching tuners, able to transform the characteristic input impedance of the network into another value at the output. The impedance matching tuners play a critical role in many RF circuits and systems, as they match the different characteristic impedances of two blocks, making it possible to cascade them without unacceptable levels of reflected power (Besser and Gilmore, 2003). The most relevant advantages of realizing an impedance matching tuner in RF MEMS technology reside in the wider achievable reconfigurability of impedance levels, and in greatly reduced losses of the network itself. Figure 4.25 shows a micro-photograph of the reconfigurable RF MEMS impedance matching tuner (surface micromachining technology and CPW configuration) reported in Iannacci *et al.* (2011). The network, realized on a 5 kΩ.cm silicon substrate, features several metal–insulator–metal (MIM) capacitors and suspended inductors. Such reactive components are placed both in series and shunt configuration, and can load or be omitted from the RF signal line, depending on the state of several cantilever-type micro-relays (also visible in figure), with a dimension of the suspended gold electromechanical transducer of 90 μm by 170 μm. Depending on the selected reactive components, the input/output impedance transformation can be changed, implementing 256 different configurations for each frequency. Several other examples of RF MEMS reconfigurable impedance matching tuners are available in the literature, showing extended capabilities in comparison to the example of Fig. 4.25. For instance, the contributions reported in Lu *et al.* (2005) and Domingue *et al.* (2010) demonstrate a nearly full coverage of the impedance Smith chart, indeed reaching a considerably elevated number of different impedance transformations between the two network terminations. Furthermore, examples of demonstrators in which the RF MEMS impedance matching tuner is interfaced to other blocks in standard technology (e.g. a CMOS PA – Power Amplifier) have been also presented in literature (Larcher *et al.*, 2009).

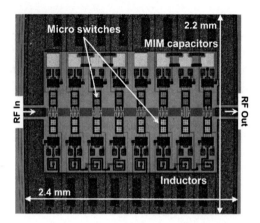

4.25 Micro-photograph of the RF MEMS reconfigurable impedance matching tuner reported in Iannacci *et al.* (2011). Series and shunt capacitors and inductors can be inserted in the RF line depending on the state of several ohmic micro-relays, manipulating the input/output characteristic impedance transformation operated by the network.

4.4.4 Other RF MEMS complex networks

The availability of RF MEMS technology enables the realization of networks with functionalities other than those discussed up to now. This concluding subsection highlights a couple of significant and successful exploitations of RF MEMS technology in the manufacturing of reconfigurable functional blocks for RF circuits and telecommunication platforms. The first example refers to RF MEMS-based phase shifters and delay lines, already mentioned in Section 4.2.2 and shown in the block diagram of Fig. 4.3. Such functional networks are suitable for electronic antennae steering, and are of particular interest for radar applications, as reported in Van Caekenberghe (2009). The scientific literature on RF MEMS technology presents several valuable examples of different realizations of phase shifters and true time delay (TTD) lines with various characteristics, in terms of reconfigurability and frequency range. A couple of examples concerning the first and the second class of devices are discussed in Reinke *et al.* (2011), Vorobyov *et al.* (2011), and in De Angelis *et al.* (2008), Van Caekenberghe and Vaha-Heikkila (2008), respectively. Furthermore, RF MEMS technology is being successfully exploited for the realization of reconfigurable RF filters (e.g. band pass and band stop) (Varadan, 2002). To this purpose, some examples of reconfigurable RF filters for various applications and working in different frequency ranges are reported in Reines *et al.* (2010), Gil *et al.* (2007) and Entesari *et al.* (2007).

4.5 Conclusion

The focus of this chapter has been on MEMS passive components for RF and microwave applications. RF MEMS technology has emerged in the past 10–15 years as a valuable solution for the realization of very high-performance passive components, such as variable capacitors (varactors) and inductors, as well as micro-relays. Moreover, RF MEMS technology has demonstrated a significant potential in the realization of high-performance and widely reconfigurable complex networks and functional sub-blocks, based on the combination of basic passive components. Some examples of this are reconfigurable impedance matching tuners, RF filters, phase shifters, switching matrices, and so on, entirely realized in RF MEMS technology. After an initial overview of the possible applications of RF MEMS components within telecommunication systems, the chapter has reported important aspects concerning the working principles and characteristics of RF MEMS devices, concerning both their electromagnetic properties and coupled electromechanical behaviour. Subsequently, the most diffused RF MEMS basic passive components (variable capacitors, inductors, and switches) have been discussed more in detail, reporting and commenting their typical behaviour and performance. Finally, starting from such basic elements, the most diverse and promising classes of RF MEMS complex networks are listed and discussed throughout the chapter, thereby completing this overview of passive components realized in RF MEMS technology.

4.6 References

Adams T M (2009), *Introductory MEMS: Fabrication and Applications*, Berlin, Springer.

Bakri-Kassem M, Fouladi S, and Mansour R R (2008), *Novel High-Q MEMS Curled-Plate Variable Capacitors Fabricated in 0.35-μm CMOS Technology*, Piscataway, IEEE, DOI: 10.1109/TMTT.2007.914657.

Bakri-Kassem M and Mansour R R (2009), *Linear Bilayer ALD Coated MEMS Varactor With High Tuning Capacitance Ratio*, Piscataway, IEEE, DOI: 10.1109/JMEMS.2008.2008626.

Besser L and Gilmore R (2003), *Practical RF Circuit Design for Modern Wireless Systems, Volume I: Passive Circuits and Systems*, Norwood, Artech House.

Blondy P, Palego C, Houssini M, Pothier A, and Crunteanu A (2007), *RF-MEMS Reconfigurable Filters on Low Loss Substrates for Flexible Front Ends*, Munich, EuMA, DOI: 10.1109/APMC.2007.4554997.

Busch-Vishniac I J (1999), *Electromechanical Sensors And Actuators*, New York, Springer.

Caekenberghe K V and Sarabandi K (2008), *A Self-Aligned Fabrication Process for Capacitive Fixed-Fixed Beam RF MEMS Components*, Piscataway, IEEE, DOI: 10.1109/JMEMS.2008.924259.

Chen P, Muller R, Shiosaki T, and White R (1979), *WP-B6 Silicon Cantilever Beam Accelerometer Utilizing a PI-FET Capacitive Transducer*, Piscataway, IEEE, DOI: 10.1109/T-ED.1979.19782.

Cho I-J, Song T, Baek S-H, and Yoon E (2005), *A Low-Voltage and Low-Power RF MEMS Series and Shunt Switches Actuated by Combination of Electromagnetic and Electrostatic Forces*, Piscataway, IEEE, DOI: 10.1109/TMTT.2005.850406.

Choi D-H, Lee H S, and Yoon J-B (2009), *Linearly Variable Inductor with RF MEMS Switches to Enlarge a Continuous Tuning Range*, Denver, IEEE, DOI: 10.1109/SENSOR.2009.5285389.

Daneshmand M, Fouladi S, Mansour R R, Lisi M, and Stajcer T (2009), *Thermally-Actuated Latching RF MEMS Switch*, Boston, IEEE, DOI: 10.1109/MWSYM.2009.5165922.

De Angelis G, Lucibello A, Marcelli R, Catoni S, Lanciano A, Buttiglione R, Dispenza M, Giacomozzi F, Margesin B, Maglione A, Erspan M, and Combi C (2008), *Packaged Single Pole Double Thru (SPDT) and True Time Delay Lines (TTDL) based on RF MEMS Switches*, Sinaia, IEEE, DOI: 10.1109/SMICND.2008.4703376.

Domingue F, Fouladi S, and Mansour R R (2010), *A Reconfigurable Impedance Matching Network Using Dual-Beam MEMS Switches for an Extended Operating Frequency Range*, Anaheim, IEEE, DOI: 10.1109/MWSYM.2010.5516995.

Entesari K, Obeidat K, Brown A R, and Rebeiz G M (2007), *A 25–75-MHz RF MEMS Tunable Filter*, Piscataway, IEEE, DOI: 10.1109/TMTT.2007.908674.

Fang D-M, Yuan Q, Li X-H, Zhang H-X, Zhou Y, and Zhao X-L (2010), *High Performance MEMS Spiral Inductors*, Xiamen, IEEE, DOI: 10.1109/NEMS.2010.5592582.

Farrington N E S and Iezekiel S (2011), *Design and Simulation of Membrane Supported Transmission Lines for Interconnects in a MM-Wave Multichip Module*, Hong Kong, EMW Publishing, DOI: 10.2528/PIERB10102709.

Fomani A A and Mansour R R (2009), *Miniature RF MEMS Switch Matrices*, Boston, IEEE, DOI: 10.1109/MWSYM.2009.5165923.

Gil I, Martin F, Rottenberg X, and De Raedt W (2007), *Tunable Stop-Band Filter at Q-Band based on RF-MEMS Metamaterials*, Herts, IET, DOI: 10.1049/el:20072164.

Gmati I, Boussetta H, Kallala M, and Besbes K (2008), *Wide-Range RF MEMS Variable Inductor Using Micro Pump Actuator*, Hammamet, SCS, DOI: 10.1109/ICSCS.2008.4746937.

Gong S, Shen H, and Barker N S (2011), *A 60-GHz 2-bit Switched-Line Phase Shifter Using SP4T RF-MEMS Switches*, Piscataway, IEEE, DOI: 10.1109/TMTT.2011.2112374.

Grajal J, Krozer V, Gonzalez E, Maldonado F, and Gismero J (2000), *Modeling and Design Aspects of Millimeter-Wave And Submillimeter-Wave Schottky Diode Varactor Frequency Multipliers*, Piscataway, IEEE, DOI: 10.1109/22.841962.

Haridas N, Erdogan A T, Arslan T, Walton A J, Smith S, Stevenson T, Dunare C, Gundlach A, Terry J, Argyrakis P, Tierney K, Ross A, and O'Hara T (2008), *Reconfigurable MEMS Antennas*, Noordwijk, ESA, DOI: 10.1109/AHS.2008.28.

Haykin S (2001), *Communication Systems*, Hoboken, John Wiley & Sons, Inc.

Hwang J (2007), *Reliability of Electrostatically Actuated RF MEMS Switches*, Singapore, IEEE, DOI: 10.1109/RFIT.2007.4443942.

Iannacci J, Faes A, Mastri F, Masotti D, and Rizzoli V (2010), *A MEMS-Based Wide-Band Multi-State Power Attenuator for Radio Frequency and Microwave Applications*, Anaheim, NSTI.

Iannacci J, Giacomozzi F, Colpo S, Margesin B, and Bartek M (2009), *A General Purpose Reconfigurable MEMS-based Attenuator for Radio Frequency and Microwave Applications*, Saint Petersburg, IEEE, DOI: 10.1109/EURCON.2009.5167788.

Iannacci J, Masotti D, Kuenzig T, and Niessner N (2011), *A Reconfigurable Impedance Matching Network Entirely Manufactured in RF-MEMS Technology*, Prague, SPIE, DOI: 10.1117/12.886186.

Kawakubo T, Nagano T, Nishigaki M, Abe K, and Itaya K (2005), *Piezoelectric RF MEMS Tunable Capacitor with 3V Operation Using CMOS Compatible Materials and Process*, Washington, IEEE, DOI: 10.1109/IEDM.2005.1609332.

Lahiri S, Saha H, and Kundu A (2009), *RF MEMS Switch: An Overview at-a-glance*, Kolkata, CODEC.

Larcher L, Brama R, Ganzerli M, Iannacci J, Margesin B, Bedani M, and Gnudi A (2009), *A MEMS Reconfigurable Quad-Band Class-E Power Amplifier for GSM Standard*, Sorrento, IEEE, DOI: 10.1109/MEMSYS.2009.4805520.

Laskar J, Matinpour B, and Sudipto C (2004), *Modern Receiver Front-ends: Systems, Circuits, and Integration*, Hoboken, Wiley-IEEE.

Lee H S, Leung C H, Shi J, and Chan S C (2004), *Micro-electro-mechanical relays-design Concepts and Process Demonstrations*, Seattle, IEEE, DOI: 10.1109/HOLM.2004.1353125.

Leidich S, Kurth S, and Gessner T (2008), *Continuously Tunable RF-MEMS Varactor for High Power Applications*, Atlanta, IEEE, DOI: 10.1109/MWSYM.2008.4633290.

Liu B, Lv Z, Li Z, He X, and Hao Y (2010), *A Surface Micromachining Process Utilizing Dual Metal Sacrificial Layer for Fabrication of RF MEMS Switch*, Xiamen, IEEE, DOI: 10.1109/NEMS.2010.5592479.

Liu C (2005), *Foundations of MEMS*, Upper Saddle River, Prentice Hall.

Lu Y, Katehi L P B, and Peroulis D (2005), *A Novel MEMS Impedance Tuner Simultaneously Optimized for Maximum Impedance Range and Power Handling*, Long Beach, IEEE, DOI: 10.1109/MWSYM.2005.1516775.

Lubecke V, Barber B, Chan E, Lopez D, and Gammel P (2000), *Self-assembling MEMS Variable and Fixed RF Inductors*, Sydney, IEEE, DOI: 10.1109/APMC.2000.925762.

Mahameed R and Rebeiz G (2010), *A High-Power Temperature-Stable Electrostatic RF MEMS Capacitive Switch Based on a Thermal Buckle-Beam Design*, Piscataway, IEEE, DOI: 10.1109/JMEMS.2010.2049475.

Mahmoud S F (1991), *Electromagnetic Waveguides: Theory and Applications*, London, Peter Peregrinus Ltd.

Martin N and Downing B (1986), *Effect of Varactor Q-factor on Tuning Sensitivity of Microwave Oscillators, Including Reverse Tuning*, Herts, IET, DOI: 10.1049/el:19860209.

Martinez J, Blondy A, Pothier A, Bouyge D, Crunteanu A, and Chatras M (2007), *Surface and Bulk Micromachined RF MEMS Capacitive Series Switch for Watt-Range Hot Switching Operation*, Munich, EuMA, DOI: 10.1109/EUMC.2007.4405424.

Meikle H (2001), *Modern Radar Systems*, Norwood, Artech House.

Mizuochi Y, Amakawa S, Ishihara N, and Masu K (2009), *Study of Air-Suspended RF MEMS Inductor Configurations for Realizing Large Inductance Variations*, Bariloche, IEEE.

Mollah M and Karmakar N (2001), *RF-MEMS Switches: Paradigms of Microwave Switching*, Taiwan, IEEE, DOI: 10.1109/APMC.2001.985292.

Montgomery C G, Henry Dicke R H, and Purcell E M (1987), *Principles of Microwave Circuits*, London, Peter Peregrinus Ltd.

Nguyen C T-C (2001), *Transceiver Front-End Architectures Using Vibrating Micromechanical Signal Processors*, Piscataway, IEEE, DOI: 10.1109/SMIC.2001.942335.

Nishino T, Kitsukawa Y, Hangai M, Lee S-S, Soda S-N, Miyazaki M, Naitoh I, and Konishi Y (2009), *Tunable MEMS Hybrid Coupler and L-Band Tunable Filter*, Boston, IEEE, DOI: 10.1109/MWSYM.2009.5165879.

Ocera A, Farinelli P, Mezzanotte P, Sorrentino R, Margesin B, and Giacomozzi F (2007), *Novel RF-MEMS Widely-Reconfigurable Directional Coupler*, Munich, EuMA, DOI: 10.1109/EUMC.2007.4405141.

Okada K, Sugawara H, Ito H, Itoi K, Sato M, Abe H, Ito T, and Masu K (2006), *On-Chip High-Q Variable Inductor Using Wafer-Level Chip-Scale Package Technology*, Piscataway, IEEE, DOI: 10.1109/TED.2006.880815.

OZENINC.COM (2011), Available from: http://www.ozeninc.com/downloads/thermo-electric%20actuator%20mems%20 robust%20design%20optimization.pdf [2011-Aug-01].

Patel C and Rebeiz G (2010), *An RF-MEMS Switch with mN Contact Forces*, Anaheim, IEEE, DOI: 10.1109/MWSYM.2010.5518064.

Peroulis D and Katehi L (2003), *Electrostatically-tunable Analog RF MEMS Varactors with Measured Capacitance Range of 300%*, Philadelphia, IEEE, DOI: 10.1109/MWSYM.2003.1210488.

Pozar D M (2005), *Microwave Engineering*, Hoboken, Wiley.

Rebeiz G M (2003), *RF MEMS: Theory, Design, and Technology*, Hoboken, Wiley-Interscience.

Reines I, Park S-J, and Rebeiz G M (2010), *Compact Low-Loss Tunable X-Band Bandstop Filter With Miniature RF-MEMS Switches*, Piscataway, IEEE, DOI: 10.1109/TMTT.2010.2050621.

Reinke J, Wang L, Fedder G K, and Mukherjee T (2011), *A 4-bit RF MEMS Phase Shifter Monolithically Integrated with Conventional CMOS*, Cancun, IEEE, DOI: 10.1109/MEMSYS.2011.5734533.

Shalaby M, Wang Z, Chow L-W, Jensen B, Volakis J, Kurabayashi K, and Saitou K (2009), *Robust Design of RF-MEMS Cantilever Switches Using Contact Physics Modeling*, Piscataway, IEEE, DOI: 10.1109/TIE.2008.2006832.

Shen H, Gong S, and Barker N (2008), *DC-Contact RF MEMS Switches Using Thin-Film Cantilevers*, Amsterdam, EuMA, DOI: 10.1109/EMICC.2008.4772309.

Shi Y, Lai Z, Xin P, Shao L, and Zhu Z (2001), *Design and Fabrication of Micromachined Microwave Transmission Lines*, Bellingham, SPIE, DOI: 10.1117/12.442983.

Stehle A, Georgiev G, Ziegler V, Schoenlinner B, Prechtel U, Schmid U, and Seidel H (2009), *Broadband Single-Pole Multithrow RF-MEMS Switches for Ka-Band*, Munich, GeMiC, DOI: 10.1109/GEMIC.2009.4815911.

TECHNICK.NET (2011), Available from: http://www.technick.net/public/code/cp_dpage.php?aiocp_dp=util_inductance_square [2011-Jul-20].

Thakur S, Sumithra Devi K, and Ranjitha I (2009), *Performance of Low Loss RF MEMS Fixed-Fixed Capacitive Switch Characterization*, Kolkata, IEEE, DOI: 10.1109/AEMC.2009.5430610.
Um D, Asiabanpour B, Foor D, Kurtz M, Tellers M, and McGregor M T (2010), *Micro Scale Silicon Dioxide Gear Fabrication by Bulk Micromachining Process*, Xiamen, IEEE, DOI: 10.1109/NEMS.2010.5592170.
Uno Y, Narise K, Masuda T, Inoue K, Adachi Y, Hosoya K, Seki T, and Sato F (2009), *Development of SPDT-structured RF MEMS Switch*, Denver, IEEE, DOI: 10.1109/SENSOR.2009.5285381.
Van Beek J, Van Delden M, Van Dijken A, Van Eerd P, Van Grootel M, Jansman A, Kemmeren A, Rijks T, Steeneken P, den Toonder J, Ulenaers M, den Dekker A, Lok P, Pulsford N, van Straten F, van Teeffelen L, de Coster J, and Puers R (2003), *High-Q Integrated RF Passives and Micromechanical Capacitors on Silicon*, Toulouse, IEEE, DOI: 10.1109/BIPOL.2003.1274955.
Van Caekenberghe K (2009), *RF MEMS on the Radar*, Piscataway, IEEE, DOI: 10.1109/MMM.2009.933596.
Van Caekenberghe K and Vaha-Heikkila T (2008), *An Analog RF MEMS Slotline True-Time-Delay Phase Shifter*, Piscataway, IEEE, DOI: 10.1109/TMTT.2008.2002236.
Varadan V K (2002), *RF MEMS and Their Applications*, Hoboken, John Wiley & Sons, Inc.
Vorobyov A, Sauleau R, Fourn E, Oberhammer J, and Baghchehsaraei Z (2011), *MEMS Based Waveguide Phase Shifters for Phased Arrays in Automotive Radar Applications*, Rome, EUCAP.
Yassini B, Choi S, Zybura A, Yu M, Mihailovich R E, and DeNatale J F (2004), *A Novel MEMS LTCC Switch Matrix*, Fort Worth, IEEE, DOI: 10.1109/MWSYM.2004.1339060.
Zahirovic N, Mansour R R, and Yu M (2009), *A Three-Step High-Q Variable MEMS Capacitor with Low Actuation Voltage*, Rome, EuMA.
Zhang Y-H, Wang C, Ouyang W-X, and Lai Z-S (2009), *Compound Sacrificial Layer Process for RF MEMS Applications*, Beijing, IEEE, DOI: 10.1109/MAPE.2009.5355590.
Zhou S, Sun X-Q, and Carr W (1997), *A Micro Variable Inductor Chip Using MEMS Relays, in Solid State Sensors and Actuators*, Chicago, IEEE, DOI: 10.1109/SENSOR.1997.635404.
Zine-El-Abidine I, Okoniewski M, and McRory J G (2004), *A Tunable RF MEMS Inductor*, Alberta, IEEE, DOI: 10.1109/ICMENS.2004.1509028.

5
RF MEMS phase shifters for wireless applications

V. PUYAL, CEA-LETI Laboratory, Minatec, France and
LAAS-CNRS, Université de Toulouse, France and
D. TITZ, Université Nice Sophia Antipolis, France

DOI: 10.1533/9780857098610.1.136

Abstract: In the introduction, the advantages and drawbacks of using radio frequency microelectromechanical systems (RF MEMS) in phase shifters compared with solid-state circuits will be presented. Then, a review of the more common phase shifter topologies will be addressed. Design equations and schematics will be given, as well as recently published papers using RF MEMS. To illustrate RF MEMS phase shifter applications such as beamforming and beamswitching, one particular architecture will be presented as a global example. Finally, we will conclude by presenting an overall summary of different architectures to enable design choice and discuss the future trends in RF MEMS phase shifters.

Key words: RF MEMS, phase shifters, phased arrays, wireless applications.

5.1 Introduction

In many wireless and mobile applications, phase shifters represent essential components of front-end circuits. They are of particular interest for communication circuits requiring beamforming techniques as key components of phased arrays. In such circuits, the beam of an antenna array is steered in different directions depending on the phase shift applied to each element (Fig. 5.1). This requires the use of precise phase shifters. Among the main domains of application are satellites, airborne or even military communications or radar applications. MEMS-based phase shifters can also be used in reflect-array designs.

RF MEMS switches have been used in phase shifter designs for more than 10 years now (Barker and Rebeiz, 1998) for their superiority in performance over traditional solid-state devices (PIN diode, FET switches) or ferrite materials. Based on the same considerations, RF MEMS phase shifters show several advantages over traditional solid-state phase shifters:

- low loss (especially at high frequencies),
- improved isolation,

RF MEMS phase shifters for wireless applications

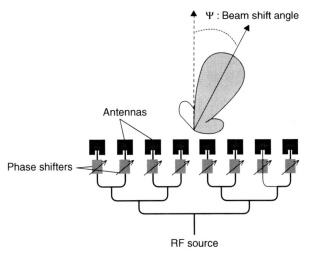

5.1 Phase shifters and antenna array in a beamforming application.

- wideband performance,
- reduction of direct current (DC) power (no consumption when the switch is OFF),
- high linearity,
- power handling,
- low parasitic effects.

However, there are still some issues which have limited the appearance of RF MEMS phase shifters on the consumer market, such as:

- low reliability,
- high switching time,
- large size,
- packaging issues,
- high actuation voltage,
- temperature stability.

A comparison between the latest published results on RF solid-state and RF MEMS phase shifters is presented in Table 5.1. RF MEMS phase shifters show an overall insertion loss of −3/−4 dB whereas solid-state phase shifters exhibit important insertion loss (around −10 dB) for passive architectures. However, for active topologies, transistor phase shifters can present good insertion loss (gain) but poor linearity and high power consumption. Note that RF MEMS phase shifters exhibit low insertion loss with very low phase error. The challenge is to design high-frequency planar phase shifters for future antenna array systems.

Table 5.1 Comparison between latest published phase shifters

Reference	Frequency (GHz)	Type/bits	Substrate	S21 (dB)	Phase error	Size
Hung et al. (2004)	75–110	MEMS/3	Glass	−2.7	3°	5 × 1.9 mm²
Hong-Teuk et al. (2004)	50–70	MEMS/2	Quartz	−4.6	5°	2.1 × 1.5 mm²
Somjit et al. (2009)	75	MEMS/4.25	HR Si	−3.5	6°	5.5 mm long
Byung-Wook and Rebeiz (2007)	30–38	0.12u BiCMOS/4	Si	+1	7°	0.9 × 0.4 mm²
Kwang-Jin and Rebeiz (2007)	18–26	0.13u CMOS/4	Si	−3.8	9.7°	0.8 × 0.6 mm²
Yu et al. (2008)	55–65	65nm CMOS/4	Si	−9.4	9.2°	/

There are two different implementations for a phase shifter: the analogue and the digital approach. The analogue phase shifter allows a continuous variable phase shift between two extreme values. Its main feature is the total achievable phase shift. As a result, a classical figure of merit (FoM) for such circuits is the phase shift divided by the insertion loss in °/dB. The digital phase shifter only allows a specific set of discrete phase delays. Its key parameters are the maximum phase shift and the number of discrete steps, often given in bits. For example, a 3-bit phase shifter with a 45/90/180° phase delays network is able to achieve 45/90/135/180/225/270/315° phase shifts. The FoM for this kind of phase shifter is the phase shift per bit in °/bit. While in theory analogue phase shifters seem to be the best choice, they are very difficult to design for large phase shifts. Thus, most published papers deal with digital-type phase shifters.

For wideband performance, a phase shifter should have a constant phase delay with frequency or a linear phase versus frequency. The former is called a true time phase shifter, while the latter is called a true time delay (TTD) phase shifter.

In this chapter, the main phase shifter architectures are presented classified into four categories:

- switched-line phase shifter,
- loaded-line phase shifter,
- reflection-type phase shifter,
- distributed-line phase shifter.

For each phase shifter type, the theory and some implementations are described. A survey of up-to-date published RF MEMS phase shifters will be drawn by categories. Specific issues prohibiting RF MEMS phase shifters from targeting the consumer market until now will be discussed. Finally, an example of a complete design and application will be given.

5.2 Switched-line phase shifter

The switched-line phase shifter is the easiest RF phase shifter to build.

5.2.1 Theory of switched-line phase shifters

A classical representation of a switched-line phase shifter is presented in Fig. 5.2. At the origin of this implementation lies a simple fact, derived from the transmission line theory that will be of use for all different categories of phase shifters: a wave travelling along a transmission line will have a phase shift between its output and input voltages, dependent on the characteristic impedance and the length of the line, described by Equation [5.1]. Considering a progressive wave on a matched line, l represents the length of the line, ω the angular frequency of the signal, γ the propagation constant, which depends on the physical characteristics of the line.

$$u(l) = u(0)e^{j\omega t - \gamma l} \qquad [5.1]$$

5.2.2 Standard implementation

There are several ways to implement a switched-line phase shifter, depending on the switch and transmission line used. The classical one already illustrated in Fig. 5.2 is to use series switches. Series switches can be positioned close to the transmission line junction (T-junction) because of their high isolation. Shunt switch design is a somewhat more complex as, when the RF MEMS is OFF, it does not result in an open circuit but in a short circuit. Hence, shunt switches must be positioned at a quarter guided wavelength

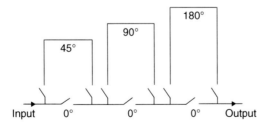

5.2 Schematic of a 3-bit switched-line phase shifter.

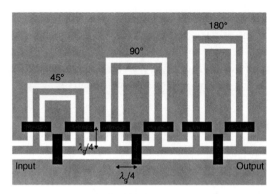

5.3 Shunt switch CPW 3-bit phase shifter implementation. MEMS switches are represented in black.

($\lambda_g/4$) from the T-junction to result in an open circuit at the T-junction. Figure 5.3 presents an example of shunt switch implementation using a coplanar waveguide (CPW) line.

When used with a microstrip line, the shunt switch implementation must use two $\lambda_g/4$ transformations, as no connection with DC ground is possible. $\lambda_g/4$ open-ended stubs are connected to the switch to result in a short circuit. Details about this implementation can be found in (Pillans *et al.*, 1999).

The architecture presented above is relatively simple to design, but presents some drawbacks:

- Large area consumption for large phase shifts (long transmission lines).
- Insertion loss depending on the length of the line, on the chosen path.

5.2.3 New implementation for size reduction

To reduce the size of the switched-line phase shifter, a simple idea was proposed in Tan *et al.* (2002). Instead of using Single Pole Double Throw (SPDT or SP2T) switches to select a delay path or the 0° path as in Fig. 5.4a, the delay path can be stacked and selected using a Single Pole Four Throw (SP4T) as in Fig. 5.4b. This is of course dependent on the performance of the SP4T itself, which was proven to be quite small and low loss in Tan *et al.* (2002). Moreover, only one 0° delay line has to be implemented for a more efficient layout. To show the benefit of an SP4T architecture in terms of insertion loss and size reduction, a comparison between two published phase shifters (Hacker *et al.*, 2003; Tan *et al.*, 2003a) is presented in Table 5.2.

Another way to improve the size of a switched-line phase shifter is to replace the transmission lines by their equivalent semi-lumped model (Fig. 5.5c) or π-network (Fig. 5.5a) (Tan *et al.*, 2003b). Equation [5.2]

Table 5.2 Comparison between published phase shifters using SP2T and SP4T architectures

4-bit designs	From Kim et al. (2001) with SP2T	From Tan et al. (2003a) with SP4T
Frequency (GHz)	DC to 40 GHz	8–12 GHz
Total phase shift	360°	360°
Phase shift step	22.5°	22.5°
Substrate	75-µm GaAs	200-µm GaAs
Number of switches	16 (8 SP2T)	16 (4 SP4T)
Size	6 × 5 mm² (30 mm²)	4.9 × 4.39 mm² (21 mm²)
Insertion loss at 10 GHz	2.2 to 2.6 dB	0.6 to 1.8 dB
Return loss at 10 GHz	Better than −20 dB	Better than −14 dB
Max phase shift	343° at 10.8 GHz	NA
Phase accuracy	NA	−0.9 to 2.3° at 9.97 GHz

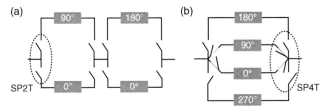

5.4 Two-bit phase shifter based on (a) SP2T architecture, (b) SP4T architecture.

represents the phase shift (ϕ) in matched conditions, which gives a maximum phase shift of −90°. To achieve a low loss phase shifter, the inductor in Fig. 5.5a is replaced by a transmission line in Fig. 5.5c. The line characteristics (Z, θ) are equivalent to the π-network in Fig. 5.5b following Equations [5.3] and [5.4], where C_t is broken into two capacitances C_0 and C_1. For a higher phase shift, several networks can be cascaded, increasing in this way the bandwidth and linearity. A comparison between two published designs (Tan et al., 2003a,b) is presented in Table 5.3 showing the miniaturization capabilities of this implementation. This architecture can also be classified as a high-pass low-pass (HPLP) architecture (Lucyszyn, 2010), as in Morton and Papapolymerou (2008).

$$\sin(\phi) = -\frac{\omega L_t}{Z_0} \quad \text{and} \quad \tan\left(\frac{\phi}{2}\right) = -\frac{\omega C_t}{Z_0} \quad [5.2]$$

$$\cos \theta = 1 - \omega^2 L_1 C_1 \quad [5.3]$$

$$\sin \theta \cdot Z^2 - \omega Z \left[Z_0^2 (2C_1 - \omega^2 C_1^2 L_1) + L_1\right] + Z_0^2 \sin \theta = 0 \quad [5.4]$$

Table 5.3 Comparison between published phase shifter using transmission lines and semi-lumped architectures

2-bit design	From Tan et al. (2003a)	From Tan et al. (2003b)
Frequency (GHz)	8–12	6–14
Total phase shift	270°	270°
Phase shift step	90°	90°
Substrate	200-μm GaAs	200-μm GaAs
Number of switches	8	6
Size	4.8 × 2.5 mm² (12 mm²)	2.49 × 1.95 mm² (5 mm²)
Insertion loss	0.31–0.94 dB	0.4–1.6 dB
Return loss	Better than −17.3 dB	Better than −14 dB
Phase accuracy	−2.2 to 2° at 10.25 GHz	−1.3 to 1° at 9.45 GHz

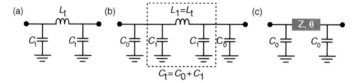

5.5 (a) π-network composed of two capacitances C_t and one inductance L_t, (b) its transformation using another π-network and (c) using a line instead of the inductance to form a semi-lumped network.

5.2.4 Comparison of switched-line phase shifters

Table 5.4 summarizes the performance of several switched-line phase shifters published in the literature. The maximum operating frequency of the proposed designs is around 77 GHz in (Buck and Kasper, 2010) and, in most of the other cases, it is centred around 10 GHz for X-band communications. Depending on the substrate, the phase shifter can be miniaturized (high resistivity silicon and GaAs). However, low loss phase shifters can benefit from organic and Low Temperature Co-fired Ceramic (LTCC) substrates, as shown in Kingsley and Papapolymerou (2006) and Yamane et al. (2008). Due to reliability issues usually encountered when using RF MEMS switches, significant effort has been put over recent years into packaged switched-line phase shifters (Kingsley and Papapolymerou, 2006; Kingsley et al., 2005; Morton and Papapolymerou, 2008). Gautier et al. (2008) show the design of a switched-line phase shifter integrated with an antenna array for the final implementation into a phased array.

5.3 Loaded-line phase shifter

Another way to design a simple phase shifter is represented by the loaded-line phase shifter. It can be of analogue or digital type.

Table 5.4 Comparison between published switched-line phase shifters

Reference	Frequency (GHz)	Substrate	Bit number	Insertion loss (dB)	Max phase error	Size (mm²)
Nordquist et al. (2006)	10	Alumina	6	1.8 ± 0.6	NA	378
Lampen et al. (2010)	6	Si	6	2 ± 1.1	NA	45
Jian et al. (2006)	10	HR Si	5	3.6 ± 0.4	5°	28
Morton and Papapolymerou (2008)	12	HR Si	5	4.5 ± 3.5	10°	9
Pillans et al. (1999)	34	NA	4	2.25 ± 0.45	13°	NA
Kim et al. (2001)	10	GaAs	4	2.4 ± 0.2	17°	30
Tan et al. (2003a)	10	GaAs	4	1.2 ± 0.5	2.3°	21
Tan et al. (2003c)	10	GaAs	4	1.47	3.3°	7
Kingsley and Papapolymerou (2006)	14	LCP	4	0.96 ± 0.25	17.1°	67
Yamane et al. (2008)	12.5	LTCC	4	0.8 ± 0.3	3.6°	130
Buck and Kasper (2010)	24	HR Si	1	2.75 ± 0.25	1.5°	NA
Hacker et al. (2003)	35	GaAs	3	2.2 ± 0.25	5°	9
Malmqvist et al. (2011)	33	GaAs	1	1.1 ± 0.3	6°	NA
Yamane and Toshiyoshi (2011)	12	SOI	1	1.7 ± 0.2	6.5°	6.8
Gautier et al. (2008)	10	HR Si	3	2	14°	NA
Al-Dahleh and Mansour (2008)	10	Alumina	3	2.5 ± 0.2	6°	6
Gong et al. (2011)	60	Quartz	2	2.5 ± 0.4	1°	4
Buck and Kasper (2010)	77	HR Si	1	3	1.5°	NA

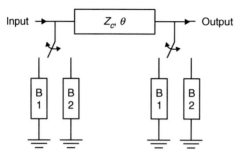

5.6 Implementation of a loaded-line phase shifter. The switch is here to choose between two lines of different length and impedance.

5.3.1 Equations

Extensive theory about loaded-line phase shifters can be found in Atwater (1985), Opp and Hoffman (1968) and Davis (1974). The general idea behind this type of phase shifter is to load a line with two different impedances, as shown in Fig. 5.5c where C_0 is varied to change the phase shift of the line. The capacitance can be varied by discrete steps (usually two) by switching the RF MEMS from its ON to OFF position, or applying a continuous voltage corresponding to different heights of the RF MEMS bridge. The mid-section line can be used as a matching network to keep the input and output impedances close or equal to Z_0. Figure 5.6 presents a global schematic of the loaded-line implementation, where B_1 and B_2 represent the two extreme values of the switched susceptance. For a fixed phase shift, $\Delta\phi$, the susceptances, the characteristic impedance, Z_c, and the electrical delay of the line, θ, assuming the phase shifter is lossless and matched, are linked via Equations [5.5], [5.6] and [5.7]. This type of phase shifter results in excellent response for small phase delays. For higher phase shifts, several phase shifters of this same type can be cascaded.

$$B_1 = Y_0 \left[\frac{\cos\theta}{\cos(\Delta\phi/2)} - \tan\left(\frac{\Delta\phi}{2}\right) \right] \qquad [5.5]$$

$$B_2 = Y_0 \left[\frac{\cos\theta}{\cos(\Delta\phi/2)} + \tan(\Delta\phi/2) \right] \qquad [5.6]$$

$$Z_c = Z_0 \frac{\cos(\Delta\phi/2)}{\sin\theta} \qquad [5.7]$$

5.3.2 Three classes for implementation

The loaded-line phase shifters can be separated into several classes (Opp and Hoffman, 1968) depending on the values of B_1 and B_2:

- Class I: general case, where $B_1 \neq -B_2$ and $B_{1,2} \neq 0$.
- Class II: load/unload case, where B_1 or $B_2 = 0$. If $B_1 = 0$, the phase shift is entirely due to B_2. $\theta = (\pi \pm \Delta\phi)/2$ and $B_2 = \pm 2Y_0 \tan(\Delta\phi/2)$.
- Class III: $\theta = 90$ and $B_1 = -B_2$. This results in a constant loss when the loads are switched.

Figure 5.7 illustrates these three classes. The vector OD represents the phase shift due to the length of the line. Switching from B_1 to B_2 rotates the vector OA from OA to OB. Figure 5.8 presents a different implementation which depends on the line (here, CPW in all the cases), the type of RF MEMS switch, and the class of the phase shifter.

Ko et al. (2003a) present a slightly different implementation using a combination of short-circuited stubs (as in Fig. 5.8) and open-circuited stubs to obtain a constant phase shift with frequency and to achieve a wideband phase shifter. Figure 5.9 shows the proposed implementation. The simulated results from (Ko et al., 2003b) with and without the open-end stub are interesting in term of phase shift constancy. Indeed, this new implementation

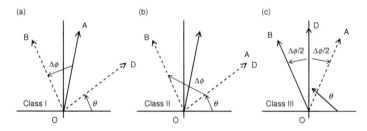

5.7 Representation of the phase shift for the three different classes of loaded-line phase shifters: (a) class I, (b) class II and (c) class III.

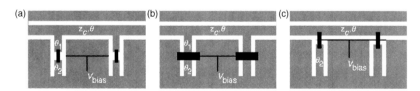

5.8 CPW implementations of a class I phase shifter (a) using series switches, (b) using shunt switches and of a class II phase shifter, and (c) using series switches. Switches are represented in black.

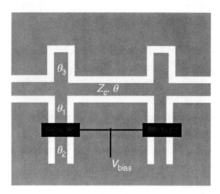

5.9 Implementation proposed for a loaded-line phase shifter in (Ko *et al.*, 2003b). An open-circuited stub is added compared to a classic architecture.

shows a reduced phase imbalance with frequency with a phase shift within 11° to 12° instead of 10° to 14°.

5.3.3 Comparison of loaded-line phase shifters

As for the switched-line phase shifter, we present here published results for loaded-line phase shifters (Table 5.5). Only two designs using analogue type loaded-line phase shifters were reported because of the unstable behaviour of RF MEMS varactors. Loaded-line phase shifters found in the literature have been designed to operate up to the W-band in Somjit *et al.* (2009) and Fritzsch *et al.* (2011).

Rock *et al.* (2009a and 2010) present a study under US Army supervision concerning affordable RF MEMS phase shifters for phased arrays manufacturing technology. A huge effort was put into the production of RF MEMS for military applications as phased arrays for both active and passive missile seekers and for on-the-move SATCOM communications systems for the warfighter. The chosen topology was a class II loaded-line phase shifter for its compromise between simplicity, low loss, compact size and easy modelling. The phase shifter was packaged and integrated with a Vivaldi antenna array. The overall circuit was measured with good beamforming capabilities in Rock *et al.* (2010). Figure 5.10 shows a picture of the global phased array with closer views on the packaged phase shifter from Rock *et al.* (2009b). It can be seen that every phase shifter was packaged separately using a glass lid and then connected to the antenna array through hermetic vias.

Another issue with loaded-line RF MEMS phase shifters is their ability to be monolithically integrated with standard integrated circuit (IC) process. Reinke *et al.* (2011) presents a way to integrate RF MEMS with BiCMOS substrates with the same process flow, thus reducing costs.

Table 5.5 Comparison between published loaded-line phase shifters

Reference	Frequency (GHz)	Substrate	Bit number	Insertion loss (dB)	Max phase error	FoM	Size
Ko et al. (2003a)	12	GaAs	5	5.25	3.5°	66.5°/dB	NA
Somjit et al. (2009)	75	HR Si	4.25	3.5	6°	71.1°/dB	5.5 mm long
Rock et al. (2009a,b)	35	HR Si	4	2.5	8.8°	NA	20 mm^2
Reinke et al. (2011)	32	BiCMOS	4	2.9 ± 1	NA	NA	4 mm long
Ko et al. (2003b)	12	GaAs	3	2	2°	39.5°/dB	25 mm^2
Somjit et al. (2009)	75	HR Si	3	4.5	NA	74°/dB	5.4 mm long
Lampen et al. (2010)	9	Duroid	1	0.56	NA	56.5°/dB	NA
Zhang et al. (2003)	26.5	Alumina	Analogue	1.45 ± 0.35	6°	22.5°/dB	NA
Puyal et al. (2009)	60	HR Si	1	1.5 ± 0.8	10.3°	NA	NA
Fritzsch et al. (2011)	76	Quartz	Analogue	2.4 ± 0.1	2°	42°/dB	NA

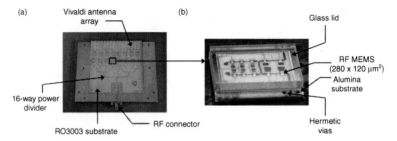

5.10 (a) Phased array module from Rock *et al.* (2009b) composed of a distribution network, phase shifters and antennas and (b) closer view on packaged loaded-line phase shifters.

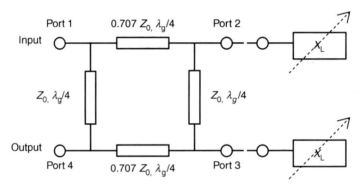

5.11 Implementation of a reflection-type phase shifter. MEMS switches can be used in the reflective loads X_L.

5.4 Reflection-type phase shifter

Reflection-type phase shifters can also use RF MEMS switches in a digital or analogue design. However, for the same reasons as for the loaded-line phase shifter, analogue implementations are not very common.

5.4.1 Theory

Two identical variable reactances, X_L, are connected to the direct (Port 2) and coupled (Port 3) ports of a 90° hybrid coupler (Fig. 5.11). The output of the phase shifter is taken at the isolated port (Port 4). Any incident signal feeding Port 1 will be reflected by both reactive loads producing a phase shift, $\Delta\varphi$, between Ports 1 and 4. If a variable reflective load is used, a variable phase shift is produced between the Ports 1 and 4 of the coupler, following Equation [5.8]. As for the loaded-line phase shifter, reflection-type phase shifters do not result in wide phase shifts. Cascaded phase shifters are often used in these cases.

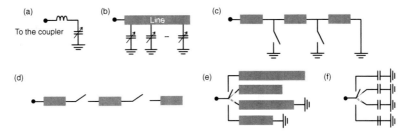

5.12 (a) Tunable capacitor with series inductor. (b) Tunable distributed loaded-line. (c) Switched reflection-line with shunt switches. (d) Switched reflection-line with series switches. (e) Switched distributed-element reactances. (f) Switched lumped-element capacitors.

$$\Delta\varphi = -2\tan^{-1}\left(\frac{X_L}{Z_0}\right) \quad [5.8]$$

5.4.2 Implementation

Two different structures have to be designed in a reflection-type phase shifter. The first is the directional coupler. In many cases, the coupler is the largest part. It must then be reduced to obtain a smaller footprint, while keeping wideband performance. This can be done using semi-lumped architectures or a multilayer of coupled lines coupler. Park *et al.* (2002) propose the same technology used for RF MEMS to realize an air-gap overlay coupler resulting in low loss and wideband performance.

The other part of the design is the reflective load itself. Its implementation depends on the type of transmission line and the RF MEMS switch used, and it can be improved for wider phase shift by adding a series inductance (Fig. 5.12a) or a π-network where the capacitance is the RF MEMS switch. A complete study of the different types of reflective loads can be found in Wu *et al.* (2008). Figure 5.12 presents some of the possible implementation for the reflective load.

5.4.3 Comparison of reflection-type phase shifters

As for the switched-line and loaded-line phase shifters, we present here published results for reflection-type phase shifters (Table 5.6). Several published reflection-type phase shifters are designed to operate in the 60 GHz band (Park *et al.*, 2002; Biglarbegian *et al.*, 2010; Kim *et al.*, 2002a) where phased arrays are useful for non-line-of-sight communications.

Table 5.6 Comparison between published reflection-type phase shifters

Reference	Frequency (GHz)	Substrate	Bit number	Insertion loss (dB)	Max phase error	Size (mm²)
Malczewski et al. (1999)	8	HR Si	4	1.4	NA	NA
Park et al. (2002)	60	Quartz	3	4.85	49.5°	7
Biglarbegian et al. (2010)	60	Alumina	3	3.9 ± 1.6	NA	22
Varian and Walton (2002)	9	HR Si	2	1.14	3.3°	NA
Kim et al. (2002)	60	Quartz	2	4.1 ± 1.4	6.3°	3
Kim et al. (2003b)	15	Quartz	2	3.1 ± 0.2	2.8°	13
Belenger et al. (2011)	25	Sapphire	2	1.8	NA	35
Lee et al. (2003)	15	Quartz	Analogue	3.5 ± 0.2	4.9°	5.5
Buck and Kasper (2010)	24	HR Si	1	2.3	3°	NA
Chung et al. (2012)	2	Rogers 4350	Analogue	1.1 ± 0.6	NA	31 cm²
Pillans et al. (2012)	15	Alumina	4	1.7 ± 0.4	7°	NA
Pillans et al. (2012)	21	Alumina	4	1.8 ± 0.5	5.3°	NA

In Park *et al.* (2002), two designs of reflection-type phase shifters are presented. The first one is a 2-bit phase shifter (45°, 90° and 135°), and the second one a 3-bit phase shifter realized departing from the first one and by cascading another one of reflection-type providing an additional 180° phase shift, as shown in Fig. 5.13.

5.5 Distributed-line phase shifter

Distributed-line phase shifters are also called distributed MEMS transmission line (DMTL) phase shifters when used with RF MEMS switches. They have been the subject of special focus since 1998 (Barker and Rebeiz, 1998). Digital and analogue topologies are used, as in the previous types.

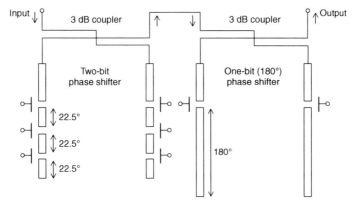

5.13 Diagram of the 3-bit reflection-type phase shifter from (Park et al., 2002). Two different Reflective-Type Phase Shifter (RTPS) are cascaded.

5.5.1 Theory

The concept of using distributed-line phase shifters with RF MEMS switches was first presented in Barker and Rebeiz (1998). The idea is to periodically load a transmission line with MEMS capacitive bridges that affect the impedance and propagation velocity of the line. This configuration often results in wideband performance and is a perfect example of a TTD phase shifter. Analytical equations have been developed in Barker and Rebeiz (1998) and Nagra and York (1999) resulting in a precise model of the phase shifter behaviour. Such modelling was then extended in Perruisseau-Carrier *et al.* (2006) and Topalli *et al.* (2006).

Figure 5.14 presents the CPW implementation of a DMTL phase shifter and its simplified equivalent circuit model (Rebeiz, 2003). Using shunt capacitive RF MEMS switches and CPW lines is the easiest approach to implement a DMTL phase shifter. The MEMS bridge is modelled as a shunt capacitor C_b, whereas L_t and C_t are the per unit inductance and capacitance of the unloaded line. If L_b and R_b are neglected, the series impedance and shunt admittance follow Equations [5.9], [5.10], [5.11] and [5.12]. This leads to an expression of the characteristic impedance of the loaded-line as shown in Equation [5.13], where ω_B is the Bragg frequency, that is, the frequency for which Z is equal to 0. Its expression is given in Equation [5.14]. Finally, if Z_{lu} and Z_{ld} are the up-state and down-state loaded-line impedance values and C_{lu} the up-state capacitance, the obtained phase shift is given by Equation [5.15]. The effective permittivity constant (ε_{eff}) appearing in Equation [5.15] means that the phase shift per length increases for larger permittivity, as well as do the losses. Hence, a silicon substrate will give a higher phase shift but also more losses than a

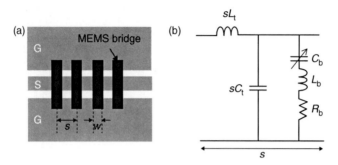

5.14 (a) CPW implementation and (b) circuit model of a DMTL phase shifter.

quartz substrate, for example. Equation [5.15] also shows that the phase shift highly depends on the capacitance ratio achievable by the MEMS switch.

$$Z_s = j\omega s L \qquad [5.9]$$

$$Y_p = j\omega(sC_t + C_b) \qquad [5.10]$$

$$L_t = C_t Z_0^2 \qquad [5.11]$$

$$C_t = \sqrt{\frac{\varepsilon_{eff}}{cZ_0}} \qquad [5.12]$$

$$Z = \sqrt{\frac{sL_t}{sC_t + C_b}}\sqrt{1 - \frac{\omega^2}{4}sL_t(sC_t + C_b)} = \sqrt{\frac{sL_t}{sC_t + C_b}}\sqrt{1 - \left(\frac{\omega}{\omega_B}\right)^2} \qquad [5.13]$$

$$\omega_B = \frac{2}{\sqrt{sL_t(sC_t + C_b)}} \qquad [5.14]$$

$$\Delta\phi = \omega\sqrt{L_t C_t}\left(\sqrt{1 + \frac{C_{lu}}{sC_t}} - \sqrt{1 + \frac{C_r C_{lu}}{sC_t}}\right) = \frac{\omega Z_0 \sqrt{\varepsilon_{eff}}}{c}\left(\frac{1}{Z_{ld}} - \frac{1}{Z_{lu}}\right) \qquad [5.15]$$

5.5.2 Analog and digital implementations

In the analog implementation, the analog control voltage varies the height of the bridge and thus the capacitive loading of the line. As for the previous analog DMTL phase shifters, the main drawback is the mechanical

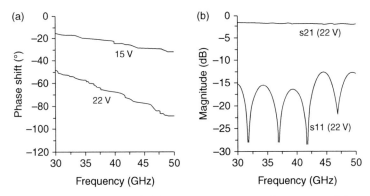

5.15 (a) Phase shift and (b) S-parameters versus frequency of the DMTL phase shifter for different applied voltages from Barker (1999).

instability of the MEMS bridge. It is also quite difficult to achieve a high capacitance tuning ratio with a single RF MEMS switch. A complete study is proposed in Barker and Rebeiz (1998) with several realizations depending on the width of the bridge, the distance between bridges, and the number of bridges. Figure 5.15 presents a typical performance for a DMTL phase shifter using 32 30-μm wide bridges spaced by 306 μm for a maximum phase shift requiring 22 V. It can be seen that for a fixed frequency the phase shift increases with the control voltage. As this is a TTD phase shifter, we can see that the phase shift also increases linearly with frequency. The insertion loss is quite low and the phase shifter is matched for the two extreme values of the control voltage.

A proposed solution in Hayden and Rebeiz (2000a) is to use a discrete capacitor (C_s) in series with the MEMS bridge to increase the total down-state capacitance (C_l) following Equation [5.16] and thereby obtain a larger capacitance ratio. However, in that case only two values (for up-state and down-state position) are used. The implementation is not analogue anymore but digital.

$$C_l = \frac{C_s C_b}{C_s + C_b} \qquad [5.16]$$

In Hayden and Rebeiz (2000b), the authors use a metal–insulator–metal (MIM) capacitance over a quartz substrate (quality factor: $Q = 14$). They are able to increase by a factor of 40–80 the down-state capacitance. MIM capacitors can be quite small (25×25 μm²), which is quite difficult to manufacture with a high quality factor for high frequencies. Figure 5.16 presents a cross-sectional view of the DMTL phase shifter with MIM capacitors as well as a circuit model for the MEMS bridge.

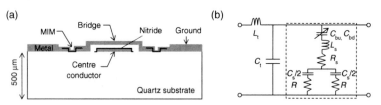

5.16 (a) Cross-sectional view and (b) circuit model of the MEMS bridge using MIM capacitors from Hayden and Rebeiz (2000b).

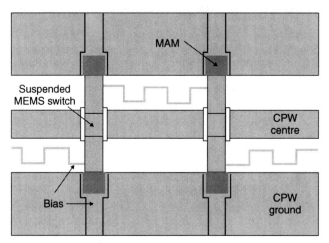

5.17 Diagram of two-units of the DMTL phase shifter from Hayden (2002).

In Hayden and Rebeiz (2003), the MIM capacitor is replaced by a metal–air–metal (MAM) capacitor. This is done to achieve even higher quality factor for the discrete capacitance ($Q = 250$) and thus a larger capacitance ratio. Moreover, MAM capacitors are larger than MIM capacitors (100 × 100 μm²), which is better for high-frequency integration. Figure 5.17 presents a picture of the realized DMTL phase shifter using MAM capacitors.

Table 5.7 presents the comparison between the two phase shifters presented in Hayden and Rebeiz (2000b, 2003). The DMTL phase shifter with MAM capacitors achieves a lower insertion loss (1.2 dB instead of 4 dB).

5.5.3 Comparison of distributed-line phase shifters

As for the switched-line, loaded-line and reflection-type phase shifters, we present here published results for distributed-line phase shifters (Tables 5.8 and 5.9). Table 5.8 presents a comparison of different digital DMTL phase shifters,

Table 5.7 Performance of DMTL phase shifters with MIM and MAM capacitors

Reference	Frequency (GHz)	Insertion loss (dB)	Phase shift	Size
Hayden and Rebeiz (2000b)	10	4 ± 2	270° by 90° steps ± 3°	21.7 mm
Hayden and Rebeiz (2003)	14	1.2 ± 0.4	270° by 90° steps ± 4°	NA

and Table 5.9 some analogue implementations. Compared to previous phase shifter architectures, an important factor is the number of bridges, which can define the size of the phase shifter. Thus, it is preferable to have a lower number of bridges for the same phase shift. This is the reason why some of the publications only give the longest dimension of the phase shifter. An important parameter for the analogue implementation is the FoM, which represents the phase shift achieved by dB of insertion loss. A larger number of references about this DMTL architecture can be found in the literature because its implementation with RF MEMS switches is the more appealing one.

In Hayden *et al.* (2001), a microstrip design is presented using open-ended stubs as in Pillans *et al.* (1999). Other line configurations are also presented in Kim *et al.* (2003a) and Van Caekenberghe and Vähä-Heikkilä (2008) using stripline design and slotline design respectively.

In Perruisseau-Carrier *et al.* (2006), a new way to achieve multi-bit operation while improving the matching properties of DMTL phase shifters is presented. Instead of cascading similar line sections of different lengths, the bridges of different capacitance values (corresponding to the different bits) are interlaced. This phase shifter is now called a variable TTD phase shifter.

5.6 Mixed-architectures and exotic phase shifters

Some phase shifters using RF MEMS are more complex and cannot be put clearly in the different categories described until now, so we present them here as mixed-architectures and exotic phase shifters.

5.6.1 Switched-loaded-line phase shifter

For a high number of bits, loaded-line phase shifters are preferred for the smaller phase shifts and switched-line phase shifters can be used for larger phase shifts. A few realizations using this technique have been found in the literature. They are reported in Table 5.10. Malmqvist *et al.* (2007) present a RF MEMS phase shifter for unmanned airborne vehicles (UAV) for communications as well as sensors. Figure 5.18 presents some conceptual

Table 5.8 Comparison between published digital-type DMTL phase shifters

Reference	Frequency (GHz)	Substrate	Bit number	Insertion loss (dB)	Max phase Error	Bridge number	Size
Du et al. (2010)	10	HR Si	5	1.54	10.66°	NA	51 mm²
Hayden et al. (2001)	18	Si	4	3	8.5°	29	NA
Kim et al. (2002)	65	Quartz	4	2.8 ± 0.8	8.3°	30	12 mm²
Liu et al. (2000)	26	Glass	3	1.7 ± 0.9	8.5°	NA	NA
Hung et al. (2004)	78	Glass	3	2.7 ± 0.5	3°	28	10 mm²
Topalli et al. (2008)	15	Glass	3	1.5 ± 0.5	2.6°	28	24 mm²
Hayden and Rebeiz (2000b)	10	Quartz	2	NA	3°	24	22 mm long
Hayden et al. (2001)	16	Si	2	2.8	8°	23	NA
Hayden and Rebeiz (2003)	14	Quartz	2	1.2 ± 0.4	4°	NA	NA
Hayden and Rebeiz (2003)	37	Quartz	2	1.5 ± 0.6	1°	21	18 mm²
Hung et al. (2004)	81	Glass	2	2.2 ± 0.3	2°	24	8 mm²
Kim et al. (2002)	60	Quartz	2	2.2 ± 0.7	15.2°	24	9 mm²
Pillans et al. (2012)	30	Alumina	4	2.4 ± 0.5	3.3°	NA	NA
Pillans et al. (2012)	35	Alumina	4	2.7 ± 0.8	6.7°	NA	NA

Table 5.9 Comparison between published analogue type DMTL phase shifters

Reference	Frequency (GHz)	Substrate	Insertion loss (dB)	Max phase shift	FoM	Bridge number	Size (mm)
Barker and Rebeiz (1998)	40	Quartz	1.8	84°	47°/dB	32	5.2
Barker and Rebeiz (1998)	40	Quartz	1.7	82°	48°/dB	16	NA
Barker and Rebeiz (1998)	40	Quartz	1.57	62°	39°/dB	32	NA
Nagra and York (1999)	20	GaAs	4.2	360°	85°/dB	15	NA
Lakshminarayanan and Weller (2002)	35	HR Si	2.4 ± 0.6	393°	242°/dB	11	8
Kim et al. (2003a)	60	Quartz	2.95	178°	74°/dB	19	4.5
McFeetors and Okoniewski (2006)	40	Quartz	1.8	NA	170°/dB	NA	5.3
Van Caekenberghe and Vähä-Heikkilä (2008)	10	Glass	4 ± 0.6	128.5°	28.2°/dB	NA	NA

Table 5.10 Comparison between published switched-loaded-line phase shifters

Reference	Frequency (GHz)	Substrate	Bit Nb	Insertion loss (dB)	Max phase error	Size (mm²)
Nordquist et al. (2008)	18	Alumina	6	1.9 ± 0.8	5°	70
Farinelli et al. (2009)	20	HR Si	5	1.3	2.4°	36
Farinelli et al. (2009)	20	HR Si	5	0.7	3.01°	21
Farinelli et al. (2009)	20	HR Si	5	0.7	8.63°	29
Malmqvist et al. (2007)	35	Quartz	4	2 ± 1	NA	55
Siegel et al. (2007)	34	Si	3	2.2 ± 1	13.25°	40
Stehle et al. (2008)	77	Si	3	5.3 ± 0.5	13.4°	7
Malmqvist et al., (2010a,b)	35	GaAs	3	4.3 ± 1.5	NA	8

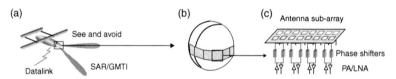

5.18 (a) Conceptual drawing of a small UAV. (b) Picture of a Ku-band conformal array antenna. (c) Sub-system architecture using MEMS phase shifters for the multifunctional radar system from Malmqvist et al. (2010b).

drawings for this application, as well as the system architecture of such a radar system. MEMS phase shifters are used in each sub-array at the edge of the UAV for communications or sense-and-avoid capabilities.

5.6.2 Dielectric phase shifter

Somjit *et al.* (2009) present a novel concept of ultra-broadband digital-type multistage binary-coded microwave MEMS phase shifters based on tuning

Table 5.11 Comparison between 7-stage dielectric-block phase shifters

Phase shifters	(a) Linear-coded 7 × 45°	(b) Binary-coded 15° + 30° + 5 × 45°	(c) Non-equidistant linear-coded 7 × 45°
Stage number	7	7	7
Distance between each stage (L_1-L_6)	10 µm	10 µm	$L_{n+1} = 10 \times 2^n$ µm, where $n = [0\text{–}5]$
Phase resolution	45°	15°	45°
Max. phase shift	315°	270°	315°
Size (length)	5.4 mm	5.5 mm	6 mm
Insertion loss*	4.2 dB	3.5 dB	5.1 dB
Return loss*	19 dB	20 dB	26 dB

*Average value at 75 GHz.
Source: Somjit (2012).

the loading of a three-dimensional (3-D) micromachined transmission line by a dielectric block placed on top of the line and moved by MEMS actuators. The performance of this phase shifter is reported in Table 5.5, as it can be considered as well as a loaded-line or distributed-line phase shifter. The working principle of a single stage phase shifter is reported in Somjit *et al.* (2009). Only one MEMS bridge is used for each single stage. Using this principle, three different single bit stages (45°, 30° and 15°) are realized. With these stages more than four bits can be achieved with 270° phase shift by 15° steps. This is another improvement. By using the same number of seven bridges, a higher resolution can be achieved by using these three stages than by using 7 45° stages. The comparison between these two implementations and the last version of Somjit (2012) is given in Table 5.11. Figure 5.19 presents pictures of the three implementations. The second achieves a better insertion loss (3.5 dB) with almost the same length of the phase shifter, whereas the third improves on the return loss (from 19 to 26 dB). The study of these phase shifters is completed in Somjit (2012), which presents their non-linearity analysis, intermodulation products, thermal behaviour and reliability. These aspects are discussed in the following section, which addresses manufacturing issues.

5.6.3 Switched-line phase shifter with rotary switches

Pranonsatit *et al.* (2011) showed the first circuit with original rotary single pole 8 throw (SP8T) RF MEMS switches. The switched-line phase shifter realized (Fig. 5.20) is composed by two SP8T switches connected by four different length lines (SP4T mode). The insertion loss is 3.4 ± 1.7 dB at 2 GHz. The return loss is less than −12 dB at the same frequency. The worst case phase error is 3.4°.

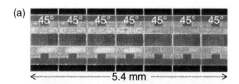

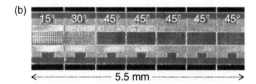

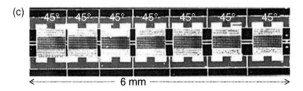

5.19 Microscope pictures of the fabricated seven-stage phase shifters from Somjit (2012): (a) linear-coded 7 × 45°, (b) binary-coded 15° + 30° + 5 × 45° and (c) non-equidistant linear-coded 7 × 45°.

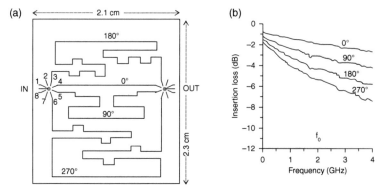

5.20 (a) Microphotograph and (b) performance of the switched-line phase shifter from Pranonsatit *et al.* (2011). The insertion loss for the different phase shifts is represented versus frequency.

5.6.4 Original slow-wave structure phase shifter

Lakshminarayanan and Weller (2006) introduce an original slow-wave transmission line concept applied to the RF MEMS distributed-line phase shifter. The realized phase shifter uses cascaded, switchable slow-wave CPW sections to achieve a large phase shift per unit length. Also, MAM capacitors

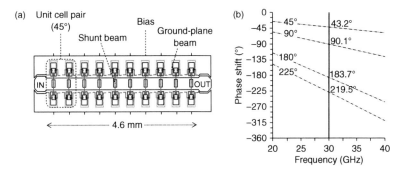

5.21 (a) Schematic and (b) measurements compared to simulation of the original slow-wave type phase shifter from Lakshminarayanan (2005).

are used to counteract the low capacitance ratio of MEMS bridges. At 30 GHz, the 4-bit phase shifter (Fig. 5.21) exhibits high return loss in both states ($S_{11} < -35\text{dB}$), low insertion loss ($S_{21} = -0.8$ dB $\pm$ 0.2 dB) and good phase error (<5.5°). This is better than previously reported DMTL phase shifter performance. Design equations are developed in Lakshminarayanan and Weller (2007).

Bakri-Kassem *et al.* (2011) shows another slow-wave structure for the RF MEMS distributed-line phase shifter as well. The ingenious principle is:

- Up-state: the switches have no effect (slow-wave mode).
- Down-state: the switches are used to shorten the series resonator (regular co-planner waveguide mode).

The V-band phase shifter designed using this technique presents a good return loss of 20 dB and a worst insertion loss of 3.21 dB at 60 GHz. The actuation voltage is 45 V. The area of the circuit is 3.8×1.5 mm². The phase shift between the two extreme cases is 126° at 60 GHz, which corresponds to 6.3° per bit.

5.7 Towards global manufacturing

This section will discuss some issues encountered when dealing with RF MEMS phase shifters for the global consumer market.

5.7.1 Linearity and intermodulation studies

Even though RF MEMS phase shifters are considered as passive components, there is a voltage controlling the actuation of the RF MEMS switch.

When the switch is actuated a non-linearity occurs depending on the stiffness of the MEMS moving parts. Thus, the phase shift depends on the input power level and an amplitude modulation (power modulation) will result in a phase modulation if the modulation frequency is below the mechanical response frequency of the device. This study in the case of the phase shifter is presented in Somjit *et al.* (2009). In order to quantify this problem, third intermodulation level and intercept point of third order (IIP3) can be defined and computed for different input powers, as is done in Somjit *et al.* (2009), Van Caekenberghe and Vähä-Heikkilä (2008) and Maury *et al.* (2009). More details can be found in Somjit *et al.* (2011).

5.7.2 Thermal study

The thermal study can be related to the power study, as the temperature rises with power. It can also be directly related to the packaging issue that will be discussed later. The limiting component for the metallic RF MEMS switch is the bridge. Such bridges are the power-limiting bottleneck of these phase shifters, since the thermal conductivity of thin suspended metal bridges to the substrate heat sink is relatively small. This limits the current handling capability of the bridges and thus of the whole phase shifter. The thermal study of the phase shifter in Somjit *et al.* (2009) is thoroughly developed in Somjit *et al.* (2011).

5.7.3 Packaging issues

As for RF MEMS switches, one of the big issues is the problem of reliability and packaging. MEMS are quite sensitive to the environment and will fail in the long term if they are not protected. One option is to use a packaged RF MEMS and to design the phase shifter architecture outside the package, but this would result in a larger footprint for the phase shifter. The choice of the package technique is also an issue between a cap and a package fabricated in the same process as the MEMS. Several phase shifters presented before are packaged phase shifters, especially in the most recent papers (Morton and Papapolymerou, 2008; Kingsley and Papapolymerou, 2006; Chen *et al.*, 2008; Chung *et al.*, 2012; Pillans *et al.*, 2012). An interesting comparison between unpackaged and packaged phase shifters is presented in Kingsley and Papapolymerou (2006). Figure 5.22 presents the phase shifter implementation and the side view of the package. The chosen phase shifter is switched type. Not all of the phase shifter was packaged. Only the MEMS switches are protected and placed into a laser drilled cavity. Here the package substrate and superstrate are made of liquid crystal polymer (LCP) material, which has very interesting electrical, thermal and mechanical properties at

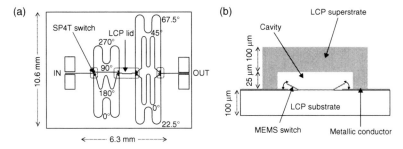

5.22 (a) Implementation of the switched-line phase shifter and (b) side view of the package from Kingsley (2007).

high frequencies. The performance of the realized phase shifter shows that packaging MEMS switches in LCP have a negligible effect. Indeed, the 4-bit phase shifter insertion loss and return loss are about constant (0.01-dB S_{21} and 1.6-dB S_{11} variations). We can note an average phase variation of 3.2°.

5.8 Applications

5.8.1 Phased array

As the targeted application for a RF MEMS phase shifter concerns phased arrays (Van Caekenberghe, 2003), its co-integration with an antenna array has to be studied, as well as its influence on the radiation pattern. Several realizations are reported in the literature (Gautier *et al.*, 2008; Topalli *et al.*, 2008; Lee *et al.*, 2006; Sundaram *et al.*, 2008; Rock *et al.*, 2010; Adane *et al.*, 2011). In Gautier *et al.* (2008), Sundaram *et al.* (2008) and Rock *et al.* (2010), the RF MEMS phase shifters are implemented on a different substrate from the antenna elements, resulting in a hybrid integration. Figure 5.23 presents the phased array from Gautier *et al.* (2008), where the phase shifters are integrated, along with the antenna array, in cavities and protected by a glass cover. Figure 5.23(b) shows the measured radiation pattern for three different phase shifts.

5.8.2 Example of design

In this sub-section, we propose a state-of-the-art RF MEMS phase shifter for future phased array satellite and radio-astronomy applications in the new 81–86 GHz band. At these millimetre wave frequencies, phase shifter design is a considerable challenge. In comparison to the standard active phase shifters used, RF MEMS technology promises to achieve THz frequencies for low-power applications with excellent RF performance.

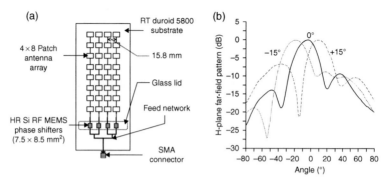

5.23 (a) X-band RF MEMS phased array from Gautier (2010). (b) Measured radiation patterns for three different phase shifts.

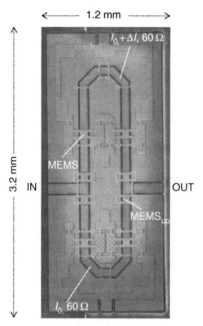

5.24 Scanning electron microscope (SEM) picture of the Laboratoire d'Analyse et d'Architecture des Systèmes (Laboratory) (LAAS) W-band switched-line phase shifter realized.

The W-band 1-bit switched-line phase shifter designed (Fig. 5.24) is based on an original SPDT switch. The phase shift $\Delta\Phi$ results from the electrical length difference between the top and bottom lines (i.e. Δl). As shown in the microphotograph, the circuit is composed of four standard RF MEMS and four up-state blocked RF MEMS ($MEMS_{up}$). The RF MEMS used are coplanar capacitive shunt switches. The fabrication technology and the model of the MEMS RF component are described with more detail in (Puyal *et al.*, 2009). The original SPDT structure that we use takes advantage of the OFF-state switch (MEMS$_{down}$) capacitance to realize a semi-distributed quarter wave line. This provides a transformation from the closed switch short circuit to an open circuit at the input.

The impedance inverter is constituted of a short high characteristic impedance line. This impedance acts as a semi-distributed inductance surrounded by two MEMS capacitors which satisfy these two equations (Dubuc *et al.*, 2003):

$$Z = Z_0 / \sin\theta \qquad [5.17]$$

$$\omega C_{MEMSup} = (1/Z_0) \cos\theta \qquad [5.18]$$

In these expressions, Z_0 is the characteristic impedance of the quarter-wavelength line, Z is the characteristic impedance of the shortened line, θ is the electrical angle of the shortened line and ω is the angular frequency. Under these conditions, a 60 Ω characteristic impedance for line (*l*) has been adopted.

A 1-bit switched-line phase shifter with a phase shift of 225° has been designed. The measurement results of this phase shifter show a low insertion loss (see S21 in Fig. 5.25): 2.3 dB (l_0) and 3.5 dB ($l_0 + \Delta l$) at 83.5 GHz. It is between 2.1 dB and 4.3 dB in the entire 81–86 GHz band. The return loss level (see S11 in Fig. 5.25) is around 20 dB for the two phase states at 83.5 GHz (19.4 dB for l_0 way and 20.2 for $l_0 + \Delta l$ way). Also, the figure shows the

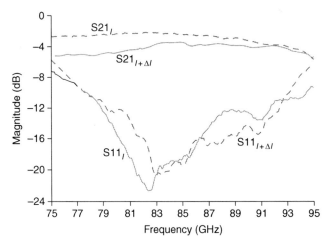

5.25 Insertion loss (S21) and return loss (S11) of the phase shifter for $\Delta\Phi = 0°$ (l_0) and $\Delta\Phi = 225°$ ($l_0 + \Delta l$) from 75 to 95 GHz.

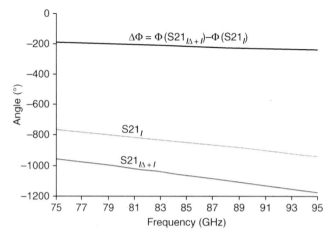

5.26 Phase shift ($\Delta\Phi$) of the phase shifter from 75 to 95 GHz.

broad band performance of the circuit (S11 less than -10dB from 77.7 GHz up to 92.9 GHz). In the useful band, the phase error is 12° (5%) at 60 GHz, 20° (9%) at 81 GHz and 5° (2%) for 86 GHz (Fig. 5.26).

Compared to other W-band RF MEMS phase shifters (Table 5.12), this phase shifter presents a good FoM of 76.8°/dB ± 15.8°/dB for a high resistivity silicon substrate based architecture at these high frequencies.

5.9 Conclusion

Within this chapter, a global overview of various RF MEMS phase shifter architectures has been shown. In Table 5.13, we summarize the different properties of each topology to help the reader in choosing the best option for a given application. To begin, the easiest design is a switched-line phase shifter with ohmic series switches, whereas it is more complex to design a DMTL phase shifter. If you want a large phase shift, the switched-line or the distributed-line are good choices. For compact designs, it is more appropriate to use loaded-line or reflection-line phase shifters. One of the key parameters for a phase shifter is the amplitude variation between the different phase states (S_{21} mismatching), which must be minimized, to assure a good coherent radiation pattern. In this case, the distributed-line topology is the best. For reliability issues, the loaded-line or reflection-line is more interesting because of the small number of switches used. For high frequencies, no universal rule exists: all topologies can be used; as for the switch element, the capacitive shunt MEMS switches often result in excellent performance. Finally, you can combine different types of phase shifters to trade off different properties and obtain a balanced performance.

Table 5.12 Comparison between W-band phase shifters

Reference	Frequency (GHz)	Type	Substrate	Bit number	Insertion loss (dB)	Max phase error	FoM	Size
Buck and Kasper (2010)	77	Switched-line	HR Si	1	3	1.5°	30.5°/dB	NA
Somjit et al. (2009)	75	Loaded-line	HR Si	4.25	3.5	6°	71.1°/dB	5.5 mm long
Somjit et al. (2009)	75	Loaded-line	HR Si	3	4.5	NA	74°/dB	5.4 mm long
Fritzsch et al. (2011)	76	Loaded-line	Quartz	Analogue	2.4 ± 0.1	2°	42°/dB	NA
Hung et al. (2004)	78	DMTL	Glass	3	2.7 ± 0.5	3°	96°/dB	10 mm^2
Hung et al. (2004)	81	DMTL	Glass	2	2.2 ± 0.3	2°	106°/dB	8 mm^2
Stehle et al. (2008)	77	Switched-loaded-line	Si	3	5.3 ± 0.5	13.4°	27.6°/dB	7 mm^2
This work	83.5	Switched-line	HR Si	1	2.9 ± 0.6	12°	76.8°/dB ± 15.8°/dB	NA

Table 5.13 RF MEMS phase shifter summary

Type	Switched-line	Loaded-line	Reflection-type	Distributed-line
Easy design	+++	++	+	+
Max. phase shift	+++	+	++	+++
Phase error	+++	++	+	+++
Insertion loss	++	++	+	+++
Amplitude variation	+	++	++	+++
Bandwidth	++	+	+	+++
Size	+	+++	+++	++
Reliability	++	+++	+++	+

Most of the recent research works described in the literature tries to demonstrate the advantage or the need to integrate RF MEMS on the phased array systems at high frequencies. Indeed, all state-of-the-art RF MEMS phase shifter found in recent publications present excellent RF performance (low insertion loss, high linearity, high quality factor, etc.) with no DC power consumption. However, a certain gap persists with the industry trust. Indeed, for the time being, existing market applications for RF MEMS are not widespread: only few RF MEMS small industrial foundries are present, such as WiSpry, Omron and Radant. Why this misgiving? Is it objective?

Yes and no. Because, despite the current advances, it is true that some key issues have still to be solved, such as reliability and actuation voltage. From the author's point of view, three main applications of RF MEMS phase shifters on phased array systems are:

- Power applications (satellite, spatial, military, etc.) where the main objective is to substitute the GaAs MMIC phase shifter to reduce the power consumption and the size of the system.
- Consumer applications (mobile, localization, automotive, etc.) for use in the active Si phase shifter for low-power and low-cost RF applications.
- Terahertz applications (imaging, high data rate link, etc.) to enable new millimetre wave applications.

To conclude, we present, as a paradigmatic example, in Fig. 5.27 a recent work using the Innovation for High Performance microelectronics (Laboratory) (IHP) CMOS-MEMS technology (Kaynak *et al.*, 2010) for applications in V-band switched-line phase shifters. A V-band single pole 3 throw (SP3T) has been designed and measured in that work and it shows the type of performance than can be expected from optimized MEMS-based phase shifters. It presents a 4 dB insertion loss and a 17 dB isolation at 65 GHz. This is an excellent example, because this type of technology will allow a perfect integration with the transceiver chip for future phased arrays.

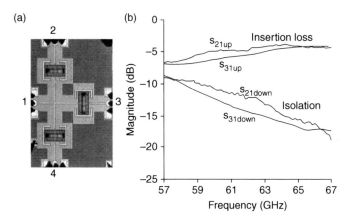

5.27 (a) SP3T V-band switch realized with IHP CMOS-MEMS technology and (b) its performance.

5.10 References

Adane, A., Gallee, F., Person, C., Puyal, V., Villeneuve, C., and Dragomirescu, D. (2011) 'Implementation of broadband microstrip-U coupled patch array on Si/BCB membrane for beamforming applications at 60 GHz', *Antennas and Propagation (EUCAP), Proceedings of the 5th European Conference on*, pp. 1263–1267.

Al-Dahleh, R. and Mansour, R.R. (2008) 'A novel via-less vertical integration method for MEMS scanned phased array modules', *Microwave Conference, 2008, EuMC 2008, 38th European*, pp. 96–99.

Atwater, H.A. (1985) 'Circuit design of the loaded-line phase shifter', *Microwave Theory and Techniques, IEEE Transactions on*, vol. 33, no. 7, pp. 626–634.

Bakri-Kassem, M., Mansour, R., and Safavi-Naeini, S. (2011) 'Novel millimeter-wave slow-wave phase shifter using MEMS technology', *Microwave Conference (EuMC), 2011 41st European*, pp. 1079–1082.

Barker, N.S. (1999) 'Distributed MEMS transmission lines', PhD thesis, University of Michigan, pp. 49–78.

Barker, N.S. and Rebeiz, G.M. (1998) 'Distributed MEMS true-time delay phase shifters and wide-band switches', *Microwave Theory and Techniques, IEEE Transactions on*, vol. 46, no. 11, pp. 1881–1890.

Belenger, B., Espana, B., Courreges, S., Blondy, P., Vendier, O., Langrez, D., and Cazaux, J.-L. (2011) 'A high-power Ka-band RF-MEMS 2-bit phase shifter on Sapphire substrate', *Microwave Integrated Circuits Conference (EuMIC), 2011 European*, pp. 164–167.

Biglarbegian, B., Bakri-Kassem, M., Mansour, R., and Safavi-Naeini, S. (2010) 'MEMS-based reflective-type phase-shifter for emerging millimeter-wave communication systems', *Microwave Conference (EuMC), 2010 European*, pp. 1556–1559.

Buck, T. and Kasper, E. (2010) 'RF MEMS phase shifters for 24 and 77 GHz on high resistivity silicon', *Silicon Monolithic Integrated Circuits in RF Systems (SiRF), 2010 Topical Meeting on*, pp. 224–227.

Byung-Wook, M. and Rebeiz, G. M. (2007) 'Ka-Band BiCMOS 4-bit phase shifter with integrated LNA for phased array T/R modules', *Microwave Symposium, IEEE/MTT-S International*, pp. 479–482.

Chen, M.J., Pham, A.-V., Evers, N., Kapusta, C., Iannotti, J., Kornrumpf, W., and Maciel, J. (2008) 'Multilayer organic multichip module implementing hybrid microelectromechanical systems', *Microwave Theory and Techniques, IEEE Transactions on*, vol. 56, no. 4, pp. 952–958.

Chung, D.J., Polcawich, R.G., Pulskamp, J.S., and Papapolymerou, J. (2012) 'Reduced-size low-voltage RF MEMS X-band phase shifter integrated on multilayer organic package', *IEEE Transactions on Components, Packaging and Manufacturing Technology*, vol. 2, no. 10, pp. 1617–1622.

Davis, W.A. (1974) 'Design equations and bandwidth of loaded-line phase shifters', *Microwave Theory and Techniques, IEEE Transactions on*, vol. 22, no. 5, pp. 561–563.

Du, Y., Bao, J., and Zhao, X. (2010) '5-bit MEMS distributed phase shifter', *Electronics Letters*, vol. 46, no. 21, pp. 1452–1453.

Dubuc, D., Rabbia, L., Grenier, K., Pons, P., Vendier, O., Graffeuil, J., and Plana, R. (2003) 'Original MEMS-based Single Pole Double Throw topology for millimeter wave space communications', *Microwave Conference, 2003, 33rd European*, vol. 3, pp. 979–982.

Farinelli, P., Chiuppesi, E., Di Maggio, F., Margesin, B., Colpo, S., Ocera, A., Russo, M., and Pomona, I. (2009) 'Development of different k-band MEMS phase shifter designs for satellite COTM terminals', *Microwave Conference, 2009. EuMC 2009. European*, pp. 1868–1871.

Fritzsch, C., Giacomozzi, F., Karabey, O.H., Goelden, F., Moessinger, A., Bildik, S., Colpo, S., and Jakoby, R. (2011) 'Continuously tunable W-band phase shifter based on liquid crystals and MEMS technology', *Microwave Conference (EuMC), 2011 41st European*, pp. 1083–1086.

Gautier, W. (2010) 'RF-MEMS based passive components and integration concepts for adaptive millimetre wave front-ends', PhD thesis, Ulm University, Germany, pp. 75–135.

Gautier, W., Stehle, A., Siegel, C., Schoenlinner, B., Ziegler, V., Prechtl, U., and Menzel, W. (2008) 'Hybrid integrated RF-MEMS phased array antenna at 10GHz', *Microwave Conference, 2008, EuMC 2008, 38th European*, pp. 139–142.

Gong, S., Hui Shen, H., and Barker, N.S. (2011) 'A 60-GHz 2-bit switched-line phase shifter using SP4T RF-MEMS switches', *Microwave Theory and Techniques, IEEE Transactions on*, vol. 59, no. 4, pp. 894–900.

Hacker, J.B., Mihailovich, R.E., Kim, M., and DeNatale, J.F. (2003) 'A Ka-band 3-bit RF MEMS true-time-delay network', *Microwave Theory and Techniques, IEEE Transactions on*, vol. 51, no. 1, pp. 305–308.

Hayden, J.S. (2002) 'High-performance digital X-band and Ka-band distributed MEMS phase shifters', PhD thesis, University of Michigan, pp. 66–99.

Hayden, J.S. and Rebeiz, G.M. (2000a) 'Low-loss cascadable MEMS distributed X-band phase shifters', *Microwave and Guided Wave Letters, IEEE*, vol. 10, no. 4, pp. 142–144.

Hayden, J.S. and Rebeiz, G.M. (2000b) '2-bit MEMS distributed X-band phase shifters', *Microwave and Guided Wave Letters, IEEE*, vol. 10, no. 12, pp. 540–542.

Hayden, J.S. and Rebeiz, G.M. (2003) 'Very low-loss distributed X-band and Ka-band MEMS phase shifters using metal-air-metal capacitors', *Microwave Theory and Techniques, IEEE Transactions on*, vol. 51, no. 1, pp. 309–314.

Hayden, J.S., Malczewski, A., Kleber, J., Goldsmith, C.L., and Rebeiz, G.M. (2001) '2 and 4-bit DC-18 GHz microstrip MEMS distributed phase shifters', *Microwave Symposium Digest, 2001 IEEE MTT-S International*, vol. 1, pp. 219–222.

Hong-Teuk, K., Jae-Hyoung, P., Sanghyo, L., Seongho, K., Jung-Mu, K., Yong-Kweon, K., and Youngwoo, K. (2004) 'V-band 2-b and 4-b low-loss and low-voltage distributed MEMS digital phase shifter using metal-air-metal capacitors', *IEEE Transactions on Microwave Theory and Techniques*, vol. 52, no. 2, pp. 600–606.

Hung, J.-J., Dussopt, L., and Rebeiz, G.M. (2004) 'Distributed 2- and 3-bit W-band MEMS phase shifters on glass substrates', *Microwave Theory and Techniques, IEEE Transactions on*, vol. 52, no. 2, pp. 600–606.

Jian, Z., Wei, Y.-Y., Chen, C., Yong, Z., and Le, L. (2006) 'A compact 5-bit switched-line digital MEMS phase shifter', *Nano/Micro Engineered and Molecular Systems, 2006. NEMS '06. 1st IEEE International Conference on*, pp. 623–626.

Kaynak, M., Ehwald, K.E., Scholz, R., Korndorfer, F., Wipf, C., Sun, Y.M., Tillack, B., Zihir, S., and Gurbuz, Y. (2010) 'Characterization of an embedded RF-MEMS switch', *Silicon Monolithic Integrated Circuits in RF Systems (SiRF), 2010 Topical Meeting on*, pp. 144–147.

Kim H.-T., Park, J.-H., Yim, J., Kim, Y.-K., and Kwon, Y. (2002a) 'A compact V-band 2-bit reflection-type MEMS phase shifter', *Microwave and Wireless Components Letters, IEEE*, vol. 12, no. 9, pp. 324–326.

Kim, H.-T., Park, J.-H., Lee, S., Kim, S., Kim, J.-M., Kim, Y.-K., and Youngwoo Kwon (2002b) 'V-band 2-b and 4-b low-loss and low-voltage distributed MEMS digital phase shifter using metal-air-metal capacitors', *Microwave Theory and Techniques, IEEE Transactions on*, vol. 50, no. 12, pp. 2918–2923.

Kim, H.-T., Lee, S., Kim, J., Park, J.-H., Kim, Y.-K., and Kwon, Y. (2003a) 'A V-band CPS distributed analog MEMS phase shifter', *Microwave Symposium Digest, 2003 IEEE MTT-S International*, vol. 3, pp. 1481–1484.

Kim, J.-M., Lee, S., Park, J.-H., Baek, C.-W., Kwon, Y., and Kim, Y.-K. (2003b) 'A 5–17 GHz wideband reflection-type phase shifter using digitally operated capacitive MEMS switches', *Transducers, Solid-State Sensors, Actuators and Microsystems, 2003, 12th International Conference on*, vol. 1, pp. 907–910.

Kim, M., Hacker, J.B., Mihailovich, R.E., and DeNatale, J.F. (2001) 'A DC-to-40 GHz four-bit RF MEMS true-time delay network', *Microwave and Wireless Components Letters, IEEE*, vol. 11, no. 2, pp. 56–58.

Kingsley, N. (2007) 'High development of miniature, multilayer, integrated, reconfigurable RF MEMS communication module on liquid crystal polymer (LCP) substrate', PhD thesis, Georgia Institute of Technology, pp. 66–120.

Kingsley, N. and Papapolymerou, J. (2006) 'Organic "wafer-scale" packaged miniature 4-bit RF MEMS phase shifter', *Microwave Theory and Techniques, IEEE Transactions on*, vol. 54, no. 3, pp. 1229–1236.

Kingsley, N., Wang, G., and Papapolymerou, J. (2005) '14 GHz microstrip MEMS phase shifters on flexible, organic substrate', *Microwave Conference, 2005 European*, vol. 1.

Ko, Y.J., Park, J.Y., Kim, H.T., and Bu, J.U. (2003a) 'Integrated five-bit RF MEMS phase shifter for satellite broadcasting/communication systems', *Micro Electro Mechanical Systems, 2003. MEMS-03 Kyoto. IEEE The Sixteenth Annual International Conference on*, pp. 144–148.

Ko, Y.J., Park, J.Y., and Bu, J.U. (2003b) 'Integrated RF MEMS phase shifters with constant phase shift', *Microwave Symposium Digest, 2003 IEEE MTT-S International*, vol. 3, pp. 1489–1492.

Kwang-Jin, K. and Rebeiz, G.M., (2007) '0.13-μm CMOS phase shifters for X-, Ku-, and K-band phased arrays', *IEEE Journal of Solid State Circuits*, vol. **4**, pp. 2535–2546.

Lakshminarayanan, B. (2005) 'Low loss rf/mm-wave mems phase shifters', PhD thesis, University of South Florida, pp. 34–68.

Lakshminarayanan, B. and Weller, T. (2002) 'Distributed MEMS phase shifters on silicon using tapered impedance unit cells', *Microwave Symposium Digest, 2002 IEEE MTT-S International*, vol. 2, pp. 1237–1240.

Lakshminarayanan, B. and Weller, T.M. (2006) 'Design and modeling of 4-bit slow-wave MEMS phase shifters', *Microwave Theory and Techniques, IEEE Transactions on*, vol. **54**, no. 1, pp. 120–127.

Lakshminarayanan, B. and Weller, T.M. (2007) 'Optimization and implementation of impedance-matched true-time-delay phase shifters on quartz substrate', *Microwave Theory and Techniques, IEEE Transactions on*, vol. **55**, no. 2, pp. 335–342.

Lampen, J., Majumder, S., Ji, C., and Maciel, J. (2010) 'Low-loss, MEMS based, broadband phase shifters', *Phased Array Systems and Technology (ARRAY), 2010 IEEE International Symposium on*, pp. 219–224.

Lee, S., Park, J.-H., Kim, H.-T., Kim, J.-M., Kim, Y.-K., and Kwon, Y. (2003) 'A 15-to-45 GHz low-loss analog reflection-type MEMS phase shifter', *Microwave Symposium Digest, 2003 IEEE MTT-S International*, vol. 3, pp. 1493–1496.

Lee, S., Kim, J.-M., Kim, J.-M., Kim, Y.-K., Cheon, C., and Kwon, Y. (2006) 'V-band single-platform beam steering transmitters using micromachining technology', *Microwave Symposium Digest, 2006. IEEE MTT-S International*, pp.148–151.

Liu, Y., Borgioli, A., Nagra, A.S., and York, R.A. (2000) 'K-band 3-bit low-loss distributed MEMS phase shifter', *Microwave and Guided Wave Letters, IEEE*, vol. **10**, no. 10, pp. 415–417.

Lucyszyn, S. (2010) *Advanced RF MEMS*, Cambridge University Press, pp. 307–337.

Malczewski, A., Eshelman, S., Pillans, B., Ehmke, J., and Goldsmith, C.L. (1999) 'X-band RF MEMS phase shifters for phased array applications', *Microwave and Guided Wave Letters, IEEE*, vol. **9**, no. 12, pp. 517–519.

Malmqvist, R., Samuelsson, C., Gustafsson, A., Boman, T., Bjorklund, S., Erickson, R., Vaha-Heikkila, T., and Rantakari, P. (2007) 'On the use of MEMS phase shifters in a low-cost Ka-band multifunctional ESA on a small UAV', *Microwave Conference, 2007. APMC 2007. Asia-Pacific*, pp. 1–4.

Malmqvist, R., Samuelsson, C., Simon, W., Rantakari, P., Smith, D., Lahdes, M., Lahti, M., Vähä-Heikkilä, T., Varis, J., and Baggen, R. (2010a) 'Design, packaging and reliability aspects of RF MEMS circuits fabricated using a GaAs MMIC foundry process technology', *Microwave Conference (EuMC), 2010 European*, pp. 85–88.

Malmqvist, R., Samuelsson, C., Carlegrim, B., Rantakari, P., Vaha-Heikkila, T., Rydberg, A., and Varis, J. (2010b) 'Ka-band RF MEMS phase shifters for energy starved millimetre-wave radar sensors', *Semiconductor Conference (CAS), 2010 International*, vol. 1, pp. 261–264.

Malmqvist, R., Samuelsson, C., Gustafsson, A., Smith, D., Vaha-Heikkila, T., and Baggen, R. (2011) 'Monolithic integration of millimeter-wave RF-MEMS switch circuits and LNAs using a GaAs MMIC foundry process technology', *Microwave Workshop Series on Millimeter Wave Integration Technologies (IMWS), 2011 IEEE MTT-S International*, pp. 148–151.

Maury, F., Pothier, A., Orlianges, J.C., Mardivirin, D., Reveyrand, T., Conseil, F., and Blondy, P. (2009) 'Ku band DMTL medium power phase shifters', *Microwave Symposium Digest, 2009. MTT '09. IEEE MTT-S International*, pp. 1153–1156.

McFeetors, G. and Okoniewski, M. (2006) 'Distributed MEMS analog phase shifter with enhanced tuning', *Microwave and Wireless Components Letters, IEEE*, vol. **16**, no. 1, pp. 34–36.

Morton, M.A. and Papapolymerou, J. (2008) 'A packaged MEMS-based 5-bit-band high-pass/low-pass phase shifter', *Microwave Theory and Techniques, IEEE Transactions on*, vol. **56**, no. 9, pp. 2025–2031.

Nagra, A.S. and York, R.A. (1999) 'Distributed analog phase shifters with low insertion loss', *Microwave Theory and Techniques, IEEE Transactions on*, vol. **47**, no. 9, pp. 1705–1711.

Nordquist, C.D., Dyck, W., Kraus, M., Reines, I.C., Goldsmith, L., Cowan, D., Plut, T.A., Austin, F., IV, Finnegan, P.S., Ballance, M.H., and Sullivan, T. (2006) 'A DC to 10-GHz 6-b RF MEMS time delay circuit', *Microwave and Wireless Components Letters, IEEE*, vol. **16**, no. 5, pp. 305–307.

Nordquist, C.D., Dyck, C.W., Kraus, G.M., Sullivan, C.T., Austin, F., Finnegan, P.S., and Ballance, M.H. (2008) 'Ku-band six-bit RF MEMS time delay network', *Compound Semiconductor Integrated Circuits Symposium, 2008. CSIC '08. IEEE*, pp. 1–4.

Opp, F.L. and Hoffman, W.F. (1968) 'Design of digital loaded-line phase-shift networks for microwave thin-film applications', *Microwave Theory and Techniques, IEEE Transactions on*, vol. **16**, no. 7, pp. 462–468.

Park, J.-H., Kim, H.-T., Choi, W., Kwon, Y., and Kim, Y.-K. (2002) 'V-band reflection-type phase shifters using micromachined CPW coupler and RF switches', *Microelectromechanical Systems, Journal of*, vol. **11**, no. 6, pp. 808–814.

Perruisseau-Carrier, J., Fritschi, R., Crespo-Valero, P., and Skrivervik, A.K. (2006) 'Modeling of periodic distributed MEMS-application to the design of variable true-time delay lines', *Microwave Theory and Techniques, IEEE Transactions on*, vol. **54**, no. 1, pp. 383–392.

Pillans, B., Eshelman, S., Malczewski, A., Ehmke, J., and Goldsmith, C. (1999) 'Ka-band RF MEMS phase shifters', *Microwave and Guided Wave Letters, IEEE*, vol. **9**, no. 12, pp. 520–522.

Pillans, B., Coryell, L., Malczewski, A., Moody, C., Morris, F., and Brown, A. (2012) 'Advances in RF MEMS phase shifters from 15 GHz to 35 GHz', *Microwave Symposium Digest (MTT), 2012 IEEE MTT-S International*, pp. 1–3.

Pranonsatit, S., Holmes, A.S., and Lucyszyn, S. (2011) 'Microwave modelling of radio frequency microelectromechanical rotary switches', *Microwaves, Antennas and Propagation, IET*, vol. **5**, no. 3, pp. 255–261.

Puyal, V., Dragomirescu, D., Villeneuve, C., Jinyu Ruan, Pons, P., and Plana, R. (2009) 'Frequency scalable model for MEMS capacitive shunt switches at millimeter-wave frequencies', *Microwave Theory and Techniques, IEEE Transactions on*, vol. **57**, no. 11, pp. 2824–2833.

Rebeiz, G.M. (2003) *RF MEMS: Theory, Design, and Technology*, Wiley, pp. 259–325.

Reinke, J., Wang, L., Fedder, G.K., and Mukherjee, T. (2011) 'A 4-bit RF MEMS phase shifter monolithically integrated with conventional CMOS', *Micro Electro Mechanical Systems (MEMS), 2011 IEEE 24th International Conference on*, pp. 748–751.

Rock, J.C., Hudson, T., Wolfson, B., Lawrence, D., Pillans, B., Brown, A.R., and Coryell, L. (2009a) 'A MEMS-based, Ka-band, 16-element sub-array', *Aerospace conference, 2009 IEEE*, pp. 1–11.

Rock, J.C., Hudson, T., Wolfson, B., Lawrence, D., Pillans, B., Brown, A.R., Coryell, L., and Milburn R. A., (2009b) 'Design, fabrication and evaluation of a MEMS-based, Ka-band, 16-element sub-array', *Technical Report RDMR-WD-09-24*.

Rock, J.C., Hudson, T., Wolfson, B., Lawrence, D., Pillans, B., Brown, A.R., and Coryell, L. (2010) 'Design, fabrication and evaluation of a MEMS-based, Ka-band, 16-element sub-array', *Aerospace Conference, 2010 IEEE*, pp.1–17.

Siegel, C., Zieglerl, V., Prechtel, U., Schonlinner, B., and Schumacher, H. (2007) 'A Ka-band RF-MEMS phase shifter approach based on a novel dual-state microstrip line', *Microwave Conference, 2007. European*, pp. 1221–1224.

Somjit, N. (2012) 'Novel RF MEMS devices for W-band beam-steering front-ends', *PhD thesis*, Royal Institute of Technology, Stockholm, Sweden, pp. 11–43.

Somjit, N., Stemme, G., and Oberhammer, J. (2009) 'Binary-coded 4.25-bit-band monocrystalline–silicon MEMS multistage dielectric-block phase shifters', *Microwave Theory and Techniques, IEEE Transactions on*, vol. **57**, no. 11, pp. 2834–2840.

Somjit, N., Stemme, G., and Oberhammer, J. (2011) 'Power handling analysis of high-power W-band all-silicon MEMS phase shifters', *Electron Devices, IEEE Transactions on*, vol. **58**, no. 5, pp. 1548–1555.

Stehle, A., Georgiev, G., Ziegler, V., Schoenlinner, B., Prechtel, U., Seidel, H., and Schmid, U. (2008) 'RF-MEMS switch and phase shifter optimized for W-band', *Microwave Conference, 2008. EuMC 2008. 38th European*, pp.104–107.

Sundaram, A., Maddela, M., Ramadoss, R., and Feldner, L.M. (2008) 'MEMS-based electronically steerable antenna array fabricated using PCB technology', *Microelectromechanical Systems, Journal of*, vol. **17**, no. 2, pp. 356–362.

Tan, G.L., Mihailovich, R.E., Hacker, J.B., DeNatale, J.F., and Rebeiz, G.M. (2002) 'A very-low-loss 2-bit X-band RF MEMS phase shifter', *Microwave Symposium Digest, 2002 IEEE MTT-S International*, vol. 1, pp. 333–335.

Tan, G.L., Mihailovich, R.E., Hacker, J.B., DeNatale, J.F., and Rebeiz, G.M. (2003a) 'Low-loss 2- and 4-bit TTD MEMS phase shifters based on SP4T switches', *Microwave Theory and Techniques, IEEE Transactions on*, vol. **51**, no. 1, pp. 297–304.

Tan, G.L., Mihailovich, R.E., Hacker, J.B., DeNatale, J.F., and Rebeiz, G.M. (2003b) 'A 2-bit miniature X-band MEMS phase shifter', *Microwave and Wireless Components Letters, IEEE*, vol. **13**, no. 4, pp. 146–148.

Tan, G.L., Mihailovich, R.E., Hacker, J.B., DeNatale, J.F., and Rebeiz, G.M. (2003c) 'A 4-bit miniature X-band MEMS phase shifter using switched-LC networks', *Microwave Symposium Digest, 2003 IEEE MTT-S International*, vol. 3, pp. 1477–1480.

Topalli, K., Unlu, M., Demir, S., Civi, O.A., Koc, S., and Akin, T. (2006) 'New approach for modelling distributed MEMS transmission lines', *Microwaves, Antennas and Propagation, IEE Proceedings -*, vol. **153**, no. 2, pp. 152–162.

Topalli, K., Civi, O.A., Demir, S., Koc, S., and Akin, T. (2008) 'A monolithic phased array using 3-bit distributed RF MEMS phase shifters', *Microwave Theory and Techniques, IEEE Transactions on*, vol. **56**, no. 2, pp. 270–277.

Van Caekenberghe, K., (2003) 'RF MEMS on the radar', *IEEE Microwave Magazine*, Oct. 2009.

Van Caekenberghe, K. and Vaha-Heikkila, T. (2008) 'An analog RF MEMS slotline true-time-delay phase shifter', *Microwave Theory and Techniques, IEEE Transactions on*, vol. **56**, no. 9, pp. 2151–2159.

Varian, K. and Walton, D. (2002) 'A 2-bit RF MEMS phase shifter in a thick-film BGA ceramic package', *Microwave and Wireless Components Letters, IEEE*, vol. **12**, no. 9, pp. 321–323.

Wu, J.-C., Chin, T.-Y., Chang, S.-F., and Chang, C.-C. (2008) '2.45-GHz CMOS reflection-type phase-shifter MMICs with minimal loss variation over quadrants of phase-shift range', *IEEE Transactions on Microwave Theory and Techniques*, vol. **56**, no. 10, pp. 2180–2189.

Yamane, D. and Toshiyoshi, H. (2011) 'Monolithic integration of passive RF components by MEMS', *VLSI Design, Automation and Test (VLSI-DAT), 2011 International Symposium on*, pp. 1–4.

Yamane, D., Yamamoto, T., Urayama, K., Yamashita, K., Toshiyoshi, H., and Kawasaki, S. (2008) 'A phase shifter by LTCC substrate with an RF-MEMS switch', *Microwave Conference, 2008. EuMC 2008. 38th European*, pp. 611–613.

Yu, Y., Baltus, P., van Roermund, A., Jeurissen, D., de Graauw, A., van der Heijden, E., and Pijper, R., (2008) 'A 60 GHz digitally controlled phase shifter in CMOS', *ESSCIRC 2008*, pp. 250–253.

Zhang, H., Laws, A., Gupta, K.C., Lee, Y.C., and Bright, V.M. (2003) 'MEMS variable-capacitor phase shifters part I: Loaded-line phase shifter', *Int J RF and Microwave Comp Aid Eng*, vol. **13**, pp. 321–337.

6
RF MEMS antennas for wireless applications

D. RODRIGO, L. JOFRE and J. ROMEU,
Universitat Politècnica de Catalunya, Spain

DOI: 10.1533/9780857098610.1.176

Abstract: Radio frequency microelectromechanical systems (RF MEMS) is an enabling technology for a new generation of intelligent antennas capable of dynamically self-adapting their properties and providing an improved performance. This chapter analyses the different reconfiguration techniques, covering external approaches based on tunable feeding networks, and internal approaches which modify the antenna radiation mechanism. The chapter also describes the main applications of RF MEMS antennas, technological perspectives, design considerations and future trends.

Key words: RF MEMS, antennas, reconfigurable architectures, adaptive systems.

6.1 Introduction

Wireless communications systems are constantly evolving towards higher data rates, longer ranges and improved robustness, together with lower costs, a lower power consumption and, in many cases, being part of compact and portable devices. Antennas, as radio-waves transceivers, play a fundamental role in this evolution. Radio frequency micro electromechanical systems (RF MEMS) are an enabling technology for a new generation of intelligent antennas with the capability of dynamically self-adapting their properties in order to maintain performance under operational or environmental variations. The tunable characteristics of MEMS can be used, for instance, to modify the antenna operation frequency or to continuously steer the antenna radiation beam towards favourable directions.

There are two main properties that make RF MEMS an excellent technology for antenna reconfiguration. The first is the superior performance of RF MEMS switches and variable capacitors compared to their corresponding semiconductor devices. For instance, a PIN diode can have insertion losses of 0.5 dB and a power consumption of 10 mW, while the insertion losses of an RF MEMS switch are below 0.1 dB and its actuation requires less than 0.1 mW (Rebeiz, 2003a). Therefore, the resulting antenna systems have higher efficiency, lower power consumption and higher linearity. The second is an exceptional integration capability, enabling antennas with better performance and lower cost.

This chapter describes the main reconfiguration techniques used by RF MEMS antennas. These techniques are divided in external solutions, which use tunable antenna feeds, and internal approaches, which interact directly with the antenna radiation mechanism. The former locates reconfiguration elements in an external feeding network, while the latter locates them in the antenna surface itself. The advantages and disadvantages of each technique are discussed and specific designs are presented to illustrate the main architectures and their performance level. The design considerations are also covered, with emphasis on the design flow and the main biasing techniques, providing also some insight on the effects of the RF MEMS losses, packaging and reliability over the antenna system.

6.2 RF MEMS antennas

This section provides a global overview of the most common applications of RF MEMS antennas as well as the main technological approaches to combine RF MEMS technology with antenna structures.

6.2.1 RF MEMS antenna applications

RF MEMS antennas can provide the existing wireless systems an improved performance by exploiting their tunability properties. The improved system performances, such as data rate, range or size, are strongly linked to the different reconfigurable parameters.

Frequency reconfiguration is particularly interesting in situations where several communication systems converge. Instead of using multiple single-function antennas, a single reconfigurable antenna can accommodate the multiple requirements. This is a very attractive approach for actual wireless devices which integrate multiple communication systems like Global System for Mobile Communications (GSM), Universal Mobile Telecommunications System (UMTS), Global Positioning System (GPS), Bluetooth or Wireless Local Area Network (WLAN). Frequency reconfiguration can also be used in portable wireless devices to implement tunable matching networks that dynamically correct frequency shifts produced by a changing environment or close-body effects. In some cases, reconfigurable frequency notches can be synthesized to filter interferences at antenna level, relaxing the specifications of subsequent filtering stages. Another important application is cognitive radio, which exploits frequency agility to dynamically select the operating frequency band according to propagation channel conditions and spectrum usage.

A classical application of radiation pattern reconfiguration is beam-steering. This consists in modifying the direction of maximum radiation in order to maximize the antenna gain and improve data rates and coverage areas. Radiation pattern reconfiguration can be used also to filter in-band interference by synthesizing patterns with nulls in the direction of arrival of the incoming interference. A recent application of radiation reconfigurability is adaptive multi-input multi-output (MIMO) (Eslami et al., 2010) which replaces the multiple static antennas of standard MIMO systems by multiple reconfigurable antennas capable of synthesizing several different radiation patterns. By combining the spatial diversity of MIMO devices with the additional degrees of freedom provided by pattern reconfiguration, the channel capacity can be significantly increased.

Finally, polarization reconfigurable antennas can be used to reduce polarization mismatch losses in portable devices. The variable orientation of portable devices can degrade transmission performance if the polarization of the transmitter and receiver are not aligned. In these cases, the use of self-orientatable antennas is recommended, especially in linearly polarized systems under line-of-sight conditions. If line-of-sight conditions do not apply, the communications channel typically presents a high non-correlation between horizontal and vertical polarizations. In this case, polarization reconfigurability can be used to enhance the performance of MIMO systems in a similar way as pattern reconfiguration.

6.2.2 RF MEMS antenna technology

The combination of RF MEMS technology with antenna structures follows different approaches which vary depending on the antenna size and frequency as illustrated in Fig. 6.1.

The first technological approach consists of manufacturing the antenna structure in a first step, then adding the RF MEMS devices in subsequent steps using wire-bonding and conductive epoxy. This is the main

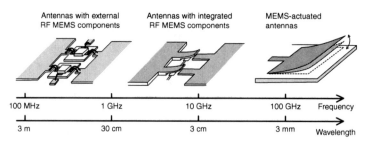

6.1 Technological approaches for the combination of RF MEMS technology with antenna structures.

technological approach at lower frequencies, typically up to a few gigahertz. The RF MEMS devices used by these antennas are switches and variable capacitors. RF MEMS switches can be used to route the RF-signal towards different ports and to physically modify the antenna structure. These modifications lead to a low number of operation modes associated with strong variations of the antenna properties. On the other hand, RF MEMS variable capacitors are used as tunable reactive loads and to implement phase-shifters. The resulting reconfiguration ranges are smaller than in the previous case but it is possible to perform continuous reconfiguration, making variable capacitors very appropriate for fine tuning capabilities.

Although RF MEMS devices maintain a good performance up to frequencies of several tens of gigahertz, the inclusion of external RF MEMS elements in the antenna surface becomes problematic as the frequency increases. This is due to the losses and parasitic effects of the interconnections and the size constraints imposed by the MEMS individual package. The preferred approach in this case is to manufacture the antenna and the micro electromechanical elements using shared microfabrication processes. Additionally, due to the higher frequency of operation, the antenna sizes are smaller, compatible with standard micromachining tools and, in many cases, several prototypes can be fabricated in the same wafer.

As the frequency approaches a hundred gigahertz, individual RF MEMS components lose performance. For a typical phase-shifter design, its insertion loss increases from 0.3 dB/bit at X-band to 1.0 dB/bit at W-band (Rebeiz, 2003b). However, the antenna size enters into the millimetre range and the complete antenna structure can be actuated using MEMS technology. At this point, the antenna itself becomes a MEMS device, falling into the group of movable antennas.

Practical examples of each of these three technological approaches can be found in the prototypes presented in the following sections.

6.3 Reconfigurable feeding networks

The use of RF MEMS components in the feeding network of a single-antenna or a multi-antenna system is an effective approach to providing reconfiguration capability. In systems with a single antenna, tunable feeds can be used to adjust the antenna input impedance or to modify its feeding point. On the other hand, in multi-antenna systems, the feeding network can be used to switch between different antennas or to adaptively combine their radiation. These techniques are illustrated in Fig. 6.2.

Strictly speaking, the resulting antennas should not be included under the label of 'reconfigurable antennas', because reconfiguration elements are

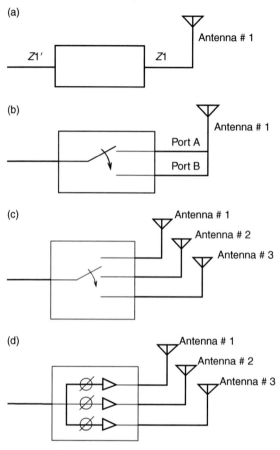

6.2 Tunable feeding networks: (a) tunable matching network; (b) multi-port antenna switching; (c) multi-antenna switching; (d) phased array.

external to the antenna surface and do not interact directly with the radiation mechanism.

6.3.1 Tunable matching networks

Tunable matching networks are used to modify the antenna input impedance, and may be used to provide frequency agility or to mitigate non-matching during the system operation (Kim *et al.*, 2001). These networks are composed of two blocks: a tunable impedance transformer and a control unit. The most common architectures for the impedance transformer are LC series circuits, stub lines and distributed MEMS transmission lines.

RF MEMS antennas for wireless applications 181

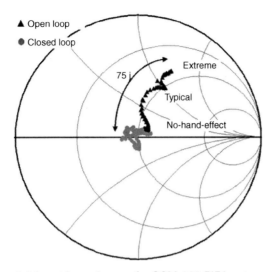

6.3 Input impedance of a GSM-900 PIFA antenna influenced by hand-effects, with and without using a tunable matching network (from van Bezooijen *et al.*, 2008). (IEEE ©).

Tunability is provided through the inclusion of RF MEMS variable capacitors. The capacitance value of these elements is determined by the control unit which monitors the reflected signal and takes decisions according to its value.

Tunable matching networks can achieve frequency reconfiguration over frequency ranges up to one or two octaves (Domingue *et al.*, 2010; Papapolymerou *et al.*, 2003). The main limitation in this case is the narrow bandwidth obtained after the impedance transformation at frequencies where the existing antenna was initially highly reactive.

Tunable matching networks can also be used in fixed frequency systems to mitigate variations on the antenna impedance. This is especially interesting for cellular and mobile applications, where the presence of artefacts in the near-field region of the antenna has a severe effect over the antenna impedance. Figure 6.3 shows the variations over the input impedance of a GSM-900 planar inverted-F antenna (PIFA) antenna produced by hand-effects and mitigated using a tunable matching network (van Bezooijen *et al.*, 2008).

6.3.2 Multi-antenna and multi-port switching

The next approach to achieving reconfiguration capability is to use MEMS-switched networks to switch between several antennas with different frequency and radiation properties. Following this approach, a specifically designed antenna is used for each operational mode. A MEMS-switched network is then used to alternatively transport the RF-signal from the input port to the corresponding antenna. Since each operational mode is located in a different physical region, the main advantage of this approach is the design flexibility. For the same reason, the main drawback is the large size occupied, especially when a high number of operational modes are required.

Pattern reconfiguration can be achieved by using a multi-antenna system composed of identical antennas with different orientations. Due to the different orientations of the antennas, the produced pattern for each operational mode is steered in a different angular direction. On the other hand, frequency properties are preserved due to the identical structure of the antennas. Figure 6.4 presents a switched multi-antenna system composed of two printed Yagi antennas orientated in opposite directions and fed through a single-pole double-throw (SPDT) MEMS switch (Cheng *et al.*, 2009b). More complex designs with a higher number of operational mode, such as the system presented in Fig. 6.5 (Cetiner *et al.*, 2007), can be found in the literature. In this design, three coplanar waveguide (CPW) slot-based antennas are used, providing additional degrees of freedom at the expense of a more complex feeding network.

Switched multi-antenna systems are also capable of providing frequency reconfiguration capability. In this case, the architecture and orientation are the same for all the antennas, but the dimensions of each antenna are different. By applying the appropriate scaling factor, each antenna can be designed to cover a different frequency band. In Fig. 6.6, a frequency-reconfigurable switched multi-antenna system is presented (Wu *et al.*, 2010).

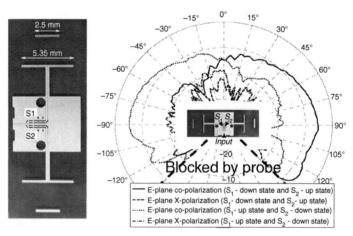

6.4 Switched multi-antenna systems composed of two printed Yagi antennas fed through a SPDT switch (from Cheng *et al.*, 2009b). (IEEE ©).

RF MEMS antennas for wireless applications 183

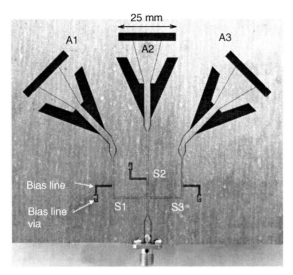

6.5 Switched multi-antenna system composed of three CPW slot-based antennas (from Cetiner *et al.*, 2007). (IEEE ©).

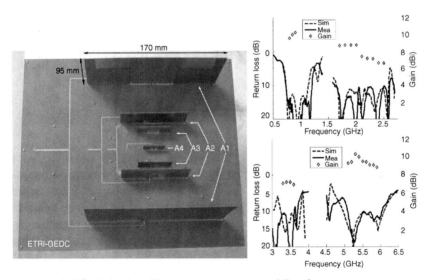

6.6 Switched multi-antenna system providing frequency reconfiguration over four different bands. The covered bands are B1 (800–900 MHz), B2 (1.7–2.5 GHz), B3 (3.3–3.6 GHz) and B4 (5.1–5.9 GHz) (adapted from Wu *et al.*, 2010). (IEEE ©).

Different scaled versions of a dipole antenna are used to provide coverage over four different frequency bands.

In some cases the multiple antennas required by the previous designs can be replaced by a single multi-port antenna. The basic idea is to use an

184 Handbook of MEMS for wireless and mobile applications

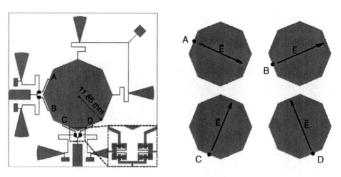

6.7 Polarization-reconfigurable antenna based on multi-port switching and the different linear-polarization modes (adapted from Grau *et al.*, 2010). (IEEE ©).

antenna structure that supports multiple modes, which are excited depending on the feed position. A MEMS-switched network is then used to feed the antenna through the different ports. These multi-port prototypes lack of the design flexibility of switched multi-antenna system but can achieve similar performance with smaller sizes.

This technique is well suited for polarization diversity applications. Figure 6.7 illustrates a multi-port octagonal patch antenna capable of creating different linear polarizations through its different ports (Grau *et al.*, 2010).

6.3.3 Phased arrays

A different approach to achieving pattern reconfiguration capability with multi-antenna systems is to combine the radiation from the multiple antennas instead of switching between them. The most common structures based on this approach are phased arrays. These consist of an antenna array in which the relative phases of the signals feeding each antenna element can be individually adjusted. By synthesizing an appropriate phase distribution the array pattern can be steered towards specific directions. Although this structure adds complexity to the feeding network, the potential reconfiguration capabilities are enhanced and a better control of the radiation pattern is obtained. The low insertion losses (between 0.3 and 1.0 dB/bit) and power consumption (<0.1 mW) of RF MEMS phase-shifters makes them excellent candidates for phased arrays (Chazelas *et al.*, 2009; Rebeiz, 2003b).

In Fig. 6.8 is shown a phased array composed of four patch antennas using distributed MEMS phase-shifters with three bits (Topalli *et al.*, 2008). The synthesized radiation patterns show beam-steering capability up to angles

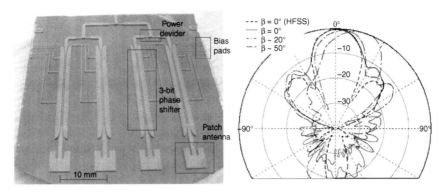

6.8 MEMS-integrated phased array composed of four patch antennas and 3-bit phase shifters (adapted from Topalli *et al.*, 2008). (IEEE ©).

of 50°. Other interesting phase-array prototypes using different antenna elements and MEMS phase-shifter architectures can be found in Kingsley *et al.* (2008) and Sundaram *et al.* (2008).

The phase-shifting structures used by RF phase arrays can also be implemented in the optical domain. Although these phase arrays require additional circuitry, such as electro-optical modulators and photo-detectors, they have significant advantages, such as smaller size, lower losses and large instantaneous bandwidth. In these cases, optical MEMS switches are excellent candidates to implement optical true time-delay feeders (Shin *et al.*, 2004).

6.4 Reconfigurable antennas

A reconfigurable antenna is an antenna structure that integrates an inner mechanism that allows the intentional redistribution of its currents, making it possible to modify its frequency or radiation properties (Huff and Bernhard, 2008). The variable electrical and mechanical properties of RF MEMS components can be effectively used as current-redistribution mechanism for reconfigurable antennas.

This approach is conceptually very different from the reconfigurable-feed designs presented in the previous section, where RF MEMS components were located outside the antenna surface without interacting directly with its radiation mechanism.

Reconfigurable antennas can be classified according to the parameter under reconfiguration. This parameter can be the frequency of operation, radiation pattern, polarization or a combination of the previous. In the next subsections, the main reconfiguration techniques using RF MEMS technology are described for each of these parameters.

6.4.1 Frequency reconfiguration

The underlying principle of operation of frequency reconfiguration is the variation of the effective length of a resonant antenna. The variations in the antenna dimensions produce shifts in the resonant frequency and, as long as the current distribution is scaled to the antenna size, the radiation pattern remains unchanged.

Although there is a common principle of operation for frequency reconfiguration, there exist very different mechanisms through which MEMS technology can be used to modify the antenna length. These mechanisms are illustrated in Fig. 6.9.

The first technique consists of using RF MEMS switches to connect or disconnect metallic sections to the antenna in order to increase or decrease its length. In Fig. 6.10, RF MEMS switches are used to tune the frequency of a slot antenna (Van Caekenberghe and Sarabandi, 2008). When the switches change to ON-state, the slot length is reduced and the resonant frequency increases. In Fig. 6.11, RF MEMS switches are used to tune the resonance frequency of a fractal antenna (Kingsley et al., 2007). It can be observed that

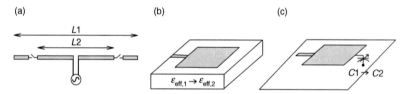

6.9 Frequency reconfiguration mechanisms: (a) physical length modification; (b) electrical length modification and (c) variable reactive loading.

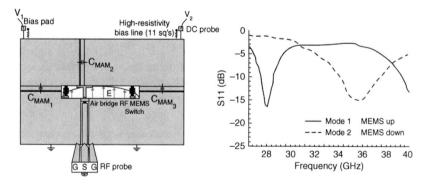

6.10 Frequency-tunable MEMS-switched slot antenna (adapted from van Caekenberghe and Sarabandi, 2008). (IEEE ©).

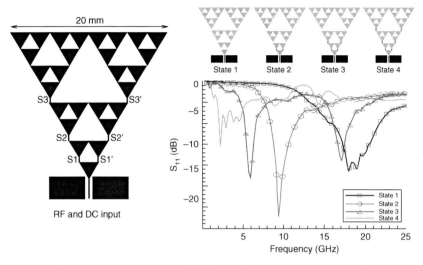

6.11 Frequency-tunable MEMS-switched fractal antenna (from Kingsley *et al.*, 2008). (IEEE ©).

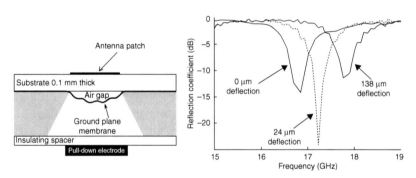

6.12 Frequency-tunable patch antenna with a MEMS actuated ground plane (from Al-Dahleh *et al.*, 2004).

the sequential activation of the RF MEMS switches shifts the antenna resonance to lower frequencies. This technique has also been applied to tune the frequency of an annular slot in Cetiner *et al.* (2010).

Frequency reconfiguration can also be provided by keeping the antenna's physical length constant but modifying its electrical length. In Fig. 6.12 a microstrip patch antenna is presented with a MEMS-actuated ground plane which achieves frequency agility using the previously mentioned technique (Al-Dahleh *et al.*, 2004). The MEMS-actuated ground plane allows the adjustment of the patch height, modifying the patch's effective permittivity and, therefore, shifting its resonance frequency. A design based on the same principle, using a fixed ground plane and a MEMS-actuated patch, is presented in (Langer *et al.*, 2003).

Another technique to design frequency-agile antennas is to load the antenna with a variable reactive load. This reactive load can be implemented using RF MEMS variable capacitors. This technique has the advantage of continuously shifting the antenna resonance frequency and, therefore, surpassing switched-reconfiguration techniques in fine tuning capability. A reactive loaded microstrip patch antenna using CPW MEMS capacitors is presented in Fig. 6.13 (Erdil *et al.*, 2007).

Although less common than resonant frequency reconfiguration, MEMS-reconfigurable antennas can also be used to provide band rejection capabilities. This is the case with the ultra-wideband (UWB) elliptical monopole presented in Fig. 6.14 (Nikolaou *et al.*, 2009). This antenna includes a MEMS-

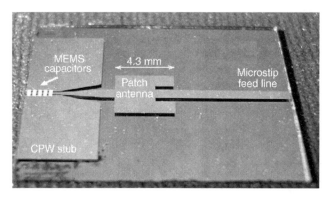

6.13 Frequency-tunable patch antenna based on variable reactive loading using MEMS capacitors (from Erdil *et al.*, 2007). (IEEE ©).

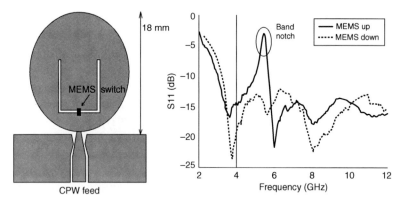

6.14 UWB elliptical monopole with a reconfigurable band notch using a MEMS-switched U-shaped slot (adapted from Nikolaou *et al.*, 2009). (IEEE ©).

switched U-shaped slot in the elliptical monopole surface. When the MEMS switch is in ON-state, the antenna behaves as a standard UWB monopole. However, when the MEMS switch turns to OFF-state, a band notch is created at 5.5 GHz rejecting the IEEE 802.11a band.

An indirect application of RF MEMS to frequency reconfiguration is reconfigurable frequency-selective surfaces (FSS). An FSS is a periodic construction that behaves as an electromagnetic wave filter. The inclusion of RF MEMS in FSSs allows the reconfiguration of the reflected and transmitted bands. Although reconfigurable FSSs are not reconfigurable antennas by themselves, they can be used as an enabling structure for other reconfigurable antennas, such as reconfigurable multiband reflectors. The interested reader can find some interesting designs in Schoenlinner *et al.* (2004) and Zendejas *et al.* (2006).

6.4.2 Radiation pattern reconfiguration

The radiation pattern of an antenna is determined by its current distribution through a Fourier transform. Therefore, radiation pattern reconfiguration can only be achieved by altering the global current distribution. There are three basic pattern reconfiguration techniques, which are illustrated in Fig. 6.15. The real challenge in this case is to keep the input impedance constant while the main currents over the antenna are modified.

The most conceptually simple technique to reconfigure the antenna pattern is to rotate the complete antenna structure by using movable antennas. The rotation of the antenna rotates its radiation pattern and leaves its reflection coefficient unaffected. In spite of the conceptual simplicity of this technique, its application often leads to bulky mechanical actuators resulting in significant drawbacks with respect to reconfiguration speed and power consumption. These disadvantages are strongly mitigated when the antennas are fabricated at microscale. At this point, MEMS technology is ideal to fabricate movable antennas with the required micro-actuators. In Fig. 6.16, a 2×2 movable patch array is presented (Kim *et al.*, 2011). Magnetic actuation is used to rotate the antenna around two orthogonal axes and thus

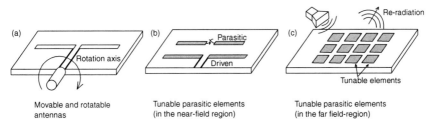

6.15 (a–c) Radiation pattern reconfiguration techniques.

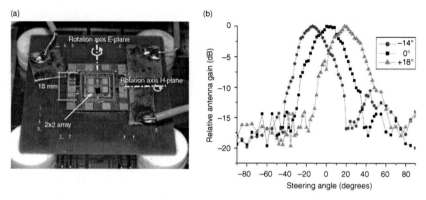

6.16 MEMS patch array rotatable around two axis using magnetic actuation (from Kim *et al.*, 2011): (a) picture of the MEMS patch array and (b) radiation patterns. (IEEE ©).

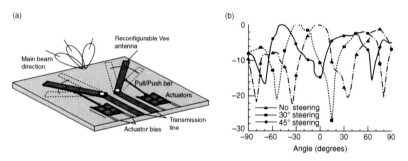

6.17 MEMS-actuated pattern-reconfigurable Vee-antenna (from Chiao *et al.*, 1999): (a) schematic of the reconfigurable Vee-antenna and (b) radiation patterns. (IEEE ©).

steer the radiation beam in both E-plane and H-plane. Another example of a MEMS-actuated movable antenna is presented in Fig. 6.17. In this case, push–pull actuators are used to rotate simultaneously the two arms of a dipole antenna, rotating its pattern along the E-plane (Chiao *et al.*, 1999).

A different strategy to reconfigure the antenna pattern consists in using switched or tunable parasitic sections. The coupled currents over these parasitic elements have a significant effect over the radiation pattern without producing drastic perturbations over input impedance. In antennas with a low number of parasitic elements, the parasitic elements need to be located into the near-field of the driven element in order to couple strong currents, which are necessary to modify the antenna pattern. Typical distances between the driven and parasitic elements are between 0.1 and 0.5 wavelengths; this distance ensures strong currents on the parasitic without damaging severely the performance of the driven antenna. In Fig. 6.18, a pattern-reconfigurable dipole antenna with switched parasitics distributed in a Yagi configuration

RF MEMS antennas for wireless applications 191

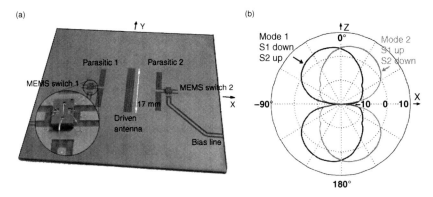

6.18 Pattern-reconfigurable antenna using switched parasitic dipoles (from Petit *et al.*, 2006): (a) picture of the switched parasitic antenna and (b) radiation patterns. (IEEE ©).

is presented (Petit *et al.*, 2006). It can be observed that the radiation pattern can be tilted by individually activating the corresponding switches. RF MEMS switches can be substituted by variable capacitors, providing additional control over the phase of the coupled currents and making it possible to fine-tune the radiation pattern of the antenna.

Parasitic elements can also be located at a higher electrical distance of the driven antenna. However, the required number of parasitic elements is much greater than in the previous case. This is the approach followed by reconfigurable reflect-arrays, transmit-arrays and lenses. In these cases, the location of the parasitic elements follows the same distribution as in conventional arrays. By controlling the phase of the re-radiated field by each element of the array, the direction of the antenna beam can be precisely controlled. It is important to note that, despite the evident similarities with phased array antennas, this method is conceptually very different. The reason is that the re-radiated field by each element of the array is not controlled by an external feeding network but by the tunable architecture of the element itself. In Fig. 6.19, a reconfigurable reflect-array antenna composed of MEMS-actuated patches is presented (Gianvittorio and Rahmat-Samii, 2006). Each patch antenna composing the reflect-array controls the phase of its re-radiated field by adjusting its height. In Fig. 6.20, the reconfiguration of a horn antenna using a lens array is presented (Cheng *et al.*, 2009a). In this case, each element of the lens is fabricated using a reconfigurable antenna-filter-antenna structure, providing beam-steering capabilities as observed in the same figure.

There exist two additional structures that are also used to provide radiation pattern reconfiguration capability; however, their usage is not as wide-spread as the previous designs. These structures are multi-mode and leaky-wave antennas. By using several switches strategically located in a multi-mode antenna, the different modes can be individually activated. Since the radiation pattern associated with each mode can be different, pattern

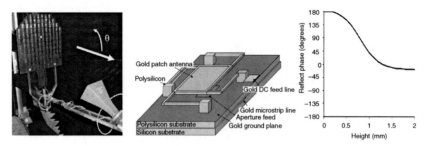

6.19 Reconfigurable reflect-array antenna and basic MEMS-actuated cell (from Gianvittorio and Rahmat-Samii, 2006). (IEEE ©).

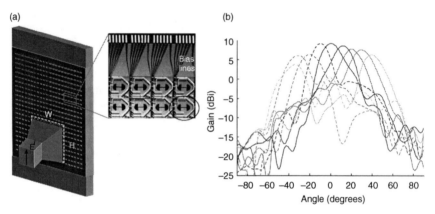

6.20 Pattern-reconfigurable lens-array for a pyramidal horn antenna (from Cheng *et al.*, 2009a): (a) schematic of the reconfigurable lens-array and (b) radiation patterns. (IEEE ©).

reconfiguration is accomplished. This concept has been applied to design a reconfigurable spiral antenna in (won Jung *et al.*, 2006). On the other hand, leaky-wave antennas can be provided with reconfiguration capability by controlling the phase velocity of the propagating wave. This can be effectively accomplished using a periodically MEMS-loaded transmission line, as presented in Zvolensky *et al.* (2011).

6.4.3 Polarization reconfiguration

The polarization of an antenna is determined by the direction of its electrical currents. There are two basic techniques to modify the direction of the antenna currents (and its polarization, as a consequence) preserving its operation frequency and radiation pattern. These techniques are illustrated in Fig. 6.21.

The first technique uses RF MEMS switches to modify the antenna structure in such a way that the resulting configuration is a symmetric version of

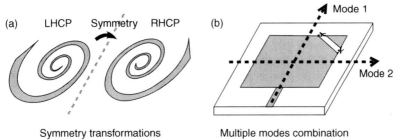

6.21 (a, b) Polarization reconfiguration techniques.

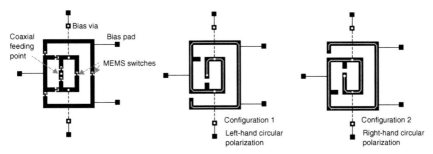

6.22 Polarization reconfigurable spiral antenna (adapted from Cetiner et al., 2006). (IEEE ©).

the original configuration. In Fig. 6.22 the application of this technique to a spiral antenna is presented (Cetiner *et al.*, 2006). It can be observed that the second configuration results from applying a symmetry respect to the horizontal axis to the previous configuration. This transformation preserves the frequency response, produces minor perturbations to the radiation pattern, and transforms left-hand circular polarization into right-hand circular polarization. The main drawback of this technique is that, as occurs in the previous design, RF MEMS switches often need to be distributed over the whole antenna surface and complex biasing networks are required.

Polarization agility can also be achieved without locating switches over the whole antenna structure by taking advantage of multi-mode antennas. In this case, the different modes of the antenna are simultaneously excited and reconfiguration is obtained by introducing minor perturbations that affect the way these modes are combined.

In Fig. 6.23, a nearly-square patch antenna achieves polarization reconfigurability by combining a horizontal and a vertical mode (Simons *et al.*, 2002). When the switch is in OFF-state the two modes are combined with equal amplitude and 90 degrees phase difference, producing circular polarization. However, switching the MEMS device to ON-state breaks the balance between the two modes and creates linear polarization.

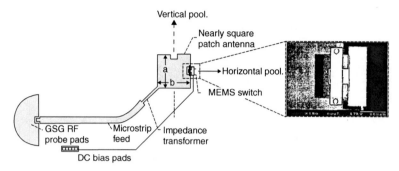

6.23 Polarization-reconfigurable multi-mode antenna with microstrip patch structure (adapted from Simons *et al.*, 2002). (IEEE ©).

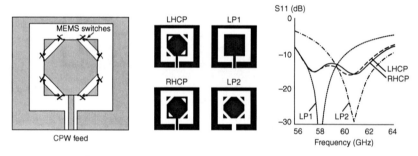

6.24 Polarization-reconfigurable multi-mode antenna with CPW patch structure (adapted from Balcells *et al.*, 2010). (IEEE ©).

In Fig. 6.24, a CPW antenna uses the same principle to switch between linear polarization, right-hand and left-hand circular polarizations (Balcells *et al.*, 2010). The excitation of the two modes for the circularly polarized configurations is evidenced by a double resonance in the reflection coefficient. The combination between different modes is very sensitive to frequency shifts and, for this reason, a narrow bandwidth regarding polarization is a common disadvantage of multi-mode polarization-agile antennas. However, this drawback is often overcome by the simplicity of the antenna structure.

6.4.4 Compound reconfiguration

The ultimate goal of MEMS-reconfigurable antennas is to provide the capability of independently adjust the frequency of operation, the antenna pattern and the polarization. The simultaneous tuning of frequency and radiation properties is known as compound reconfiguration.

While single-parameter reconfiguration is a deeply studied problem, the situation is quite different when considering compound reconfiguration. In this case, the interdependence between the different antenna parameters constitutes a much greater obstacle than in the single-parameter reconfiguration. The main progress towards compound reconfiguration has followed two basic approaches, which are depicted in Fig. 6.25.

The first approach consists in combining in the same structure different single-parameter reconfiguration techniques. A frequency and radiation pattern-reconfigurable patch antenna based on this approach is presented in Fig. 6.26. Four switched parasitic patches are included to reconfigure the antenna pattern, and these patches are loaded with slots of tunable length to adjust their resonance frequency (Yang *et al.*, 2007). By combining parasitic elements with frequency tuning techniques, the antenna can steer the beam towards three different directions for different frequencies of operation between 9.3 and 10.9 GHz. However, the three radiation modes are not all available for each frequency.

Compound reconfigurable antennas following this approach are relatively simple in structure, but their reconfiguration capabilities are significantly limited. This is due to compatibility problems between different one-dimensional techniques, leading to small frequency ranges and a low number of operation modes.

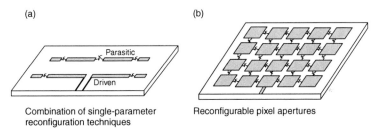

6.25 (a, b) Compound reconfiguration techniques.

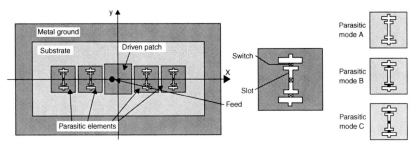

6.26 Frequency and radiation pattern-reconfigurable Yagi patch antenna (adapted from Yang *et al.*, 2007). (IEEE ©).

The second approach is based on using structures with an inherent capability of modifying simultaneously both frequency and radiation properties. These structures are based on a dense distribution of electrically small metallic sections interconnected by switches. The most common architecture is a uniform grid of square metallic patches (Fig. 6.27), known by the name of 'reconfigurable apertures' or 'pixel antennas'. Instead of introducing specific perturbations over the antenna surface, as is done by other reconfiguration methods, pixel antennas reshape the complete antenna surface by activating a specific switch configuration. This configuration is determined by discrete optimization algorithms, such as particle swarm optimization or genetic algorithms.

A 5 by 5 pixel antenna fed through capacitive coupling is presented in Fig. 6.28 (Rodrigo *et al.*, 2011). The antenna can operate at 9 and 10 GHz, being capable of switching at each frequency between three patterns steered to different angular directions.

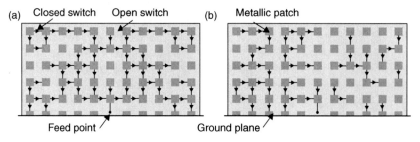

6.27 Pixel reconfigurable antenna with planar monopole architecture. (a) Broadband, bidirectional, broadside configuration. (b) Narrowband, unidirectional, end-fire configuration (adapted from Pringle *et al.*, 2004). (IEEE ©).

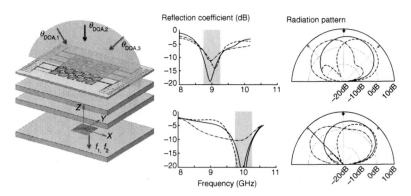

6.28 Frequency and pattern-reconfigurable pixel antenna fed through capacitive coupling (adapted from Rodrigo *et al.*, 2011). (IEEE ©).

Pixel antennas are extremely flexible from reconfiguration perspective due to the possibility of synthesizing a rich variety of antenna shapes. On the other hand, they involve an extremely large complexity, typically requiring beyond a hundred switches, and producing severe impacts over the antenna cost and efficiency. Recently some advances have been reported in the complexity minimization by using multiple-sized pixels (Rodrigo and Jofre, 2012).

6.5 Design considerations

RF MEMS devices have excellent circuit characteristics regarding insertion losses, isolation and linearity. However, the non-idealities of RF MEMS produce noticeable effects over the antenna performance that need to be taken into account during the design phase. In this section, design guidelines for RF MEMS antennas are provided. Additionally, the different biasing techniques for antenna applications are presented and the effects of losses, packaging and reliability over the antenna performance are evaluated.

6.5.1 Design flow and simulation

During the first steps in the design and optimization of a RF MEMS antenna, a numerical simulation model with ideal switches is usually used. A first decision is taken about the antenna structure and the location of the RF MEMS devices. To validate the frequency and radiation parameters of the antenna, hard-wired prototypes implementing the different configurations are fabricated and measured. These prototypes replace MEMS variable capacitors by equivalent lumped capacitors, and MEMS switches are replaced by wires or gaps depending on status.

In the next step, the exact parameters of the RF MEMS device are included in the antenna numerical model. It is important to notice that electromagnetic simulators cannot capture the complete circuital parameters of the MEMS device. For instance, in the case of a MEMS switch, electromagnetic (EM) simulators typically provide accurate values of its isolation but fail in simulating its insertion losses, which involve metal-contact physics at microscale. For this reason, the parameters of the RF MEMS device have to be determined independently, either using multi-physics software or through direct measurements. Taking into account these values, an equivalent circuit model is adjusted and included in the antenna model in order to perform the necessary fine tuning in the design.

There are different ways to include the MEMS circuit model in EM simulation. For example, in simulators based on the finite element method, MEMS can be modelled using impedance boundaries. For other methods, such as methods-of-moments (MoM) or finite-differences in the time-domain

(FDTD), a general technique consists of replacing each MEMS device by a port. By computing the complete S-parameter matrix and the radiation pattern associated with each port, the antenna parameters can be computed in a post-processing step (Mehmood and Wallace, 2010). In antennas with a high number of configurations, this method can reduce significantly the simulation time. Indeed, just a single electromagnetic simulation is required, while the post-processing step, which is executed as many times as there are different configurations, has a low computational complexity.

A final step prior to the fabrication of the RF MEMS antenna is the design and modelling of the biasing lines and circuitry. These structures need to be designed properly in order to minimize mutual coupling with the radiating elements of the antenna. By accurately modelling the biasing network and performing the corresponding full-wave simulations, their effect over the antenna performance can be assessed and final adjustments can be performed.

6.5.2 Biasing network

A clever design of the switch biasing network is of great importance in antenna applications. Since electromagnetic radiation enhances coupling, the perturbations produced by the induced currents over the biasing lines are much more intense in antenna elements that in other devices, such as amplifiers, where electromagnetic fields are confined. These effects are especially important in MEMS-reconfigurable antennas where MEMS elements are literally inside the antenna structure. The different coupling mitigation techniques are depicted in Fig. 6.29.

The first approach is to use quarter-wavelength radial stubs to force an RF high-impedance condition at the intersection points between the antenna and the biasing lines. This technique is effective in microstrip antennas; however, this is a narrowband solution and the radial stubs often occupy a prohibitively large area.

An alternative to radial stub are high-resistive lines. Since the DC-current consumption of MEMS devices is almost negligible, the high-resistance of biasing lines does not affect the MEMS performance but attenuates significantly the RF coupled currents. High-resistive materials, such as tantalum

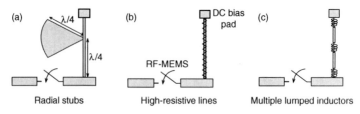

6.29 (a–c) Coupling mitigation techniques for biasing lines.

nitrate (TaN) or silicon chrome (SiCr), require specific deposition processes (sputtering or evaporation, typically) which makes them suitable for microfabricated antennas but hard to implement in designs with external individually packaged MEMS.

The preferred approach in antennas with non-integrated MEMS is the location of several lumped inductors uniformly distributed over the biasing lines. These inductors, which have low impedance for DC currents, split the biasing lines into small non-resonant sections, thereby mitigating RF currents.

Although all the previous methods are effective in reducing the effects of biasing lines over the antenna performance, a clever biasing design is still fundamental to ensure the good performance of the antenna. Some useful guidelines for the bias design are the minimization of the length of the biasing lines and the reduction of the number of required lines by using common grounds or taking advantage of existing antenna parts for biasing. The location and orientation of the biasing lines is also important. It is preferable to choose locations with a less intense near-field, such as behind ground planes, and orienting the biasing lines orthogonally to the existing electric field.

6.5.3 Insertion losses, packaging and reliability effects

In this section an initial insight is given about the effect of the RF MEMS insertion losses, packaging and reliability over the antenna performance. Although the exact quantization of the perturbations produced by the MEMS non-idealities requires a case-by-case analysis, the presented results provide an initial insight useful for the proper design of RF MEMS antennas.

The insertion losses of the MEMS device affect the antenna efficiency and, as a consequence, its gain. The gain reduction depends on the number of RF MEMS and, more importantly, on the current driven by these devices. An exact quantization of the gain reduction for a reconfigurable aperture is shown

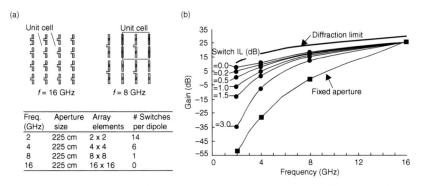

6.30 Gain analysis for a reconfigurable aperture with lossy switches (adapted from Brown, 2001): (a) configurations of the reconfigurable aperture and (b) reconfigurable aperture gain. (IEEE ©).

in Fig. 6.30 (Brown, 2001). It can be observed that the gain reduction can be much higher than the switch insertion losses and, actually, this is the typical situation when several switches are serially interconnected. In the example presented, the low-frequency configurations interconnect a higher number of RF MEMS switches per dipole and, for this reason, the impact of the switch losses over the aperture gain is more pronounced than in high-frequency configurations. For typical values of insertion losses in RF MEMS switches (below 0.2 dB), the gain reduction is relatively small, usually less than 1dB reduction.

The effects of RF MEMS packaging have also been studied in the literature (Huff and Bernhard, 2006). External individually packaged RF MEMS devices are usually fabricated over a different substrate than that used by the antenna, and interconnections are usually made using wire-bonding, which has a parasitic inductive effect. It has been observed that these characteristics produce a small mismatch at the interconnection point and a virtual lengthen of the RF path. Simple matching networks and minor size readjustments of around one-twentieth of a wavelength can mitigate the previous effects.

Another property of RF MEMS devices, which has a major impact on antenna performance, is their reliability and fabrication yield. For instance, the fabrication yield of MEMS switches is often around 95% and, although RF MEMS switches performing over a hundred billion cycles have already been reported, their life expectancy can be much shorter depending on the package hermeticity or on the operational conditions. To mitigate the effects of fabrication yield and reliability, some added redundancy is sometimes included in the antenna design to keep the antenna operative even when one or more MEMS fail. Interesting analyses of antenna performance degradation depending on the redundancy level and the MEMS reliability have been carried out for reflect-arrays (Salti *et al.*, 2010) and phased arrays (Teti and Darreff, 2004). Figure 6.31 presents a reflect-array cell optimized

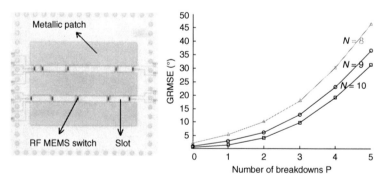

6.31 Reflect-array cell optimized to maximize robustness against MEMS breakdowns and the resulting performance degradation. Performance is evaluated as the phase error in the reflected wave (adapted from Salti *et al.*, 2010). (IEEE ©).

to maximize robustness against MEMS breakdown. The performance degradation in terms of the reflected wave phase error is evaluated for different redundancy and reliability levels. For instance, the reflect-array cell with eight MEMS can tolerate up to one breakdown without exceeding a phase error of five degrees. However, if two additional MEMS are included, this cell can tolerate an additional breakdown for the same error levels.

6.6 Conclusion and future trends

Wireless communications are evolving towards multi-application systems where multiple communication protocols, such as WiFi, WiMax, GPS, Bluetooth or DVB-H, converge. The future trend is toward the implementation of flexible systems capable of accommodating multiple applications and protocols, and providing scalability for future changes (Chun, 2010). Progress towards system-level flexibility requires the development of reconfigurable antennas, in which RF MEMS technology plays a fundamental role. Some of the future trends in RF MEMS antennas are described below.

The increasing demand for flexibility in multi-application systems will require reconfigurable antennas to provide strong reconfiguration capabilities over both frequency and pattern properties. New reconfigurable antenna architectures would be required in order to provide rich compound reconfiguration. MEMS-reconfigurable pixel apertures can efficiently serve this purpose. Additionally, the natural redundancy of these structures mitigates the effect of RF MEMS reliability and makes these structures compatible with medium-yield fabrication processes.

The possibility of providing strong reconfiguration capabilities while keeping a low cost will require the application of antenna-level packaging techniques. Since individually packaged RF MEMS devices are prohibitively costly for high-volume applications, the complete antenna would need to be packaged using wafer-level packaging. For this reason, future RF MEMS antennas will need to take this packaging into account and even improve the antenna performance by taking advantage of its presence, for example by applying superstrate-loading concepts.

The continuous improvement of the antenna reconfiguration capabilities would also require exploring new technological approaches beyond common electrostatic or thermal RF MEMS actuation. In this direction, some initial work has been already developed using different actuation mechanisms, such as microfluidic actuation. These antennas are partially composed of liquid metal and can be mechanically reconfigured through the actuation of micropumps or electrodes. An example of a microfluidic reconfiguration is illustrated in Fig. 6.32, where a circular Yagi antenna rotates its pattern using movable liquid-metal parasitics controlled by a micropump actuator (Rodrigo et al., 2012).

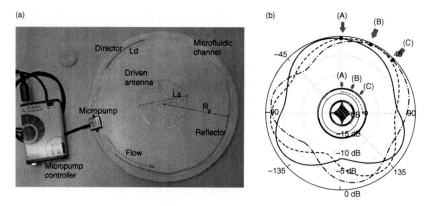

6.32 Circular Yagi-Uda antenna with micropump-actuated parasitics composed of liquid metal (Hg) (adapted from Rodrigo *et al.*, 2012): (a) picture of the microfluidic Yagi antenna and (b) radiation patterns. (IEEE ©).

According to these observations, the natural evolution of RF MEMS antennas is toward structures with rich multi-parameter reconfiguration capabilities, taking advantage of antenna-level packaging materials and applying improved actuation mechanisms.

6.7 Sources of further information and advice

The interested reader can find information about the theory, design and technology of RF MEMS in Rebeiz (2003a). A comprehensive library of RF MEMS devices is also provided, together with equivalent circuit models useful for RF MEMS antenna design.

Basic concepts about general antenna structures can be reviewed in Balanis (2005) and Krauss and Marhefka (2001).

Further information about the basics of antenna reconfiguration can be found in Bernhard (2007) and Huff and Bernhard (2008), which provide additional reconfigurable antenna examples using both electromechanical and electronic components.

Further prototypes and details of RF MEMS antenna elements, arrays and feeding networks, as well as antenna micromachining, are presented in (Pan *et al.*, 2008).

6.8 References

Al-Dahleh, R., Shafai, C., and Shafai, L. (2004), 'Frequency-agile microstrip patch antenna using a reconfigurable MEMS ground plane', *Microwave and Optical Technology Letters* **43**, 64–67. DOI: 10.1002/mop.20376

Balanis, C. A. (2005), *Antenna Theory: Analysis and Design*, New Jersey, Wiley-Interscience.

Balcells, J., Damgaci, Y., Cetiner, B. A., Romeu, J., and Jofre, L. (2010), Polarization reconfigurable MEMS-CPW antenna for mm-wave applications, in 'Proc. Fourth European Conf. Antennas and Propagation (EuCAP)', pp. 1–5.

Bernhard, J. T. (2007), *Reconfigurable Antennas, Synthesis Lectures on Antennas*, California, Morgan & Claypool Publishers.

Brown, E. (2001), 'On the gain of a reconfigurable-aperture antenna', *IEEE Transactions on Antennas and Propagation* **49**(10), 1357–1362. DOI: 10.1109/8.954923

Cetiner, B., Akay, E., Sengul, E., and Ayanoglu, E. (2006), 'A MIMO system with multifunctional reconfigurable antennas', *IEEE Antennas and Wireless Propagation Letters* **5**(1), 463–466. DOI: 10.1109/LAWP.2006.885171

Cetiner, B. A., Crusats, G. R., Jofre, L., and Biyikli, N. (2010), 'RF MEMS integrated frequency reconfigurable annular slot antenna', *IEEE Transactions on Antennas and Propagation* **58**(3), 626–632. DOI: 10.1109/TAP.2009.2039300

Cetiner, B. A., Jofre, L., Qian, J., Liu, S., Li, G. P., and De Flaviis, F. (2007), 'A compact broadband MEMS-integrated diversity system', *IEEE Transactions on Vehicular Technology* **56**(2), 436–444. DOI: 10.1109/TVT.2007.891418

Chazelas, J., Ziaei, A., Dolti, D., and Merlet, T. (2009), 'Potential technological breakthroughs for phased array antennas', *IEEE Aerospace and Electronic Systems Magazine* **24**(11), 22–27. DOI: 10.1109/MAES.2009.5344178

Cheng, C.-C., Lakshminarayanan, B., and Abbaspour-Tamijani, A. (2009a), 'A programmable lens-array antenna with monolithically integrated MEMS switches', *IEEE Transactions on Microwave Theory and Techniques* **57**(8), 1874–1884. DOI: 10.1109/TMTT.2009.2025422

Cheng, S., Rantakari, P., Malmqvist, R., Samuelsson, C., Vaha-Heikkila, T., Rydberg, A., and Varis, J. (2009b), 'Switched beam antenna based on RF MEMS SPDT switch on quartz substrate', *IEEE Antennas and Wireless Propagation Letters* **8**, 383–386. DOI: 10.1109/LAWP.2009.2018712

Chiao, J.-C., Fu, Y., Chio, I. M., DeLisio, M., and Lin, L.-Y. (1999), MEMS reconfigurable vee antenna, in 'Proc. IEEE MTT-S Int. Microwave Symp. Digest', Vol. 4, pp. 1515–1518. DOI: 10.1109/MWSYM.1999.780242

Chun, A. (2010), 'Key lessons from the scalable communications core: a reconfigurable wireless baseband', *IEEE Communications Magazine* **48**(12), 101–109. DOI: 10.1109/MCOM.2010.5673079

Domingue, F., Fouladi, S., and Mansour, R. R. (2010), A reconfigurable impedance matching network using dual-beam MEMS switches for an extended operating frequency range, in 'Proc. IEEE MTT-S Int. Microwave Symp. Digest (MTT)', pp. 1552–1555. DOI: 10.1109/MWSYM.2010.5515472

Erdil, E., Topalli, K., Unlu, M., Civi, O., and Akin, T. (2007), 'Frequency tunable microstrip patch antenna using RF MEMS technology', *IEEE Transactions on Antennas and Propagation* **55**(4), 1193–1196. DOI: 10.1109/TAP.2007.893426

Eslami, H., Sukumar, C. P., Rodrigo, D., Mopidevi, S., Eltawil, A. M., Jofre, L., and Cetiner, B. A. (2010) 'Reduced overhead training for multi reconfigurable antennas with beam-tilting capability', *IEEE Transactions on Wireless Communications* **9**(12), 3810–3821. DOI: 10.1109/TWC.2010.091510.100267

Gianvittorio, J. P. and Rahmat-Samii, Y. (2006), 'Reconfigurable patch antennas for steerable reflectarray applications', *IEEE Transactions on Antennas and Propagation* **54**(5), 1388–1392. DOI: 10.1109/TAP.2006.874311

Grau, A., Romeu, J., Lee, M.-J., Blanch, S., Jofre, L., and De Flaviis, F. (2010), 'A dual-linearly-polarized MEMS-reconfigurable antenna for narrowband MIMO communication systems', *IEEE Transactions on Antennas and Propagation* **58**(1), 4–17. DOI: 10.1109/TAP.2009.2036197

Huff, G. H. and Bernhard, J. T. (2006), 'Integration of packaged RF MEMS switches with radiation pattern reconfigurable square spiral microstrip antennas', *IEEE Transactions on Antennas and Propagation* **54**(2), 464–469. DOI: 10.1109/TAP.2005.863409

Huff, G. H. and Bernhard, J. T. (2008), *Modern Antenna Handbook*, New Jersey, John Wiley & Sons, Inc., chapter Reconfigurable Antennas, pp. 369–398.

Kim, H.-T., Jung, S., Kang, K., Park, J.-H., Kim, Y.-K., and Kwon, Y. (2001), 'Low-loss analog and digital micromachined impedance tuners at the Ka-band', *IEEE Transactions on Microwave Theory and Techniques* **49**(12), 2394–2400. DOI: 10.1109/22.971626

Kim, Y., Kim, N., Kim, J., Lee, S., Kwon, Y., and Kim, Y. (2011), '60 GHz full MEMS antenna platform mechanically driven by magnetic actuator', *IEEE Transactions on Industrial Electronics* **58**(10), 4830–4836 DOI: 10.1109/TIE.2011.2114317

Kingsley, N., Anagnostou, D. E., Tentzeris, M., and Papapolymerou, J. (2007), 'RF MEMS sequentially reconfigurable sierpinski antenna on a flexible organic substrate with novel DC-biasing technique', *Journal of Microelectromechanical Systems* **16**(5), 1185–1192. DOI: 10.1109/JMEMS.2007.902462

Kingsley, N., Ponchak, G. E., and Papapolymerou, J. (2008), 'Reconfigurable RF MEMS phased array antenna integrated within a liquid crystal polymer (LCP) system-on-package', *IEEE Transactions on Antennas and Propagation* **56**(1), 108–118. DOI: 10.1109/TAP.2007.913151

Krauss, J. D. and Marhefka, R. J. (2001), *Antennas For All Applications*, New York, McGraw-Hill Science.

Langer, J.-C., Zou, J., Liu, C., and Bernhard, J. (2003), 'Micromachined reconfigurable out-of-plane microstrip patch antenna using plastic deformation magnetic actuation', *IEEE Microwave and Wireless Components Letters* **13**(3), 120–122. DOI: 10.1109/LMWC.2003.810123

Mehmood, R. and Wallace, J. W. (2010), Exploring beamforming performance versus complexity in reconfigurable aperture antennas, in 'Proc. Int Smart Antennas (WSA) ITG Workshop', pp. 383–389. DOI: 10.1109/WSA.2010.5456399

Nikolaou, S., Kingsley, N. D., Ponchak, G. E., Papapolymerou, J., and Tentzeris, M. M. (2009), 'UWB elliptical monopoles with a reconfigurable band notch using MEMS switches actuated without bias lines', *IEEE Transactions on Antennas and Propagation* **57**(8), 2242–2251. DOI: 10.1109/TAP.2009.2024450

Pan, B., Papapolymerou, J., and Tentzeris, M. M. (2008), *Modern Antenna Handbook*, New Jersey, John Wiley & Sons, Inc., chapter MEMS integrated and micromachined antenna elements, arrays and feeding networks, pp. 829–865.

Papapolymerou, J., Lange, K. L., Goldsmith, C. L., Malczewski, A., and Kleber, J. (2003), 'Reconfigurable double-stub tuners using MEMS switches for intelligent RF front-ends', *IEEE Transactions on Microwave Theory and Techniques* **51**(1), 271–278. DOI: 10.1109/TMTT.2002.806513

Petit, L., Dussopt, L., and Laheurte, J.-M. (2006), 'MEMS-switched parasitic-antenna array for radiation pattern diversity', *IEEE Transactions on Antennas and Propagation* **54**(9), 2624–2631. DOI: 10.1109/TAP.2006.880751

Pringle, L., Harms, P., Blalock, S., Kiesel, G., Kuster, E., Friederich, P., Prado, R., Morris, J., and Smith, G. (2004), 'A reconfigurable aperture antenna based on switched links between electrically small metallic patches', *IEEE Transactions on Antennas and Propagation* **52**(6), 1434–1445. DOI: 10.1109/TAP.2004.825648

Rebeiz, G. M. (2003a), *RF MEMS: Theory, Design, and Technology*, John Wiley & Sons, Inc., New York, NY, USA.

Rebeiz, G. M. (2003b), RF-MEMS switches: status of the technology, in 'Proc. 12th International Conference on Solid State Sensors, Actuators and Microsystems', Vol. 2 pp. 1726–1729. DOI: 10.1109/SENSOR.2003.1217118

Rodrigo, D., Damgaci, Y., Unlu, M., Cetiner, B. A., Romeu, J., and Jofre, L. (2011), Antenna reconfigurability based on a novel parasitic pixel layer, in 'Proc. 5th European Conf. Antennas and Propagation (EuCAP)', pp. 3497–3500.

Rodrigo, D. and Jofre, L. (2012), 'Frequency and radiation pattern reconfigurability of a multi-size pixel antenna', *IEEE Transactions on Antennas and Propagation* **60**(5), 2219–2225. DOI: 10.1109/TAP.2012.2189739

Rodrigo, D., Jofre, L., and Cetiner, B. A. (2012), 'Circular beam-steering reconfigurable antenna with liquid metal parasitics', *IEEE Transactions on Antennas and Propagation*. **60**(4), 1796–1802. DOI: 10.1109/TAP.2012.2186235

Salti, H., Fourn, E., Gillard, R., and Legay, H. (2010), 'Minimization of MEMS breakdowns effects on the radiation of a MEMS based reconfigurable reflectarray', *IEEE Transactions on Antennas and Propagation* **58**(7), 2281–2287. DOI: 10.1109/TAP.2010.2048861

Schoenlinner, B., Abbaspour-Tamijani, A., Kempel, L. C., and Rebeiz, G. M. (2004), 'Switchable low-loss RF MEMS Ka-band frequency-selective surface', *IEEE Transactions on Microwave Theory and Techniques* **52**(11), 2474–2481. DOI: 10.1109/TMTT.2004.837148

Shin, J.-D., Lee, B.-S., and Kim, B.-G. (2004), 'Optical true time-delay feeder for x-band phased array antennas composed of 2 × 2 optical mems switches and fiber delay lines', *IEEE Photonics Technology Letters* **16**(5), 1364–1366. DOI: 10.1109/LPT.2004.826083

Simons, R. N., Chun, D., and Katehi, L. P. B. (2002), Polarization reconfigurable patch antenna using microelectromechanical systems (MEMS) actuators, in 'Proc. IEEE Antennas and Propagation Society Int. Symp', Vol. 2, pp. 6–9. DOI: 10.1109/APS.2002.1016015

Sundaram, A., Maddela, M., Ramadoss, R., and Feldner, L. M. (2008), 'MEMS-based electronically steerable antenna array fabricated using pcb technology', *Journal of Microelectromechanical Systems* **17**(2), 356–362. DOI: 10.1109/JMEMS.2008.916291

Teti, J. G., and Darreff, F. P. (2004), 'MEMS 2-bit phase-shifter failure mode and reliability considerations for large X-band arrays', *IEEE Transactions on Microwave Theory and Techniques* **52**(2), 693–701. DOI: 10.1109/TMTT.2003.822017

Topalli, K., Civi, O. A., Demir, S., Koc, S., and Akin, T. (2008), 'A monolithic phased array using 3-bit distributed RF MEMS phase shifters', *IEEE Transactions on Microwave Theory and Techniques* **56**(2), 270–277. DOI: 10.1109/TMTT.2007.914377

van Bezooijen, A., de Jongh, M. A., Chanlo, C., Ruijs, L., van Straten, F., Mahmoudi, R., and van Roermund, A. (2008), 'A GSM/EDGE/WCDMA adaptive series-LC matching network using RF-MEMS switches', *IEEE Journal of Solid-State Circuits* **43**(10), 2259–2268. DOI: 10.1109/JSSC.2008.2004334

Van Caekenberghe, K. and Sarabandi, K. (2008), 'A 2-bit Ka-band RF MEMS frequency tunable slot antenna', *IEEE Antennas and Wireless Propagation Letters* **7**, 179–182. DOI: 10.1109/LAWP.2008.921390

won Jung, C., jer Lee, M., Li, G., and De Flaviis, F. (2006), 'Reconfigurable scan-beam single-arm spiral antenna integrated with RF-MEMS switches', *IEEE Transactions on Antennas and Propagation* **54**(2), 455–463. DOI: 10.1109/TAP.2005.863407

Wu, T., Li, R. L., Eom, S. Y., Myoung, S. S., Lim, K., Laskar, J., Jeon, S. I., and Tentzeris, M. M. (2010), 'Switchable quad-band antennas for cognitive radio base station applications', *IEEE Transactions on Antennas and Propagation* **58**(5), 1468–1476. DOI: 10.1109/TAP.2010.2044472

Yang, X.-S., Wang, B.-Z., Wu, W., and Xiao, S. (2007), 'Yagi patch antenna with dual-band and pattern reconfigurable characteristics', *IEEE Antennas and Wireless Propagation Letters* **6**, 168–171. DOI: 10.1109/LAWP.2007.895292

Zendejas, J. M., Gianvittorio, J. P., Rahmat-Samii, Y., and Judy, J. W. (2006), 'Magnetic MEMS reconfigurable frequency-selective surfaces', *Journal of Microelectromechanical Systems* **15**(3), 613–623. DOI: 10.1109/JMEMS.2005.863704

Zvolensky, T., Chicherin, D., Raisanen, A. V., and Simovski, C. (2011), 'Leaky-wave antenna based on microelectromechanical systems-loaded microstrip line', *IET Microwaves, Antennas and Propagation* **5**(3), 357–363. DOI: 10.1049/iet-map.2010.0168.

7
RF MEMS-based wireless architectures and front-ends

P. RÖJSEL, Lund University, Sweden

DOI: 10.1533/9780857098610.1.207

Abstract: Future demands for increasing capacity, increasing complexity, miniaturization and cost reduction of mobile communication devices are driving radio frequency (RF) technology towards the use of MEMS-based components to replace standard RF components currently used. MEMS is a technology that readily lends itself to be integrated into modules or even directly on to the RF-chips of silicon or other materials suited for the active RF components. New innovative transceiver architectures will be made possible when MEMS components are available for integration. Ultimately, MEMS technology could enable the design and manufacturing of a complete transceiver on a chip.

Key words: RF MEMS, mobile communication, transceiver, RF technology, RF-switch.

7.1 Introduction

All cellular telephones use one or more parts of the radio frequency (RF) spectrum. The particular frequency band in use locally is determined by international standards and sometimes by historical or protectionist reasons. The result is more or less local 'standards' determining where in the world the telephone can be used. Cellular telephones are evolving towards the use of more and more frequency bands so that more and more true global mobility is achieved. This of course increases the complexity of the RF circuitry in the telephone, making the use of new technologies such as MEMS desirable in order to keep the physical size and power consumption of the mobile device at a reasonable level.

On top of these existing frequencies additional bands for 4G are being introduced.

Some of these frequency bands are shared with other services, such as television, Wi-Fi and Bluetooth. The television bands are in some regions, such as the UK, Germany and Japan to mention a few, being at least in part transferred to cellular use. The reason is the system change from analogue

Table 7.1 At present, the GSM system uses these frequencies

System	Band	Uplink (MHz)	Downlink (MHz)
T-GSM-380	380	380.2–389.8	390.2–399.8
T-GSM-410	410	410.2–419.8	420.2–429.8
GSM-450	450	450.6–457.6	460.6–467.6
GSM-480	480	479.0–486.0	489.0–496.0
GSM-710	710	698.2–716.2	728.2–746.2
GSM-750	750	747.2–762.2	777.2–792.2
T-GSM-810	810	806.2–821.2	851.2–866.2
GSM-850	850	824.2–849.2	869.2–894.2
P-GSM-900	900	890.0–915.0	935.0–960.0
E-GSM-900	900	880.0–915.0	925.0–960.0
R-GSM-900	900	876.0–915.0	921.0–960.0
T-GSM-900	900	870.4–876.0	915.4–921.0
DCS-1800	1800	1710.2–1784.8	1805.2–1879.8
PCS-1900	1900	1850.2–1910.2	1930.2–1990.2

Table 7.2 The UMTS (3G) system uses these frequencies

Region	Band	Uplink (MHz)	Downlink (MHz)
I	2100	1920–1980	2110–2170
II	1900	1850–1910	1930–1990
III	1800	1710–1785	1805–1880
IV	1700	1710–1755	2110–2155
V	850	824–849	869–894
VI	800	830–840	875–885
VII	2600	2500–2570	2620–2690
VIII	900	880–915	925–960
IX	1700	1749.9–1784.9	1844.9–1879.9
X	1700	1710–1770	2110–2170
XI	1500	1427.9–1447.9	1475.9–1495.9
XII	700	698–716	728–746
XIII	700	777–787	746–756
XIV	700	788–798	758–768

to digital television transmissions in these countries requiring less spectrum space, which frees up parts of the spectrum.

The large number of bands is mostly due to historical reasons. The frequencies used for cellular networks differ between the Americas, Europe, Africa and Asia. More precise information on regional frequency use is provided by standardization bodies, such as ETSI, FCC and ITU.

7.1.1 Frequency bands: brief historical review

The first commercial standard for mobile communication in the United States was AMPS, which was in the 800 MHz frequency band. In the Nordic countries of Europe, the first widespread automatic mobile network, the NMT-450, was as the name suggests in the 450 MHz band. As mobile telephones became affordable for everyone and increasingly popular, service providers soon encountered a capacity problem. This created a need to develop existing networks and to introduce new standards to keep a backward compatibility and the possibility for the new standards to coexist with the old ones (Fig. 7.1). The new standards are often based on new frequency bands which are added to the communication standards system.

The GSM standard, which appeared in Europe as a successor to NMT-450, initially used the 900 MHz band. As demand grew, providers acquired licenses in the 1800 MHz band, which is mostly used in urban areas with high capacity demands (Table 7.1). The frequencies used by the UMTS (3G) system are shown in Table 7.2. Higher frequencies have a shorter physical range, and each base station cell covers a smaller area, creating the possibility of building denser and higher capacity networks.

In a multiband handset receiver there is a fixed bandpass filter needed for each frequency band. To switch the single antenna and often single input to the receiver chip, an antenna switch is used. At present PIN-diode or field-effect-transistor (FET) switches are used, which can, for size and practical reasons, accommodate a maximum of about five frequency bands. The use of more frequency bands requires a more compact and complex antenna switch, and this is one requirement where MEMS comes into use. MEMS RF switches will be discussed further in the following sections.

7.2 Communication standards

In the USA, the analogue AMPS standard that used the 800 MHz band was replaced by a number of digital systems. Initially, systems based upon the

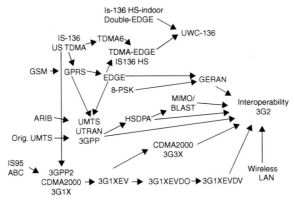

7.1 This rather complex figure shows a small part of the mobile standards evolution.

AMPS mobile phone model were popular, including IS-95 – often known as CDMA after the radio technology it uses – and IS-136, known as D-AMPS, Digital AMPS, or time division multiple access (TDMA) – after the radio technology it uses. Eventually, IS-136 on these frequencies was replaced by most operators with GSM (GSM is also a TDMA system). GSM had already been running for some time on the US PCS band on 1900 MHz.

Some NMT-450 analogue networks have been replaced with digital networks reusing the same frequency band. In Russia and some other countries, local carriers received licenses for 450 MHz frequency to provide CDMA mobile coverage. In the Nordic countries the 450 MHz band and existing base station locations from the NMT-450 network are reused as a wireless broadband network for lightly populated areas, giving fairly good bit rates of up to 3.1 Mbit/s and transparent coverage throughout the Nordic countries.

Many GSM-only phones support three bands (900/1800/1900 MHz or 850/1800/1900 MHz) or four bands (850/900/1800/1900 MHz), and are usually referred to as triple band and quad-band phones, or 'world phones'. Users with such a phone can travel internationally and use the same handset. This portability is not as extensive with IS-95 phones however, as IS-95 networks do not exist in most of Europe.

Mobile networks based on different standards may use the same frequency range; for example, AMPS, D-AMPS, N-AMPS and IS-95 all use the 800 MHz frequency band. Moreover, one can find both AMPS and IS-95 networks in use on the same frequency in the same area and they do not interfere with each other. This is achieved by the use of different channels to carry data. The actual frequency used by a particular phone can vary from place to place, depending on the settings of the carrier's base station.

Often the requirements for different standards are such that physically different receivers and transmitters are needed, one for each standard. For example, some systems require a highly linear receiver and transmitter, while others can use a class C transmitter and a less linear receiver. This increases the complexity of the antenna and RF paths, further increasing the need to switch to MEMS technology in the antenna switch and RF components such as filters.

7.3 Receivers, transmitters and transceivers: basic architectures

There are two basic types of receiver architectures used in mobile phones, heterodyne and homodyne, which will be discussed, together with transmitters, antenna switches and filters.

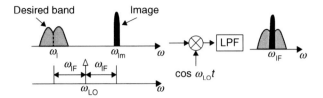

7.2 Basic principle of heterodyne receiver.

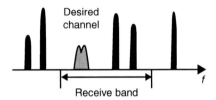

7.3 Typical example frequency spectrum received by the antenna of a handset.

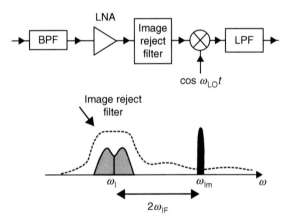

7.4 Frontend of a heterodyne receiver with filter to suppress the image frequency.

7.3.1 Heterodyne receiver

In a heterodyne receiver (Fig. 7.2) the incoming (antenna) frequency is mixed to a usually lower intermediate frequency (Fig. 7.3) where the entire RF signal processing and filtering is performed. This signal processing can be either analogue or digital. In the digital case the signal is digitized and fed into a signal processor, which extracts the desired information and suppresses the unwanted information. Digital signal processing will not be discussed in this chapter. In the analogue case the processing takes place with channel-wide bandpass filters (Fig. 7.4) and additional mixing to extract the I and Q quadrature signals. Most radio sets are of the heterodyne type.

7.3.2 Homodyne receiver

In a homodyne receiver (Fig. 7.5) the incoming signal is mixed with the signal carrier frequency directly down to the baseband. This technique eliminates the image frequencies and the intermediate frequency bandpass channel filter. Instead a simple low pass filter with the knee frequency of the channel width can be used. This lowpass filter can be realized either integrated on chip or as a software digital filter. However, there is a very high isolation between the input signal and the local oscillator (LO). This requirement is most pronounced in the mixer between the RF input and the LO input. With modern RF chip technology, this is not an impossible problem to overcome and has been in use in high volume handsets since the late 1990s. Even in single chip RF transceivers, including both the low power transmitter circuits, mixers, LOs and low noise amplifiers (LNA), by providing the LO in quadrature the I and Q baseband signals can be extracted in the receiver, yielding a much simpler (and cheaper) receiver chain.

In Fig. 7.6, the lower box shows a module containing the power amplifiers (PA) and its matching networks, the antenna switch, and a diplexer to connect the low- and high- frequency bands to the antenna.

To the left outside the boxes are the four receiver band bandpass filters. This shows a quad-band mobile device. The upper box shows the LNAs, the mixers, and the baseband amplifiers. The frequency synthesizer and voltage controlled oscillator (VCO) for receiving, and the VCO for transmitting, are also shown, together with the buffers that drive the PAs. The circuits in the upper box have been realized as a single chip. The receivers are of the homodyne type.

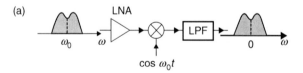

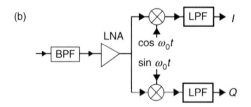

7.5 (a) Frontend of a homodyne receiver and (b) quadrature frontend of a homodyne receiver.

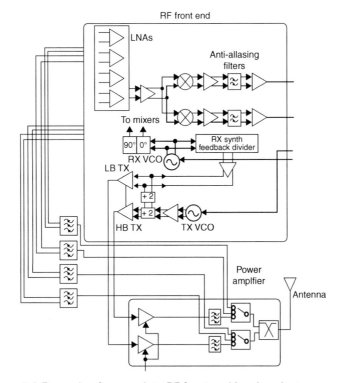

7.6 Example of a complete RF front end in a handset.

7.4 Conventional component technology

There are several components in a receiver front end that can benefit from being realized using MEMS technology when the complexity increases. Even at lower complexity levels MEMS competes with conventional technologies.

7.4.1 Antenna switches

In a conventional antenna switch, active elements such as PIN-diode switches or GaAs FET switches are used. As mentioned above, the antenna switch which, in addition to the switching between different receive bandpass filters, must switch the handset's single antenna also to the transmitter as GSM, is a TDMA system where the handset switches between receiving and transmitting with a period of a little less than 5 ms.

In Fig. 7.7, a conventional antenna switch using PIN diodes and quarter wave chokes is shown to the right. Only one RX/TX branch is shown. For a multiband antenna switch at least one branch is needed for each frequency

(a)

Current consumption	10 mA max
Switching device	PIN diode
Dimensions	4.5 × 3.2 × 1.5 mm
TX1 loss	824.869 MHz 1.2 dB max 880.915 MHz 1.2 dB max
TX1 attenuation	2fo 35 dB min 3fo 30 dB min
TX2 loss	1710..1785 MHz 1.4 dB max 1850..1910 MHz 1.4 dB max
TX2 attenuation	2fo 30 dB min 3fo 30 dB min
RX1 loss	869..894 MHz 1.1 dB max 925..960 MHz 1.1 dB max
RX2 loss	1805..1880 MHz 1.3 dB max 1930..1990 MHz 1.3 dB max

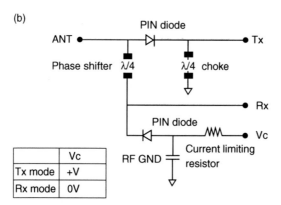

(b)

	Vc
Tx mode	+V
Rx mode	0V

7.7 Conventional antenna switch in a cell phone. (a) Example specification. (b) Simplified schematic of one branch.

band. The data shown are typical values for a two-band switch with ports for one antenna and two receiver chains and two transmitter chains. Note that the PIN-diode is 'on' when DC current is flowing through it. That is why the switch consumes current when operating. A MEMS switch can operate virtually without any power consumption.

7.4.2 Band select filters

Until recently the dominant technology for band select filters has been surface acoustic wave (SAW) filters (Fig. 7.8), based on the principle of an acoustic (mechanical) wave travelling on a structure on the surface of a chip made of a piezoelectric material. This makes the SAW structure rather large and the SAW chip technology differs significantly from normal semiconductor chip technology, which makes it almost impossible to integrate into a silicon or GaAs radio chip.

In Fig. 7.9, note the rather large area used by the SAW filters and their matching components. If replaced by bulk acoustic wave (BAW) filters (see Section 7.5.2) using MEMS technology the filters could be integrated into the transceiver chip saving a significant amount of printed circuit board (PCB) area.

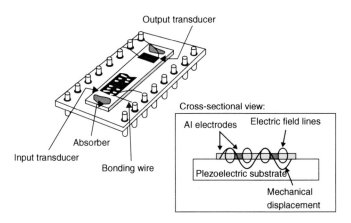

7.8 Example of a SAW-filter structure.

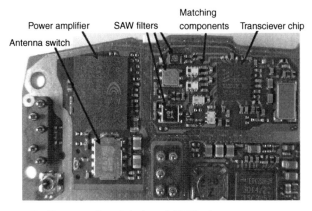

7.9 Radio part of a triple band GSM phone.

7.5 MEMS-based technology: filters, duplexers, switches, tunable devices and architecture

We now look at examples of how MEMS technology can be applied to wireless communication.

7.5.1 RF MEMS switches

A basic switch element in MEMS technology (Fig. 7.10) is the single-pole single-throw (SPST) switch. There have been lines of research trying to achieve metallic contact switches, but the tendency of the switch contacts to stick is difficult to overcome, especially if some RF power, such as in the transmit branch, is to be passed through the switch. Other lines of research have come up with a capacitive switch, where a change in capacitance between a fixed and a moving plate is used (see Fig. 7.11b). Since the plates are covered with a thin isolating layer there is no direct current passing through the switch and there is less tendency to stick. The actuation of a capacitive switch can be done in various ways but the most common and simple is to apply a DC voltage exceeding the maximum peak signal voltage across the switch element. This causes the moving plate to be attracted by electrostatic force to the fixed plate and the switch element is closed. It is important to design the switch and its control circuitry in such a way that the actuation voltage is at all times greater than the signal voltage, since self-actuation by the signal could otherwise occur.

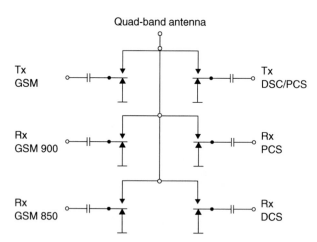

7.10 Schematic of a quad-band antenna switch to be realized with MEMS.

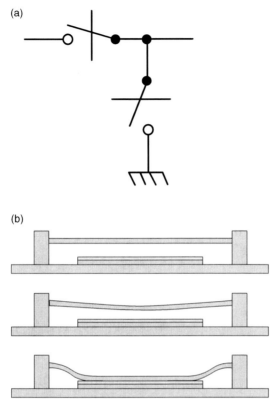

7.11 (a) An SPDT switch made out of two SPST switches and (b) a sketch of a capacitive membrane MEMS SPST switch.

The easiest way to make a single-pole double-throw (SPDT) switch when using MEMS technology is using SPST switches are shown in Fig. 7.11a. Figure 7.11b shows a MEMS switch from the side. At the top, the switch is inactive, at middle the switch is moving, and at bottom the switch is closed. On this particular switch there is an oxide layer on top of the fixed electrode to prevent stiction. Stiction is a phenomenon whereby the two switch surfaces stick to each other, even after the actuation is removed. Since this particular switch is designed for RF, the oxide layer will act as a dielectric layer and the movement of the switching electrode will vary the capacitance between a very low value of less than a pF and a high enough value, in the range of a few pF, to provide a low impedance path for the RF.

Figure 7.12 is an example of the layout of an early prototype MEMS antenna switch developed in an EU project together with imec and KU-Leuven. Each triangle shape is one switch element. Image courtesy of Jeroen De Coster, imec.

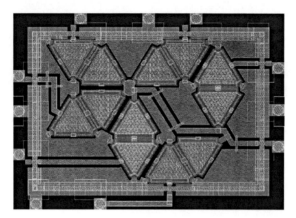

7.12 Example of layout of an early prototype MEMS antenna switch developed in an EU project together with imec and KU-Leuven. Each triangle shape is one switch element. Image courtesy of Jeroen De Coster, imec.

A properly designed MEMS switch works as a completely linear device, since there are no PN-junctions in the signal path and thus no non-linearities that generate harmonics and distortion to the switched RF signal. This reduces the need for low pass filtering to remove harmonics. The MEMS switch also has very low insertion loss of typically 0.1–0.5 dB compared to a PIN-diode switch, which has about 1.5–2.5 dB insertion loss. The isolation is also better in a MEMS switch, typically 20–35 dB compared to 15–25 dB for a PIN-diode switch.

7.5.2 Band select filters using MEMS

BAW filters are classified as MEMS devices. Just as in SAW filters, an electrical signal is converted to a mechanical vibration in a mechanically resonant structure. The BAW filter contains the vibration in the bulk of an AlN layer, whose shape and thickness sets the frequency and bandwidth of the filter. The mechanically vibrating AlN layer is mechanically isolated from the bulk of the silicon chip by layers forming a $\lambda/4$ Bragg reflector acting as a mirror (Fig. 7.13).

The BAW filter can rather easily be integrated onto a silicon chip with just the addition of a few extra processing steps.

Let us now compare a thin film bulk acoustic resonator (FBAR) filter with a conventional SAW-filter resonator (Table 7.3).

RF MEMS-based wireless architectures and front-ends

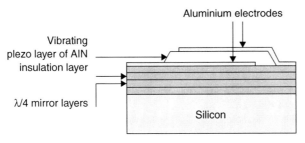

7.13 Example of physical design of a BAW, bulk acoustic filter. The thickness of each layer is about 1 μm. The λ/4 layers constitute a Bragg reflector.

Table 7.3 Comparison of FBAR and SAW filters

FBAR filter	SAW-filter
Frequency range of technology 10 MHz–10 GHz	Frequency range of technology 10 MHz to ~3 GHz
Passband loss < 1 dB	Passband loss ~ 2 dB
Out of band attenuation > 50 dB	Out of band attenuation ~ 35 dB
High power handling > 2 W	Limited power handling capacity ~ 100 mW
Can be manufactured in a RFIC compatible process with a few added process steps.	Manufactured in a dedicated non-silicon compatible process
Fairly small area on chip	Large area, often several mm²

7.5.3 Transmitter matching

Maximum power transfer to the antenna requires matching of the transmitter output impedance to the complex conjugate of the impedance of the antenna.

Present technology using fixed low Q matching of the transmitter, in such devices as a mobile phone, to the antenna over a whole transmission frequency band gives a power efficiency of roughly 47% in a class C PA, resulting in a total transmission power efficiency of about 35% in the mobile phone. Thus 65% of the DC power drawn from the battery during transmit becomes heat losses inside the mobile phone.

To minimize the current consumption of a transmitter we need to maximize its efficiency. This can be done by having a relatively high Q in the LC-network matching the transmitter's transistors (typically 2 ohms) to the antenna (50 ohms), making it necessary to tune the circuit inside the transmit frequency band to the actual frequency channel in use at the moment. The matching network must also be able to quickly change its frequency,

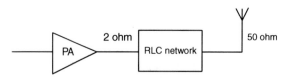

7.14 Between the PA and the antenna an impedance matching network is needed.

usually in less than about a millisecond, since the mobile device must support roaming between different base-stations which operate at different frequency channels. This can be done by using low loss MEMS switches switching in or out high Q MEMS-inductors and/or capacitors, or by having continuously adjustable low loss capacitors, or a combination of these.

A MEMS switch of the capacitive type (Fig. 7.11) consists of a fixed electrode and a spring-loaded moveable electrode. A variable MEMS capacitor is very similar in construction. By changing the separation between the electrodes, the capacitance is varied. The distance can be controlled by electrostatic forces created, for instance, with a DC voltage across the capacitor.

Using an RF MEMS tunable high Q channel bandwidth matching network the power efficiency in a class C PA can approach the theoretical value of 80%, giving a total power efficiency in the phone of about 60%. This almost doubles the talk time compared to using a low Q fixed matching network covering the whole frequency band, without increasing the battery capacity.

A tunable channel bandwidth RLC network can be integrated onto the PA chip or incorporated into a PA module (Fig. 7.14). To be able to select channels the high Q network must be tunable. The matching network will benefit greatly from being designed using low loss MEMS components.

7.6 Diversity in receivers and transmitters

In a mobile communications system, the radio signal path through the air is subject to multiple reflections, and the signal from the transmitter to the receiver can travel different distances and thus the same signal can reach the receiver with different strengths and delays in time. In addition, both the transmitter and receiver can be moving, both with respect to each other and relative to the surrounding reflecting objects. This creates fading. In a faded signal, the signal strength can reach almost zero for certain moments in time at certain positions in space. This leads to loss of information if a significant amount of redundant data is added to the transmitted information. The receiver and, to a certain degree, the transmitter architecture determines how much fading the communication link can cope with.

Antenna diversity, which is the use of multiple antennas and receivers/transmitters, helps reduce deep fading. The simplest way is just to double the antenna and receiver. When the receiver circuitry is doubled all the RF circuitry must also be doubled. To cope with this, we need to increase the miniaturization level which leads to **RF MEMS**.

In Fig. 7.15a we see two approaches to receiver diversity.

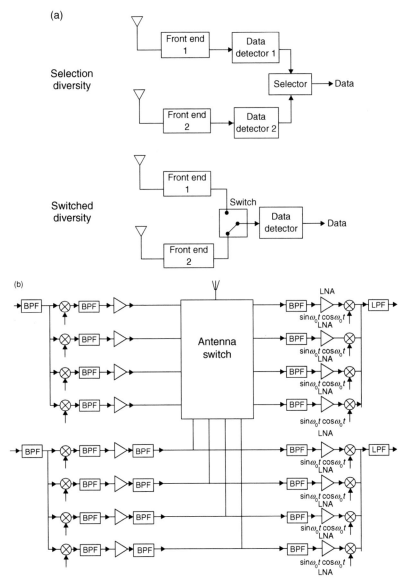

7.15 (a) Approaches to receiver diversity. (b) Example of frontend complexity for a quad-band diversity system.

Selection diversity uses only one antenna signal to the receiver at any given time. The antenna chosen, however, is based on the best signal-to-noise ratio (SNR) among the received signals. This requires that a pre-measurement takes place and that all antennas have established connections (at least during the SNR measurement). The actual selection process can take place in between received packets of information. This ensures that a single antenna connection is maintained as much as possible. Switching can then take place on a packet-by-packet basis if necessary. This works with slow fading. In a switching receiver, the signal from only one antenna is fed to the receiver for as long as the quality of that signal remains above some prescribed threshold. If and when the signal degrades, another antenna is switched in. Switching is the easiest and least power consuming of the antenna diversity processing techniques, but periods of fading and desynchronization may occur while the quality of one antenna degrades and another antenna link is established.

In Fig. 7.15b we see a block schematic of the RF parts of one receiver/transmitter for a quad-band system. For each added diversity channel, all the blocks shown must be added to the system.

7.7 Multi-input multi-output (MIMO) systems

A multi-input multi-output (MIMO) system uses many signal paths between transmitters and receivers to create a type of spatial multiplexing. The system measures the transfer parameters of the various channels α_{11}, α_{12} and so on to create a matrix **H** that describes the system transfer function. This is an expansion of the diversity concept but, in addition, the transfer matrix allows the system itself to optimize the transfer capacity of the transmission system. In an ideal MIMO system with high separation between the signal paths in the system, the diagonal elements of the matrix **H** will dominate and it is desirable to strive towards this in the design of a real world system. The more orthogonal the matrix **H** is, the more decoupled the MIMO channels are from each other and the higher the system transfer capacity will be.

The signal from each transmitter antenna is received slightly differently by each receiving antenna. How the signal from a transmitter antenna Tx_1 is received by a receiver antenna Rx_1 is described in α_{11}, the signal from a transmitter antenna Tx_1 to a receiver antenna Rx_2 is described in α_{21}, and so on, making up the transfer matrix **H**.

In a well-designed and well-functioning MIMO system (Fig. 7.16) the capacity can reach N (or M, whichever is smaller) times the capacity of a single channel system. Normally N = M and the matrix **H** is quadratic.

To cope with the high number of receivers and transmitters in a MIMO system, RF MEMS is needed to provide necessary miniaturization of RF-filters, antenna switches, matching networks for the transmitters, and so on, as described in Section 7.5.

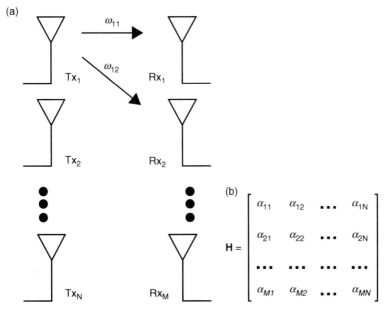

7.16 (a) Array of transmitters and receivers and (b) the resulting transfer matrix **H**.

7.8 Systems-on-a-chip

When systems become more and more complex, physical space needs to be used more and more efficiently in order to hold more components in the available space without making the mobile device impracticably large. To integrate all RF components on a single chip or in a module increases the component density significantly. To do this, RF MEMS is a most useful and perhaps even necessary technology. Figure 7.17 shows an example of what could be a large block of the communication parts in a mobile telephone. It is worth mentioning that MEMS is already used in the form of an accelerometer in many mobile devices to sense the orientation in which the device is held, for example, to be able to show the image on a smart phone display in the correct orientation.

7.9 Conclusion

Future demand for increasing capacity, miniaturization and cost reduction of mobile communication devices are driving the RF technology towards the use of MEMS for RF components. It is a technology that readily lends itself to be integrated into modules or even directly onto the RF-chips of silicon or other materials suited for the active RF components. Some devices, such

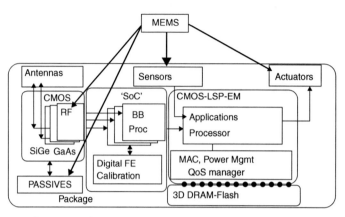

7.17 Example of a possible system in a package using MEMS.

as BAW filters, are already in production and packaged as discrete components or to be inserted in modules as bare chips. RF MEMS and other MEMS devices help significantly to achieve the performance needed from high functionality devices and to keep cost and size at a manageable level, so that these devices can be in everybody's hands.

7.10 Bibliography

Fisher G. *et al*. RF-MEMS and SiC/GaN as Enabling Technologies for a Reconfigurable Multi-Band/Multi-Standard Radio.

Razavi B., *RF Microelectronics*. Prentice-Hall, first ed., 1998 ETSI TS 125 102 V3.8.0 Universal Mobile Telecommunications System (UMTS); UTRA (UE) TDD; Radio Transmission and Reception (3GPP TS 25.102 version 3.8.0 Release 1999).

EN-Digital Cellular Telecommunications System (Phase 2+); Radio Transmission and Reception-3GPP TS 05.05 Version 8.9.0 Release 1999.

Loebl H. P., Metzmacher C., Milsom R. F., Tuinhout A., Lok P., and van Straten F., Solidly Mounted Bulk Acoustic Wave Filters, 2003 MRS Fall Meeting.

Mitsubishi Electric, Datasheets on various RF switches.

Mems2tune, private communication.

ISSCC 2005 feb 7, conference proceedings Design and characterization of RF-MEMS components', Katholieke Universiteit Leuven with ISBN number 978-90-5682-758-8.

8
RF MEMS technology for next-generation wireless communications

F. GIACOMOZZI and J. IANNACCI,
Fondazione Bruno Kessler, Italy

DOI: 10.1533/9780857098610.1.225

Abstract: This chapter discusses the use of microelectromechanical systems (MEMS) technology for the realization of next-generation microwave devices for wireless communications. This technology allows the fabrication of both improved performance lumped elements and newer tunable or reconfigurable complex networks, adding extra functionality in modern wireless systems. After an overview, the salient technological features of lumped element components, such as ohmic and capacitive switches, as well as variable capacitors and inductors, are presented. A technological platform for the fabrication of complex networks is then illustrated in detail, together with some examples of fabricated devices.

Key words: radio frequency microelectromechanical systems (RF MEMS) technology, RF passive components, RF MEMS switches, variable capacitors, varactors, inductors.

8.1 Introduction

In modern wireless and telecommunication applications, the requirements for high-performance radio frequency (RF) components and sub-systems are becoming more and more demanding, as the remarkable characteristics of such basic elements represent a critical key-point in enabling the integration of more functionality implemented in the same hardware, as well as in boosting their quality. Given such a scenario, microelectromechanical systems (MEMS) technology finds room as a valuable and real solution, enabling the manufacture of RF passive components and networks, characterized by very high performance and remarkable characteristics that cannot be achieved with the currently diffused solutions based, for instance, on standard semiconductor technology platforms (e.g. complementary metal oxide semiconductor (CMOS)). Beside the very high performance enabled by MEMS devices for RF applications, referred to as RF MEMS, another important characteristic makes them very interesting for application in wireless and telecommunication systems, namely their reconfigurability. Networks and components based on RF MEMS technology indeed enable the implementation of a significant number of different states and configurations, as well as tuning one or more of their characteristics within wide ranges and with a typically pronounced linearity. These characteristics, namely large reconfigurability and tunability, represent the *Holy Grail* in modern and next-generation wireless applications, as the trend followed in the design and realization of new RF platforms and devices is clearly oriented towards the integration of more and more functionalities in the same hardware. In synthesis, RF MEMS technology possesses the critical features of both high performance and reconfigurability, making it a very good candidate for reaching a wide and capillary exploitation in next-generation wireless systems, on a mass market production basis. The exploitation of RF MEMS technology in wireless and telecommunication systems can be framed at two different levels. On one level, such a technology enables the manufacture of lumped components with very high performance. The most relevant lumped elements enabled by RF MEMS technology fall into the categories of switches (or relays), variable capacitors (also referred to as varactors), and inductors. The most relevant characteristics they show are good isolation, low losses and very high quality factor (Q factor), wide tuning range, good linearity and very low (virtually zero) power consumption. By following an increasing complexity trend, these basic elements can be exploited for the realization of RF networks, sub-blocks and functional circuits, of which they represent the constitutive bricks. Consequently, by putting together micro-switches, varactors and inductors, it is possible to assemble impedance matching networks, filters, phase shifters, switching matrices, RF power splitters, and so on, entirely based on RF MEMS technology. On the other level, these devices are also characterized by a very wide reconfigurability, making them critical components for the integration of additional functionalities in modern wireless systems. Given all these considerations, it is straightforward to understand that RF MEMS technology holds the potential to make the difference in next-generation wireless communication systems. However, some relevant aspects related to such a technology are still limiting its diffusion into large volume market applications, and can be summarized in three key words: reliability, packaging, and integration. RF MEMS devices, being characterized by movable micro-parts and membranes, are subjected to several sources of malfunctioning and failure that are typical of mechanical structures, and nearly totally unknown, on the other hand, for standard semiconductor components. The most relevant are fatigue, creep, plastic deformation, ageing, and delamination.

The presence of electrical fields and RF signals also affects MEMS operation, such as malfunctioning of RF MEMS electrostatically controlled switches caused by the stiction, which is the non-release of the movable structure when the biasing voltage is removed, due to the charge entrapped in the dielectric layer, as well as caused by the micro-welding of metal contacts. The latter phenomenon is more frequent in the case of large RF signals (power handling). Besides the critical failure due to stiction, the malfunctioning of an RF MEMS switch has to be identified also in the performance drifts, as happens with the charge entrapment phenomenon. In this, the unwanted potential caused by the charge acts as a spurious direct current (DC) bias, causing the shift of the actuation (pull-in) and release (pull-out) voltages, also referred to as screening phenomena. Finally, RF MEMS structures are rather sensitive towards the conditions of the environment where they are operating. To this end, moisture, dust particles, and contaminants in general, are common sources of partial malfunctioning as well as of irreversible failure. Several strategies are available and pursuable to mitigate and/or eliminate one or more of these failure mechanisms, making, in turn, the RF MEMS devices more robust and reliable. Indeed, it is possible to act at the technology level by developing materials and processes that are less prone to induce failure. For example, insulating layers of better quality, in which the charge entrapment is less pronounced can be tested and employed. Moreover, it is also possible acting at design level, by appropriately shaping the structural MEMS parts, as well as the contacts, in such a way as to mitigate mechanical and electrical device failure, for example, by avoiding stress concentrations. Another possible strategy to improve reliability is to act at operation level, controlling the MEMS devices by keeping them in a safe regime of functioning. For instance, an appropriate shaping of the waveform applied to the device, in order to actuate it, can prevent abrupt contacts with the movable parts and their mechanical degradation. The second additional aspect is the packaging, which is closely related to the issue of reliability. RF MEMS devices, because of their mechanical fragility, cannot be included as they are within an RF circuit or system, but need to be encapsulated at first. The package is a protective lid applied to RF MEMS devices, ensuring their mechanical protection from shocks, as well as their isolation from contaminants, dust particles, moisture, and so on. Besides, the package has also to be carefully designed and realized, in order to ensure the redistribution of the electrical signals, from the RF MEMS devices to the external world.

The goal of this chapter is to provide the reader with useful information about the critical aspects that must be addressed in order to reach the outstanding performance of RF MEMS devices mentioned above, as well as about their solutions at technology and design level. The chapter is arranged as follows: Section 8.2 gives a brief overview. Section 8.3 presents the salient features of electrostatically activated devices and of lumped RF MEMS components, such as ohmic and capacitive switches, varactors and inductors, as well as some of the most relevant issues at manufacturing level. Section 8.4 presents the fabrication process developed at Fondazione

Bruno Kessler (FBK), to give the reader a detailed example of a technological platform for the fabrication of both lumped components and complex RF circuits. The chapter is concluded by Section 8.5, where some examples of high-performance devices, such as single-pole double-throw (SPDT) and single-pole four-throw (SP4T) switches, switching matrices and phase shifters are presented.

8.2 RF MEMS technology

MEMS technology is well developed and extensively used for the manufacture of sensors and actuators, such as pressure sensors, accelerometers, gyroscopes, micro-mirrors, ink jet printers and hard disk-head fine positioning. The basic fabrication process is derived from monolithic planar technology, adding mechanical to electrical functionality and is potentially CMOS compatible, even if some materials are incompatible and therefore cannot be processed in the same facility. When using MEMS technology to realize devices working at high frequency (up to hundreds of GHz) dimensions are comparable with the signal wavelength, and interaction between adjacent components becomes important. This induces additional constraints, not only in the design but also in fabrication.

For the realization of RF MEMS devices there is not a well-defined and standardized fabrication technology as for CMOS, but rather several fabrication processes customized for specific purposes. Some basic fabrication steps are common, despite different materials, deposition technologies and patterning methods being used. In order to reduce the fabrication cost and to improve the throughput, batch semiconductor processing and related equipment are used, adding movable structures such as cantilever and clamped-clamped beams obtained by micromachining techniques. RF circuits and control electronics can be realized on the same substrate, yielding high flexibility at the expense of an increasing process complexity.

The definition of the most appropriate RF MEMS fabrication flow must be done, accounting for the different types of structures that must be manufactured, and for the critical aspects they introduce. With regard to this, the most common RF MEMS basic elements are fixed and variable capacitors, inductors and switches. Highly conductive RF signal lines connect different components, realizing input and output terminations for the intrinsic MEMS devices. Additional signal lines, working in DC or low-frequency regimes, are required for delivering biasing signals and for controlling, in turn, the micro-devices.

Switches can be realized in many different configurations (Tilmans, 2002). The RF signal can be transmitted by a resistive (ohmic) metal-to-metal contact, or by the capacitive coupling between two metal plates across an

RF MEMS technology for wireless communications   229

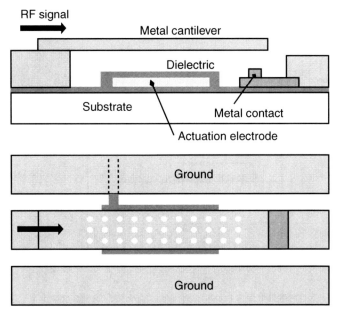

8.1 Schematic of a cantilever-based series ohmic metal-to-metal contact switch. In the rest (up) position, represented in the figure, the signal line is open. When a voltage is applied to the actuation electrode, the electrostatic force moves down the suspended cantilever realizing an ohmic metal-to-metal contact closing the signal line.

insulating (dielectric) layer. The switch can operate in series when it opens or closes a contact on a signal line, or in shunt configuration when the switch connects or disconnects the signal line to ground. The movable parts of the switch can be actuated in different ways. The most common is the electrostatic actuation (Rebeiz, 2003) where an attractive Coulomb force is generated by a voltage drop imposed across a fixed and a movable electrode. Devices can be operated by using negligible power, but they require a high voltage that is often not directly available on wireless devices, and therefore additional voltage multiplier circuits are needed. The fabrication process is relatively simple in concept, because many of the steps used are similar to standard integrated circuit (IC) fabrication.

Other diffused actuation mechanisms are piezoelectric, electro-thermal and electro-magnetic (Lisec, 2010). In piezoelectric devices, a piezoelectric film and a top electrode are deposited on the movable structure. By applying a voltage, the piezoelectric material deforms, inducing beam bending.

The piezoelectric actuation requires low actuation voltage and allows fast response and reasonable power consumption, but the fabrication technology is more complex and frequently the deposition temperature required to

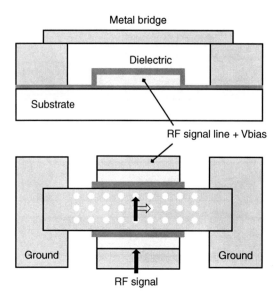

8.2 Schematic of a capacitive shunt switch. In the rest (up) position the RF signal flows through the signal line under the grounded suspended bridge. When the bias voltage is applied to the bottom electrode, the bridge is pulled down by the electrostatic force, touching the dielectric over the underpass line and the high-capacitance shorts to ground the RF signal opening, in turn, the line.

obtain good quality piezoelectric material is high and not compatible with the high-conductivity metal layers needed for RF circuits.

In electro-thermal devices the actuation is induced by the heat produced by the current flowing in a resistor. The thermal expansion generated by the change in temperature induces a movement or displacement (Blondy *et al.*, 2001). It requires a simple technology and low actuation voltage, but the response is slow and thermally inefficient (all the heat is not converted into actuation) and the high actuation power required is not suitable for wireless communications.

In electro-magnetic switches (Tilmans *et al.*, 1999) the current flowing in coils will induce a magnetic field that can actuate the switch. Typically, the fabrication is quite complex and the power consumption can be high.

Among all the possible configurations, the most widely used and the most suitable for wireless applications is represented by electrostatically actuated series ohmic and shunt capacitive switches (Tilmans *et al.*, 2002). The schematic of the two kinds of switches is presented in Figs 8.1 and 8.2.

The main difference is in the frequency behaviour. In ohmic switches the isolation reduces with increasing frequency, being very high from DC to a few GHz and still acceptable up to tens of GHz. On the contrary, shunt capacitive switches are not effective at DC and low frequency and start working at some GHz. The isolation increases with frequency up to a maximum, depending on the device capacitive and inductive behaviour, which has to be suitably dimensioned at design level.

8.3 RF MEMS technology for high-performance passive components

This section reports about the relevant technological features for the fabrication of high-performance passive lumped components. For each device, namely electrostatically actuated switches, capacitors and inductors and their basic parts, the main technological requirements and the materials to be used are analysed.

8.3.1 Electrostatically actuated devices

In electrostatically actuated switches a voltage is applied between two electrodes, one of which is movable, generating an attraction force that deflects the beam (Rebeiz, 2003). When the voltage is removed the beam returns to the rest position, due to the elastic restoring force. The actuation voltage depends on the electrode configuration, beam geometry and material, as well as on the distance between the electrodes (Rebeiz, 2003). By reducing the switch stiffness it is possible to design switches that can be actuated using a low voltage, despite this implying a low restoring force that increases the probability of stiction. Considering actuation speed (decreasing the spring constant will increase the switching time), repeatability of the contact and reliability, it is usually necessary to use a high actuation voltage; 30 to 50 V is common, but it can be up to 100 V. Because the current involved in the operation is very low the dissipated power is minimal, allowing the use of electrostatic actuated devices in battery-powered systems. The required actuation voltage can be obtained by a charge pump circuit (Aaltonen and Halonen, 2009).

Many different RF MEMS switch configurations have been demonstrated, but from the fabrication point of view there are some features and technology solutions in common between them, such as the movable membrane with contacts, suspended structures (air bridges), dielectric layers for isolation and, to realize capacitors, highly conductive metal lines for RF signal transmission, including the underpass lines, that is, the part of signal line under the movable membrane, actuation electrodes and biasing lines.

8.3.2 RF signal lines and biasing lines

The RF signal lines, either in coplanar waveguide (CPW) or microstrip configuration, are usually made of aluminium, aluminium-based alloys or gold, although in some cases copper has been used (Morris *et al.*, 2003). To have low resistance, high thickness is required, usually a few microns. Aluminium is deposited by sputtering and dry etching, while gold and copper are usually deposited by electroplating inside a photoresist moulding mask. To reduce losses it is important to minimize coupling with closer structures and substrate. In particular on high-resistivity silicon substrate, the charging phenomenon at the interface between the silicon surface and the insulating silicon oxide can induce a conductive channel that can introduce a few dB of losses in the signal lines. To avoid this effect, different solutions have been considered, such as high temperature annealing after thermal oxidation, or the deposition of a layer of non-doped polycrystalline silicon (Gamble *et al.*, 1999) or amorphous silicon (Rong *et al.*, 2004) before oxide deposition. Ion implantation of the Si–SiO$_2$ interface, to create traps in order to reduce mobility of charges, has proven to be useful too (Jansman *et al.*, 2003).

The underpass line is the part of signal line that runs beneath the suspended structures, and it consists of electrodes and contacts as well. To avoid or reduce non-planarization effects on the movable membranes above, due to vertical steps on buried layers, the underpass lines must be thin. Moreover, they have to be flat and smooth in order to realize a good contact when the switch is actuated, particularly in the case of capacitive contact where an intimate contact between electrodes is necessary to achieve the desired high-capacitance value. In ohmic switches it is preferable to have a hard surface to reduce the wear of the contacting surfaces. On the other hand, in capacitive contact switches the underpass has to be covered by a dielectric film and therefore its material must not be negatively affected by the dielectric deposition temperature avoiding roughness increase. Sometimes the underpass is fabricated by depositing a thinner layer of the same material used for the signal line, but frequently a different material is used to optimize the contact area. Because the underpass is relatively short, resistivity is not so critical and refractory materials such as W, Mo, Ru and Pt have been used for their thermal stability.

To apply the actuation voltage to the electrodes, biasing lines are required. Because they are very close to, or cross, the RF lines, coupling effects can induce significant loss. High resistances are required to decouple the RF from the AC/DC signals. The biasing lines can be either fabricated by high-resistivity materials such as polysilicon or, most commonly, realized by Al or Au metal lines adding lumped resistors to realize the decoupling.

8.3.3 Movable structures

The movable structures are the key parts of the switches and have both electric and mechanical functions. They must be highly conductive to transmit the RF signal, elastic in order to deform, and stiff enough to provide the restoring force when the actuation voltage is removed. The structures have to be flat and present a low internal stress and stress gradient to reduce distortion. Both the fabrication process and the design have to be tailored to meet these specifications.

Either clamped–clamped beam or cantilever configuration are used, possibly with suitably designed anchoring parts to reduce the effects of stress accumulation and temperature gradients. Cantilevers are very compact and, because they are free on one side, can deform to compensate the stress, despite inducing a change in the air gap, thereby modifying the actuation voltage.

Double-clamped beams are more robust and present higher restoring force, reducing stiction problems, but their stiffness can be strongly influenced by residual stress that can significantly change the actuation voltage. Moreover, they are more sensitive to temperature, due to the difference in thermal expansion coefficients between beam and substrate. Careful design of the anchoring system and bridge geometry will reduce these effects (Nieminen et al., 2004), but the fabrication process has to provide a low, uniform and repeatable tensile stress.

Usually the same high-conductivity metal of the signal lines, such as gold, aluminium or aluminium alloys, is used, but copper (Balaraman et al., 2002) and nickel (Pacheco et al., 2000; Zavracky et al., 1997) have been used too. Palego et al. (2009) used molybdenum membrane because, due to its reduced thermal expansion coefficient, it is less sensitive to temperature changes. In some cases the movable membranes are realized in silicon or polysilicon, or by using dielectric films, such as silicon nitride, with metal areas for contacts and actuation electrodes. WiSpry used three-layer gold-silicon oxide-gold to obtain a stress-compensated bridge (Morris et al., 2003).

The movable and suspended structures are generally fabricated by surface micromachining, that is, they are deposited over a sacrificial layer that is later removed to release the membrane. To facilitate the process, a matrix of uniformly distributed holes is typically realized on the movable membrane. This contributes to increase the actuation speed too, by reducing the air viscous damping. Many combinations of membrane materials, sacrificial layer and release technique are reported in the literature. One of the simplest technological solutions is to use photoresist or other polymers, such as polyimide, and deposit over it a metal layer by sputtering or electroplating. Oxygen plasma can easily remove the polymer. The process is simple and compatible with standard microelectronic technology, but there are limitations to the maximum temperature that can be used, and planarization can be difficult.

Aluminium and copper (Zavracky *et al.*, 1997) have also been used as sacrificial layers and removed by wet etching. To avoid sticking problem during liquid evaporation, supercritical drying is required. Copper allows obtaining very flat structures by planarization using chemical mechanical polishing (CMP). Silicon oxide is frequently used in MEMS sensors and sometimes in RF MEMS too, and it can be easily removed by hydrofluoric acid (HF) vapour or dry etching.

8.3.4 RF MEMS ohmic metal-to-metal contact switches

Ohmic switches (Fig. 8.3) are based on a resistive metal-to-metal contact. In the actuated state the signal is transmitted through the ohmic contact. At low frequency the insertion loss is mainly due to the contact resistance. On the other hand, at higher frequency parasitic capacitance and inductance contribute to the losses and have to be minimized by proper design. In the non-actuated state the contact is open and the isolation is very good both in DC and low RF frequency. Increasing the frequency, the capacitance of the switch in the up-position, and other residual capacitance and inductance contributions, play a role in transmitting some signal and reducing, in turn, the isolation. The isolation is still good enough for practical applications up to a few tens of GHz.

The metal-to-metal contact is the critical part. It should be highly conductive to have low insertion loss, and it must be highly reliable. Wear, corrosion and contamination can deteriorate the RF performance, and adhesion and stiction phenomena can lead to device failure. In the simplest configuration the contact is made directly between the movable structure and the underpass line. Consequently, materials and deposition process have to be chosen in order to have a good contact. In some cases to optimize performance a dedicated metal layer has been deposited under the bridge or over the underpass line. As an example, Almeida *et al.* (2006) presented a laterally actuated switch with 20 μm electroplated Ni as structural material, covered by electroplated gold to improve the contact resistance.

Oxidation of the surface of the materials in contact will lead to a poor contact and therefore such metals as aluminium and copper, frequently used in microelectronics, are not appropriate. Gold is a good candidate and is largely used, due to its high conductivity and its chemical inertness, but it is expensive and quite soft. If the contact is not well designed it can deform and wear after a relatively small number of actuation cycles and micro-welding can induce failure by permanent stiction, particularly in the case of 'hot switching'. Contact between two hard metals, or between gold and a hard metal such as tungsten or ruthenium (Broue *et al.*, 2010), has been shown to enhance mechanical resistance, but at the expense of an increased contact resistance.

To improve hardness and Young's modulus, gold alloys were tested, adding other metals such as ruthenium, rhodium (Lee *et al.*, 2006), nickel (Yang *et al.*, 2009), palladium and platinum (Chen *et al.*, 2007).

Another possibility is to use multi-layered structures (Mulloni *et al.*, 2012), stacking many alternate layers of gold and a harder metal and inducing partial alloying by controlled thermal treatment. The presence of interfaces is a barrier for mechanical dislocation migration and induces further hardening. Gold can be left on external surfaces to preserve its low resistance characteristics.

The contact resistance depends not only on the materials in contact but on the contact force (the higher the force the lower the resistance) and area too. Internal stress induces distortion of movable structures and the contact area can be not reproducible from device to device. A good solution to have a well-defined contact area despite bridge distortion is to design small contact dimples, either on the fixed or the movable part. To better control the contact force, the movable part can be constituted of parts with different rigidities, either by design or by changing the thickness. As an example concerning the FBK ohmic switches, in order to have a reproducible contact force and position, the area is defined by small diameter 600 nm thick polysilicon dimples under the metal signal line. As shown in Fig. 8.3 the central part of the movable membrane over the actuation electrode is made thicker, in order to be rigid and remain flat during displacement, while the part close to the contact area is thinner, in order to have a controlled deflection. The contact force is defined by the dimple thickness and by the elastic constant of the tip (Farinelli *et al.*, 2007).

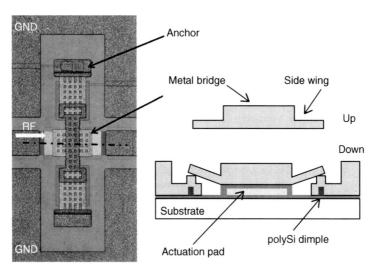

8.3 Picture and schematic cross-section of an electrostatic actuated ohmic switch. The metal-to-metal contact is obtained by a movable clamped–clamped beam. The contact force is controlled by the deflection of side wings over the contact dimples.

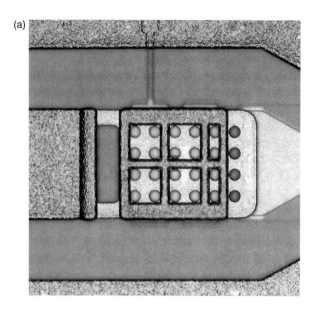

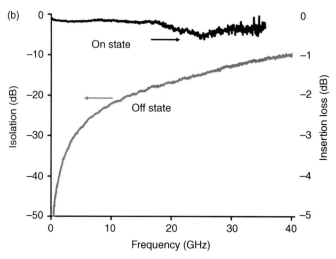

8.4 (a) Picture of an electrostatically actuated cantilever ohmic switch. The cantilever is anchored to the signal line by two narrow legs on the left side, while it is free to move on the right side. (b) Typical transmission parameters: isolation in the OFF state and insertion loss in the ON state of a cantilever ohmic switch.

An image of a cantilever ohmic switch is shown in Fig. 8.4a. The switch is 170 μm long, 110 μm wide, and has an air gap of 3 μm. The cantilever is anchored on the left side while the right side is free to move and touches the metal underpass line in correspondence to the contact dimples. The central part, over the actuation electrode, is made more rigid by thicker gold, in order to reduce stress-induced distortions. Figure 8.4b reports the typical behaviour of a cantilever switch with the isolation in the OFF state decreasing with frequency. In the actuated state the insertion loss is less than 0.2 dB up to 20 GHz, and better than 0.5 dB up to 40 GHz. The contact resistance is 0.9 ohms.

8.3.5 RF MEMS capacitive contact switches

On capacitive shunt switches the movable armature is connected to ground (Fig. 8.5). In the non-actuated position it is separated from the signal line by an air gap realizing a small capacitance, that is, high impedance, and the RF signal flows through the line with a minimum loss. When the movable membrane is actuated, the two metal electrodes are ideally separated only by the thin dielectric film covering the bottom contact, realizing a high capacitance that induces a low impedance path, and the RF signal flows from the line to ground through the capacitor.

In contrast to an ohmic device, in a capacitive switch there is no metal contact between the termination, and the RF signal passes through a (variable) capacitive coupling. This means that a shunt capacitive switch in the ON state shorts to ground RF signals (i.e. open switch), but passes to the output termination DC and low-frequency signals, regardless of the state

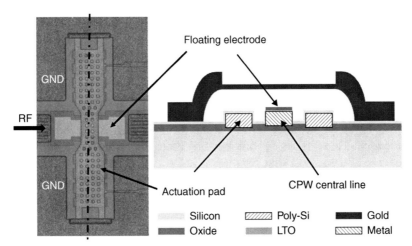

8.5 Picture and schematic cross-section of a capacitive shunt switch using separated electrodes for contact and actuation (four-terminal configuration). Electrostatic actuation is obtained by applying a voltage to the lateral electrodes while the capacitive contact is realized between the movable bridge and the isolated metal underpass constituting the central line of a CPW. A gold floating electrode is deposited over the dielectric on the lower contact in order to have a well-defined and repetitive capacitance value independently of stress-induced distortions of the movable bridge.

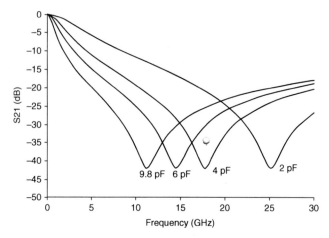

8.6 Simulated isolation parameters of a capacitive shunt switch in the actuated position. The value of capacitance in the actuated position (C_{on}) strongly influences the frequency behaviour, and therefore it is important that the fabrication process allows obtaining a highly repeatable and uniform value.

of the MEMS micro-switch. In the DC and low-frequency regimes, indeed, the capacitive coupling to ground is not sufficient to create a low impedance path to ground.

The higher isolation is obtained at the LC series resonant frequency (Rebeiz, 2003) defined by

$$f = \frac{1}{2\pi}\frac{1}{\sqrt{LC_{on}}} \qquad [8.1]$$

where C_{on} is the capacitance in the actuated state and L is the inductance of the switch. These types of switches are therefore suited only for high frequencies, and the working frequency range can be defined by design, as indicated in Fig. 8.6. From the graph it appears clear that to obtain the desired RF performances the capacitance in the actuated state has to be accurate and reproducible from device to device.

Due to the presence of the dielectric, it is also possible to use the contact as the actuation electrode (Fig. 8.2). The biasing signal is applied directly to the RF signal line, realizing a two-terminal configuration (Tilmans, 2002). Decoupling capacitors and/or choke inductors, either external or on-chip, are required to avoid the biasing signal from flowing along the RF lines. A four-terminal configuration with separate electrodes for contact and actuation, as in Fig. 8.5, is more bulky and requires a longer fabrication process but adds much more design flexibility.

The main parameter to consider for the fabrication of capacitive switches is the ratio between the capacitance in the actuated and non-actuated positions. To obtain low capacitance in the up-position, small electrodes and high electrode distance (air gap) are required. Because the actuation voltage depends on the initial air gap (Rebeiz, 2003), it has to be limited. Typical values of the air gap are in the range from 1.5 to 4 µm. To have high capacitance in the actuated position, large electrodes and a thin dielectric with high relative dielectric constant (ε_r) are needed. The minimum thickness of the dielectric is limited because it must provide DC isolation without breakdown. Typical values are 100–200 nm, depending on the characteristics of the material used.

A critical aspect for reliability is the dielectric charging that modifies the actuation voltage and induces switch sticking. Therefore, this aspect must involve careful consideration in the choice of the dielectric material and its deposition method. The charging effects are strongly correlated to the dielectric structure. Stoichiometric films with low crystallographic defects exibit reduced charging phenomena, but to obtain this kind of film, usually high deposition temperatures, not compatible with the fabrication, are required.

Many different dielectrics can be used, the most common being silicon oxide ($\varepsilon_r \approx 4$) and nitride ($\varepsilon_r \approx 7$–8), which can be easily deposited, even at the low temperature required for the MEMS fabrication, by using standard microelectronic process such as low temperature oxide (LTO) chemical vapour deposition and plasma-enhanced chemical vapour deposition (PECVD). The film obtained at low temperature presents a high number of defects and lower quality. The PECVD silicon nitride has higher dielectric constant but usually, due to the high hydrogen content and defects in the film, it suffers from higher charging effects that reduce reliability.

High- ε_r dielectrics, such as lead zirconium titanate (PZT) ($\varepsilon_r = 150$–200), barium strontium titanate (BST) ($\varepsilon_r > 200$) and tantalum oxide (Ta_2O_5) ($\varepsilon_r \approx 25$) (Lisec et al., 2004), have been tested but deposition of good quality film at low temperature is difficult and high charging is frequently found. A promising material seems to be sputtered AlN ($\varepsilon_r \approx 10$); a deposition process has been developed using dedicated equipment allowing densely packed grains with reduced defects to be obtained (Lisec et al., 2004).

To reduce charging phenomena and improve reliability it is possible to use the dielectric-less approach (Blondy et al., 2004; Mardivirin et al., 2009). By placing stoppers, either on the movable bridge or on the underpass, direct contact is avoided and a thin air layer remains acting as a dielectric. The air layer must be thick enough to avoid breakdown and, therefore, the obtainable capacitance is limited.

On the four-terminal configurations, where the electrodes for electrostatic actuation and the RF contacts are separated, it is possible to optimize separately the dielectrics. A thin dielectric layer on the contact is optimized for RF performance while, on the actuation electrode, it is possible to use the dielectric-less configuration or a thicker dielectric to better sustain the actuation voltage reducing the electric field and the charging phenomena.

Due to surface roughness, internal stress that deforms the movable membrane, and topological problems, the contact of the two electrodes is not perfect and a residual equivalent air gap remains, reducing the capacitance in the actuated state with respect to the designed value. This effect is not uniform, and the capacitance changes from die to die modifying the performance and the working frequency band. To mitigate the problem, both smart design and accurate control of the fabrication process to reduce roughness and stress are required.

A good solution was developed at imec, by adding a floating metal electrode over the dielectric. The value of the capacitance is defined by the overlap of floating electrode and the signal line underpass, and not by the movable membrane. It is therefore possible to obtain a uniform capacitance close to the theoretical value. The movable membrane has just to touch the floating electrode to realize an ohmic metal-to-metal contact. The dimensions of the membrane can be strongly reduced obtaining a much smaller capacitance in the non-actuated state and therefore a much higher capacitance ratio in the so-called boosted configuration (Rottemberg *et al.*, 2002). Figure 8.7 represents a boosted capacitive switch fabricated at FBK. The movable membrane is modified in order to have just three narrow bars over the contact area, touching the floating electrode on contact dimples. The capacitance ratio is close to 200, but it can be easily increased by acting at design level. The RF measured behaviour results to be very close to the simulated one and repeatability from device to device is quite high.

8.3.6 RF MEMS variable capacitors

Capacitors are a key element in RF circuits. Fixed capacitors can be easily realized by interposing a dielectric, either an insulator (MIM) or air (MAM) between two conductive metal layers. Because there are no moving parts, charging is not an issue and high ε_r dielectrics can be used.

RF MEMS technology allows changing the capacitance by realizing either switchable capacitors (Palego *et al.*, 2006) or tunable varactors. Furthermore, it is possible to use switches to connect or disconnect any element of a fixed capacitor bank. Brank *et al.* (2001) and Entesari and Rebeiz (2005) presented tunable filters realized by using capacitive switches to connect series-fixed capacitors. WiSpry is fabricating antenna tuners for cell phones with digital capacitors (Natarajan *et al.*, 2011).

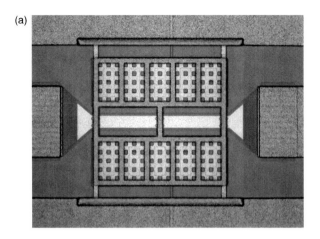

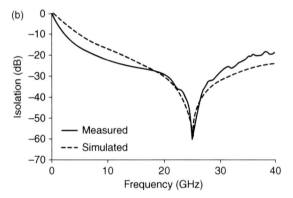

8.7 (a) Picture of a capacitive shunt switch in 'boosted' configuration. In the actuated position the movable membrane touches the floating metal realizing a high capacitance defined by the floating metal-dielectric-underpass line MIM capacitor that is independent of bridge distortions or surface roughness, and therefore highly repeatable. In the up-position only three narrow bars overlap the underpass inducing a very small metal-air-metal (MAM) capacitance. (b) The measured isolation parameter is similar to the simulated one, indicating that the capacitance in the actuated state is close to the designed value.

Parallel-plate capacitive contact switches are basically variable capacitors. By applying or removing a fixed voltage the capacitance switches between two values. The higher one in the actuated state is defined by the dimension of the contact electrodes and the thickness and dielectric constant of the dielectric material. When the switch is released the air gap that is in series with the dielectric defines the lower value of capacitance.

Tunability can be obtained by applying an analogue control voltage. By increasing the applied voltage the force induced by the electric field deflects the beam, reducing the air gap and therefore increasing the capacitance. When the displacement is one-third of the initial gap the electrostatic force becomes higher than the elastic force induced by the deformation, and the beam snaps down (Tilmans, 2002). The theoretical tunability range is therefore limited to a maximum increase of 50% with respect to the low capacitance value in the up-position. In fabricated devices fringing field and parasitic capacitance introduce other limitations, and capacitance ratios in the range 1.42–1.27 were reported (Rebeiz, 2003).

A higher capacitance ratio can be obtained by using a four-terminal configuration with the air gap between contact electrodes smaller than the air gap between actuation electrodes, in order to reach the full excursion before the actuation electrode reaches the one-third limit (Nieminen *et al.*, 2002). Zou *et al.* (2001) fabricated devices on Pyrex glass using evaporated gold as the bottom electrode. The sacrificial layer was made from evaporated copper in two steps in order to obtain the 2 and 3 µm variable height spacer. The movable membrane was realized by electroplated Permalloy. Afterwards copper wet etching supercritical carbon dioxide dryer was used to avoid stiction.

Three-plate variable capacitors were also reported by Dec and Suyama (2000), using a process with three layers of polysilicon separated by silicon oxide. The oxide was removed by HF wet etching followed by supercritical carbon dioxide drying. Gold was deposited over the top polysilicon layer to reduce resistance.

Variable capacitors can also be obtained by modifying the electrode-overlap area. Rockwell demonstrated interdigitated structures where a movable suspended electrode is moved on the plane by electrostatic forces modifying the overlapping area with respect to a fixed electrode, obtaining a tuning ratio of 3 (Yao *et al.*, 1998). The devices were made of silicon, starting from silicon on insulator (SOI) wafer having 30 µm of silicon over a silicon oxide interlayer. The interdigitated structure was obtained by deep reactive ion etching (DRIE) stopping on the oxide. To reduce parasitic losses the substrate was removed selectively on the back side of the device by a second DRIE step. The silicon oxide was removed by HF and supercritical drying.

By using an adhesive bonding process and design improvements, performances were further enhanced. After deposition and patterning of the aluminium layer on the back side of the device, the SOI wafers were epoxy-bonded to a carrier glass wafer and the silicon substrate and buried oxide completely removed. Aluminium was deposited and patterned on the top side and the silicon etched by DRIE. The structures were released by isotropic etching of the epoxy in oxygen plasma (Borwick *et al.*, 2003). Due to DRIE process improvements it was possible to increase the thickness of the capacitor finger up to 80 µm. A capacitance ratio of 8.4 was obtained with a voltage of 8V.

8.3.7 RF MEMS inductors

Inductors integrated in the substrate are required for many RF circuits, but losses and parasitic capacitance induced by the substrate can reduce the Q factor and the maximum frequency. This effect can be quite high on low resistivity silicon.

Meandered ribbon inductors (Fig. 8.8a) can be easily fabricated in planar technology by using just a metal layer. Spiral inductors present higher

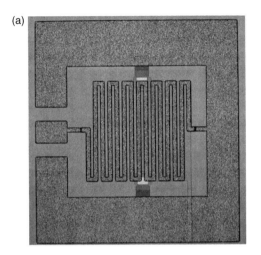

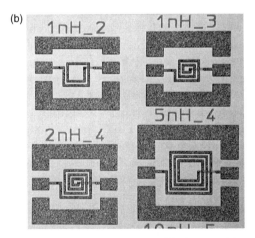

8.8 Pictures of air-suspended inductors (a) meander ribbon, and (b) spiral based. The inductors, realized by surface micromachining, present 5 μm thick gold lines suspended in air over the substrate, after removing 4,5 μm thick sacrificial photoresist. On spiral inductors, a metal underpass connects the spiral central point to the output.

inductance and therefore are preferable, but the need to connect the central point to the outside requires a second metal layer to realize either an air bridge crossover or an underpass line (Fig. 8.8b). To obtain low resistance, thick layers of high-conductive metal are required and therefore electroplated copper or gold are frequently used.

Different approaches have been used to reduce the substrate influence and to obtain higher Q inductors, either increasing the distance to substrate or removing the substrate.

By using DRIE or anisotropic wet etching with potassium hydroxide (KOH) or tetramethylammonium hydroxide (TMAH), the Si substrate can be completely removed by bulk micromachining from the back side, leaving the device suspended on a thin dielectric membrane (Chi and Rebeiz, 1995; López-Villegas *et al.*, 2000). As an alternative, a deep hole in the silicon can be realized from the front side under the spiral (Sun *et al.*, 1999).

A frequently used solution is to fabricate the inductor over a very thick dielectric layer or suspended in air. Sun and Miao (2005) fabricated inductors over a 20 μm thick oxide layer obtained by DRIE etching an array of 2 μm spaced 2 μm wide trenches inside the silicon substrate and then oxidizing the remaining Si. A more common and simple procedure is to use a thick polymer-like polyimide or benzocyclobutene (BCB) (Pieters *et al.*, 2000).

Spiral inductors suspended in air on two very thick signal posts were realized by KAIST using three-dimensional (3D) lithography (Yoon *et al.*, 2002). A very thick resist, up to 100 μm, was spun over the bottom Cu electrodes and exposed twice with different masks and exposure times. With a reduced time, only the top part of the resist was exposed defining the mould for the suspended coils, while with a full time exposure the holes for the posts were realized. The posts were then filled by Cu electroplating and a Cu seed layer was deposited. After removing the topmost seed metal by mechanical polishing, the coil was realized with 10 μm thick electroplated Cu. The sacrificial resist layer was removed with acetone.

With a similar process, tridimensional solenoid structures were also fabricated (Yoon *et al.*, 2003). Thick posts were realized over each end of parallel Cu lines on the substrate, while a second series of Cu lines were electroplated over the sacrificial resist to complete the solenoid spirals. Leblond *et al.* (2006) realized 3 μm thick gold suspended inductors over a 10 μm thick resist sacrificial layer.

8.4 Technology platform for the fabrication of RF MEMS complex circuits

After introducing and describing the salient features of lumped RF MEMS components, such as varactors, switches and inductors, as well as some of the most relevant issues at manufacturing level, a technology platform suitable for their fabrication is next discussed. The specific process is the surface micromachining technology available at FBK, specifically optimized for the fabrication of RF MEMS lumped components and complex networks.

For frequencies up to 40 GHz, high-resistivity silicon substrates are used. For higher frequencies, quartz (fused silica) wafers are preferable, because they present lower substrate losses. Quartz is very brittle and must be handled with care, particularly when thin substrates (300 μm) are needed for microstrip structures. To reduce the number of wafers broken during fabrication, the internal stress is reduced by a preliminary thermal treatment at 1050°C, followed by a very slow cooling.

The movable and suspended structures are realized by means of 1.8 μm electroplated gold, while the thicker (>5 μm) signal line and the anchoring structures are realized by adding a second electroplated gold layer. Underpass lines are made by a multilayer composed of Al 1% Si alloy and Ti–TiN diffusion barrier and capping layer to avoid diffusion of Al in polysilicon and the formation of hillocks during the subsequent deposition of silicon oxide (LTO).

Biasing lines and actuation electrodes are realized using high-resistivity polysilicon to reduce RF losses. Polysilicon allows high temperature processing and therefore good quality silicon oxide (TEOS) can be deposited over it. The actuation electrodes can be isolated by using both TEOS and LTO to sustain the actuation voltage without breakdown, while on the capacitive contacts only the thinner LTO is used, to have higher capacitance. As an alternative, it is possible to realize dielectric-free actuation electrodes removing all the dielectric over the polysilicon and building some posts that prevent the movable bridges from touching the electrode (short circuit). In this way it is possible to drastically reduce the pull-in voltage shift induced by charging (Solazzi et al., 2011).

A scheme of the process flow is illustrated in Fig. 8.9. The fabrication process starts on high-resistivity silicon wafers with the realization of an insulating layer consisting of 1 μm of silicon oxide grown by wet thermal oxidation at 975°C. The charges trapped at the silicon oxide interface can induce a conductive channel that increases the losses on the substrate by capacitive coupling. Annealing at 975°C for 50 min in nitrogen atmosphere is performed in order to reduce the trapped charge. On quartz wafer those steps are obviously not required.

To realize the electrodes for electrostatic actuation and the corresponding DC signal bias lines as well as resistors, a 630 nm thick layer of polysilicon is deposited by low pressure chemical vapour deposition (LPCVD) at 630°C. The polysilicon layer is used also to create small dimples (usually 4 × 4 μm) to define exactly the number and position of contact points between the movable membrane and the underpass line (Fig. 8.9a).

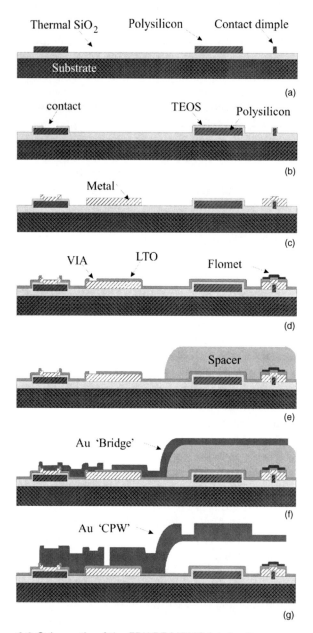

8.9 Schematic of the FBK RF MEMS fabrication process flow: (a) silicon substrate thermal oxidation and polysilicon deposition and patterning, (b) TEOS deposition and contact opening, (c) metal deposition and patterning, (d) LTO deposition, vias opening and floating metal deposition, (e) spacer deposition and backing, (f) seed layer and first gold 'bridge' electroplating and (g) second gold 'CPW' electroplating and release of suspended structures. The picture represents the fabrication of a capacitive contact switch. To realize ohmic switches the dielectric (LTO) over the metal underpass is removed allowing a metal-to-metal contact.

To obtain the required resistivity the polysilicon layer is implanted with boron ions (BF_2) at energy of 120 keV. Typically a 6.2×10^{14} B/cm² dose is used to obtain a sheet resistance of about 1600 ohm/sq. If a different resistivity is required the corresponding dose can be easily calculated. The first lithography step will define the polysilicon structures that are obtained by dry etching using Cl based chemistry plasma. After removing the photoresist layer with oxygen plasma, the implanted B ions are diffused and electrically activated by annealing at 925°C for 1 h in nitrogen atmosphere to obtain the required doping profile. A 300 nm thick insulating layer of SiO_2 is deposited by LPCVD using tetra-ethyl-ortho-silicate (TEOS) at 718°C.

When devices, such as phased array antennas or microstrip lines, require a backside conductive layer, an aluminium film is sputtered on the back side, defined by lithography (using a front side alignment) and dry etched. A PECVD silicon oxide or silicon nitride is used for isolation and to protect from scratches and corrosion.

The process continues on the front side with a lithography step and a dry etching (using F-based chemistry) to define the opening in the TEOS for the contacts between polysilicon and metal (Fig. 8.9b).

To realize the underpass line and other conductors a metal layer (Al 1%Si) is then deposited by sputtering. A diffusion barrier (Ti/TiN) is used to avoid spiking by Al diffusion at the polysilicon interface and hillocks formation on the top during dielectric deposition. The resulting multilayer is composed of 30 nm Ti, 50 nm TiN, 410 nm Al 1%Si, 60 nm Ti and 80 nm TiN. The thicknesses of the multimetal underpass and of the polysilicon actuation electrodes have to be the same in order to avoid distortion in the actuated bridge. The metal layer is defined by lithography and dry etched (Fig. 8.9c).

A 100 nm thick SiO_2 dielectric layer LTO is deposited by LPCVD at 430°C using silane. It is used both to isolate the metal from other conductors and as a dielectric for capacitive contacts.

Holes in the LTO are defined by a lithography step and dry etched (Fig. 8.9d) to realize the vias that contact the metal underpass with the gold signal line and to prepare the areas of metal-to-metal contacts for ohmic switches. If dielectric-less actuation electrodes are required, the same step is used to remove both LTO and TEOS over the polysilicon electrodes by increasing the etching time.

In this case, to avoid short circuits, a matrix of mechanical stoppers is distributed over the electrodes (Fig. 8.10), designed by superimposing TEOS, metal, LTO and floating metal in order to obtain an air gap of 550 nm, thick enough to ensure isolation at the actuation voltage levels normally used.

5 nm Cr–150 nm Au layer is deposited by electron beam gun to be used both to realize electrically floating metal layer for capacitive contact switches and to realize the bottom part of the gold-to-gold contact for ohmic switches.

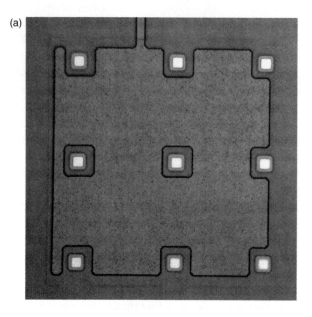

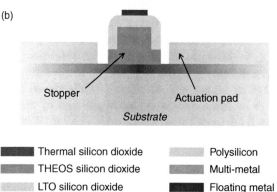

8.10 Picture (a) and schematic of pillars (b) used as stoppers to avoid short circuits between electrodes and movable membranes in dielectric-free actuation electrodes.

The Cr is used as adhesion layer because gold has very poor adhesion over silicon oxide. The floating metal is defined by a lithography step and wet etched (Fig. 8.9d).

Photoresist was chosen as sacrificial layer (spacer) for the fabrication of movable membranes and suspended air bridges, because it can be easily removed by oxygen plasma. The drawback is that only a partial planarization of the underlying structure's topography is obtained, and the top surface is not completely flat. The standard thickness is 3 µm but, depending on device requirements, different thicknesses are used, ranging from 1.6 to 4.5 μm. Photoresist is spun over the wafers and the sacrificial spacers are defined by lithography (Fig. 8.9e). The resist is backed at 200°C, a temperature much higher than the usual one, in order to round the edges by reflow, and to improve step coverage, as well as to increase the photoresist chemical and mechanical resistance. After this treatment the resist is not dissolved by the solvents used in the next steps, and further lithography can be performed without damaging the spacer.

The conductive seed layer, required for the electroplating process, is then evaporated all over the wafers. This layer is composed of 2.5 nm of Cr, to have good adhesion to the substrate, 25 nm of Au as conductive layer and a sacrificial top layer of 2 nm of Cr, to increase the adhesion of the photoresist mask during electroplating. A lithography step, using a 6 μm thick AZ 4562 positive resist, defines the pattern where the first Au film, called the 'bridge', will be grown. After wet etching of the top Cr layer, a 1.8 μm thick Au film is electroplated using cyanide-based chemistry (Fig. 8.9f). The deposition parameters have been chosen in order to obtain a slightly tensile residual stress. After photoresist removal, a further lithography step defines the pattern of a second thicker (3.5 μm) Au layer called the 'CPW', which is also grown by electroplating. The thinner 'Bridge' layer is used mainly to fabricate the suspended and movable structures while low resistance RF signal lines, ground areas and the anchor points of movable structures, are fabricated by superimposing both the gold layers. Frequently, the 'CPW' layer is deposited over selected areas of movable bridges in order to have stiffer parts that move rigidly while deformation is localized on thinner suspension spring legs.

The seed layer is removed by wet etching, and gold sintering at 190°C is performed to increase the gold adhesion to substrate and the bondability of pads for external connections. In addition, this step leads to a more homogeneous and reproducible (tensile) stress in the gold membranes. The last process step is the release of suspended structures by removal of sacrificial resist with oxygen plasma (Fig. 8.9g). The process temperature and the etching parameters were optimized in order to reduce the structural deformations induced by stress and the stress gradient along the thickness of the films (Mulloni *et al.*, 2010).Using a process variant, it is possible to remove locally the Si substrate to realize devices such as inductors and interdigitated capacitors on very thin suspended dielectric membranes. Before removing the seed layer on the front side, holes are realized on the silicon oxide on the back side, and the substrate is selectively removed either by deep RIE or by anisotropic Si etching using TMAH in a wafer holder that protects the front side. With the same technique it is possible to realize vias through the wafer that can be filled with copper by electroplating to electrically connect the front and backside of the wafer.

8.5 Some examples of high-performance devices enabled by the RF MEMS technology

As a concluding section of this chapter, a brief overview of some of the relevant realizations of lumped elements and complex networks in RF MEMS technology will be discussed.

Single switches are used to open or close a signal line but in many applications it is required to connect an input to different outputs, such as to switch between different antennas or insert different filters. This can be easily obtained by combining more switches, as in the SPDT devices presented in Fig. 8.11 (DiNardo *et al.*, 2006). In this case to obtain isolation better than 30 dB up to 40 GHz, a combination of ohmic series and capacitive shunt switches is used on each arm. The ohmic switch alone (upper curve with shunt not actuated in Fig. 8.11b) gives high isolation on the lower frequency range, starting from DC. The shunt switch was designed to have a maximum isolation at about 18 GHz and when actuated (lower curve) it increases the isolation at higher frequency. The insertion loss is higher than using a single switch, reaching 1.5 dB at 40 GHz, of which about 0.4 dB due to the input and output lines that are longer than in the case of a single switch.

When more connections are required, other switches can be added as in the SP4T shown in Fig. 8.12, where the incoming signal is split into the four output lines oriented at 60° (Casini *et al.*, 2010). To obtain a compact device, series ohmic cantilever switches have been used due to their small dimension. The shape and dimensions of the junction area have been optimized to minimize mutual coupling. In the working frequency band from DC to 6 GHz, the return loss is better than 20 dB and the insertion loss better than 0.5 dB, while the isolation between ports is better than 30 dB. To increase the frequency range and isolation, it is possible to cascade a second cantilever switch in shunt configuration.

When many input and output lines have to be connected together independently, reconfigurable switching matrices are required (Braun *et al.*, 2008; Daneshmand and Mansour, 2011). One of the easier solutions is to use a modular approach, connecting together some building blocks like the 2 × 2 matrix shown in Fig. 8.13. The two input and the two output ports are perpendicular, in order to avoid crossing of signal lines, which reduces insulation. Depending on the switch configuration, the signal on each input line can be independently connected to one or both of the output terminations, or can be disconnected. To obtain non-blocking higher-order matrices, the switching elements have to be assembled in a configuration that always allows each input port to be connected to each output port by a smart routing of the signals. Increasing the number of the elements increases the complexity of the signal lines network and many crosses are required. The fabrication of cross-overs integrated on the same substrate is possible

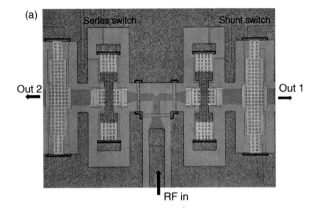

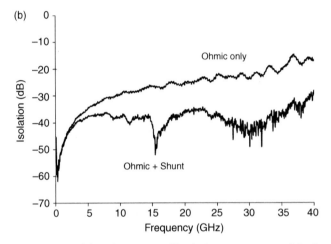

8.11 Picture (a) and measured isolation parameters (b) of an SPDT switch realized by combining series ohmic and shunt capacitive switches to increase the high isolation frequency band.

but requires additional levels of metals, with insulating dielectric layers in between, increasing the process complexity. Moreover, the coupling between crossing lines can be non-negligible. Assembling the switching elements on a separate board, such as by using low temperature cofired ceramics (LTCC) technology, allows to realize the RF connection on different highly conductive layers connected by vias and separated by ground planes. A further conductive layer can be used to realize the complex DC biasing network for the independent actuation of each switch (DiNardo *et al.*, 2005).

Switches are also the key element to fabricate reconfigurable or tunable circuits by selectively connecting components such as capacitors, varactors, inductors or delay lines. Many examples are reported in literature about

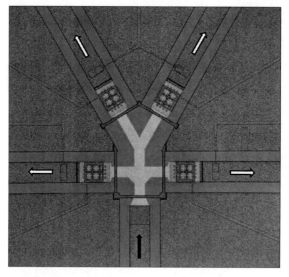

8.12 SP4T switch obtained by using compact cantilever ohmic switches.

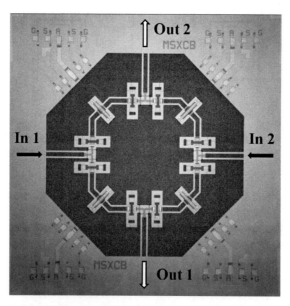

8.13 Building block for switching matrices. By assembling together two input–two output switching elements, high order non-blocking matrices can be realized.

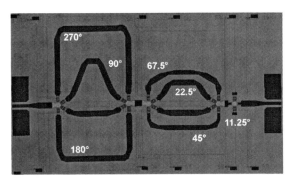

8.14 Picture of a 5-bit switchable phase shifter. The cantilever switches in SP4T configuration connect alternatively microstrip lines of different lengths.

impedance matching tuners, phase shifters, couplers, power splitters, reconfigurable LC tanks to tune oscillation frequency, and tunable filters (Rebeitz *et al.*, 2009).

Figure 8.14 shows a programmable 0–360° 5-bit K-band phase shifter (Farinelli *et al.*, 2009). Depending on the switches position, a shift from 0° to 360° in steps of 11.25° can be obtained. The less significant bit, on the right, is obtained by a microstrip line loaded by a shunt capacitive switch having a capacitance ratio of 5, while the other four bits are obtained by alternately connecting microstrip lines of different appropriate length by ohmic cantilevers disposed in an SP4T configuration. To have the appropriate impedance of the microstrip lines, the substrate is 200 μm thick high-resistivity silicon with a metal layer on the back side.

8.6 Conclusion

This chapter has discussed the exploitation of MEMS technology for the realization of next-generation microwave devices for wireless communications, taking as technology reference the RF MEMS surface micromachining process available at the micro-fabrication facility of FBK in Italy. First of all, the main functional and technological characteristics of electrostatically driven RF MEMS based lumped components, such as ohmic and capacitive switches, varactors and inductors, have been mentioned and reviewed. Subsequently, a comprehensive description of the FBK fabrication flow, including specific features, issues, and on-purpose developed technology modules, was presented, providing the reader with a deep insight into manufacturing of RF MEMS devices and components. Finally, the chapter was completed with a review of a few significant examples of RF MEMS lumped components and complex networks.

8.7 References

Aaltonen L and Halonen K (2009), *On-chip charge-pump with continuous frequency regulation for precision high-voltage generation*, Research in Microelectronics and Electronics. PRIME 2009.

Almeida L, Ramadoss R, Jackson R, Ishikawa K, and Yu Q (2006), Study of the electrical contact resistance of multi-contact MEMS relays fabricated using the MetalMUMPs process, *Journal of Micromechanics and Microengineering*, Vol. 16, 1189–1194.

Balaraman D, Bhattacharya S K, Ayazi F, and Papapolymerou J (2002), Low-cost low actuation voltage copper RF MEMS switches, *IEEE MTT-S International Microwave Symposium*, 2002.

Blondy P, Crunteanu A, Champeaux C, Catherinot A, Tristant P, Vendier O, Cazaux J L, and Marchand L (2004), Dielectric less capacitive MEMS switches, *IEEE MTT-S International Microwave Symposium* 2004.

Blondy P, Mercier D, Cros D, Guillon P, Rey P, Charvet P, Diem B, Zanchi C, Lapierre L, Sombrin J, and Quoirin J B (2001), *Packaged millimeter wave thermal MEMS switches*, 31st European Microwave Conference, London, UK, Sept. 2001.

Borwick R L, Stupar P A, DeNatale J, Anderson R, Tsai C, Garrett K, and Erlandson R (2003), A high Q, large tuning range MEMS capacitor for RF filter systems, *Sensors and Actuators A*, Issues 103(1–2), 33–41.

Brank J, Yao J, Eberly M, Malczewsk A, Varian K, and Goldsmith C (2001), RF MEMS-based tunable filters, *International Journal of RF and Microwave Computer-Aided Engineering*, 11(5), 276–284.

Braun S, Oberhammer J, and Stemme G (2008), Single-chip MEMS 5×5 and 20×20 double-pole single-throw switch arrays for automating telecommunication networks, *Journal of Micromechanics and Microengineering*, 18(1), 015014.

Broue A, Dhennin J, Courtade F, Charvet P L, Pons P, Lafontan X, and Plana R (2010), *Thermal and topological characterization of Au, Ru and Au/Ru based MEMS contacts using nanoindenter*, IEEE 23rd International Conference on Micro Electro Mechanical Systems (MEMS) 2010.

Casini F, Farinelli P, Mannocchi G, DiNardo S, Margesin B, De Angelis G, Marcelli R, Vendier O, and Vietzorreck L (2010), *High performance RF-MEMS SP4T switches in CPW technology for space applications*, 40th European Microwave Conference, Paris, France 2010.

Chen L, Lee H, Guo Z J, McGruer N E, Gilbert K W, Leedy K D, and Adams J J (2007), Contact resistance study of noble metals and alloy films using a scanning probe microscope test station, *Journal of Applied Physics*, 102, 074910-1 to 074910-7.

Chi C Y and Rebeiz G M (1995), Planar microwave and millimeter-wave lumped elements and coupled-line filters using micro-machining techniques, *IEEE Transactions on Microwave Theory and Techniques*, 43(4), 730–738.

Daneshmand M and Mansour R R (2011), RF MEMS satellite switch matrices, *Microwave Magazine, IEEE*, 12(5), 92–109.

Dec A and Suyama K (2000), Microwave MEMS-based voltage-controlled oscillators, *IEEE Transactions on Microwave Theory and Techniques*, 48(11), 1943–1949.

DiNardo S, Farinelli P, Giacomozzi F, Mannocchi G, Marcelli R, Margesin B, Mezzanotte P, Mulloni V, Russer P, Sorrentino R, Vitulli F, and Vietzorreck

L (2006), *Broadband RF-MEMS based SPDT*, IEEE 36th EuMC, European Microwave Conference, Manchester, UK.

DiNardo S, Farinelli P, Giacomozzi F, Mannocchi G, Marcelli R, Margesin B, Mezzanotte P, Mulloni V, Russer P, Sorrentino R, Vitulli F, and Vietzorreck L (2005), *RF MEMS based switch matrices for complex switching networks*, IEEE Microwave Theory and Techniques and 5th ESA Round Table on Micro/Nano Technologies for Space, ESA ESTEC Netherlands, 3–5 Oct. 2005.

Entesari K and Rebeiz G M (2005), A Differential 4-bit 6.5–10-GHz RF MEMS tunable filter, *IEEE Transactions on Microwave Theory and Techniques*, 53(3), 1103–1110.

Farinelli P, Chiuppesi E, Di Maggio F, Margesin B, Colpo S, Ocera A, Russo A, and Pomona I, (2009), *Development of different K-band MEMS phase shifter designs for satellite COTM terminals*, IEEE European Microwave Conference (EuMC 2009), Rome, Italy.

Farinelli P, Margesin B, Giacomozzi F, Mannocchi G, Catoni, S, Marcelli R, Mezzanotte P, Vietzorreck L, Vitulli F, Sorrentino R, and Deborgies F (2007), A low contact-resistance winged-bridge RF-MEMS series switch for wide-band applications, *Journal of the European Microwave Association*, 3(3), 268–278.

Gamble H S, Armstrong B M, Mitchell S J N, Wu Y, Fusco V F, and Stewart J A C, (1999), Low-loss CPW lines on surface stabilized high-resistivity silicon, *IEEE Microwave and Guided Wave Letters*, 9(10), 395–397.

Jansman A B M, van Beek J T M, Van Delden M H, Kemmeren A L, den Dekker A, and Widdershoven F P, (2003), '*Elimination of accumulation charge effects for high-resistivity silicon substrate*', Proc. ESSDERC 2003.

Leblond H, Blondy P, and Baillargeat D, (2006), *On-chip spiral inductors and metal-air-metal capacitors in suspended technology*, IEEE 36th EuMC, European Microwave Conference, Manchester, UK.

Lee H, Coutu R A, Mall S, and Leedy K D (2006), Characterization of metal and metal alloy films as contact materials in MEMS switches, *Journal of Micromechanics and Microengineering*, 16, 557–563.

Lisec T (2010), 'Switches and their fabrication technologies' in *Advanced RF MEMS*, Cambridge University Press, 55–57.

Lisec T, Huth C, and Wagner B (2004), *Dielectric material impact on capacitive RFMEMS reliability*, IEEE EuMC, European Microwave Conference, Amsterdam, The Netherlands.

López-Villegas J M, Samitie J, Cané C, Losantos P, and Bausells J (2000), Improvement of the quality factor of RF integrated inductors by layout optimization, *IEEE Transactions on Microwave Theory and Techniques*, 48(1), 76–83.

Mardivirin D, Pothier A, Crunteanu A, Vialle B, and Blondy P (2009), Charging in dielectricless capacitive RF-MEMS switches, *IEEE Transactions on Microwave Theory and Techniques*, 57(1), 231–236.

Morris A S, Cunningham S, Dereus D, and Schropfer G (2003), *High-performance integrated RF-MEMS: Part 1-The process*, 33rd European Microwave Conference, Munich 2003.

Mulloni V, Giacomozzi F, and Margesin B (2010), *Controlling stress and stress gradient during the release process in gold suspended micro-structures*, Sensors and actuators A, Physical, 162(1), 93–99.

Mulloni V, Iannacci J, Bartali R, Micheli V, Colpo S, Laidani N, and Margesin B (2012), Gold-based thin multilayers for ohmic contacts in RF-MEMS switches, *Microsystem Technology*, 18(7–8), 965–971.

Natarajan S P, Cunningham S J, Morris A S, and Dereus D R (2011), *CMOS integrated digital RF MEMS capacitors*, IEEE 11th Topical Meeting on Silicon Monolithic Integrated Circuits in RF Systems (SiRF), 2011.

Nieminen H, Ermolov V, Nybergh K, Silanto S, and Ryhanen T (2002), Microelectromechanical capacitors for RF applications, *Journal of Micromechanics and Microengineering*, 12, 177–186.

Nieminen H, Ermolov V, Silanto S, Nybergh K, and Ryhänen T (2004), Design of a temperature-stable RF MEM capacitor, *Journal of Microelectromechanical Systems*, 13(5), 705–714.

Pacheco S P, Katehi L, and Nguyen C T C (2000), *Design of low actuation voltage RF MEMS switch*, IEEE MTT-S International Microwave Symposium 2000.

Palego C, Deng J, Peng Z, Halder S, Hwang J, Forehand D, Scarbrough D, Goldsmith C L, Johnston I, Sampath S K, and Datta A (2009), Robustness of RF MEMS capacitive switches with molybdenum membranes, *IEEE Transactions on Microwave Theory and Techniques*, 57(12), 3262–3269.

Palego C, Pothier A, Gasseling T, Crunteanu A, Cibert C, Champeaux C, Tristant P, Catherinot A, and Blondy P (2006), *RF-MEMS switched varactor for high power applications*, IEEE MTT-S International Microwave Symposium Digest, 2006.

Pieters P, Vaesen K, Diels W, Carchon G, Brebels S, De Raedt W, Beyne E, and Mertens R P (2000), *High-Q integrated spiral inductors for high performance wireless front-end systems*, IEEE Radio and Wireless Conference RAWCON 2000.

Rebeiz G, Entesari K, Reines I, Park S, El-tanani M, Grichener A, and Brown A (2009), Tuning in to RF MEMS, *Microwave Magazine*, IEEE, 10(6), Oct. 2009.

Rebeiz G M (2003), *RF MEMS: theory, design, and technology*, Hoboken, Wiley-Interscience.

Rong B, Burghartz J N, Nanver L K, Rejaei B, and van der Zwan M (2004), Surface-passivated high-resistivity silicon substrates for RFICs, *IEEE Electron Device Letters*, 25(4), 176–178.

Rottenberg X, Jansen H, Fiorini P, De Raedt W, and Tilmans H (2002), *Novel RF-MEMS capacitive switching structures*, IEEE 32nd European Microwave Conference EuMC, 23–26 September 2002.

Solazzi F, Resta G, Mulloni V, Margesin B, and Farinelli P (2011), *Influence of beam geometry on the dielectric charging of RF MEMS switches*, 2011 European Microwave Integrated Circuits Conference (EuMIC) 10–11 Oct. 2011.

Sun J and Miao J (2005), High performance MEMS inductors fabricated on localised and planar thick SiO_2 layer, *Electronics Letters*, 41(7), 446–447.

Sun Y, Tauritz J L, and Baets R G F (1999), Micromachined RF passive components and their applications in MMICs, *International Journal of RF and Microwave Computer-Aided Engineering*, 9(4), 310–325.

Tilmans H A C (2002), *MEMS components for wireless communications*, 16th European Conference on Solid-State Transducers EUROSENSORS, 15–18 September 2002, Prague, Czech Republic.

Tilmans H A C, De Raedt W, and Beyne E (2003), MEMS for wireless communications: 'from RF-MEMS components to RF-MEMS-SiP', *Journal of Micromechanics and Microengineering*, 13(4), S139-S163.

Tilmans H A C, Fullin E, Ziad H, Van de Peer M D J, Kesters J, Van Geffen E, Bergqvist J, Pantus M, Beyne E, Baert K, and Naso F (1999), *A Fully packaged electromagnetic microrelay*, 12th IEEE International Conference on Micro Electro Mechanical Systems, MEMS 99.

Yang Z, Lichtenwalner D J, Morris A S, Krim J, and Kingon A I, (2009), Comparison of Au and Au–Ni alloys as contact materials for MEMS switches, *Journal of Microelectromechanical Systems*, 18(2), 287–295.

Yao J J, Park S, and DeNatale J (1998), *High tuning-ratio MEMS-based tunable capacitors for RF communications applications*, Tech. Digest, Solid State Sensor and Actuator Workshop.

Yoon J B, Choi Y S, Kim B, Eo Y, and Yoon E (2002), CMOS-compatible surface-micromachined suspended-spiral inductors for multi-GHz silicon RF ICs, *IEEE Electron Device Letters*, 23(10), 591–593.

Yoon J B, Kim B, Choi Y S, and Yoon E (2003), 3-D construction of monolithic passive components for RF and microwave ICs using thick-metal surface micromachining technology, *IEEE Transactions on Microwave Theory and Techniques*, 51(1), 279–288.

Zavracky P M, Majumder S, and McGruer N E (1997), Micromechanical switches fabricated using nickel surface micromachining, *Journal of Microelectromechanical Systems*, 6(1), 3–9.

Zou J, Liu C, and Schutt-Ainé J E (2001), Development of a wide-tuning-range two-parallel-plate tunable capacitor for integrated wireless communication systems, *International Journal of RF and Microwave Computer-Aided Engineering*, 11(5), 322–329.

9
Wafer-level packaging technology for RF MEMS

S. SEOK, IEMN CNRS, France

DOI: 10.1533/9780857098610.1.258

Abstract: This chapter discusses the wafer-scale packaging technology for radio frequency microelectromechanical systems (RF MEMS) devices. First, the need for the wafer-level packaging of RF MEMS devices and the electrical effect of the packaging cap are assessed. This chapter shows examples of different types of packaging techniques, with emphasis on wafer-level bonding using hard cap materials, such as silicon and glass, and polymer cap materials, based on benzo-cyclobutene and PerMX.

Key words: wafer-level packaging, polymer, BCB, PerMX, RF MEMS.

9.1 Introduction

As microelectromechanical systems (MEMS) packaging is being recognized as an essential technique for successful commercialization of MEMS products, it is attracting increased interest. It must be cost-effective, because packaging is the highest cost within the whole manufacturing and commercialization processes, similar to integrated circuits (IC) packaging in microelectronics. Therefore, wafer-level packaging technology becomes a key technique to develop, along with wafer-level MEMS release, as has been demonstrated.[1,2] For radio frequency (RF)-MEMS devices, packaging faces more constraints, due to detuning effects that the packaging materials may have on the performance of the packaged RF device.

In Section 9.2, the zero-level packaging of RF MEMS is defined and various packaging approaches based on different technologies such as thermal wafer-to-wafer bonding, thin-film deposition, polymer capping and nanoporous materials are introduced. Section 9.3 presents an analytical solution for the packaging cap illustrating the detuning effect on the packaged coplanar waveguide (CPW) using conformal mapping and the partial capacitance method. The effective dielectric constant and characteristic impedance before and after packaging are investigated as a function of air-cavity height. Section 9.4 deals with the packaging method using hard materials such as silicon and glass caps. These packaging caps are bonded through metal-to-metal bonding and polymer sealing ring bonding. The measured S-parameters before and after packaging are compared, to investigate the packaging effect on performance characteristics. Section 9.5 presents polymer cap packaging. The different capping methods using benzo-cyclo-butene (BCB) caps and PerMX (PerMX™ of DuPont™) caps are explained, and the S-parameters before and after packaging are measured to evaluate the packaging effect.

9.2 Wafer-level zero-level packaging for RF MEMS

RF MEMS components contain movable fragile parts that should be encapsulated and protected during wafer handling, wafer dicing or plastic moulding. The packaging technique that is carried out at wafer-scale, or wafer-level packaging is preferred in the aspects of manufacturability and cost-effectiveness. According to the definition, zero-level packaging identifies non-repairable parts, such as ICs, transistors, resistors, and so forth. Therefore, the encapsulation of the (RF-) MEMS components is also categorized as zero-level packaging. Figure 9.1 shows examples of different methods of zero-level packaging. There exist two major approaches; thermal wafer-to-wafer bonding and thin-film deposition/growth bonding.[3–5] The thermal wafer-to-wafer bonding is realized through wafer bonding between a cap wafer and a device wafer. The conventional packaging cap materials are Si,[6] glass,[7] and low-temperature co-fired ceramic (LTCC)[8] due to their compatibility with the wafer-to-wafer bonding process. Frequently used bonding techniques are anodic bonding,[9] metal-to-metal bonding,[10] glass frit bonding[11] and polymer bonding.[12] Polymer bonding is attracting an increased interest because polymer materials have excellent electrical properties, such as low dielectric constant, and mechanical properties, such as low moisture uptake, and minimal outgassing. Also, the polymer bonding process is basically performed at lower temperature than the other processes. For thin-film packaging, the packaging caps are poly-Si[13] or nitride/oxide film.[14] The process temperature for the thin-film packaging is higher than wafer-to-wafer bonding because the deposition temperature is 1000°C for poly-Si and 850°C for low pressure chemical vapour deposition (LPCVD) nitride film. Some channels are needed for a sacrificial etch release of MEMS structures inside the packaging caps. It should be noted that the process temperature is a critical parameter for RF MEMS packaging because RF MEMS devices are generally realized using metallic materials. Therefore, wafer-to-wafer bonding, using a polymer sealing ring and a metallic sealing ring, has been frequently used for RF MEMS devices packaging. As a new thin-film package, nanoporous packaging caps with alumina and chromium materials have been recently

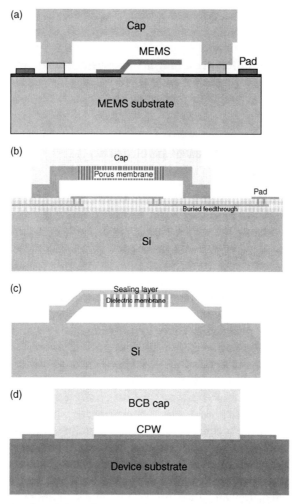

9.1 Examples of zero-level packaging: (a) hard material cap packaging; (b) porous material cap packaging; (c) dielectric material packaging and (d) polymer material cap packaging.

reported. The maximum process temperature is approximately 350°C.[15,16] Both metallic sealing ring and metal-sealed nanoporous cap need to be grounded to minimize their parasitic effect on the packaged RF MEMS components. Finally, polymer cap encapsulation, combining the merits of wafer-to-wafer bonding and thin-film packaging, has been reported.[17–21] It consists of a polymer membrane as a packaging cover and a polymer sealing ring. The polymer caps can be implemented through sacrificial etching and a wafer-level transfer technique. The effect of the polymer cap on the packaged device is regarded as minimal due to its low dielectric

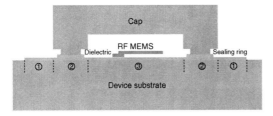

9.2 Cross-section of RF MEMS package.

constant and the polymer capping reduces the need for a deep cavity (as required for Si capping) to minimize its effect on the packaged devices. Also, its optical transparency is helpful for the optical inspection of packaged MEMS devices.

As mentioned earlier, it is important to take the effect of the capping materials on packaged RF devices into account. Figure 9.2 shows a cross-sectional drawing of a typical RF MEMS package. The packaging cap has three different regions for electrical-design consideration: ① input and output port ② packaging cap part with sealing ring on RF line, and ③ packaging cap with air-cavity housing the RF MEMS. The transmission line under the sealing ring has to be carefully designed for impedance matching depending on the sealing ring material. In the case of a metallic sealing ring, the dielectric layer between the sealing ring and the RF line should be also considered. The packaging cap with a housing cavity has a detuning effect on the packaged RF MEMS devices due to its proximity. This will be explained later in more detail using the partial capacitance technique.

9.3 Electrical effects of the packaging material on the packaged devices

It is important to study the effect of the packaging cap on the packaged devices. As mentioned earlier, the packaging cap has some electrical influence on the packaged RF elements, including the microstrip line, the CPW, filters and resonators, etc. It is known that the characteristic impedance Z_c and effective dielectric constant ε_{eff} of the CPW transmission line can be expressed in closed form expressions derived from conformal mapping techniques as shown below. It assumes a quasi-static transverse electromagnetic (TEM) mode of propagation along the line, and the partial capacitance technique is used to find the corresponding capacitances.[22]

$$\varepsilon_{eff} = \frac{C_{CPW}}{C_{air}}$$

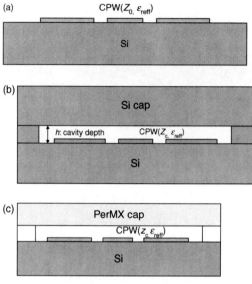

9.3 Test structures: (a) CPW, (b) Si cap-packaged CPW and (c) PerMX cap-packaged CPW.

$$Z_c = \frac{1}{cC_{air}\sqrt{\varepsilon_{eff}}}$$

where c is the velocity of light in free space, C_{CPW} is the total capacitance of the CPW and C_{air} is the partial capacitance of the CPW in the absence of all the dielectric layers.

Similarly, the influence of the packaging cap materials can be also investigated in terms of the characteristic impedance Z_c and effective dielectric constant ε_{reff} of the packaged CPW. The packaged CPW is divided into separate partial regions based on the partial capacitance method to find the corresponding capacitance C_{CPW} and C_{air} of the packaged CPW. For comparison, three different test structures are used, as shown in Fig. 9.3: (a) CPW on Si, (b) Si cap-packaged CPW and (c) PerMX cap-packaged CPW. The 50 Ω CPW is designed to have a central conductor width of 85 μm and a slot width of 15 μm. The dielectric constants are 12 for Si and 3 for PerMX, respectively. Also, it is assumed that the I/O interfaces at the bonding area are suitably designed to be 50 Ω. The packaging cap thicknesses are assumed to be 100 μm for the Si cap and 50 μm for the PerMX cap.

Figure 9.4 shows the characteristic impedance and effective dielectric constant as functions of cavity depth for the three different structures. As a reference, the unpackaged coplanar is designed to have characteristic impedance of 50.3 Ω and effective dielectric constant of 6.45. The silicon

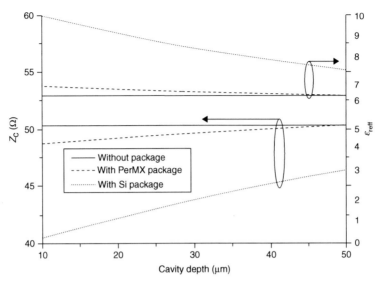

9.4 Z_c and ε_{eff} as a function of cavity depth.

capped CPW gives the impedance of 40.5 Ω and 46.4 Ω at 10 μm and 50 μm cavity depth, respectively, while the PerMX capped has 48.7 Ω and 50.3 Ω at each depth. It is found that the silicon cap must have higher cavity depth to minimize its influence on the packaged device, due to its relatively high dielectric constant. It needs more than 50 μm cavity depth to reach the impedance of the unpackaged CPW. Also, it is found that the Si cap and the PerMX cap result in impedance change per cavity depth of 0.15 Ω/μm and 0.04 Ω/μm, respectively. As seen in Fig. 9.4, the effective dielectric constant of the Si capped CPW is higher than that of the PerMX capped; the Si packaged CPW has 9.96 at 10 μm cavity height and 7.59 at 50 μm, while PerMX packaged line has 6.88 and 6.45 at each cavity height. In conclusion, a package cap with low dielectric constant has better RF transparency in terms of characteristic impedance and effective dielectric constant of the packaged CPW.

9.4 Packaging with hard cap materials

As a capping material, silicon and glass are the most frequently used materials because they are widely used as a substrate for semiconductor and MEMS devices. In this section, silicon-cap packaging with metal-to-metal bonding[23] and Si cap (or glass-cap) packaging with BCB polymer bonding[7,24] will be described. Also, Si cap packaging with a PerMX sealing ring[25] will be presented. Additionally, the difference in package design between a metallic sealing ring and a non-metallic sealing ring will be assessed.

9.4.1 Si cap packaging with a AuSn sealing ring

Figure 9.5 shows the concept of the Si cap packaging using the gold–tin–gold bonding technique. It consists of the Si cap wafer, the AuSn sealing ring, and the nitride/oxide passivation layer between the sealing ring and CPW. A 508 µm-thick high resistivity (2 kΩ · cm) silicon is used for both the cap and the device substrate. A 50 Ω CPW on the Si substrate wafer is designed to have a centre conductor width of 98 µm and a gap of 55 µm. The thickness of the AuSn sealing ring is 7 µm after the bonding process and its width is 50 µm. The sealing ring is connected to the CPW ground to avoid possible parasitic resonances, and the Si cavity height of 60 µm is made to minimize the packaging effect to the packaged transmission line. The packaged CPW lines on 6 inches of wafer after pad opening are shown in Fig. 9.6. Figure 9.7 shows the fabricated sealing ring before the packaging. As mentioned earlier, the CPW line under the sealing ring is redesigned to minimize capacitive coupling with the RF signal; the conductor width is 20 µm and the gap is 60 µm.

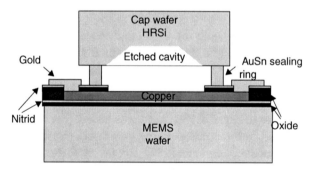

9.5 Concept of Si cap packaging with AnSn sealing ring.

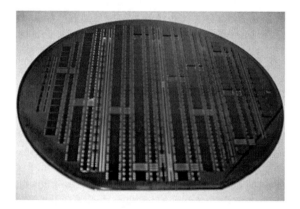

9.6 Packaged CPW lines.

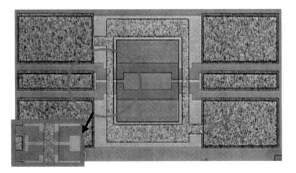

9.7 Fabricated sealing ring before packaging.

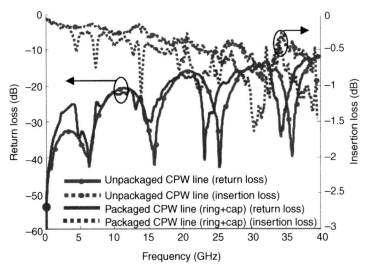

9.8 Measured S-parameters before and after Si cap packaging with AnSn sealing ring.

The measured S-parameters before and after packaging are shown in Fig. 9.8. The insertion loss has resonances at certain frequencies, and it can be suppressed with more contacts between the sealing ring and the ground. The average measured packaged insertion loss is about 0.2 dB higher than the unpackaged one. The return loss of the package is mainly determined by the gold ring transition and is better than 15 dB from direct current (DC) up to 30 GHz.

9.4.2 Glass-cap packaging with a BCB sealing ring

This consists of Pyrex glass cap, BCB sealing ring, and Pyrex glass substrate as shown in Fig. 9.9. The Pyrex glass has been widely used as a packaging

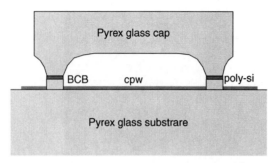

9.9 Concept of glass-cap packaging with BCB sealing ring.

material for other MEMS devices, such as gyroscopes and accelerometers. Also, it is known that Pyrex glass has good RF characteristics and hence it is used as a packaging cap and a RF substrate.

The conventional BCB coating process suffers from a topography problem due to housing cavities and hence a BCB sealing ring has been defined before glass wet etching. It makes it possible to get a flat BCB sealing ring that is essential to the quality of the bonding.

The packaging process is shown in Fig. 9.10; (a) a 0.1 μm thick poly-silicon was deposited by LPCVD on 525 μm-thick Pyrex glass – BCB 4020–40 was coated and patterned by a conventional photo-lithography process and then 1.2 μm thick photoresist (AZ1512) was coated to pattern poly-Si and to protect the BCB sealing ring when hydrofluoric acid (HF) etching the glass-cap wafer, (b) AZ1512 was patterned and then poly-Si was dry-etched, (c) Pyrex glass was wet-etched to make a cavity for MEMS devices and pad access, (d) AZ1512 was removed by acetone and plasma O_2, (e) residual poly-Si outside the sealing ring was removed by dry etching, and (f) after bonding with another glass substrate, a dicing was performed to make pad accesses. Figure 9.11a shows the fabricated glass cap with the BCB sealing ring and additional rectangular BCBs at each corner after step (e).

BCB bonding has been performed using Karlsuss SB6 bonder at the condition of 250°C bonding temperature and 2 bars applied pressure. Additional rectangular BCBs are used to increase BCB bonding strength. The BCB sealing ring is 45 μm in width and 5.14 μm in thickness after fabrication. A CPW on a glass wafer has been also encapsulated using the packaging process. It has a entre conductor width of 85 μm and gap of 15 μm. The glass cap thickness is 200 μm and the cavity is 80 μm. The packaged CPW line and the measured S-parameters before and after the packaging are shown in Figs 9.11b and 9.12, respectively. The insertion loss change from the packaging was not observed up to 40 GHz, while the return loss of the packaged CPW was always better than 20 dB up to 60 GHz.

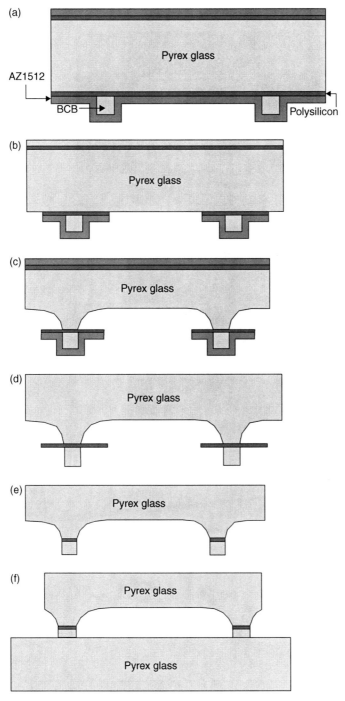

9.10 Packaging process flow: (a) etch masks formation, (b) AZ1512, poly-silicon patterning, (c) glass wet etching, (d) removal AZ1512, (e) removal of poly-silicon, and (f) bonding and dicing.

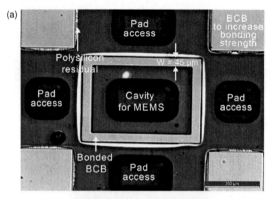

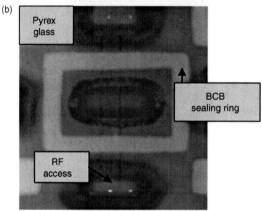

9.11 Fabricated glass cap and glass-cap packaged CPW: (a) glass cap with BCB sealing ring, (b) glass-capped CPW.

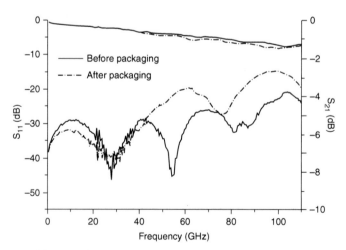

9.12 Measured S-parameters before and after glass-cap packaging with a BCB sealing ring.

9.4.3 Si cap packaging with a BCB sealing ring

The package concept and the designed BCB sealing ring are shown in Fig. 9.13. The BCB ring consists of two layers; the first is hard-cured at 250°C, and the second one is soft-cured at 110°C. Similar to the previous glass-cap packaging, a flat BCB sealing ring is defined before Si cavity dry etching to accomplish uniform bonding and high bonding strength. The ring width on the RF signal line is 100 µm to minimize the influence of the dielectric material at higher frequencies, and the sealing ring on the ground (GND) plane is 200 µm wide to increase the bonding strength of the package. The second BCB ring is designed to be slightly narrower than the first. The thickness of both the Si cap and the Si substrate is 530 µm, and the cavity height is 65 µm. The CPW has a centre conductor width of 100 µm and gap of 80 µm.

Figure 9.14 shows the packaging process with photosensitive BCB polymer; (a) the first BCB sealing ring is patterned on the Si cap wafer using the

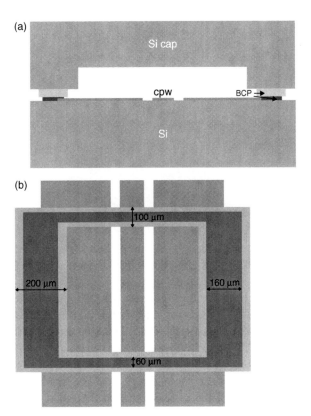

9.13 Concept of silicon-cap packaging with a BCB sealing ring: (a) cross-sectional view and (b) top view of BCB sealing ring on CPW.

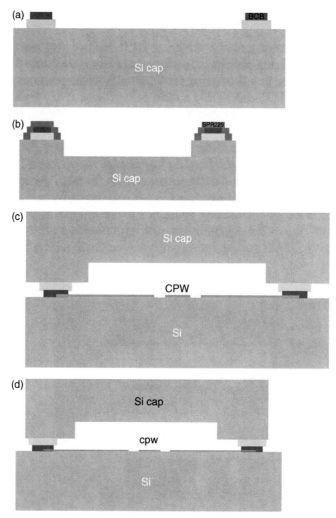

9.14 Packaging process flow: (a) BCB ring patterning; (b) ICP Si etch with PR protection of BCB ring; (c) wafer bonding and (d) dicing.

lithography process, and then it is hard-cured at 250°C – the second BCB is patterned on top of the first BCB layer, and then it is soft-baked at 110°C, (b) Si is deep-etched for the cavity with SPR220 etching mask, (c) the Si cap wafer is bonded to the CPW target wafer, and (d) the pad access is obtained through dicing.

The fabricated package is shown in Fig. 9.15a. The scanning-electron microscopy (SEM) pictures of the cross-section of the package are shown in Figs 9.15b and c. The sealing widths bonded to the RF signal path and the GND plane are 50 μm and 155 μm, respectively, and its thickness is

Wafer-level packaging technology for RF MEMS 271

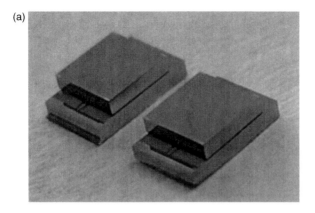

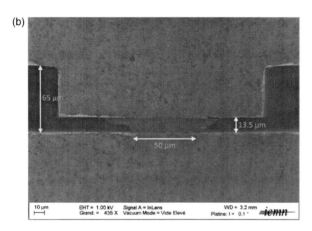

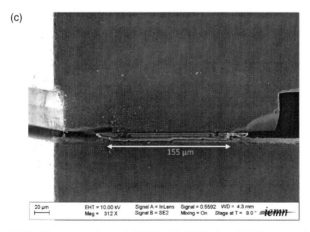

9.15 Si cap-packaged CPW with BCB ring: (a) Si capped CPW; (b) cross-section of the package (RF signal path) and (c) cross-section of the package (ground plane).

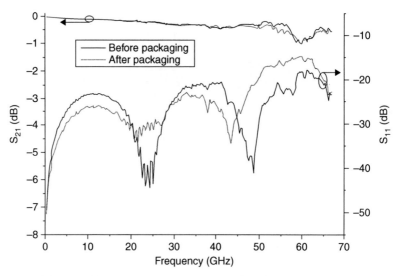

9.16 Measured S-parameters before and after Si cap packaging with a BCB sealing ring.

13.5 μm. Also, the conformal bonding on gold ground plane is as shown in Fig. 9.15b.

The packaged CPW line is measured to find the influence of the developed packaging. The measured S-parameters before and after packaging are shown in Fig. 9.16. The insertion loss change of the packaged CPW is less than 0.1 dB up to 67 GHz, while the return loss is better than 15 dB at the measured frequency range.

9.4.4 Si cap packaging with a PerMX sealing ring

The two packaging methods explained earlier have the BCB sealing ring coated and patterned on packaging cap wafers with housing cavities, and thus they need a specific process to get flat sealing rings. The photosensitive film-type PerMX polymer can be a solution for the sealing ring on a high topographic cap wafer because it can be processed through lamination. It is of interest for RF applications, due to its low dielectric constant of 3.2. The commercially available PerMX films from Dupont Company are PerMX 3014, PerMX 3020 and PerMX 3050, having thicknesses of 14 μm, 20 μm and 50 μm, respectively.[24] PerMX 3050 is selected for the Si cap packaging. The packaging process is shown in Fig. 9.17; (a) PerMX is laminated on the Si cap wafer and photo-lithographically patterned. The process condition of PerMX patterning is detailed in Table 9.1, (b) the Si cap wafer is bonded to a target Si substrate at 150°C – note that the PerMX bonding temperature

Table 9.1 PerMX 3050 process conditions

Step	Conditions
Lamination	Hot roll at 65°C
Soft bake	4 min at 95°C
Expose	400 mJ
PEB	10 min at 60°C
Develop	PGMEA, 5 min
Hard bake	30 min at 150°C

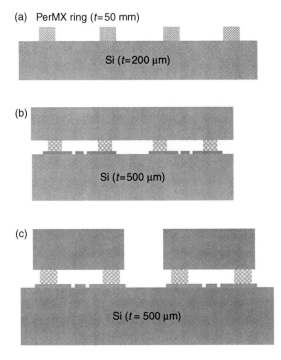

9.17 Process flow of Si cap packaging using a PerMX sealing ring: (a) PerMX ring patterning; (b) Si cap bonding and (c) Si cap dicing.

is less than that of the BCB bonding, and (c) the Si cap is diced to get pad access, and then the Si substrate is diced to separate the packaged chips.

The fabricated package is shown in Fig. 9.18a. The CPW has a centre conductor width of 100 µm and gap of 80 µm. The metal pattern on top of the Si cap is for the dicing process. It does not have a hosing cavity in the Si cap, because the 50 µm-thick PerMX sealing ring provides enough space to avoid the detuning effect of the cap for the packaged CPW. Also, a PerMX sealing ring is implemented on an Si cap with a cavity as shown in Fig. 9.18b.

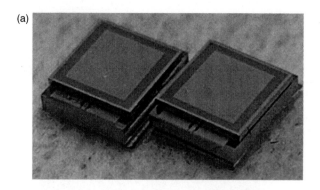
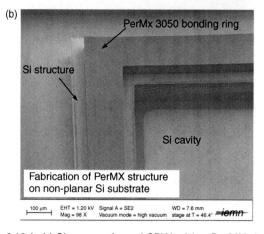

9.18 (a,b) Si cap-packaged CPW with a PerMX ring.

Figure 9.19 shows the measured *S*-parameters of the CPW before and after packaging. The insertion loss change is less than 0.1 dB up to 30 GHz, while the return loss is better than 25 dB for both cases.

9.5 Packaging with a polymer cap

Polymer cap packaging has been reported to have a negligible influence on the packaged device, the so-called RF transparent cap, due to its low dielectric constant and low loss tangent. In addition, its optical transparency makes it possible to perform optical inspection after the packaging process. Polymer cap packaging can be implemented through sacrificial etching as a thin-film package,[21] wafer-level transfer technique,[17,18] or film-type polymer lamination.[19,20,25] Both the wafer-level transfer technique and film-type polymer lamination technique will be described in this section. This packaging technique is different from the ones reported ones in References 26–30.

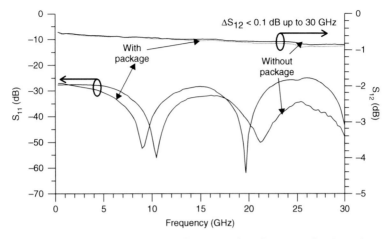

9.19 Measured S-parameters before and after Si cap packaging with PerMX sealing ring.

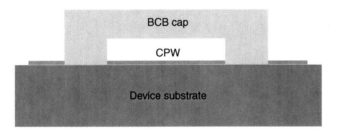

9.20 Concept of BCB cap packaging.

9.5.1 BCB cap packaging

The concept of BCB cap packaging is shown in Fig. 9.20. The height of the BCB cap is limited to approximately 30 μm because of its polymeric properties and its residual stress issues. The housing cavity of the BCB cap is 15 μm. As mentioned earlier, the cavity depth is a critical parameter for the packaging effect on the packaged devices. Therefore, the BCB cap deformation based on ANSYS modelling is first investigated to find the BCB cap deflection due to the BCB residual stress.[25,31] The three principal parameters of the BCB cap are the BCB sealing ring width, the BCB sealing ring height, and the BCB membrane height. BCB cap deflection and chip deflection have been monitored as a function of each parameter and the ambient temperature effect on the BCB cap deflection has been also studied, as shown in Fig. 9.21. It is found that the BCB cap deflection is proportional to the BCB sealing ring height and the

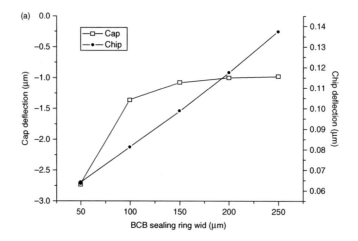

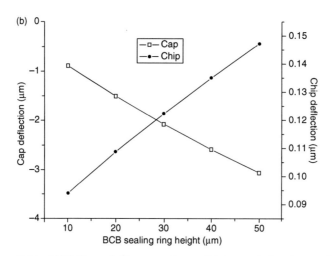

9.21 ANSYS modelling results on BCB cap deflection and chip deflection: (a) cap and chip deflection vs BCB ring width; (b) cap and chip deflection vs BCB ring height; (c) cap and chip deflection vs BCB membrane height and (d) maximum cap deflection vs temperature.

BCB membrane height, and inversely proportional to the BCB sealing ring width. Also, the BCB cap deflection can be significant to the performance of the packaged device below zero temperature rather than higher temperature.

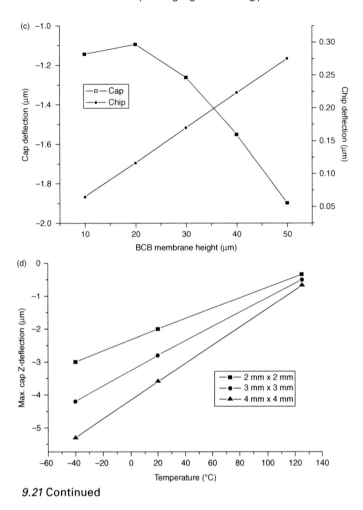

9.21 Continued

The BCB cap packaging can be fabricated through sacrificial etching and the wafer-level BCB cap transfer technique. The wafer-level BCB cap transfer technique with photosensitive BCB[32] provides an opportunity to realize the packaging after the release of the (RF-) MEMS devices. In general, it uses an Si carrier wafer to transfer the BCB cap to a target wafer using the BCB polymer bonding technique. The packaging process is completed when the Si carrier wafer is removed, using grinding process and the Si dry or wet etching process. The Si carrier wafer removal is a significant barrier to a high success rate for the packaging process. Therefore, a wafer-level BCB cap transfer technique based on an anti-adhesion layer assisted bonding–debonding has been reported.

The packaging process is shown in Fig. 9.22; (a) the Si carrier wafer is surface-modified with a monolayer for easier debonding after packaging, (b) the BCB caps are fabricated on the Si carrier wafer through the conventional photo-lithography process, (c) the BCB cap wafer is BCB-bonded to the device wafer at 250°C, and (d) the Si carrier wafer is released from the BCB cap after the bonding process through blade insertion between the two wafers.

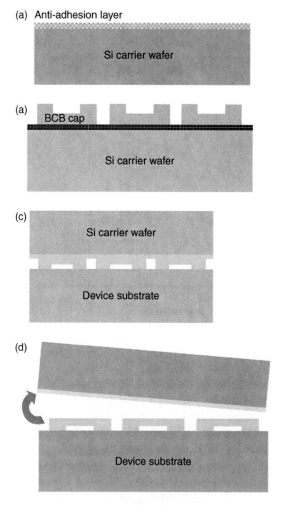

9.22 Process flow of BCB cap packaging: (a) anti-adhesion coating of Si carrier wafer; (b) BCB cap formation; (c) wafer bonding and (d) peel-off Si carrier wafer.

The BCB cap-packaged CPW wafer and the diced BCB-capped CPW chip are shown in Fig. 9.23. Three differently sized BCB caps of 1.4×1.1 mm^2, 2.1×2.1 mm^2 and 5.1×5.1 mm^2 have been successfully implemented. The measured BCB cap profiles are shown in Fig. 9.24. The S-parameters of the CPW before and after the BCB cap packaging have been measured and compared, as shown in Fig. 9.25. The insertion loss change of the CPW before and after packaging is negligible up to 67 GHz, while e return loss is better than 20 dB.

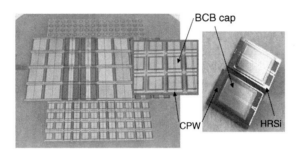

9.23 BCB cap-packaging results.

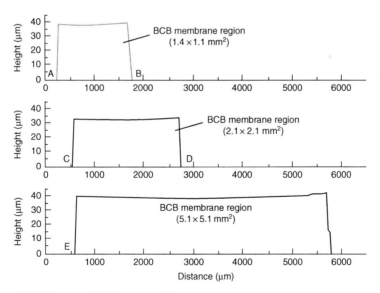

9.24 Measured BCB cap profiles.

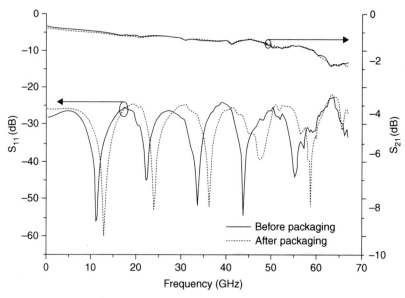

9.25 Measured S-parameters of BCB-capped CPW.

9.5.2 BCB cap packaging with vertical interconnect

A flip-chip compatible BCB cap packaging has also been implemented using an electroplating gold plug as a vertical interconnect RF line. The packaging process is shown in Fig. 9.26; (a) gold plugs were electroplated using a thick photoresist (AZ9260) mould, (b) the photoresist (PR) mould was removed after the electroplating process, (c) the BCB cap was fabricated through a multi-layer BCB coating process, (d) the thermo-compressive BCB bonding was performed, (e) the silicon carrier wafer was removed and (f) the packaging was completed after the seed metal layer etching.

The fabricated prototype BCB polymer packaging and the SEM photograph of electroplated gold plugs are shown in Fig. 9.27.

Test patterns, a gold-plugged CPW line, and a gold-plugged CPW covered with a BCB sealing ring, as shown in Fig. 9.28, have been prepared to investigate the effect of the gold plug interconnect.

The measured S-parameters with the test patterns are shown in Fig. 9.29. The measured insertion losses of the 50 Ω CPW and the gold-plugged CPW are compared with HFSS (high frequency structural simulator) simulation results in Fig. 9.29a. Insertion losses of 0.35 dB/mm at 80 GHz were measured for both the CPW line and a gold-plugged CPW line. Return losses of less than 20 dB at the same frequency were obtained for both lines. The

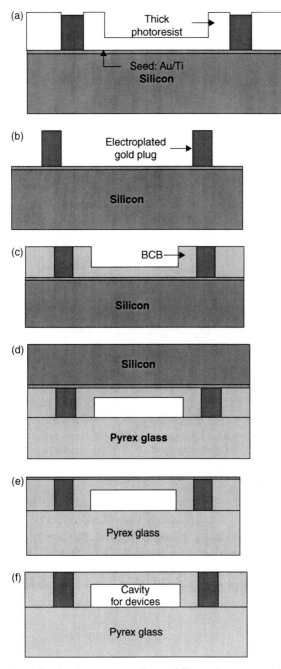

9.26 Packaging process flow of flip-chip compatible BCB cap packaging: (a) gold plug electroplating, (b) removal of PR mould, (c) formation of the BCB cap, (d) bonding with device wafer, (e) removal of the carrier wafer and (f) removal of e layers.

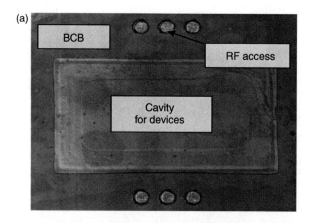
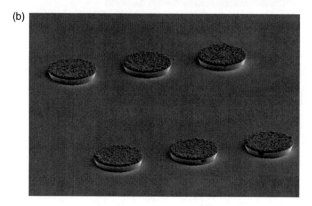

9.27 Fabrication results: (a) fabricated flip-chip compatible BCB package and (b) gold plugs for vertical interconnection.

resonant frequency of the gold-plugged CPW line was decreased due to the series inductance from the gold plug. The effect of the BCB polymer on the gold-plugged CPW has been also measured, as shown in Fig. 9.29b and the insertion loss does not change up to 80 GHz. From 80 to 110 GHz, the insertion loss increased by 0.1 dB. The return loss increased by a few dB over the whole frequency range and the resonant frequency was also increased by a few GHz due to increased shunt capacitance from the BCB ring.

9.5.3 PerMX cap packaging

The PerMX cap packaging is fabricated based on a multi-layer lamination of the film-type PerMX polymer. The packaging has been implemented

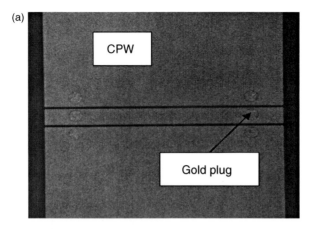

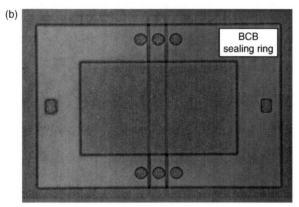

9.28 RF test patterns: (a) CPW with gold plug and (b) gold-plugged CPW with BCB sealing ring.

with PerMX 3050 polymer. The packaging process is shown in Fig. 9.30; (a) the PerMX sealing ring formation, (b) lamination PerMX on the patterned sealing ring, (c) photo-lithography and PEB, (d) develop and hard bake. The thickness of PerMX at step (a) and (b) is 50 μm. One of the significant advantages of the PerMX polymer is the low process temperature. The process condition of the PerMX is given in Table 9.1. The PerMX film is first laminated on a substrate at 65°C and then it is soft-baked at 95°C for 4 min. The laminated PerMX is patterned by a conventional photo-lithography process. The exposure energy was 400 mJ, developed using PGMEA after 10 minutes PEB. Finally, it is hard-baked for 30 min. The maximum process temperature is 150°C. Figure 9.31 shows the wafer-level PerMX cap packaging result on 3-inch Si substrate. The packaging cap sizes are 1.4 × 1.1 mm^2, 2.1 × 2.1 mm^2, and 5.1 × 5.1 mm^2. The measured profiles of the fabricated PerMX caps are shown in Fig. 9.32. The cap height is 100 μm. The maximum

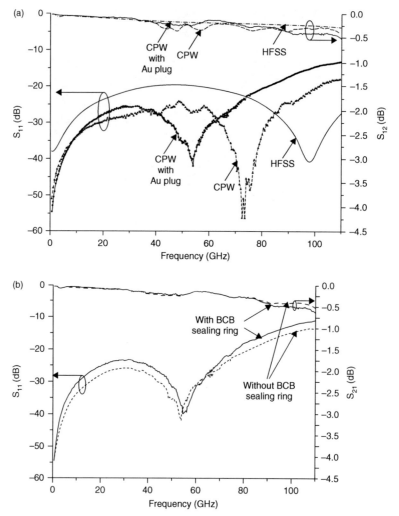

9.29 Measured S-parameters of RF test patterns: (a) HFSS simulation and measurement of CPW and a gold-plugged CPW and (b) S-Parameter measurement of a gold-plugged coplanar with/without BCB sealing ring.

deflection of the PerMX cap is approximately 6.2 μm for 5.1 × 5.1 mm² at its centre, due to the residual stress effect.

To estimate the PerMX cap packaging effect on the transmission line, a 50 Ω coplanar on high resistivity silicon (HRS) was measured before and after packaging. Figure 9.33 shows the PerMX cap-packaged test coplanar lines. The insertion loss change was negligible up to 67 GHz while the return loss was better than 20 dB at the whole frequency range, as shown in Fig. 9.34. Note that the proposed PerMX cap packaging has a competent RF performance with the earlier BCB cap packaging.

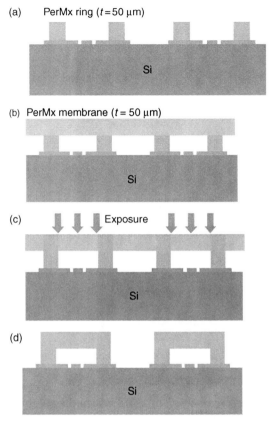

9.30 PerMX packaging process: (a) PerMX sealing ring formation, (b) lamination PerMX on the sealing ring, (c) photo-lithography and PEB and (d) develop and hard bake.

9.6 Conclusion

Wafer-level packaging of RF MEMS plays a major role in MEMS development and commercialization, because all MEMS devices are extremely sensitive to such environmental conditions as humidity and particles etc. Also, hermetic packaging is preferable, to protect MEMS devices from these environmental conditions. Such a packaging can be realized by using thermal wafer-to-wafer bonding and thin-film deposition/growth bonding. Wafer-to-wafer bonding adopts Si, glass and LTCC as packaging caps that are generally bonded by using anodic bonding, metal-to-metal bonding, and polymer bonding. For thin-film packaging, poly-Si and nitride/oxide film caps are used as packaging caps. The high process temperature is one of the biggest drawbacks of these packaging methods. Concerning RF MEMS packaging, the effect on the packaged device from the packaging materials and

286 Handbook of MEMS for wireless and mobile applications

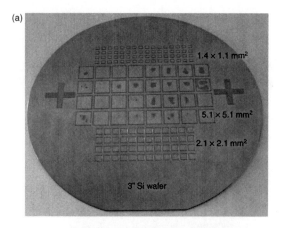

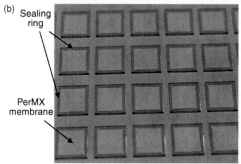

9.31 PerMX packaging results: (a) PerMX cap-packaged wafer and (b) enlarged view of PerMX caps.

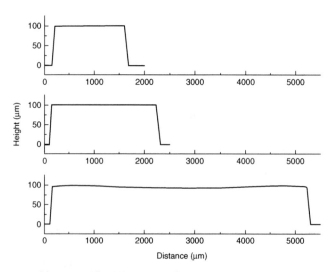

9.32 Measured PerMX cap profiles.

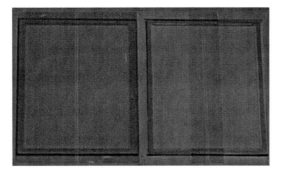

9.33 PerMX cap-packaged coplanar.

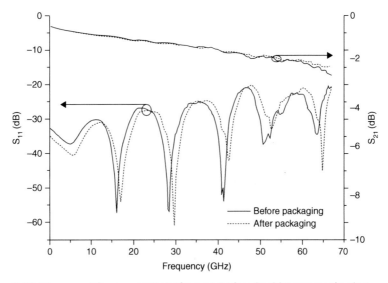

9.34 Measured S-parameter before and after PerMX cap packaging.

the sealing ring should be taken into account. In other words, the parasitic effect of the sealing ring and the detuning effect of the packaging cap in the proximity are the main design issues of the RF MEMS package. Therefore, whole polymer cap packaging provides the great advantage of a negligible cap effect, due to its low dielectric constant. BCB, SU8 and PerMX can be realized as a packaging cap-using wafer-level transfer technique, sacrificial etching and lamination process, respectively. The packaging is performed at a temperature lower than 250°C, which is also good for the packaging of MEMS components integrated with complementary metal oxide semiconductor (CMOS) or monolithic microwave integrated circuit (MMIC) circuits. RF characterization of the polymer cap packaging has been shown to have an insertion loss change less than 0.01 dB up to 70 GHz, while return loss is better than 20 dB. The weakness of the polymer cap packaging is its non-hermeticity. Hermetic package is significant for the packaged (RF-) MEMS devices. It can be improved using dielectric passivation or metallic material overcoat, at the cost of process complexity and loss of optical transparency of the cap in the case of metallic overcoat. Furthermore, environment and reliability tests are required for commercial products.

9.7 References

1. B. Lee, S. Seok, and K. Chun, 'A study on wafer level vacuum packaging for MEMS devices', *Journal of Micromechanics and Microengineering*, **13**(5) (2003), pp. 663–669.
2. H. Hemmi, S. Shoji, Y. Shoji, and M. Esashi, 'Vacuum packaging for microsensors by glass–silicon anodic bonding', *Sensors and Actuators*, **A 43** (1994), pp. 243–248.
3. H. Guckel and D. W. Burns, 'Planar processed polysilicon sealed cavities for pressure transducer arrays,' *International Electron Devices Meeting (IEDM)* (1984), pp. 223–225.
4. L. Lin, R. T. Howe, and A. P. Pisano, 'Microelectromechanical filters for signal processing,' *IEEE/ASME Journal of Microelectromechanical Systems*, **7** (1998), pp. 286–294.
5. K. S. Lebouitz, R. T. Howe, and A. P. Pisano, 'Permeable polysilicon etch-access windows for microshell fabrication,' Transducers'95 (1995), pp. 224–227.
6. A. Jourdain, H. Ziad, P. D. Moor, and H. A. C. Tilmans, 'Wafer-scale 0-level packaging of (RF-)MEMS devices using BCB', *Design, Test, Integration and Packaging of MEMS/MOEMS* (2003), pp. 239–244.
7. S. Seok, N. Rolland, and P.-A. Rolland, 'A novel packaging method using wafer-level BCB polymer bonding and glass wet-etching for RF applications', *Sensors and Actuators A-Physical*, **147**(2) (2008), pp. 677–682.
8. K. Kim, J. Kim, G. Hwang, C. Baek, and Y. Kim, 'Packaging for RF MEMS devices using LTCC substrate and BCB adhesive layer', *Journal of Micromechanics and Microengineering*, **16**(1) (2006), pp. 150–156.
9. J. Wei, H. Xie, M. L. Nai, C. K. Wong, and L. C. Lee, 'Low temperature wafer anodic bonding', *Journal of Micromechanics and Microengineering*, **13** (2003), pp. 217–222.
10. C. C. Lee, C. Y. Wang, and G. S. Matijasevic, 'A new bonding technology using gold and tin multilayer composite structures', *IEEE Transactions on Components, Hybrids, and Manufacturing Technology*, June (1999), pp. 407–412.
11. R. Knechtel, 'Glass frit bonding: a universal technology for wafer level encapsulation and packaging' *Microsystem Technologies*, **12** (2005), pp. 63–68.
12. F. Niklaus, P. Enoksson, E. Kalvesten, and G. Stemme, 'Void-free full wafer adhesive bonding', Micro Electro Mechanical Systems 2000 (MEMS2000), 23–27 Jan. (2000), pp. 247–252.
13. A. Höchsta, R. Scheuerera, H. Stahla, F. Fischera, L. Metzgera, R. Reichenbacha, F. Lärmera, S. Kronmüllera, S. Watchamb, C. Rusuc, A. Witvrouwc, and R. Gunn, 'Stable thin film encapsulation of acceleration sensors using polycrystalline silicon as sacrificial and encapsulation layer', *Sensors and Actuators A: Physical*, **114**(2–3) (2004), pp. 355–361.

14. Q. Li, J. F. L. Goosen, J. T. M. van Beek, F. van Keulen, K. L. Phan, G. Q. Zhang, 'Failure analysis of a thin-film nitride MEMS package', *Microelectronics Reliability*, **48** (2008), pp. 1557–1561.
15. J. Zekry, D. S. Tezcan, J.-P. Celis, R. Puers, C. Van Hoof, and H. A. C. Tilmans, 'Wafer-level thin film vacuum packages for MEMS using nanoporus anodic alumina membranes', Transducers'11, Beijing, China, 5–9 June (2011), pp. 974–977.
16. B. Lee, D. Choi, and J. Yoon, 'Use of nanoporous columnar thin film in the wafer-level packaging of MEMS devices', *Journal of Micromechanics and Microengineering*, **20** (2010), pp. 1–9.
17. S. Seok, N. Rolland, and P. -A. Rolland, 'Packaging methodology for RF devices using a BCB membrane transfer technique', *Journal of Micromechanics and Microengineering*, **16**(11), Nov. (2006), pp. 2384–2388.
18. S. Seok, N. Rolland, and P. -A. Rolland, 'Design, fabrication and measurement of BCB polymer zero-level packaging for millimeter-wave applications', *IEEE Transaction on Microwave Theory and Techniques*, May (2007), pp. 1040–1045.
19. S. Seok, J. Kim, N. Rolland, and P.-A. Rolland, 'Low-temperature zero-level packaging technique using photosensitive film type PerMX polymer' Transducers'11, Beijing, China, June (2011), pp. 334–337.
20. J. Kim, S. Seok, N. Rolland, and P.-A. Rolland, 'Low loss 0-level packaging for high frequency RF applications by using PerMX film photoresist' European Microwave Conference 2011, Oct. (2011), pp. 273–276.
21. I. Zine-El-Abidine and M. Okoniewski, 'A low-temperature SU-8 based wafer-level hermetic packaging for MEMS devices', *IEEE Transactions on Advanced Packaging*, **32**(2) (2009), pp. 448–452.
22. Z. Wand and Z. Liu, 'An analytical method for optimization of RF MEMS wafer level packaging with CPW detuning consideration' Progress in Electromagnetics Research Symposium Proceedings, Moscow, Russia, 18–21 August (2009), pp. 479–483.
23. H. El Gannudi, P. Farinelli, I. Pieper, E. Chiuppesi, and R. Sorrentino, 'Design and manufacturing of wideband buried RF feedthroughs for wafer-level RF MEMS package', The 5th European Microwave Integrated Circuits Conference (EuMIC), 27–28 September (2010), Paris, France, pp. 321–324.
24. S. Seok, M. Fryziel, N. Rolland, and P. -A. Rolland, 'Enhancement of bonding strength of packaging based on BCB bonding for RF devices', *Microsystem Technologies* (2012), DOI: 10.1007/s00542-012-1530-0.
24. DuPont™ PerMX™ 3000 Photodielectric Dry Film Adhesive Technical data sheet.
25. J. Kim, S. Seok, and N. Rolland, 'Low-temperature, low-loss zero level packaging technique for RF applications using a photopatternable dry film', *Journal of Micromechanics and Microengineering* (2012), 065032.
26. A. Jourdain, P. D. Moore, K. Baert, I. D. Wolf, and H. A. C. Tilmans, 'Mechanical and electrical characterization of BCB as a bond and seal material for cavities housing (RF-)MEMS devices', *Journal of Micromechanics and Microengineering*, **15**(7) (2005), pp. 89–96.
27. H. A. C. Tilmans, H. Ziad, H. Jansen, O. D. Monaco, and A. Jourdain, 'Wafer-level packaged RF-MEMS switches fabricated in a CMOS Fab', IEEE International Electron Devices Meeting (2001), pp. 921–924.

28. J. Oberhammer, F. Niklaus, and G. Stemme, 'Sealing of adhesive bonded devices on wafer level', *Sensors and Actuators A: Physical*, **110**(1–3) (2004), pp. 407–412.
29. J. Oberhammer, F. Nickaus, and G. Stemme, 'Selective wafer-level adhesive bonding with benzocyclobutene for fabrication of cavities', *Sensors and Actuators*, **A 105** (2003), pp. 297–304.
30. J. Oberhammer and G. Stemme, 'BCB contact printing for patterned adhesive full-wafer bonded 0-level package', *Journal of Microelectromechanical systems*, **14**(2), April (2005), pp. 419–425.
31. S. Seok, N. Rolland, and P. -A. Rolland, 'A theoretical and experimental study of BCB thin-film cap zero-level package based on FEM simulations', *Journal of Micromechanics and Microengineering* (2010), pp. 1–7.
32. Dow Chemical Company, Processing Procedures for CYCLOTENE 4000 Series Photo BCB Resins, February 2005.

10
Reliability of RF MEMS

I. DE WOLF, P. CZARNECKI, J. DE COSTER,
O. V. PEDREIRA, X. ROTTENBERG and
S. SANGAMESWARAN, imec, Belgium

DOI: 10.1533/9780857098610.1.291

Abstract: After a brief overview of possible failure mechanisms and failure defects that can occur in radio frequency microelectromechanical systems (RF MEMS), this chapter focuses on three specific reliability issues: charging, because it remains the most important problem for capacitive RF MEMS; electrostatic discharge, because it is less known as a possible failure cause for MEMS; and package hermeticity, because this is an often underestimated problem for RF MEMS.

Key words: reliability, failure mechanisms, MEMS, RF MEMS, switches, charging, ESD, hermeticity.

10.1 Introduction

Microelectromechanical systems (MEMS) or nanoelectromechanical systems (NEMS) can only take their place on the market if their reliability is proven. For RF MEMS, this is one of the main hurdles that are still to be taken. Not only do the devices themselves suffer from seemingly unavoidable failure mechanisms, such as unintended electrical charging, but also the reliability of the package required for keeping the MEMS in a well-controlled, stable environment is far from established. There are various, mostly product dependent, packaging solutions for MEMS. Because of this large variation, reported numbers on the percentage cost the package takes within the entire manufacturing also vary, from 30% up to 95%. This cost can be reduced substantially by developing the MEMS package together with the MEMS. At the same time, such a co-development would result in better reliability. The specifications on pressure and pressure stability are defined for most applications, but it is not clear how to test these, that is, how to qualify the reliability of the MEMS package.

Reliability can be defined as '*the probability that an item will perform a required function under stated conditions for a stated period of time*'. It involves both short term (early failures) and long term (wear-out) MEMS stability studies. A 100% reliable MEMS device probably does not exist, not only because reliability can only be 'predicted', but also because some failure mechanisms cannot be avoided, only delayed. As a consequence, it is important to fabricate devices that are 'just reliable enough', that is, that remain within specification during their intended life for a certain application. For a mobile phone application, this would be shorter than for an automotive application. It is also important to realize that some component-level reliability issues can be suppressed at system level. Design for reliability should not only address the device and the package, but also the complete system around it. For example, the effect of electrical charging in capacitive RF MEMS switches, which leads to an increase in pull-in voltage and eventually to stiction, can be reduced by alternating between two RF MEMS, allowing for one that is not being used to discharge (a kind of redundancy), or by using bipolar actuation or discharging the device regularly by applying actuation with the opposite polarity. In any case, in order to have an optimal design for reliability and to be able to make 'reliable-enough' RF MEMS, it is mandatory that the physics underlying the failure mechanisms affecting them is understood.

In this chapter, we first list a number of possible failure mechanisms, or 'failure defects' that can occur in RF MEMS. Most of these have been already extensively addressed in De Wolf (2010). For this reason, we focus in the remainder of the chapter on only three specific reliability issues: *charging*, because it still remains the most important problem for capacitive RF MEMS; *electrostatic discharge* (ESD), because it is less well known as a possible failure cause; and *package hermeticity*, because this is an often underestimated problem for RF MEMS, especially for resonators, and there do not exist clear test methods or standards.

10.2 Overview of failure mechanisms in RF MEMS

There are many possible failure mechanisms in MEMS, and specifically in RF MEMS. The major known ones are as follows.

10.2.1 Dielectric charging

Dielectric charging appears in a capacitor when strong electric fields are applied across the thin dielectric layer, or when it is exposed to ionizing radiation. In RF MEMS switches containing a dielectric, charging of this dielectric constitutes a major problem, especially when the capacitive RF MEMS switch is in the down position, that is, touching the dielectric. Charging results in a shift of the pull-in and pull-out voltages, and eventually in stiction of the device. Resonators may suffer from charges that can build up near actuation electrodes or in the substrate.

10.2.2 Dielectric breakdown of the dielectric

When a large amount of charge is built up in an insulator, it can form a conductive path leading to breakdown of the insulator. Also a very high electrical field can cause breakdown.

10.2.3 Dielectric breakdown of the air gap

If the gap between two conductors is or becomes small, and a high voltage is present between them, breakdown of the air gap can occur. Another effect that can take place for small gaps is electron emission from one electrode to the other. When separating contacts under load, electrons and ions tend to keep the contact closed and metallic ions are emitted from anode to cathode. This phenomenon, called the Townsend arc, is an important wear mechanism in micro-relays. All these effects can result in charging, fusion or breakdown of the device.

10.2.4 Stiction

An important problem in MEMS is stiction. Because the structures are so small, surface forces can dominate all others, and cause structures to stick together when their surfaces come into contact. The most important surface forces in MEMS are the capillary force (due to condensed water between the surfaces), the molecular van der Waals force, micro-welding, and electrostatic forces (charging). Recently it was shown that the capillary forces not only depend on humidity level and the roughness/shape of the devices, but also on the applied bias (Zaghloul *et al.*, 2011a). It is important to mention that stiction is not necessarily permanent. It can, for example, cause small delays in the pull-out voltage (Ling *et al.*, 2011a,b).

10.2.5 Fatigue

Fatigue is crack initiation and growth during cyclic loading. It is a time-dependent phenomenon that can lead to a drift in device parameters and eventually to complete failure of the device due to fracture. Fatigue typically starts at locations in the material where a high local stress concentration is present, for example at hinges of a bridge or at the anchor point. It is probably not a real threat as long as local stresses at these points remain relatively small. This is highly dependent on the mechanical properties of the materials used (metals are typically more sensitive than, e.g. silicon).

10.2.6 Creep

This is a time-dependent deformation of a sample caused by external loads. High local stresses or stress gradients may result in microscopic material changes through dislocation glide and climb, and diffusion mechanisms. Aluminium is often used as a bridge metal in RF MEMS switches, because its properties and deposition parameters are well known in the integrated circuit (IC) industry and it allows easy processing. Unfortunately, it turns out that pure Al has very undesirable creep properties. Creep can manifest in the form of a kind of 'memory effect' (Douglass, 1998). This may, after a while, result in a non-functional device, due to the fact that the restoring force is lowered. In addition, it can result in a shift of device parameters, such as the pull-in voltage and the capacitance swing. Even if one can assume that at room temperature creep is not a major problem, it can become a major reliability problem during hot switching of the devices, especially for high-power applications. Creep is mostly associated with high mechanical stress and high temperatures. But stress-induced plastic deformation can also occur at low temperatures. Due to very high CTE mismatches, a MEMS component might experience very high loads at low temperatures, causing it to deform plastically or even to fracture.

10.2.7 Temperature-induced plastic deformation

Every metal has a critical temperature T_c above which it deforms plastically. This can result in a permanent deformation of the metal component, for example an RF MEMS bridge. Temperatures higher than T_c can occur during packaging, be caused by the environment, or be RF-induced in high-power applications.

10.2.8 Temperature-induced elastic deformation

Another source of deformation is the temperature itself. Even if the material remains elastic and does not change properties, a high temperature might cause buckling of the moving element of a MEMS, due to differences in CTE between the element and the substrate or package, or even due to non-uniform temperature differences within the element. This is especially important also for high-power RF MEMS. Internal temperature changes, depending on signal power and frequency, can have a severe impact.

10.2.9 Micro-welding and wear

This only affects metal layers coming into contact. It mainly concerns ohmic switches. Depending on the contact force (e.g. shock loading) and temperature (e.g. current-flow induced heating), welding or material transport between the two contacting materials (wear) can occur, resulting in stiction or surface degradation.

10.2.10 Friction

Sliding of two materials during contact can cause wear effects, particles, increased temperature or even charging. There are not many reports on friction problems in RF MEMS. The exception, for resonators, is the so-called fly-catching effect: due to friction of the resonating beam with the surrounding medium, charging of the beam might occur. This can not only directly affect the functioning, but it can also result in attraction of particles from the air, with a consequent mass increase and a shift of the resonance frequency.

10.2.11 Corrosion

The most general definition of corrosion is 'a process in which a metal is deteriorated by a chemical or electrochemical reaction with its environment'. Oxidation is a form of corrosion and is certainly a reliability problem for resonators. Small changes in stiffness or mass, due to oxidation, can have a high effect on the resonance frequency.

10.2.12 Electromigration

Electromigration is the movement of ions under the influence of an electrical potential difference. At first sight, it is not expected to be a problem for RF MEMS and, as such, it is mostly not mentioned in literature. But the RF current will not flow homogeneously in devices. Due to field concentrations at edges, skin effect and resonance nodes, locally high current densities can be expected and might cause electromigration effects.

10.2.13 Self-biasing

Self-actuation is the motion of the MEMS mobile structure leading to an actuated state without actuation voltage being applied. This can be due to Lorentz forces or due to the RF power. It should be addressed especially for high-power RF signals. Devices with a low mechanical stiffness will have a higher sensitivity to self-biasing.

10.2.14 Fracture

Fracture of mechanical parts of the MEMS structure can occur during large shock loading combined with local stress concentration. Because MEMS are thin and light, they can be expected to resist large shock and vibration tests. But their sensitivity to fracture depends on the fracture strength of the used materials. For some applications, it might be an important issue.

10.2.15 Electrical short

Electrical contact can occur between (movable) conductive layers, leading to breakdown, or functional or actuation failures. Temperature, particles, shock loadings, ESD, plastic deformation and Lorentz forces can cause electrical shorts.

10.2.16 Fusing

Fusion is a destructive local evaporation/explosion of a metal line or contact. This effect is related to high local power dissipation in the metallic path, for example due to a high voltage pulse (e.g. ESD). The high temperatures or local high electric fields vaporize the metal, creating opens in conductors.

10.2.17 Outgassing and adsorption

Outgassing of molecules or gases from materials surrounding a packaged resonator or from the resonator itself can affect the pressure in the package or affect the mass of the resonator. These are important reliability concerns, often underestimated and not well studied. They can also affect the contact properties in ohmic RF MEMS. On the other hand, adsorption of, for example, water can have similar effects and, in addition, affect stiction properties.

10.2.18 Mechanical or acoustic coupling

The resonance frequency of RF MEMS can be, depending on its design, highly sensitive to mechanical stress – from the package, for example. If this stress changes over time, due to creep or other effects, this will cause a drift and, as such, a reliability problem. Acoustic coupling is a well-known effect, where the resonating of one device affects a nearby device. There might even be coupling with the package. These problems can in general be avoided through an optimal design.

Most of these failure mechanisms have been described in detail in the Chapter 'Reliability' in the book 'Advanced RF MEMS' (De Wolf, 2010). For this reason, in the following we focus on only three reliability issues: charging, ESD, and package hermeticity.

10.3 Charging in RF MEMS

Charging is recognized as the main failure mechanism for MEMS. Actually, any MEMS using electrical actuation can suffer from this problem. In the following, this problem is discussed in detail using the capacitive RF MEMS switch as an example.

10.3.1 The RF MEMS capacitive switch: a special-purpose switched capacitor

The electrostatically driven capacitive RF MEMS switch is a device fabricated in MEMS technology. The function of the device is to switch (route) RF signals. The operation of the switch is based on capacitance changes due to motion of the movable armature by an externally applied electrostatic force.

A typical example of a capacitive switch is shown in Fig. 10.1. A coplanar waveguide (CPW) line is fabricated on an insulation substrate, for example, high resistivity Si or glass. A beam is suspended above the signal line and is anchored in the ground planes of the CPW to form a bridge. An interposer dielectric is deposited on the signal line under the bridge. To first order, the switch can be modelled as a capacitor between the grounded bridge and the signal line. In the RF ON state the bridge is up, hence the switch capacitance is small, hardly affecting the impedance of the line. By applying a direct current (DC) bias to either bridge or signal line, the switch capacitance charges, giving rise to electrostatic forces that tend to close the device. When these forces overcome the mechanical stiffness of the bridge, the latter pulls-in and contacts the dielectric. The switch capacitance becomes high and the switch is OFF or in the isolation state.

The interposer dielectric layer has two main functions in a capacitive switch. On the one hand, it improves the capacitive contrast between up- and down-states, an important figure of merit for switches. On the other hand, it prevents ohmic contact between the beam and the signal line upon device actuation. It is easy to see that this interposer dielectric will be subjected, during the lifetime of a switch, to repeated electrical, mechanical and electromechanical stress.

As mentioned in the Introduction, dielectric charging is widely accepted as the major yield and reliability issue for electrostatically actuated (RF) MEMS switches such as that shown in Fig. 10.1 (De Natale *et al.*, 2002; Goldsmith *et al.*, 2001; Lisec *et al.*, 2004; McClure *et al.*, 2002; Melle *et al.*, 2003; Reid, 2002; Wibbeler, 1998).

The physics behind charging in RF MEMS capacitive switches is not straightforward. The problem is that many different charging mechanisms can take place, and which one dominates depends highly on the dielectrics

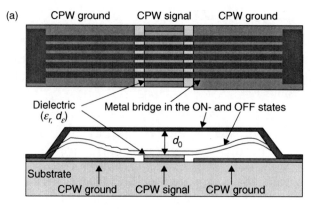
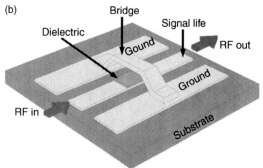
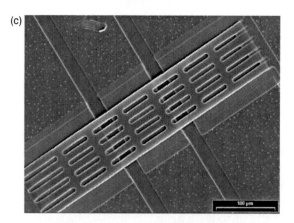

10.1 (a,b) Schematics and (c) SEM image of a capacitive electrostatically driven RF MEMS switch. (a): © 2007, IEEE. Reprinted, with permission, from Rottenberg *et al.* (2007b); (b) © 2008, IEEE. Reprinted, with permission, from Czarnecki (2008b)).

used and on the processing conditions (Zaghloul, 2011; Zaghloul *et al.*, 2011b). Charging mechanisms can be related to surface and bulk charges, but also to polarization related charges (Papaioannou *et al.*, 2005, 2010). Dipole related charging can even occur without direct contact between the movable top electrode and the MEMS dielectric. In addition, for a small gap and high electric field, electron emission or air gap breakdown can also cause non-contact charging (Czarnecki *et al.*, 2008b, 2009; Yuan *et al.*, 2004).

The main processes that are identified as responsible for charge injection in MEMS are the Poole–Frenkel effect and trap assisted tunnelling. The first is a thermal emission of charges from traps in the bulk of a dielectric, enhanced by an electric field. The second is the motion of charges between traps. Mostly these effects can take place in combination (Zaghloul, 2011).

Charges trapped or displaced during the processing, during the actuation, and by irradiation of the devices can result in a shift of the pull-in and pull-out voltages, self-biasing or latching. To avoid these problems, not only an understanding of the physics behind the charge trapping is required, but also the impact of these charges on the functioning of the MEMS has to be understood. This is discussed in the next sections, where measurement methods and experiments are discussed, and analytical models are proposed that can be used to predict/understand the observed effects and provide guidelines for obtaining optimal reliability.

10.3.2 Experimental charging evaluation

The study of charging in RF MEMS can be performed in various ways. Closest to the real application is the technique that consists in monitoring the effect of charging on the S-parameters of the device (Melle *et al.*, 2003). This is, however, neither the easiest nor the most efficient technique, as it requires fully functional RF MEMS devices as well as expensive and delicate RF measurement equipment. Especially for reliability studies, which are in general time consuming, simpler test methods are mandatory. The most commonly used approaches consist in monitoring the capacitance–voltage (C–V) characteristic of RF MEMS switches, or the resonance frequency and Q factor of MEMS resonators, and check for any shift or deformation of these characteristic curves.

As an alternative to the C–V method for capacitive switches, metal insulator metal (MIM) capacitors can be realized and measured to study the charging and breakdown properties of the dielectric used within the actual microelectromechanical (MEM) devices. In this case, possible electrical measurements include I–V and C–V measurements, charge/discharge current transient measurements (C/DCT) and thermally stimulated depolarization current measurements (TSCD). Scanning-probe-based techniques

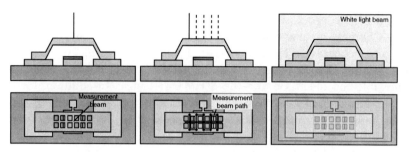

10.2 Motion measurement of a MEMS beam using either a laser Doppler vibrometer in one point (left) or by scanning over the surface (centre); or by using WLI (right).

can further be implemented to gain insight in the local reliability of MEM switched capacitors. For example, Kelvin probe force microscopy (KPFM) can be applied to directly assess local charging either on the dielectric itself or through a thin metal film (KPFM-TF) coated on the dielectric. Also force–distance curves (based on AFM) can provide important information on local charging in MEMS (Zaghloul, 2011; Zaghloul *et al.*, 2010).

The movement of the MEMS armature and the impact of charging on that motion can be monitored by optical methods if the moving surface is larger than a few microns. For example, laser Doppler vibrometry (LDV) and optical interferometry (e.g. white light interferometry (WLI)) are commonly used (Fig. 10.2). LDV uses a focused laser beam and allows for fast measurement (the response of the beam in real time), but only at one point at a time. Under certain conditions, out-of-plane displacements in the pico-scale sensitivity can be measured with this technique, with a bandwidth up to 20MHz. Observation of the movement of the whole device is possible by scanning the beam across the surface during a sequence of actuations. This, however, requires that the MEMS motion is not modified during the duration of the scan. In comparison, WLI gives access to a complete height map of a (quasi-) static device, but in general does not allow fast measurements and is less accurate, giving out-of-plane displacement at best at nm scale. There exist WLI solutions using a stroboscopic LED for the illumination that allow motion analysis with a frequency bandwidth of the order of 2 MHz (Chen *et al.*, 2007).

In this section we focus on capacitance measurements, mainly because they are the simplest and cheapest way to study the charging problem in RF MEMS capacitive switches. Indeed, from the charging point of view, the electrostatically driven RF MEMS capacitive switch is a movable beam that responds to the applied actuation voltage. The function of the device, switching, is an outcome of the beam displacement. Charge trapped in the switch changes the electric field in the vicinity of the beam. Thereupon, it influences the relation between the applied voltage and the electrostatic force actuating the beam. Observations of the changes of the beam response to the applied actuation voltage can thus provide valuable information.

The capacitance measurement techniques allow obtaining one of the most basic characteristic of the device: the C–V characteristic. Observation of the changes of the C–V characteristic allows fast and non-invasive study of charge trapped in the switch. However, there is one main problem with this technique: charging can also occur during the C–V measurement, that is, the measurement technique affects the measurement result. To avoid this, van Spengen *et al.* (2003) presented a dedicated system for testing the reliability of capacitive RF MEMS switches. This electrical lifetime test (ELT) system allows acquiring actuation characteristics equivalent to C–V curves. It is not the real capacitance that is measured, but the impact of changes of the capacitance on an applied high frequency signal. Depending on the implementation, the system allows observation of capacitance changes in the order of 10 fF with a bandwidth of a few hundreds of kHz; voltages of nearly any waveform up to 100 V can be applied. These fast C–V measurements allow observation charging mechanisms and reduce the impact of the measurement on the charge trapped during stressing. A typical result of a conventional and a fast C–V measurement is shown in Fig. 10.3.

Figure 10.4 defines some of the main parameters of a C–V measurement result: the down- (on) and up-state (off) capacitance and the pull-in and pull-out voltages.

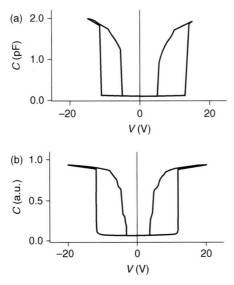

10.3 Examples of C–V characteristic measurements. (a) Standard, performed with an RLC meter. (b) Fast with the ELT system.

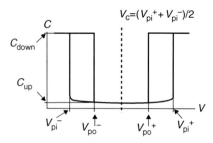

10.4 Definition of C_{down} (the down (on)) and C_{up} (the up-state (off)) capacitance and V_{pi} (the pull-in) and V_{po} (the pull-out) voltages. The centre of the C–V curve V_c can be calculated as $V_c = (V_{pi}^+ + V_{pi}^-)/2$.

Test structures

A reliability study does not always require fully processed devices as these are expensive and time consuming. When performing failure-driven reliability testing (De Wolf, 2010), often simple test structures can be used. The simplified structures have to be representative from the point of view of the assessed problem.

In the charging studies, MIM capacitors are often proposed. They allow testing of the charging properties of dielectrics. However, they do not fully represent the MEMS devices. The main difference is in the interfaces. In MIM capacitors, both top and bottom electrodes are in physical contact with the dielectric layer (Fig. 10.5). The MEMS devices are usually more asymmetric. The top surface of the dielectric layer is free (exposed to ambient gas, vacuum, etc.) and has (limited) contact with the beam. This can allow different or additional charging mechanisms (gas breakdown, electron emission), which are not seen in MIM capacitors.

We have proposed a simplified test structure that allows testing the charging properties of dielectric materials in conditions very similar to those occurring in the fully processed devices: the movable beam is deposited on a non-patterned stack of bottom metal and dielectric layers (Fig. 10.6). Actuation of the device requires scratching through the dielectric layer in order to contact the metal layer underneath. That metal sheet plays the role of one of the actuation electrodes. The second electrode is the beam. This test structure requires much fewer processing steps than a fully functional RF MEMS capacitive switch, but allows testing of the charging sensitivity of the dielectric in conditions very close to those of the real device.

Reliability testing techniques for charging assessment

Numerous techniques can be implemented to test the sensitivity of a MEMS device to charging. The first is based on monitoring the up- and down-state

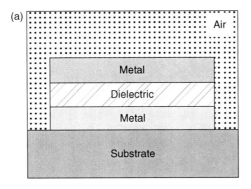

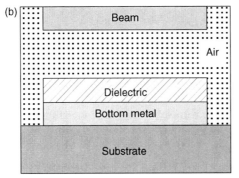

10.5 The main difference between the MIM (a) and MEMS (b) devices is the different top dielectric interface.

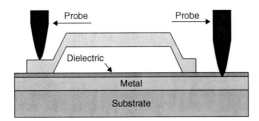

10.6 A simplified MEMS structure allows a charging study in conditions similar to those occurring in the fully processed devices. Probing the bottom electrode requires scratching through the dielectric layer.

capacitance of the switch during stressing (cycling) of a device. An actuation waveform (e.g. rectangular) causes actuation of the tested device. The changes of the capacitance values reflect the movement of the beam. If charging occurs when cycling a device, its on- and off-state capacitances vary from their initial values (Fig. 10.7). Once these values go out of specification, with stiction or not closing in the extreme case, end-of-life (EOL)

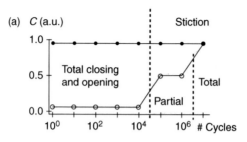

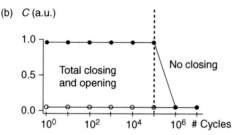

10.7 Monitoring of the down-state (full symbols) and up-state (open symbols) capacitance of a switch allows distinguishing two failure modes: stiction (a) and no closing (no actuation) (b).

is reached. This method takes a lot of time, because the effect of charging is not always immediately observable in changes of C_{down} or C_{up} and long duration stressing might be required. It is possible to accelerate the experiments by using higher actuation voltages (Goldsmith *et al.*, 2001). However, some failure mechanisms may be overlooked in this way. It has been shown, for example, that for certain devices, different charging mechanisms can take place at low or high voltages (Czarnecki, 2010).

Since the C–V characteristic can provide information about charge build-up in the switch, observation of changes of the *complete* C–V curve, so not only C_{down} and C_{up}, can provide more detailed information on how the charge changes in time, for example, during stressing or idling. The simplest case would be to measure the C–V characteristics just before and immediately after stressing (Fig. 10.8). The amount of charge is related to the voltage shift (V_S) and/or narrowing of the C–V curve.

Accelerated testing

As mentioned before, the charging mechanism can be accelerated by using higher actuation voltages for the MEMS (Goldsmith *et al.*, 2001). The lifetime of the switch can be determined from capacitance measurements during stressing (e.g. cycling). The EOL is reached when the measured values (C_{up}, C_{down}, ΔC, C_{up}/C_{down}) go out of specification as shown in Fig. 10.7. However, this methodology may be time consuming. On top of that, increasing the actuation

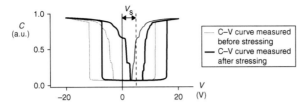

10.8 An example of the voltage shift between two C–V curves measured before and after stressing.

voltage may not be possible in some cases. The higher actuation voltage may trigger additional mechanisms. Observation of the full C–V characteristic evolution is a better alternative, not only before and after as shown in Fig. 10.8. The C–V characteristics can be measured during stressing using the fast C–V method described before (van Spengen *et al.*, 2003) and the pull-in and pull-out voltages can be extracted (Czarnecki *et al.*, 2008b; Herfst *et al.*, 2006; van Spengen *et al.*, 2004). Figure 10.9 shows an example of a result of such an experiment. Capacitance measurements during stressing (a) do not show any changes after 5000 cycles, however, the C–V curve measurements (b) reveal charging, visible as a voltage shift of the pull-in (V_{pi}^+ and negative V_{pi}^-) and pull-out (positive V_{po}^+ and negative V_{po}^-) voltages. This is even more visible when the evolution of the C–V curve is presented as the changes of the centre V_c (c) (mean voltage between positive V_{po}^+ and negative V_{po}^-).

As mentioned in the introduction on charging, various charging mechanisms can take place at the same time in a MEMS device. Periodical C–V measurements performed during stressing (Czarnecki *et al.*, 2006; Herfst *et al.*, 2006; van Spengen *et al.*, 2004) can reveal this because they can provide insight into the dynamics of the charging mechanisms. Figure 10.10 shows an example of a measurement that revealed two co-existing mechanisms with different polarities and time constants (τ_1 and τ_2) (Czarnecki *et al.*, 2008b).

This monitoring method during voltage stressing of MEMS can be used for a relatively fast evaluation and comparison of different devices, different processing recipes, composition of materials, design, etc. Figure 10.11 shows the evolution of the positive pull-in voltage of two different devices (devices 1 and 2) during stressing. The goal of the experiment was to evaluate which one of the two devices' processing recipes can provide more reliable devices from a charging point of view. Therefore, both devices were stressed under the same conditions (amplitude, frequency and duty cycle of the actuation voltage, atmosphere, etc.) and the evolution of the C–V characteristic was monitored. It was assumed that EOL is reached when the positive pull-in changes more than 2 V from the initial value, even though the switch is still switching, that is, the C_{down}/C_{up} ratio is still relatively high. The lifetime of the two tested devices obtained with that method is 4500 and 12000 cycles as

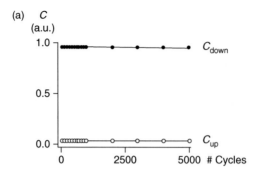
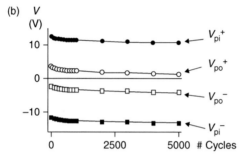
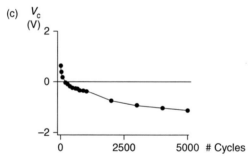

10.9 (a) Capacitance measurements showing C_{up} and C_{down} evolution; (b) evolution of C–V pull-in and pull-out voltages; and (c) the extracted change of the centre voltage, V_c.

indicated in the figure. This technique allows obtaining detailed information on charging in a very rapid way as compared to the conventional C_{down}/C_{up} ratio testing. Even more, as the experiment can be set in such a way that it lasts only a few seconds, obtaining statistical data does not take a lot of time and allows for a statistically relevant evaluation of, for example, different processing recipes or materials (Czarnecki, 2010; González et al., 2011). In conclusion, the observation of the evolution of the C–V characteristic is a powerful tool that allows studies of charging mechanisms in the switch in a relatively easy and non-invasive way.

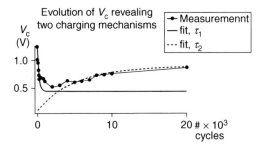

10.10 Two charging mechanisms with two different time constant (τ_1 and τ_2) observed with C–V curve measurements performed during stressing.

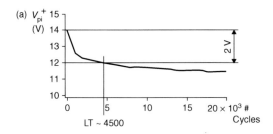

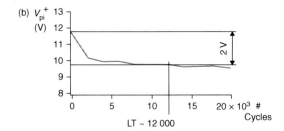

10.11 The shift of V_c in function of the number of switching cycles of a capacitive RF MEMS. The lifetime of two different devices can be compared in a short time: (a) device 1 and (b) device 2.

Localization of the charging mechanisms

The previous methods allowed distinguishing charging mechanisms in the time domain. However, a switch (MEMS) may contain more than one dielectric material that can trap charges. In that case, a method to localize the most dominant mechanism is needed. It has, for example, been reported (Czarnecki *et al.*, 2008a; Rottenberg *et al.*, 2007a) that not only the interposer dielectric but also the substrate can trap charges.

One way to distinguish between these different charging locations consists in a combination of dedicated stressing methods and C–V characteristic measurements. Figure 10.12 shows an example of such a dedicated biasing scheme. Two actuation waveforms, V_{beam} and V_{elec}, were applied simultaneously to the beam and bottom electrode, respectively. The component waveforms (V_{beam} and V_{elec}) and the resulting virtual voltage sources, generating an electric field across the dielectric and substrate (V_{diel} and V_{sub}), are presented in Fig. 10.13. Even though two unipolar (positive or negative) waveforms are used, the electric field across the interposer dielectric is similar to that generated by a single bipolar waveform applied to the bottom electrode and grounded beam. Since the back side of the substrate is grounded, the polarity of the electric field across the substrate is constant during stressing. It depends on the polarity of the component waveforms.

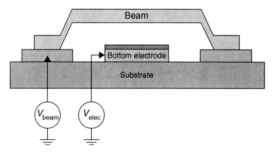

10.12 Using two actuation sources allows stressing different dielectric materials in the switch at the same time with a different electric field.

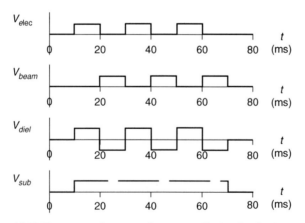

10.13 Two actuation waveforms applied to both electrodes of the switch (bottom electrode and beam) allow obtaining different stressing conditions for the interposer dielectric and the substrate.

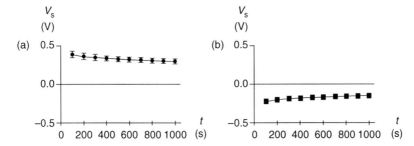

10.14 The results of an experiment where two sources of actuation waveforms were used. The voltage shift of the C–V curve depends on the polarity of the component waveforms ((a) negative and (b) positive) pointing to the substrate charging as dominant charging mechanism (Czarnecki, 2010).

The distribution of the field changes: the potential is switched between the bottom electrode and the beam. As a result, the substrate can be stressed with either positive or negative voltage. Simultaneously, the interposer dielectric is stressed with a bipolar voltage in both cases and, as a result, stressed less. A number of devices were stressed using this combination of two positive or negative component waveforms. The C–V characteristic was observed during idling after the stressing was finished. Figure 10.14 shows the results of the experiment.

The polarity of the voltage shift of the measured C–V curves on the switch was always related to the polarity of the used component actuation waveforms. That shows that the substrate charge trapping is the dominant mechanism in this test. If the voltage shift was dominated by the interposer dielectric charging, then the polarity of the voltage shift should not depend on the polarity of the component waveforms. In this way, substrate charging can be studied independently of interposer dielectric charging, or vice versa by choosing different voltage combinations.

10.4 Analytical modelling

There exist various analytical models describing charging effects and their impact on, for example, C–V characteristics of MEMS switches, starting from a simple parallel plate system to more complicated deformable plates. These models are discussed in the following sections.

10.4.1 Uniform charge in parallel-plate approximation

Wibbeler *et al.* (1998) described the impact of the dielectric charging on the actuation of electrostatic MEMS devices, considering the device of Fig. 10.15a.

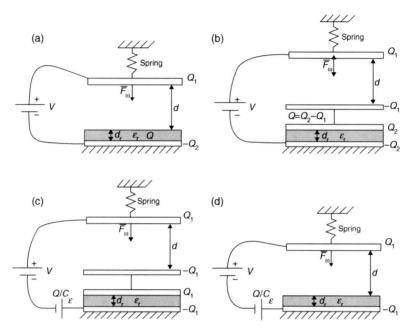

10.15 (a–d) Schematic development of Wibbeler's model (Wibbeler et al., 1998), taking into account a uniform surface charge on the dielectric coating the actuation electrode of an electrostatic actuator.

The system can be seen as a fixed capacitor C_ε and a variable air capacitor C_{air}. They demonstrated that the presence of a uniform charge distribution (Q) at the surface of the dielectric layer shifts the symmetric C–V actuation characteristic as a whole along the voltage axis as shown in Fig. 10.16. The direction of this shift depends both on the sign of the trapped charges and on the way the voltage source is connected to the device, that is, top or bottom electrode grounded and respectively bottom or top electrode biased.

Figure 10.15 sketches the progressive development of Wibbeler's model and clearly expresses the equivalence of a parasitic trapped charge in the device with a series parasitic DC-bias in the actuation path. Chan *et al.* (1998) in particular explored through extensive measurements and simulations the importance of the contact force and progressive zipping of the non-ideal MEMS devices on the profile of their C–V characteristic. They further coupled in Chan *et al.* (1999) a charging model in their electromechanical simulation and showed the crucial role of the contact time in determining the built-up charge in the device and thus the shift of the pull-in voltage over the lifetime of the device.

Reid *et al.* (2002) complemented these studies, demonstrating the possible dynamic latching – stiction – of an electrostatically actuated MEMS device due to dielectric charging. Indeed, should a pull-out voltage have

Reliability of RF MEMS

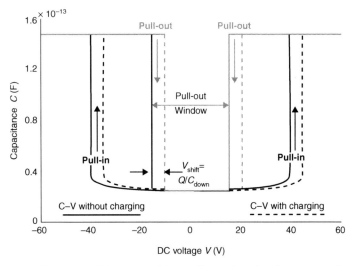

10.16 Simulated C–V curve with a uniform charging (i.e. zero variance). (© 2011, IEEE. Reprinted, with permission, from Rottenberg et al. (2004).)

drifted across the origin of the voltage axis, the successive actuations and de-actuations of the MEMS could be too fast compared to the mechanical response time of the device for this to release. This situation results in an apparent stiction that is switching-time dependent.

Besides lowering the actuation voltage in an attempt to minimize the stress on the dielectric layer and the resulting built-in charges, various complex actuation schemes, such as shaped actuation-pulses (Goldsmith *et al.*, 2001) and bipolar actuation voltages (Rebeiz, 2003) have been proposed. These techniques tend to keep the C–V characteristics more centred on the bias origin at 0 V, preserving the normal actuation of the switches.

Nevertheless, the shift of the C–V curve does not succeed in explaining, among other phenomena, the narrowing of the pull-out window shown in Fig. 10.17 and the resulting vanishing of the pull-out bias that leads to an irreversible stiction (Czarnecki *et al.*, 2005; Melle *et al.*, 2003; van Spengen *et al.*, 2004; Yuan *et al.*, 2004).

The narrowing of the overall C–V actuation characteristic is often observed when using bipolar actuation. It can be explained by the effect of non-uniform charging, as is discussed in the following section.

10.4.2 Non-uniform charge distribution in parallel-plate and generalized distributed plates approximations

This section summarizes an analytic description of the actuation of electrostatic devices in the presence of non-uniform dielectric charging. We use

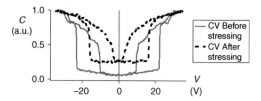

10.17 Measured fast C–V characteristic before and after 20 million cycles of bipolar actuation at +/−35 V under a 1 bar N_2 atmosphere at 25°C with 50% duty cycle for an Al-based switch using SiN_x as dielectric material (Czarnecki *et al.*, 2005).

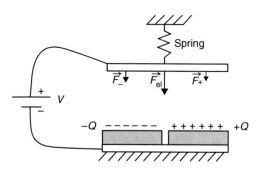

10.18 Stiction thought experiment. (© 2011, IEEE. Reprinted, with permission, from Rottenberg *et al.* (2004).)

remarkably simple formalisms and concepts to take a fixed three-dimensional (3D) charge distribution into account. Our model, which is described in detail in Rottenberg *et al.* (2007b) and Rottenberg (2008), extending our work presented in Rottenberg *et al.* (2004), proposes an explanation for the shift of the actuation characteristics and the deformation of the C–V curves leading to a failure but also to an increase of the up-capacitance without assuming any trapping/de-trapping model. We further show the impact of the curvature of the electrodes on the deformation of the actuation characteristic. We pinpoint the important role played by the spatial covariance of the charge and capacitance distributions. This covariance can break the symmetry of the actuation characteristic. In this case, the capacitances and displacements at pull-in or after pull-out differ when ramping up or down the bias voltage.

Thought experiment

Consider the set-up sketched in Fig. 10.18. A fixed metal plate is covered with a dielectric layer split in two parts with equal areas. The two dielectric islands have uniform fixed surface charges of opposite sign (+/−Q). A movable metal plate is fastened with a spring above the dielectric layer. A DC

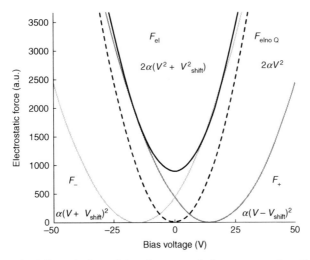

10.19 Description of the electrostatic force exerted on the moving plate at a given and fixed position as a function of the applied voltage V, in the stiction thought experiment of the figure. © 2011, IEEE. Reprinted, with permission, from Rottenberg et al. (2004).)

voltage is applied across the two plates. The $+/-Q$ charges shift the local voltage-force characteristics, that is, $F_{+/-}(V)$, by $+/-V_{shift}$, opposite quantities for the two dielectric islands.

Figure 10.19 describes the electrostatic force $F_{el}(V)$ exerted on the top plate of Fig. 10.18 as a function of the applied voltage V and for a given and fixed position. As $F_{el}(V) = F_+(V) + F_-(V)$ and $F_{+/-}(V)$ define the light and dark grey parabolas crossing at $V = 0$, $F_{el}(V)$ describes another narrower black parabola centred on $V = 0$. It shows a simple force offset compared to the dashed characteristic, that is, $F_{el,no\,Q}(V)$, obtained in total absence of trapped charge. However, the top plate carries no net charge at $V = 0$; the charged dielectric islands induce on this plate charges of opposite polarity that produce this force offset $F_{el}(0)$.

It is thus striking to observe that although the net dielectric charge is zero, the resulting electrostatic force $F_{el} = F_+ + F_-$ is not zero, even at zero applied voltage.

2D+ model description

Using what we have learned from the simple thought model of Fig. 10.18, we now extend the model to a more realistic situation. Consider the set-up in Fig. 10.20, generalizing the model presented in Wibbeler (1998). A fixed non-flat metal plate of area A is covered with a dielectric layer of uniform thickness d_ε, dielectric constant ε_r and volume charge density $\psi(x,y,z)$. A

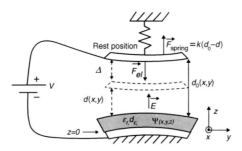

10.20 Model of a MEMS device with non-uniform trapped charge and air-gap distributions. (© 2011, IEEE. Reprinted, with permission, from Rottenberg et al. (2004).)

rigid but non-flat movable metal plate is fastened with a linear spring k to a fixed wall above the dielectric layer at a rest position $d_0(x,y)$. A DC voltage source of amplitude V is applied to the two plates. The set-up is placed in vacuum.

The equilibrium positions of this system are described by:

$$\frac{2\varepsilon_0 k \Delta}{A} = (V\mu_\alpha - \mu_\beta)^2 + V^2 \sigma_\alpha^2 + \sigma_\beta^2 - 2V \, \mathrm{cov}_{(\alpha,\beta)} \quad [10.1]$$

where μ, σ^2 and cov denote respectively the mean, variance and covariance of the capacitance distribution (subscript α) and the induced charge distribution (subscript β). The capacitance distribution, $\alpha(x,y,\Delta)$, in the set-up of Fig. 10.20 and the charge distribution, $\beta(x,y,\Delta)$, induced on the top electrode due to the charges trapped in the dielectric in the same set-up (Rottenberg, 2008), are expressed as

$$\alpha(x,y,\Delta) = \frac{\varepsilon_0}{(d_0(x,y) - \Delta) + (d_\varepsilon / \varepsilon_r)} \quad [10.2]$$

$$\beta(x,y,\Delta) = \frac{d_\varepsilon}{\varepsilon_0 \varepsilon_r} \Psi_{eq}(x,y) \alpha(x,y) \quad [10.3]$$

where

$$\Psi_{eq}(x,y) = \int_0^{d_\varepsilon} \int_\chi^{d_\varepsilon} \frac{\Psi(x,y,z)}{d_\varepsilon} dz\, d\chi \quad [10.4]$$

is an *equivalent surface charge distribution*. It is defined as the charge distribution located at the surface $z = d_\varepsilon$, that would produce the same F_{el} as the actual $\Psi(x,y,z)$. Note that a charge Q placed at the surface of the dielectric has an equivalent $Q_{eq} = Q$, while the same charge placed at the bottom of the dielectric has an equivalent $Q_{eq} = 0$. This means that the closer the charges are to the free surface of the dielectric, the larger their impact will be on the actuation characteristics of the switch.

The 'equivalent charge distribution', and especially its mean value, $\overline{\Psi_{eq}}$, and its variance, $\sigma^2(\Psi_{eq})$, are values that play an important role in explaining the observed shift and narrowing, respectively, of the C–V curves of capacitive RF MEMS, as will be discussed further on.

The details of the model are described in Rottenberg et al. (2007b) and Rottenberg (2008). The key assumption is that the device can be locally described as a parallel-plate capacitor with the electric field everywhere aligned with the z-axis. This is only valid for low capacitance and charge gradients in x and y. For the latter, this means that the charge distribution is assumed to be locally uniform in x and y and only distributed in z. This allows analytical expression of the electric field in the system and defining $\Psi_{eq}(x,y)$. As a second consequence, the parallel-plate approximation can be locally used to compute the electrostatic force. In particular, the assumption becomes more accurate when closing the air gap $d(x,y) = d_0(x,y) - \Delta$.

Model implications

Let us first assume that the movable electrode and dielectric remain parallel, that is, there is a uniform air gap, $d_0(x,y) = d_0$; the equilibrium position then simplifies to

$$F_{el} = \frac{A}{2\varepsilon_0}\left[(V\mu_\alpha - \mu_\beta)^2 + \sigma_\beta^2\right]$$

$$= \frac{\varepsilon_0 A}{2}\left(\frac{1}{d_0 - \Delta + (d_\varepsilon/\varepsilon_r)}\right)^2\left[\left(V - \frac{\overline{\Psi_{eq}}d_\varepsilon}{\varepsilon_0\varepsilon_r}\right)^2 - \left(\frac{d_\varepsilon}{\varepsilon_0\varepsilon_r}\right)^2\sigma^2(\Psi_{eq})\right] \quad [10.5]$$

where $\overline{\Psi_{eq}}$ and $\sigma^2(\Psi_{eq})$ are the mean and variance of the equivalent surface charge distribution $\Psi_{eq}(x,y)$.

The electromechanical equilibrium positions of the movable plate are thus expressed by

$$V = \frac{\overline{\Psi_{eq}}d_\varepsilon}{\varepsilon_0\varepsilon_r} \pm \sqrt{\frac{2k}{\varepsilon_0 A}(d_0 - d)\left(d + \frac{d_\varepsilon}{\varepsilon_r}\right)^2 - \frac{d_\varepsilon^2\sigma^2(\Psi_{eq})}{\varepsilon_0^2\varepsilon_r^2}} \quad [10.6]$$

While the mean equivalent surface charge shifts the C–V as a whole, like the uniform distribution did in Wibbeler's case (1998), the variance of $\Psi_{eq}(x,y)$ affects the shape of the actuation characteristics. The non-zero variance has the effect of a force offset depending on the air-gap height, but not on the polarity of the actuation voltage or on the sign of the trapped charges. Note for example that a non-zero variance forbids the rest position of the spring $d = d_0$ as an equilibrium position for the system. This case constitutes therefore a generalization of our thought experiment where we had just as an example considered a very specific charge distribution.

The pull-out and pull-in voltages, V_{PO} and V_{PI}, are obtained from Equation [10.6] and given by

$$V_{PO} = \frac{\overline{\Psi_{eq}} d_\varepsilon}{\varepsilon_0 \varepsilon_r} \pm \sqrt{\frac{2kd_0 d_\varepsilon^2}{\varepsilon_0 \varepsilon_r^2 A} - \frac{d_\varepsilon^2 \sigma^2(\Psi_{eq})}{\varepsilon_0^2 \varepsilon_r^2}} \qquad [10.7]$$

$$V_{PI} = \frac{\overline{\Psi_{eq}} d_\varepsilon}{\varepsilon_0 \varepsilon_r} \pm \sqrt{\frac{8k}{27\varepsilon_0 A}\left(d_0 + \frac{d_\varepsilon}{\varepsilon_r}\right)^3 - \frac{d_\varepsilon^2 \sigma^2(\Psi_{eq})}{\varepsilon_0^2 \varepsilon_r^2}} \qquad [10.8]$$

Increasing the variance of $\Psi_{eq}(x,y)$, the two symmetric V_{PO} and V_{PI} shift towards each other as shown in Fig. 10.21 in the case of a zero mean charge. The pull-out window narrows, as measured and reported in Melle *et al.* (2003) and Czarnecki *et al.* (2005), and vanishes for a variance of $\Psi_{eq}(x,y)$, independent of the dielectric layer parameters and given by

$$\sigma^2_{no\_PO} = \frac{2kd_0 \varepsilon_0}{A} \qquad [10.9]$$

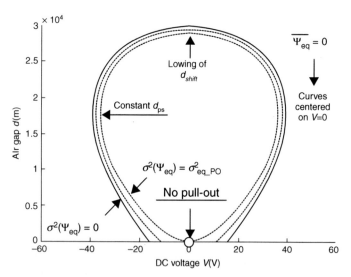

10.21 Simulated narrowing of the d–V curve for the system of Fig. 10.20 $\sigma^2(\Psi_{eq})$ increasing until $\sigma^2_{no\_PO}$; $k = 10$ N/m, $A = 10^4$ μm², $d_0 = 3$ μm $\varepsilon_r = 5$ and $d_\varepsilon = 3$ μm. © 2011, IEEE. Reprinted, with permission, from Rottenberg *et al.* (2004).

As the movable plate cannot be released anymore, the structure fails by stiction on the dielectric, due only to the variance of $\Psi_{eq}(x,y)$. Note that the pull-in voltage V_{PI} hardly changes in comparison to V_{PO} when $\sigma^2(\Psi_{eq})$ varies from 0 to $\sigma^2_{no\_PO}$.

V_{PI} can also disappear due to the variance of $\Psi_{eq}(x,y)$. The critical variance for the pull-in is given by

$$\sigma^2_{no\_PI} = \frac{8k\varepsilon_0 d_\varepsilon}{27 A \varepsilon_r}\left(\frac{\varepsilon_r d_0}{d_\varepsilon}+1\right)^3 \qquad [10.10]$$

Increasing $\sigma^2(\Psi_{eq})$ from $\sigma^2_{no\_PO}$ to $\sigma^2_{no\_PI}$, the whole C–V characteristic gradually vanishes. For variances larger than $\sigma^2_{no\_PI}$, there is no more stable position for the movable armature. The device fails by self-actuation due only to the variance of the equivalent surface distribution.

Remarkably, only the variance of $\Psi_{eq}(x,y)$ is needed to explain the irreversible stiction phenomenon. The dependency of the two branches of V_{PO} and V_{PI} vs the charging variance is illustrated in Fig. 10.22 from Equations [10.9] and [10.10]. As $|V_{PO}|<|V_{PI}|$ in absence of charge, the pull-out disappears earlier than the pull-in. Note that imposing $\sigma^2_{no\_PI} = \sigma^2_{no\_PO}$ implies $d_\varepsilon = 2\varepsilon_r d_0$ using Equations [10.9] and [10.10]. This condition is equivalent to $|V_{PO}| = |V_{PI}|$ and to the condition derived in Seeger et al. (1997) for a continuously stable actuation from $d = d_0$ to $d = 0$.

All other things being equal, a larger spring constant per unit area k/A, a larger rest air gap d_0, a thinner dielectric layer d_ε, and a higher dielectric constant ε_r make a switching device less sensitive to the variance and mean of

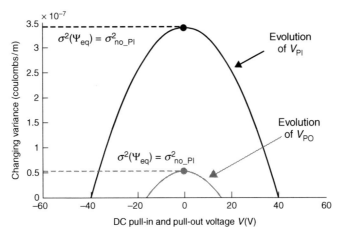

10.22 Evolution of V_{PO} and V_{PI} vs $\sigma^2(\Psi_{eq})$. (© 2011, IEEE. Reprinted, with permission, from Rottenberg et al. (2004).)

$\Psi_{eq}(x,y)$. In this view, assuming the equivalent surface charge distribution is independent of k, A, d_e, ε_r, and d_0, large capacitance ratio ($\varepsilon_r d_0/d_e$) switches with large V_{PO} and V_{PI} are expected to be more reliable.

This case offers an explanation for all the reported phenomena attributed previously to the dielectric charging but lacking until now a comprehensive model (Czarnecki *et al.*, 2005; Melle *et al.*, 2003; van Spengen *et al.*, 2004; Yuan *et al.*, 2004). In particular, this model predicts the irreversible stiction failure and the increase of the up-state capacitance during the cycling of switched RF MEMS capacitors.

Not only shift, narrowing or a combination of both can be observed during cycling measurements of switched MEMS capacitors, as shown in Fig. 10.23. The actuation characteristic as a whole can eventually deform and lose its symmetry, as visible in the figure. This phenomenon can be explained by extending the model already presented.

Indeed, let us as a second, more general, case assume combined gap and charge non-uniformities. The model then shows that the C–V and d–V actuation characteristics deform and become asymmetric. As a simple example, we assume the non-uniform gap and the charge distribution as shown in Fig. 10.24. The resulting C–V characteristic is shown in Fig. 10.25. There is a combined shift and deformation: positive and negative pull-in/out events

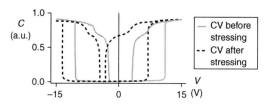

10.23 Charging induced asymmetry of the C–V characteristic observed in case of cycling under bipolar actuation.

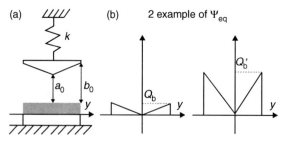

10.24 (a,b) Example of corresponding linear variations of air gap and equivalent charge distributions; the maximum value of the charge distribution, that is, Q_b, is the only parameter of the family of devices. (© 2011, IEEE. Reprinted, with permission, from Rottenberg *et al.* (2004).)

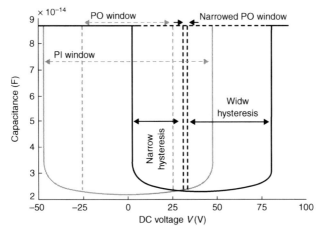

10.25 Stable C–V characteristics computed for the family of devices presented in the figure with small and large air gaps at rest, a_0 and b_0, respectively equal to 3 μm and 4 μm, a total area $A = 10^4$ μm², $\varepsilon_r = 5$, $D_\varepsilon = 3$ μm and a spring constant $k = 10$ N/m. Grey, without charge; black, with a charge amplitude slightly lower than $Q_{b\_no\_PO}$. (© 2011, IEEE. Reprinted, with permission, from Rottenberg *et al.* (2004).)

occur at different capacitance, displacements, and voltage values. The centres of the pull-in and pull-out voltage windows do not coincide and both differ further from the voltage of maximum opening. For a given set of device parameters, the asymmetry of the actuation characteristics can even be strong enough for the device to be continuously tunable until full closure on one side of its C–V characteristic while preserving its unstable characteristics on the other side of its C–V. Such an extreme case is shown in Fig. 10.26.

These examples show that not only charge distribution, but also non-flat and deformable actuation electrodes, for example, typical clamped–clamped and clamped–free beams with uniform cross-sections, can seriously affect the C–V characteristic of (RF) MEMS switched capacitors, varicaps and switches. To avoid such effects, it is better to ensure that the actuation gap between mobile electrodes and dielectric remains always uniform over the whole surface of the structure (Czarnecki *et al.*, 2008b). This is often not the case. Low-stiffness MEMS bridges especially will typically first touch the dielectric in the centre, and only at higher actuation voltages at the edges.

10.5 Electrostatic discharge

Compared to better-studied reliability issues in MEMS, such as charging, stiction and fatigue, one of the newer and less understood problems is the

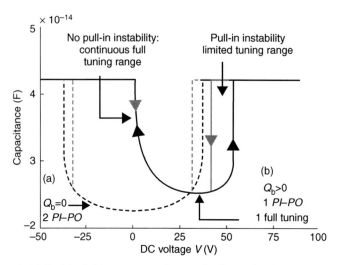

10.26 Stable C–V corresponding to the figure in the case where a_0 and b_0 are equal respectively to 1.5 μm and 6 μm. (© 2011, IEEE. Reprinted, with permission, from Rottenberg *et al.* (2004).)

impact of ESD. ESD as a reliability threat is very well investigated for complementary metal oxide semiconductor (CMOS) devices (Amerasekara and Duvvury, 2002), whereas for MEMS, it only started gathering interest among researchers from the year 2000 on (Walraven *et al.*, 2000). However, the number of studies of the impact of ESD on MEMS is still very small. The main MEMS test structures investigated in this context are ohmic (Tazzoli *et al.*, 2007) and capacitive RF MEMS switches (Ruan *et al.*, 2009), electrostatically actuated torsional micromirrors (Sangameswaran *et al.*, 2008), and a few other similar structures (Walraven *et al.*, 2000).There are very few ESD solutions for MEMS proposed in literature (Acquaviva *et al.*, 2009; Ikehashi *et al.*, 2009), whereas the challenge is expected to become of greater significance for smaller low-power MEMS applications with increasing functionalities.

ESD, is defined as a single-event, rapid transfer of electrostatic charge when two objects at a large potential difference come in close proximity or into direct contact with each other. Electrostatic charge build-up can occur most commonly through 'triboelectric charging' (Harper, 1967).

Most common existing ESD test models and techniques were developed for ICs and not for MEMS. They are the human body model (HBM), machine model (MM), charged device model (CDM), human metal model (HMM) and the transmission line pulsing (TLP) technique (Amerasekara and Duvvury, 2002). The HBM test is very commonly used for device qualification and replicates the real life event where a charged human operator discharges by touching an IC pin (or MEMS in this case) causing a current flow through the device to the ground and destroying it (ESDA, 2010).

10.5.1 The effect of electrostatic discharge on MEMS

A MEMS device can typically be subject to ESD during many stages of its production, for instance processing, assembly, packaging, shipping and handling, and even during normal operation. Since MEMS have movable components across air gaps during regular operation, unlike semiconductor ICs, two possible effects can occur during an ESD event. The high voltage build-up across the air gap during ESD might make the component move, causing the air gap to reduce and eventually close. When the gap closes during the ESD event, breakdown and resulting thermal damage between the electrodes can occur, causing catastrophic failure of the MEMS. When the electrical contact remains 'open' during the ESD event, air gap breakdown or field emission can occur, causing charging of the device or even permanent damage. Which of these effects occurs depend a lot on the robustness/stiffness of the MEMS. For robust MEMS, an ESD event often results in an electrical voltage overstress (EOS) due to the typically high impedance of the device.

Figure 10.27 shows results from wafer-level HBM ESD tests performed on poly-SiGe micromirrors and capacitive RF MEMS switch test devices to measure their ESD sensitivity (Scholz et al., 2007). Normally, the current through the device under test (DUT) is used to monitor the failure, as in semiconductor devices, but here the voltage during ESD was used to characterize the MEMS because of the electrically open behaviour of these devices, as in Fig. 10.27c. Based on electrical measurements which detected a change in the DUT resistance during failure, the HBM ESD failure level of the micromirrors (Fig. 10.27a) was measured to be 40 V (Sangameswaran et al., 2008) and that for Al-based switches (Fig. 10.27b) with a 200 nm Si_3N_4 dielectric was measured to be 120 to 180 V (Sangameswaran et al., 2009). All these test devices suffered catastrophic damage upon failure and, if we were to follow the same classification as is used for ICs, they could be classified as Class 0, that is, extremely ESD-sensitive devices with a failure level < 250 V (ESDA, 2010).

However, since most MEMS exist with different non-electrical functionalities, such as optical, mechanical, motion-based, chemical, thermal, etc., the correct point of failure can be determined only by comparing their functionality before and after ESD stress of increasing amplitude. It was noticed through measurements that RF MEMS switches often suffered functional failure at ESD stress levels lower than the catastrophic failure detected electrically (Sangameswaran et al., 2010a). It is therefore

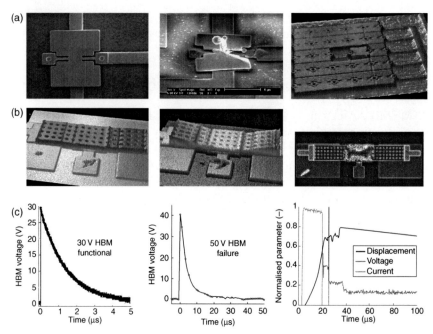

10.27 Damage caused by ESD to MEMS: (a) Single micromirror before failure, after failure, micromirror array after failure; (b) RF MEMS switch before and after failure (functional failure or catastrophic damage); (c) HBM voltage across micromirrors showing faster discharge during failure and measurements with customized set-up.

recommended to perform functionality tests on MEMS during and after ESD to conclusively detect failure. Customized test setups were built for this purpose by integrating a portable probe-mountable HBM ESD tester with a laser Doppler vibrometer for out-of-plane motion measurements. Simultaneous measurements of out-of-plane displacement, current and voltage in the MEMS DUT were performed (as in Fig. 10.27c) *in situ* during ESD stress using this set-up, which enabled improved failure detection and deeper understanding of the failure mechanisms in MEMS during ESD (Sangameswaran *et al.*, 2010a). The test set-up can also be used, together with a pressure-controlled vacuum chamber, to study the effect of pressure on the ESD sensitivity, which is of importance when testing, for example, resonators which have to function in vacuum. For example, the ESD reliability of capacitive MEMS switches was found to be worse at vacuum as compared to atmospheric pressure.

Designing ESD protection or adapting from conventional CMOS ESD protection structures is challenging in such cases because MEMS operate at high voltages and in both voltage polarities, have unique packaging and processing requirements, and impose severe area and cost constraints on the ESD protection designer. Moreover, MEMS sometimes operate as stand-alone devices, without any CMOS circuitry, for which effective ESD protection is virtually unknown. Thus, it is equally important to understand the correct ESD failure level and failure mechanisms for unprotected MEMS devices and also to develop strategies to improve the ESD robustness of MEMS and implement ESD protection devices.

One way to improve the intrinsic ESD robustness of MEMS is by varying the design parameters to increase their mechanical stiffness, since a direct correlation was found between the mechanical robustness of the MEMS, the pull-in voltage, and the ESD failure level (Sangameswaran *et al.*, 2010b). However, this goes together with an increased pull-in voltage and can reduce the performance of the MEMS. Commonly implemented customer requirements in industry require at least 2 kV HBM robustness for the shipped product in the case of consumer applications. For MEMS integrated in a CMOS chip or package to survive this high amount of ESD stress, design improvements alone above are insufficient. An dedicated ESD protection is therefore essential. An example how this can be implemented is shown in Fig. 10.28. ESD protection was implemented on a MEMS-on-CMOS process by adapting the silicon controlled rectifier (SCR), commonly used for ESD protection in CMOS devices (Ker *et al.*, 2005), to a high trigger voltage and connected in parallel with a MEMS switch. The fabricated device improved the MEMS ESD robustness from 140 V (Class 0) to 5 kV (Sangameswaran *et al.*, 2011).

Other advanced bi-directional ESD protection devices with high turn-on voltages may be used in a similar manner taking advantage of slower turn-on time requirements for MEMS and lower area constraints. However, in stand-alone MEMS applications, MEMS-based ESD protection will be required.

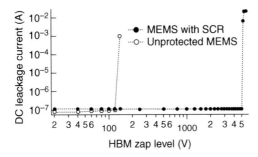

10.28 DC leakage measurements on unprotected MEMS (failure level 140 V) and MEMS with SCR protection (ESD failure level >5 kV) performed after every HBM stress show that MEMS can be protected with >5 kV HBM robustness with an on-chip SCR.

10.6 Reliability issues of MEMS packages

The package is an essential part of any MEMS. It can prevent reliability problems, but it can also generate issues. The focus of this section is on one important aspect of MEMS packages: hermeticity. A hermetic package is essential for the reliable functioning of RF MEMS, especially resonators.

10.6.1 Device parameters affected by ambient conditions

Many functional parameters of MEMS devices are dependent on ambient conditions such as pressure, humidity, presence of chemical compounds, etc. (De Wolf et al., 2005, 2009). A hermetic package is thus required in those cases where a stable operation of the MEMS device is desired, regardless of fluctuations in the ambient.

A first example is given in Fig. 10.29, which shows the measured response of an RF MEMS switch when the actuation voltage V_b is toggled off (at $t = 0$ μs) and on (16 V, at $t = 250$ μs). Measurements of the displacement z were performed using a laser Doppler vibrometer and results are shown for ambient pressures of 50, 100, 200, ..., 600 mbar. The switch behaviour clearly changes with ambient pressure. The closing time obtained from this figure is shown as a function of ambient pressure in Fig. 10.30. The opening time varies between 20 μs and 50 μs. This shows that maintaining the pressure in the package at a constant level is required in order to ensure a predictable switching time.

A second parameter that is strongly dependent on ambient pressure is the Q factor of mechanical resonators. As depicted in Fig. 10.31, the Q factor

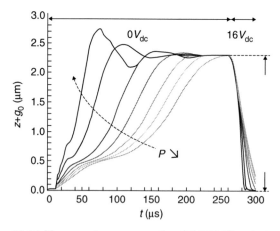

10.29 Measured response of an RF MEMS switch at different ambient pressures. At $t = 0$ μs, the actuation voltage is removed and the switch opens. At $t = 250$ μs, the actuation voltage is applied and the switch closes again.

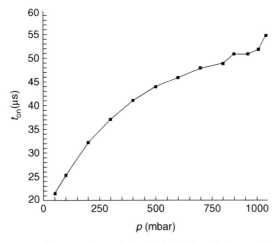

10.30 Closing time of the RF MEMS switch as a function of ambient pressure.

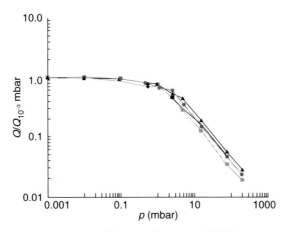

10.31 Measured Q factor of several MEMS resonators as a function of pressure. At low pressures, Q is limited by mechanisms such as anchor losses, material damping and thermoelastic damping. As pressure increases, air damping gradually becomes the dominant loss mechanism.

reaches a stable plateau at low pressures where the dominant loss mechanisms are a combination of anchor losses, material damping, thermoelastic damping, etc. At higher pressures, air damping becomes more important and the Q factor drops as a result.

Also, thermal effects in MEMS devices are very much pressure dependent. An example of this is shown in Fig. 10.32, where results of a four-point

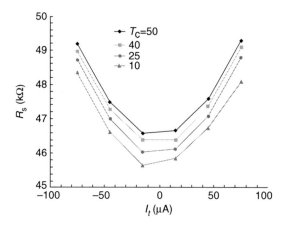

10.32 Measured resistance R_s of a suspended beam, as a function of the test current I_t that flows through the beam. The measurement was performed at 10^{-5} mbar. Results are given for different chuck temperatures T_c.

resistance (R_s) measurement of a freestanding, clamped–clamped beam are shown. The measurement was performed at an ambient pressure of 10^{-5} mbar. A test current I_t is forced through the beam and R_s is calculated from the resulting voltage drop. Due to Joule losses, the beam's temperature (and thus resistance) increases quadratically with I_t. As seen in the figure, the effect of the self-heating due to Joule losses is far more significant than increasing the ambient temperature T_c from 10°C to 50°C. At atmospheric pressure though, this effect completely vanishes due to convective heat transfer and no dependence of R_s on I_t is observed.

As a last example, the presence of humidity in the ambient and its effect on the operation of a MEMS device is illustrated for a torsional micromirror in Fig. 10.33. When the torsional mirror is pulled in, it comes into mechanical contact with a landing electrode. As a result, the adhesion force between the mirror and the landing electrode will affect the mirror's pull-out voltage V_{po}. Figure 10.33 shows that the pull-in voltage V_{pi} remains constant (i.e. the mechanical properties of the mirror do not change) whereas the pull-out voltage V_{po} changes by more than 20% between 5% RH and 95% RH. Similar effects can be expected for any MEMS making contact upon actuation, so also RF MEMS switches.

For all the reasons mentioned above, MEMS devices need to be encapsulated in a hermetic cavity that ensures a constant ambient pressure and excludes contaminants that might otherwise affect the performance of the device. However, hermeticity alone is not sufficient to guarantee a constant pressure in the cavity. This will be briefly explained in the next section.

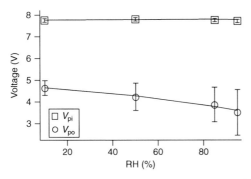

10.33 Measured pull-in (V_{pi}) and pull-out (V_{po}) voltage of a micromirror, as a function of relative humidity (© 2011, IEEE. Reprinted, with permission, from Ling *et al*. (2011b).)

It is often mentioned in literature that packaging takes a large amount of the development cost of MEMS. This is certainly the case if the development of the package is done after the development of the MEMS. Costs can be reduced considerably if, from the design phase on, the packaging aspects are also taken into account, that is, if MEMS and package are co-developed. This is not only valid from a design and processing point of view, but also from a reliability point of view. Especially when hermeticity has to be guaranteed, the package and the MEMS should be considered as two extremely interdependent parts in the development. Issues such as outgassing and hermeticity can be prevented by correct material choice. Many packaging-related reliability issues should be tackled in a very early stage of the development, and often can be studied using simple test structures such as cavities with different size, splits in the processing using different material, tests of films consisting of materials used in the packaging process, etc. Packaging can be made cheaper and more reliable by, where possible, making it part of the MEMS processing instead of seeing it as consequent step after the MEMS device is finished. For example, wafer-level packaging methods, where a cap is processed on top of the MEMS using similar processing steps as used for the MEMS themselves, is a very promising technique both from a cost and from a reliability point of view (Guo *et al*., 2012). The cap has holes to allow releasing the MEMS (etching the sacrificial layer). They are closed after the release step, providing optimal hermeticity and reliability.

10.6.2 Mechanisms degrading the atmosphere in the cavity

Figure 10.34 gives a schematic representation of different processes that might be on-going in a MEMS package. A first mechanism that affects the

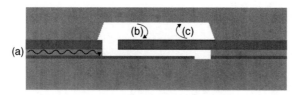

10.34 Schematic cross-section of a MEMS resonator in a wafer-level package.

internal pressure is diffusion of gases through the bulk or along the interfaces between layers. This is depicted as (a) in the figure and is driven by an imbalance between the partial pressures of an element inside and outside the cavity. Silicon oxide for instance is known to allow helium to pass through, and moisture can slowly diffuse through polymers like benzocyclobutene (BCB).

Outgassing from the capping layer (or e.g. the sacrificial layer) can also lead to a build-up of cavity pressure (b). In addition, the released molecules can deposit on the surface of the packaged MEMS device. In case of resonators, this will affect both the mass and the Q factor of the device. Alternatively, the structural layer itself might outgas (c) – in which case, not only the cavity pressure changes, but also the mass of the MEMS device. Again, this is especially relevant for resonators. Rather than outgassing, some materials in the package may act as a getter – leading to a decrease in cavity pressure.

Lastly, elements present in the cavity atmosphere may chemically react with the packaged device (e.g. oxidation). In ohmic switches, for instance, this will affect the properties of the contact. In the case of resonators, the effective stiffness can be affected, as well as the overall mass density and Q factor.

10.6.3 Hermeticity testing of packages

Measuring hermeticity can be done in a different number of ways but the concept is the same: a pressure difference between the internal volume of the package and the external environment causes gas or liquid to diffuse through the sealing material.

Classical hermeticity testing is divided into two main categories: gross leak testing (for leaks > 10^{-4} mbar·L/s) and fine leak testing (for leaks > 10^{-9} mbar·L/s). Both methods are described in the standard: MIL-STD-883H, Method 1014.13 (Military Standard, 2010). This way of testing is not always appropriate for MEMS packages because the standard is defined for package volumes that are typically >0.05 cm^3, that is, much larger than those often used for MEMS. For smaller volumes, the allowed leak rate is much smaller than can be measured by a typical He leak tester (Jourdain et al., 2002). So, there is a need for alternative test methods (De Wolf et al., 2007). In the following, we discuss some alternatives, based on either electrical or optical methods.

Electrical measurements: capped resonator

As shown in Fig. 10.31, a resonator exhibits a strong dependence of its quality factor Q on the ambient pressure. The critical pressure, above which the sensitivity is greatest, depends on the design of the resonator and can thus be tuned to the requirements of the packaging process.

Once the relationship between the Q factor and the pressure for a test structure has been established, the Q factor can thus be used as a metric for pressure (De Coster et al., 2005). Measuring the Q factor can be done in several ways, one of which is an S-parameter measurement. This is illustrated in Fig. 10.35a, which shows a complex plot of the measured S_{21} of a resonator for frequencies around its resonance frequency. By fitting a resonator model to this measurement, one can extract all device parameters, including Q. Figure 10.35b gives the extracted Q for a device, measured continuously during 100 h and at regular intervals between 100 and 1500 h. The fluctuations that are seen illustrate what was discussed in Section 10.6.2: because several phenomena are on-going simultaneously, their combined effect on the Q factor can result in a complex behaviour.

Electrical measurements: helium leak rate

This section shows how a good design for test can provide information on leak tightness of a capping material. Although it is known that He diffuses through SiO_2, which is present in this MEMS package, exactly this property is used for the test. In the example, a polycrystalline silicon germanium (poly-SiGe) capping layer is deposited on top of a silicon dioxide sacrificial layer (Helin et al., 2011). This is depicted in the top part of Fig. 10.36. In the experiment, the test structure is placed in a pure He atmosphere of 1000 mbar for 12 h. Since it is known that He will diffuse through the SiO_2 layer, the He pressure in the cavity is 1000 mbar after this dwell time. Next, the chamber is evacuated (10^{-5} mbar) and the Q factor of the sealed resonator is monitored over time. As the He diffuses out of the cavity (either through the poly-SiGe cap which is to be studied or through the SiO_2), the pressure drops and thus the Q increases. The result of this experiment is shown in the bottom part of Fig. 10.36 for two test structures, one with a short and one with a longer He diffusion path through SiO_2. For the structure with a short diffusion path, it roughly takes 20 h for the measured Q to reach the expected value at 10^{-5} mbar. For the device with the longer diffusion path, the pressure only reaches the critical pressure of about 1 mbar after

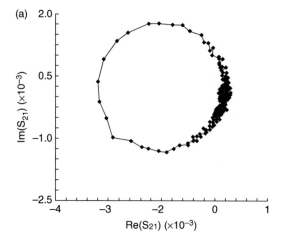
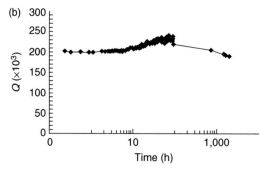
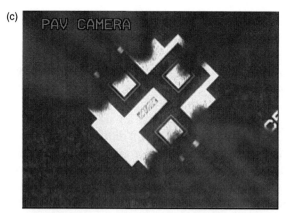

10.35 (a–c) Measured *Q* factor of a capped resonator during storage in N_2 at room temperature. The *Q* factor is extracted from the measured S_{21} parameter. (c) The test structure with two RF probes and 1 DC probe for biasing.

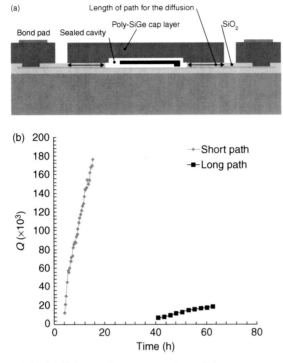

10.36 (a) Schematic cross-section of the test structure, (b) Measured Q as a function of time during evacuation of a He-filled cavity, for two different lengths of the diffusion path. (© 2011, IEEE. Reprinted, with permission, from (Helin et al., 2011).)

about 50 h. Since the dimensions of the poly-SiGe cap are equal for both structures, and only the length of the SiO_2 diffusion path is different, it is concluded that diffusion of He only takes place through the SiO_2. The poly-SiGe cap has thus been verified to be He leak tight.

Electrical measurements: Outgassing: opening packages in vacuum

The effect that impurities in the ambient (released into the cavity by outgassing, for instance) can have on the Q factor of a resonator is illustrated by the measurement shown in Fig. 10.37. The figure shows measured Q factors of a sealed resonator, placed in a vacuum test chamber at 10^{-4} mbar. Due to the high pressure in the cavity, the Q factor is relatively low. When the cavity is opened (by mechanically breaking the seal), the pressure drops to 10^{-4} mbar and the Q rises accordingly. The Q factor is then monitored over time and is seen to drop significantly due to impurities that are present in the vacuum test chamber and that contaminate the resonator (this is not an ultra-high vacuum chamber and is opened and exposed to normal ambient at regular

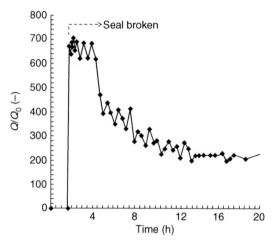

10.37 Measured Q on a sealed resonator, before and after breaking the seal in a N_2 environment at 10^{-4} mbar.

times). This illustrates the importance of maintaining a clean atmosphere at low pressure in a MEMS package, especially for MEMS resonators.

Optical measurement: capped resonator

As mentioned above, Q factors can be measured in several ways. Figure 10.38a shows an example of an optical measurement on a device that is packaged with a transparent Pyrex cap (Bogaerts *et al.*, 2011). Using a laser Doppler vibrometer, the mechanical frequency response of the device is measured. The device is excited mechanically by placing it on a piezoelectric shaker; the whole assembly is placed in a pressure-controlled chamber and the laser is pointed at the packaged MEMS device through a window. A differential measurement using two laser beams (one beam is pointed at the armature of the device, the second beam is pointed at the substrate) is performed so as to obtain the relative velocity of the MEMS device with respect to the substrate. Figure 10.38b gives the measured frequency response, which shows several resonance modes. The Q factor of each mode can be calculated and measured as a function of ambient pressure. This is shown in Fig. 10.38c for the first mode at 14.3 kHz. Since the capped device gives the same Q as an uncapped reference, it is concluded that the package is not hermetic in this case.

Optical measurement: cap deflection

This test measures the cap deflection in response to a change in ambient pressure. If the device has a good hermetic seal, then the cap will deflect

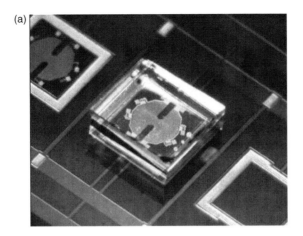
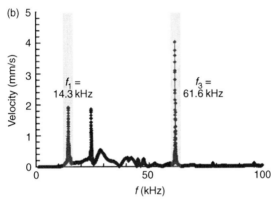
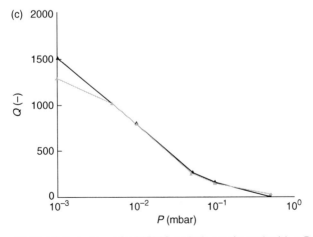

10.38 (a) Top view of a MEMS switch, packaged with a Pyrex cap, (b) measured frequency response and (c) Q extracted from the first mode for a capped device and an uncapped reference.

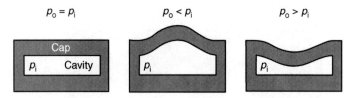

10.39 Deflection response to a change in pressure. Left: If $p_i = p_o$ the cap shows no deflection. Centre: If $p_o < p_i$ the cap deflects upwards. Right: If $p_o > p_i$ the cap deflects inwards.

in response to the pressure difference between the cavity and the outside atmosphere. Ideally, if the pressure inside the package is equal to the pressure outside the package, then the cap will show no deflection (Fig. 10.39, left). On the other hand, if the pressure outside (p_o) is different than the pressure inside (p_i) the cap would deflect upwards, when $p_o < p_i$ (Fig. 10.39, centre) or inwards, when $p_o > p_i$ (Fig. 10.39, right).

This technique is possible only if the cap is flexible enough to show any deflection with changes of pressure. That demands the use of optical techniques with a high sensitivity for small packages; the leak rate resolution depends on the resolution of the system and the size and thickness of the package.

Interferometry is the most common technique used to measure cap deflection, and one important advantage is that it is a non-destructive test that can be used directly on the sealed package.

Optical measurement: cap deflection in vacuum/air

A fast method to determine whether the packages have a gross leak or not is by measuring the cap deflection in vacuum and air. The packages are placed in a vacuum chamber that has a viewport. The deflection is measured (using the interferometer) first at atmospheric pressure and then at vacuum.

A gross leak will be indicated by a lack of deflection when the pressure inside the package and the pressure of the chamber come to equilibrium quickly. On the other hand, a difference in the deflection under the two different pressures would indicate that the package is air-tight.

Figure 10.40a shows the top view of an array of 18 poly-silicon germanium thin-film packages sealed with a microcrystalline silicon germanium porous layer (Claes, 2011; González *et al.*, 2011). In six of these packages (inside the white square) a hole was drilled by focusing ion beam (FIB).

Only two packages (DUT in the figure) were measured in vacuum–air, one package with the hole and the other without it. Figure 10.40b shows the package deflection measured by interferometry of two membranes. The one with the FIB hole shows no difference in deflection when changing the

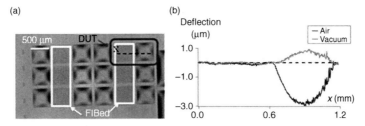

10.40 (a) Top view picture of 18 empty packages, in 6 of them (inside white square) a hole was drilled by FIB (González *et al.*, 2011) (reproduced with permission). (b) Membrane deflection of two packages (with and without hole) measured by interferometry in vacuum and air. The package in the left has the drilled hole and shows a lack of deflection as expected, while the package on the right shows a difference in the deflection under the two pressures indicating that it is air-tight.

pressure in the chamber from air to vacuum, indicating that it is leaky, as expected. The one without the FIB hole does change deflection, indicating that there is no large leak path. In order to determine whether there might be a small leak path, the sample should remain in the chamber and be measured regularly. Another option to check for fine leak paths is to use a variation on the fine leak testing using He, as is done in the MIL-STD-883H, Method 1014.13 (Military Standard, 2010). This is discussed in the following.

Optical measurement: helium pressurization

With this method one can determine the presence of small (fine) leaks. To perform this test, the samples are placed in a chamber that allows storing in helium at a certain pressure (e.g. 3 bar) to stress the sample. This kind of test is also called the 'He bomb'. Helium is chosen amongst other gases, for example, nitrogen, due to the smaller molecule size, which would allow an easier penetration inside the cavity than air.

The shape of the cap of the packages is measured by interferometry in atmospheric pressure before and after He storage.

In the case that the package is hermetic, the shape of the cap should not change. On the other hand, if the package is leaky to He, the cap should deflect upwards indicating the presence of He inside the cavity.

Figure 10.41 shows the results of fine leak test on a thin-film SiGe package. Two measurements were performed in atmospheric pressure before He pressurization to check the stability of the membrane deflection. Then the packages were stored during 10 days in He at a pressure of 3 bar. After

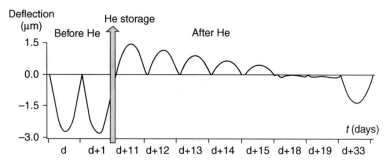

10.41 Deflection measurements before and after He storage of a sealed package leaky for He.

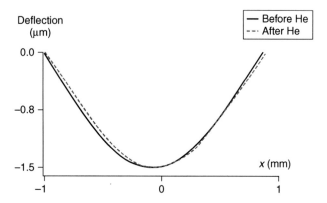

10.42 Result of He fine leak test performed on a Si package. The sample was stored in He for 11 days and shows no He leak.

10 days, the packages were then measured again in atmospheric pressure and monitored over a period of 20 days.

Looking at the membrane deflection, it can be concluded that He was able to penetrate in the cavity, resulting in a very high deflection after the He bomb. The deflection decreases over time, indicating that the He escapes from the inside.

Figure 10.42 shows the result of the He bomb test performed on a Si package (González et al., 2011) over 11 days. In the graph we can see that the deflection before and after storage stays the same, meaning that the sample is not leaky for He.

One must be very careful when making conclusions based on this fine leak test. We need to consider the so-called 'dwell time', that is, the time necessary to transport the samples from the 'He bomb' to the optical tool (interferometer). It can happen that the leakage is faster than the dwell time and that He escapes during transportation, so the deflection before and after He would be the same and the conclusion that the package is He tight would be wrong. One solution for this issue would be to try to minimize the dwell time as much as possible, in the extreme case to use the 'He bomb' also as a test chamber for the optical measurements, which requires a window that allows interferometry and can withstand the pressure differences. Other solutions are being investigated (Pham et al., 2011).

10.7 Conclusion

The most important reliability issue for capacitive RF MEMS remains electrical charging. The electrical fields associated with electrons or holes, trapped in the dielectric, will affect the functioning of the MEMS. Pull-in and pull-out voltages of switches will shift, and eventually stiction might occur. This charging can take place in the interposer dielectric, but also in the substrate or any dielectric that sees an electrical field. In this chapter, various measurement methods and analytical models were discussed.

Charging is not only a problem for capacitive RF MEMS switches. Any MEMS where due to its actuation principle, an electrical field is present across a dielectric, can suffer from charging. Often such charging cannot be prevented, but its impact on the MEMS can be reduced by a well-chosen design, meaning the charging should take place far from the movable parts, such that the associated electrical fields do not affect its functioning. As discussed in this chapter, studying charging can be done using the normal actuation scheme of the MEMS. However, often new insights can be gained by using alternative actuation schemes. The influence of dielectric charging on the reliability of the MEMS can only be reduced if there is an in-depth understanding of the impact of this charging on the MEMS functionality. For this reason, a profound theoretical study demonstrating the impact of charging on the MEMS electrical characteristics is also presented in this chapter. It offers an explanation for all the reported effects of dielectric charging and of non-flat and deformable actuation electrodes on the switching characteristics of capacitive (RF) MEMS switched capacitors, varicaps and switches, and gives guideline for reducing the charging sensitivity of these devices.

RF MEMS can suffer from various reliability issues. At the start of the chapter an overview is given, and for more details reference is made to De Wolf (2010). One problem that was not discussed in De Wolf (2010) is 'electrostatic discharge'. This is not really a failure mechanism as such, but more a failure cause, which can result in welding, fracture, shorts and charging. MEMS turn out to be very sensitive to ESD, and it is clear that both during handling and use they should be protected against ESD and EOS events. Depending on their design, MEMS might react slowly to an ESD event and, as such, withstand the high short-duration voltage pulse. But even if they are not damaged during the ESD event, they might during the following EOS. The sensitivity of MEMS to ESD can be reduced by making them more robust. But this mostly results in an increased stiffness and, for example, higher pull-in voltages. This enhances their sensitivity to charging. For this reason a better solution might consist in protecting the MEMS against ESD events by MEMS or CMOS-based protection devices.

A third topic that was addressed in this chapter is the hermeticity of the MEMS package. This is of great importance for most RF MEMS devices. RF MEMS switches were proven to have a better reliability in a controlled atmosphere such as dry nitrogen gas (De Wolf et al., 2005). Resonators in general require vacuum to have a high Q factor. Pressure variations inside the package cavity, either due to leaks, diffusion processes or outgassing, will affect the functioning and reliability of the MEMS. Several measurement methods were demonstrated in this chapter. Which to apply highly will depend on various factors, such as the presence of a MEMS device, the thickness of the cap, the volume of the cavity, the roughness of the top surface, etc. With the on-going research for cheap and reliable packaging solutions for RF MEMS, this topic will remain of high importance and other innovative measurement solutions and reliability assessment methodologies will have to be addressed.

10.8 References

Acquaviva D, Tsamados D, Coronel D P, Skotnicki T, and Ionescu A M (2009), 'Micro-electro-mechanical metal-air-insulator-semiconductor (MEM-MAIS) diode: a novel hybrid device for ESD protection', *Proc. IEEE 22nd International Conference on Micro Electro Mechanical Systems (MEMS)*, 132–135.

Amerasekara A and Duvvury C (2002), *ESD in Silicon Integrated Circuits*, John Wiley & Sons.

Bogaerts L, Phommahaxay A, Rottenberg X, Naito Y, De Coster J, Varela Pedreira O, Van Hoovels N, Cherman V, Helin P, Onishi K, and Tilmans H A (2011), 'MEMS 0-level packaging technology based on CuSn/Cu chip capping bonding', *Proc. Micromechanics Europe Workshop, MME*.

Chan K, Garikipati K, and Dutton R W (1999), 'Characterization of contact electromechanics through capacitance-voltage measurements and simulations', *Journal of Microelectromechanical Systems*, **8**(2), 208–217.

Chan K, Garikipati K, Hsiau Z K, and Dutton R W (1998), 'Characterization of electrostatically-actuated beams through capacitance-voltage measurements and simulations', *Proc. of Modeling and Simulation of Microsystems*, 180–185.

Chen L-C, Huang Y-T, and Fan K-C (2007), A dynamic 3D-surface profilometer with nanoscale measurement resolution and MHz bandwidth for MEMS characterization', *IEEE/ASME Transactions on mechatronics*, **12**(3), 299–307.

Claes G (2011), 'Poly-silicon germanium thin-film package: study of structural features enabling CMOS-MEMS integration', Leuven, Katholieke Universiteit Leuven, PhD thesis.

Czarnecki P (2010), 'Impact of charging mechanisms on the reliability of RF MEMS devices', Leuven, Katholieke Universiteit Leuven, PhD thesis.

Czarnecki P, Rottenberg X, Puers R, and De Wolf I (2006), 'Effect of gas pressure on the lifetime of capacitive RF MEMS switches', *Proc. of the IEEE 19th International Conference on Microelectromechanical System – MEMS*, 890–893.

Czarnecki P, Rottenberg X, Puers R, and De Wolf I (2005), 'Impact of biasing scheme and environment conditions on the lifetime of RF-MEMS capacitive switches', *Proc. MEMSWAVE*, 133–136.

Czarnecki P, Rottenberg X, Soussan P, Ekkels P, Muller P, De Raedt W, Tilmans H A C, Puers R, Marchand L, and De Wolf I (2009), 'Effect of substrate charging on the reliability of capacitive RF MEMS switches', *Sensors and Actuators A*, **154**, 261–268.

Czarnecki P, Rottenberg X, Soussan P, Ekkels P, Muller P, Nolmans P, De Raedt W, Tilmans H A C, Puers R, Marchand L, and De Wolf I (2008a), 'Influence of the substrate on the lifetime of capacitive RF MEMS switches', *Proc. of the 21st IEEE International Conference on Micro Electro Mechanical Systems – MEMS*, 172–175.

Czarnecki P, Rottenberg X, Soussan P, Nolmans P, Ekkels P, Muller P, Tilmans H A C, De Raedt W, Puers R, Marchand L, and De Wolf I (2008b), 'New insights into charging in capacitive RF MEMS switches', *Proc. IEEE 46th Annual International Reliability Physics Symposium (IRPS)*, 496–505.

De Coster J, Jourdain A, Puers R, and Tilmans H A C (2005), 'A method to evaluate internal cavity pressure of sealed MEMS devices', *Proc. IMAPS EMPC2005*, 599–603.

De Natale J, Mihailovich R, and Waldrop J (2002), 'Techniques for reliability analysis of MEMS RF switch', *Proc. IEEE Annual International Reliability Physics Symposium (IRPS)*, 116–117.

De Wolf I (2010), 'Reliability', in Lucyszyn S, ed., *Advanced RF MEMS*, Cambridge, Cambridge University Press, 109–133.

De Wolf I, Czarnecki P, Jourdain A, Modlinski R, Puers R, Tilmans H A C, van Beeck J T M, and van Spengen W M (2005), 'The influence of the packaging environment on the functioning and reliability of capacitive RF-MEMS switches', *Proc. 43rd Annual IEEE International Reliability Physics Symposium 2005*.

De Wolf I, De Coster J, Cherman V, Czarnecki P, Kalicinski S, Varela Pedreira P, Sangameswaran S, and Vanstreels K (2009), 'New methods and instrumentation for functional, yield and reliability testing of MEMS on device, chip and wafer level', *Proc. SPIE*, 7362, 73620N-1-73620N-9.

De Wolf I, Jourdain A, De Moor P, Tilmans H A C, and Marchand L (2007), 'Hermeticity testing and failure analysis of MEMS packages', *Proc. 14th IPFA*, 147–154.

Douglass M R (1998), 'Lifetime estimates and unique failure mechanisms of the DigitalMicromirror Device (DMD)', *Proc. International Reliability Physics Symposium (IRPS)*, **31**, 9–16.

ESDA Standard 2010–46 (2010), *For Electrostatic Discharge Sensitivity Testing – Human Body Model (HBM) – Component Level*, ANSI-ESDA-JEDEC JS-001-2010.

Goldsmith C, Ehmke J, Malczewski A, Pillans B, Eshelman S, Yao Z, Brank J, and Eberly M (2001), 'Lifetime characterization of capacitive RF MEMS switches', *Proc. of the 2001 IEEE MTT-S Int. Microwave Symp.*, **1**, 227–230.

González P, Guo B, Varela Pedreira O, Severi S, De Meyer K, and Witvrouw A (2011), 'Sealing of poly-SiGe surface micromachined cavities for MEMS-above-CMOS applications', *Journal of Micromechanics and Microengineering*, **21**, 115019–115031.

Guo B, Wang B, Wen L, Helin P, Claes G, De Coster J, Du Bois B, Verbist A, Van Hoof R, Vereecke G, Haspeslagh L, Tilmans HAC, Decoutere S, Osman H, Puers R, De Wolf I, Tanaka S, Severi S, and Witvrouw A (2012), 'Poly-SiGe-based MEMS thin-film encapsulation', *Journal of Microelectromechanical Systems*, **21**, 110–120.

Harper W R (1967), *Contact and Frictional Electrification*, United Kingdom, Oxford University Press.

Helin P, Verbist A, De Coster J, Guo B, Severi S, Witvrouw A, Haspeslagh L, Tilmans H A W, Naito Y, Nakamura K, and Onishi K (2011), 'A wafer-level poly-sige-based thin film packaging technology demonstrated on a SOI-based high-Q MEM resonator', *Proc. Solid-State Sensors, Actuators and Microsystems Conference (TRANSDUCERS)*, 982–985.

Herfst R W, Huizing H G A, Steeneken P G, and Schmitz J (2006), 'Characterization of dielectric charging in RF MEMS capacitive switches', *Proc. of the IEEE Int. Conf. Microelectr. Test Struct.*, 133–136.

Ikehashi T and Saito T (2009), 'An ESD protection device using normally-on MEMS switch,' *Proc. IEEE International Solid-State Sensors, Actuators and Microsystems Conference (TRANSDUCERS)*, 1774–1777.

Jourdain A, De Moor P, Pamidighantam S, and Tilmans H A C (2002), 'Investigation of the hermeticity of BCB-sealed cavities for housing (RF-)MEMS devices', *Proc. MEMS, 2002*, 677–680.

Ker M D and Hsu K C (2005), 'Overview of on-chip electrostatic discharge protection design with SCR-based devices in CMOS integrated circuits', *IEEE Transactions on Device and Materials Reliability*, **5**(2), 235–249.

Ling F, De Coster J, Beernaert R, Witvrouw A, Celis J-P, and De Wolf I (2011a), 'An investigation of stiction in Poly-SiGe micromirror'. *Proc. IEEE 61st Electronic Components and Technology Conference – ECTC*.

Ling F, De Coster J, Lin W, Witvrouw A, Celis J-P, and De Wolf I (2011b), 'Investigation of temporary stiction in poly-SiGe micromirror arrays', *Proc. Solid-State Sensors, Actuators and Microsystems Conference (TRANSDUCERS), 2011 16th International*, 2378–2381.

Lisec T, Huth C, and Wagner B (2004), 'Dielectric material impact on capacitive RF MEMS reliability', *Proc. of the 12th European Gallium Arsenide and other Compound Semiconductors Application Symposium*, 471–474.

McClure S S, Edmonds L D, Mihailovich R, Johnston A H, Alonzo P, De Natale J, Lehman J, and Yui C (2002), 'Radiation effects in micro-electromechanical systems (MEMS): RF Relays', *IEEE Transactions on Nuclear Science*, **49**(6).

Melle S, Flourens F, Dubuc D, Grenier K, Pons P, Pressecq F, Kuchenbecker J, Muraro J L, Bary L, and Plana R (2003), 'Reliability overview of RF MEMS devices and circuits', *Proc. of the 33rd European Microwave Conf.*, 37–40.

Military Standard (2010), *'Test Methods and Procedures for Microelectronics'*, MIL-STD-883H, 2010–54.

Papaioannou G J, Exarchos M, Theonas V, Wang G, and Papapolymerou J (2005), 'On the dielectric polarization effects in capacitive RF-MEMS switches', *Proc. of the 2005 IEEE MTT-S Int. Microwave Symp.*

Papaioannou G J and Plana R (2010), 'Advanced microwave and millimeter wave technologies semiconductor devices, circuits and systems: Physics of charging in dielectrics and reliability of capacitive RF-MEMS switches' in M. Mukherjee, InTech, Rijeka, Croatia.

Pham N P, Limaye P, Czarnecki C, Varela Pedreira O, Cherman V, Tezcan D S, and Tilmans H A C (2011), 'Metal-bonded, hermetic 0-level packaging for MEMS', *Proc. 12th IEEE Electronics Packaging Technology Conference*, 1–6.

Rebeiz G M (2003), 'RF MEMS. Theory, Design and Technology', Hoboken – New Jersey, J. Wiley & Sons, 12185–12192.

Reid J R (2002), 'Dielectric charging effects on capacitive MEMS actuators', *IEEE MTT-S Int. Microwave Symp. Digest*, RF MEMS workshop, June 2002.

Rottenberg X (2008), '*Electrostatic Switching RF-MEMS Devices in Thin-Film Technology*', Leuven, Katholieke Universiteit Leuven, PhD Thesis.

Rottenberg X, Brebels S, Ekkels P, Czarnecki P, Nolmans P, Mertens R P, Nauwelaers B, Puers R, De Wolf I, De Raedt W, and Tilmans H A C (2007a), 'An electrostatic fringing-field actuator (EFFA): application towards a low-complexity thin film RF-MEMS technology', *Journal of Micromechanics and Microengineering*, **17**, 204–210.

Rottenberg X, De Wolf I, Nauwelaers B, De Raedt W, and Tilmans H A C (2007b), 'Analytical model of the DC-actuation of electrostatic MEMS devices with distributed dielectric charging and non-planar electrodes', *IEEE J. Microelectromechanical Systems*, **16**(5), 1243–1253.

Rottenberg X, Nauwelaers B, De Raedt W, and Tilmans H A C (2004), 'Distributed dielectric charging and its impact on RF MEMS devices', *Proc. of the 34th European Microwave Conf.*, 77–80.

Ruan J, Nolhier N, Papaioannou G J, Trémouilles D, Puyal V, Villeneuve C, Idda T, Coccetti F, and Plana R (2009), 'Accelerated lifetime test of RF-MEMS switches under ESD stress', *Microelectronics Reliability*, **49**(9–11), 1256–1259.

Sangameswaran S, De Coster J, Cherman V, Czarnecki P, Linten D, Thijs S, Scholz M, Groeseneken G, and De Wolf I (2010a), 'Behavior of RF MEMS switches under ESD stress', *32nd Annual EOS/ESD Symposium Proceedings*, 1–8.

Sangameswaran S, De Coster J, De Wolf I, and Groeseneken G (2010b), 'Impact of design factors and environment on the electrostatic discharge sensitivity MEMS micromirrors', *Microelectronics Reliability*, **50**(9–11), 1383–1387.

Sangameswaran S, De Coster, Linten D, Scholz M, Thijs S, Haspeslagh L, Witvrouw A, Van Hoof C, Groeseneken G, and De Wolf I (2008), 'ESD reliability issues in microelectromechanical systems (MEMS): a case study on micromirrors,' *EOS/ESD Symposium Proceedings*, 249–257.

Sangameswaran S, De Coster J, Linten D, Scholz M, Thijs S, Van Hoof C, De Wolf I, and Groeseneken G (2009), 'Mechanical response of electrostatic actuators under ESD stress,' *Proc. IEEE International Solid-State Sensors, Actuators and Microsystems Conference, (TRANSDUCERS)*, 2110–2113.

Sangameswaran S, Thijs S, Scholz M, De Coster J, Linten D, Groeseneken G, and De Wolf I (2011), 'A silicon-controlled rectifier-based ESD protection for MEMS – merits and challenges,' *33rd Annual EOS/ESD Symposium Proceedings*, Anaheim, CA, USA.

Scholz M, Thijs S, Linten D, Trémouilles D, Sawada M, Nakaei T, Hasebe T, Natarajan M, and Groeseneken G (2007), 'Calibrated wafer-level HBM measurements for quasi-static and transient device analysis,' *EOS/ESD Symposium Proceedings*, 89–94.

Seeger J I and Crary S B (1997), 'Stabilization of electrostatically actuated mechanical devices', *Proc. Transducers '97*, 2, 1133–1136.

Tazzoli A, Peretti V, and Meneghesso G (2007), 'Electrostatic discharge and cycling effects on ohmic and capacitive RF-MEMS switches', *IEEE Trans. Device and Materials Reliability*, **7**(3), 429–437.

van Spengen M W, Puers R, Mertens R, and De Wolf I (2004), 'A comprehensive model to predict the charging and reliability of capacitive RF MEMS switches', *Journal of Micromechanics and Microengineering*, **14**, 514–521.

van Spengen M W, Puers R, Mertens R, and De Wolf I (2003), 'A low frequency electrical test set-up for the reliability assessment of capacitive RF MEMS switches', *Journal of Micromechanics and Microengineering*, **13**, 604–612.

Walraven J A, Soden J M, Tanner D M, Tangyunyong P, Cole Jr E I, Anderson R R, and Irwin L W (2000), 'Electrostatic Discharge/electrical overstress susceptibility in MEMS: a new failure mode,' *Proceedings of SPIE*, **4180**, 30–39.

Wibbeler J, Pfeifer G, and Hietschold M (1998), 'Parasitic charging of dielectric surfaces in capacitive microelectromechanical systems (MEMS)', *Sensors and Actuators*, **A71**, 74–80.

Yuan X, Cherepko S, Hwang J, Goldsmith C L, Nordquist C, and Dyck C (2004), 'Initial observation and analysis of dielectric-charging effects on RF MEMS capacitive switches', *Proc. of the 2004 IEEE MTT-S Int. Microwave Symp.*, **3**, 1943–1946.

Zaghloul U (2011), *Nanoscale and macroscale characterization of the dielectric charging phenomenon and stiction mechanisms for electrostatic MEMS/NEMS reliability*, Toulouse, University of Toulouse III, Paul Sabatier, PhD dissertation.

Zaghloul U, Bhushan B, Pons P, Papaioannou G J, and Plana R (2011a), 'On the influence of environmental gases, relative humidity and gas purification on dielectric charging processes in electrostatically driven MEMS/NEMS devices', *Nanotechnology*, **22** (3), 035705.

Zaghloul U, Koutsoureli M, Wang H, Coccetti F, Papaioannoua G J, Pons P, and Plana R (2010), 'Assessment of dielectric charging in electrostatically driven MEMS devices: A comparison of available characterization techniques,' *Journal of Microelectronics Reliability*, **50**, 1615–1620.

Zaghloul U, Papaioannou G J, Bhushan B, Coccetti F, Pons P, and Plana R (2011b), 'On the reliability of electrostatic NEMS/MEMS devices: Review of present knowledge on the dielectric charging and stiction failure mechanisms and novel characterization methodologies', *Microelectronics Reliability*, **51**, 1810–1818.

Part II
Wireless techniques and applications of wireless MEMS

11
Energy harvesters for powering wireless systems*

G. DE PASQUALE, Politecnico di Torino, Italy

DOI: 10.1533/9780857098610.2.345

Abstract: This chapter focuses on the strategies and devices used to convert the energy present in the environment into electricity to supply wireless and mobile systems. The 'energy harvesting' discipline is proving to be the first relevant response to the need for power supply without wire connections and batteries. Many transduction principles were investigated, and a number of design solutions were described in the literature. This chapter aims to provide the tools for static and dynamic design of energy harvesters, with focus on kinetic generators. Some innovative design solutions are introduced, and the most attractive modelling and simulation strategies are described.

Key words: energy harvesting, non-linear vibrations, random vibrations, dynamic response, resonance tuning, analytic modelling, reduced order modelling, modal analysis, Fourier transform, finite element method (FEM), magnetic levitation, microelectromechanical systems (MEMS).

11.1 Introduction

The power supply of wireless and mobile devices requires local sources that replace wires and cabling connections. The common approach is to use energy reservoirs (batteries) directly connected to the device or embedded in the same package. More recently, many studies and prototypes have demonstrated the possibility of generating the power needed by converting energy available in the environment into electricity directly on site; this discipline, known as 'energy harvesting', is facilitated by the diffusion of sensors and devices with very low power consumption, such as microelectromechanical systems (MEMS). The challenge to fabricate energetically autonomous transceiver sensors, which is attracting the efforts of many researchers worldwide, is finally receiving its first promising responses.

---

* The publishers wish to point out that some of the figures in this chapter are hand drawn by the author. These have been included unaltered in the chapter at the specific request of the author.

This chapter discusses the research advances in the design of energy harvesters, including original contributions and experimental results. Particular focus is given to kinetic energy conversion, which is the most attractive source for autonomous devices associated with machines. The most important generating strategies are then described, such as photovoltaic, radiofrequency, and thermoelectric. The crucial aspects of static and dynamic dimensioning are analysed, including analytic, numerical, and reduced order modelling, as well as strategies for resonance tuning and bandwidth amplification. The concept of levitating suspensions is applied to energy harvesters to improve their performance, with relevant preliminary results.

The next part of the chapter is divided into three sections, respectively dealing with the transduction principles for kinetic energy conversion, the design of generators converting vibrations into electricity, and the other typologies of energy harvesters.

11.2 Kinetic energy harvesters

Vibrations are the most attractive source of energy suitable for harvesting purposes. Many systems provide abundant kinetic energy to be converted into electricity and stored in batteries, even if some challenges make this goal quite complicated. Depending on the application field, the characteristics of vibration may differ greatly, introducing some uncertainties about the typology of the transducer to be used and its dimensioning. Three main generation strategies, among others, are described in this section: piezoelectric, electromagnetic, and capacitive.

11.2.1 Piezoelectric energy harvesting

Properties and typologies

This typology of generators is based on the deformation of mechanical parts made of (or coated with) piezoelectric materials, which are able to produce an electric power proportional to the applied strain.

Piezoelectric materials are formed by dipoles that have been aligned during manufacture by using a large electrical field. Due to this property, when the material in operative conditions is subjected to a mechanical strain along the direction of the dipoles' orientation, there is an electrical charge separation that produces a voltage difference along the material. Similarly, if a voltage is applied in the same direction, an elongation of the material is produced. The described effect is called 'piezoelectricity', and it has been exploited for many years to build sensors and actuators.

For piezoelectric generators, the directions of the load application and voltage generation are precisely identified by the rules reported in the normative (IEEE, 1997). The operation mode is identified by two indexes, i,

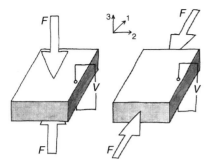

11.1 Examples of piezoelectric materials operation modes: 33 mode (left) and 31 mode (right).

j, where i is the direction of voltage difference and j is the direction of the mechanical load, as reported in Fig. 11.1 as an example. The same rule is applicable to define all the electromechanical properties, which are strongly anisotropic due to the internal structure of piezoelectric materials. The properties of piezo materials are described by the following main parameters: the piezoelectric charge constant (or strain coefficient) d, defining the polarization generated in direction i per unit of mechanical stress applied in direction j; the piezoelectric voltage constant g, giving the electric field generated in direction i per unit of mechanical stress applied in direction j; the permittivity (or dielectric constant) of piezo material ε_p; and the Young's module (E).

The constitutive equations of piezo materials are:

$$\varepsilon = \frac{\sigma}{E} + d\overline{E} \qquad [11.1]$$

$$D = \varepsilon_p \overline{E} + d\sigma \qquad [11.2]$$

where $\overline{E}$ is the electric field, D is the charge density, σ is the mechanical stress, and ε is the mechanical strain. Another important parameter is the electro-mechanical coupling coefficient k, which is a valid indicator of the effectiveness of the material in generating electrical energy (along direction i) by converting mechanical energy (applied along direction j); it is defined as

$$k = d\sqrt{\frac{E}{\varepsilon_p}} \qquad [11.3]$$

The mechanical resistance of the material is limited by its ultimate tensile strength (σ_{UTS}) in single static actuation, and by its fatigue limit (σ_L) in cyclic

Table 11.1 Properties of common piezoelectric materials for energy harvesters

	PZT	BaTiO$_3$	PVDF
d_{31} (10^{-12} C/N)	27.0 ÷ 320	78.0	23.0
d_{33} (10^{-12} C/N)	71.0 ÷ 650	149	33.0
g_{31} (10^{-3} Vm/N)	7.50 ÷ 13.7	5.00	216
g_{33} (10^{-3} Vm/N)	8.50 ÷ 42.0	14.1	330
k_{31}	0.14 ÷ 0.44	0.21	0.12
k_{33}	0.37 ÷ 0.75	0.48	0.15
$\varepsilon_p/\varepsilon_0$	425.0 ÷ 3800	1700	12.00
T_C (°C)	193 ÷ 350	120	~150
E (GPa)	63 ÷ 99	67	2.0
ρ (kg/m^3)	7400 ÷ 7750	6000	1770

excitation, which is the common operative condition for power generators. The Curie temperature (T_C) is also crucial, because it preludes the modification of the crystal structure and the loss of piezoelectricity. Ikeda (1990) presents a more in-depth description of piezoelectric material properties.

The most commonly used piezoelectric materials are polycrystalline ceramics (also called piezoceramics), such as lead zirconate titanate (PZT), which are brittle materials with good conversion properties, or polymers such as polyvinylidene fluoride (PVDF). Table 11.1 reports the properties of piezo materials commonly usable for energy harvesters (Jaffe and Berlincourt, 1965; NASA, 1998; Sakakibara *et al.*, 1994; Starner, 1996).

Basics on transduction principle

To optimize the output power, the cantilever shape with proof mass on the tip is usually preferable (Fig. 11.2a). In this case, the piezo material is actuated in the 31 mode, and the ratio between mechanical strain and applied force is maximized. By introducing a spacer material at the centre of the beam, the expansion and compression of piezo surfaces provide the maximum output voltage when the cantilever bends; this agrees with the stress distribution along a cross-section of the cantilever under bending moment, as reported in Fig. 11.2b. The power generated by piezo harvesters is a function of the resistive load: Fig. 11.3 (De Pasquale *et al.*, 2011a) reports some typical output power curves coming from experimental measurements on a piezo beam with variable proof mass on the tip. A general expression of the optimal load resistance for the power maximization in resonance condition is

$$R_{\text{load,opt}} = \frac{2\zeta_m}{\omega_n C \sqrt{4\zeta_m^2 + k^4}} \qquad [11.4]$$

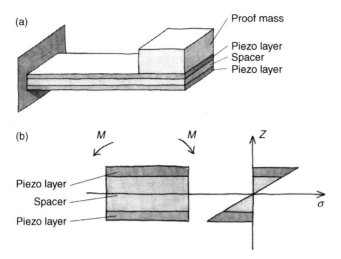

11.2 Piezoelectric cantilever for energy harvesting applications. The schematic view (a) includes a spacer between two piezo layers and the proof mass; the axial stress distribution under the applied bending moment is maximized at the upper and lower surfaces (b) in correspondence to the piezoelectric material.

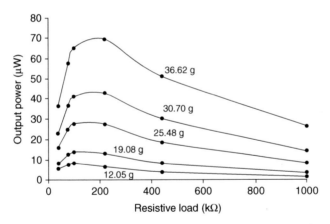

11.3 Experimental values of the output power measured on a piezoelectric generator with variable resistive load at 0.2 g acceleration in resonance condition (ranging from 5.71 to 11.77 Hz). The generator characteristics are 55 × 35 × 0.2 mm³ size, 90 nF capacitance, 23.3 GPa Young's module and variable proof mass on the tip (indicated near each curve).

where ζ_m is the mechanical parasitic damping ratio (arising from material, anchors, surrounding fluid, etc.), C is the capacitance of the piezo material, ω_n is the natural frequency of the undamped system, and k is the electro-mechanical coupling coefficient. The electric damping coefficient of the generator is

$$c_e = \frac{m\omega_n^2 k^2}{\sqrt{\omega_n^2 + \frac{1}{(R_{load}C_{load})^2}}} \qquad [11.5]$$

where m is the oscillating mass, and R_{load} and C_{load} are the resistive load and load capacitance, respectively. The maximum power corresponds to the condition $\zeta_e = \zeta_m$ where $\zeta_e = c_e/(2m\omega_n)$ is the electric damping ratio. Some expressions for the calculation of the output power are reported in the literature; they are usually complicated, and sometimes the lack of knowledge about the electro-mechanical parameters of the material may limit their application. For instance, for a cantilever with proof mass on the tip and two piezo layers separated by a central shim, the equation by Roundy et al. (2003a) to calculate the output power is

$$P = \frac{1}{x^2 \omega_n^2} \frac{R_{load,opt} C^2 \left(2dt E \varepsilon / \alpha \varepsilon_p\right)^2 a^2}{(4\zeta_m^2 + k^4)(R_{load,opt}C\omega_n)^2 + 4\zeta_m k^2 (R_{load,opt}C\omega_n) + 2\zeta_m^2} \qquad [11.6]$$

where t is the thickness of each piezo layer, a is the acceleration of the environment, α is a parameter assuming value 1 if piezo layers are connected in series, and 2 if they are connected in parallel, and x is the tip displacement.

For more details about the analytic description of the piezo transduction principle, the reader is referred to Roundy et al. (2003a) and Beeby and White (2010).

11.2.2 Electromagnetic energy harvesting

Properties and typologies

Electromagnetic generators have been developed in two configurations: linear generators (to harvest energy from vibrations) and rotating generators. They are based on Faraday's law of electromagnetic induction concerning the relative motion between a conductor and a magnet. By focusing on the first configuration (Fig. 11.4), the generator is composed of a conductive wire coil and a magnet; when the environmental vibration induces the relative motion between these parts, a potential difference (or electromotive force) is induced between the ends of the coil. Different design solutions have been proposed in the literature, with fixed coil and oscillating magnet or vice-versa. The most important parameters to be considered in the dimensioning are the size and the material of the magnet, responsible for the magnetic field intensity, and the coil parameters (number of turns, length, coil area, wire diameter), responsible for the electric output. For

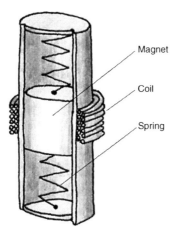

11.4 Schematic of a linear electromagnetic generator: a permanent magnet suspended on elastic springs moves through a conductive coil.

generators in the centimetre scale, a small wire diameter (ranging from 0.1 to 0.5 mm) is usually needed to provide the necessary number of coils; on the other hand, the wire diameter is proportional to the coil resistance and directly influences the output current. The magnets with the best performances are rare earth permanent magnets, especially the neodymium iron boron (NdFeB) type, which produce the strongest available magnetic field.

Basics on transduction principle

By considering a magnet moving with velocity $\dot{x}$ in a coil with N turns and the average orthogonal flux linkage per turn φ, the voltage induced in the coil is

$$V = -N\frac{d\varphi}{dt} = -N\frac{d\varphi}{dx}\dot{x} \qquad [11.7]$$

if the flux density is uniform on the coil area A and the magnetic field B varies during the time, the voltage induced is

$$V = -NA\frac{dB}{dx}\dot{x} \qquad [11.8]$$

According to El-Hami *et al.* (2001), the electromagnetic damping caused by the magnetic field induced by the current flowing in the coil and opposing the magnet's motion can be expressed as

$$c_e = \frac{(NlB)^2}{R_{load} + R_{coil} + j\omega L_{coil}} \qquad [11.9]$$

where l is the coil axial length, and R_{coil} and L_{coil} are the resistance and inductance of the coil, respectively. Similarly to piezoelectric generators, the output power of electromagnetic harvesters can be maximized by introducing an optimum load resistance (condition verified for $\zeta_e = \zeta_m$), given by the equation

$$R_{load,opt} = C_{coil} + \frac{(NlB)^2}{c_m} \qquad [11.10]$$

where C_{coil} is the coil capacitance and c_m is the mechanical damping coefficient (Stephen, 2006). The current generated in the coil is related to the relative velocity with the magnet by the equation

$$i = \frac{(NlB)}{R_{load} + R_{coil}} \dot{x} \qquad [11.11]$$

the maximum average output power can be expressed as

$$P_{max} = \frac{mA^2}{16\zeta_m \omega_n}\left(1 - \frac{R_{coil}}{R_{load}}\right) \qquad [11.12]$$

where m is the magnet mass (Stephen, 2006). Some procedures to maximize the output power of electromagnetic generators can be found in the literature (Saha et al., 2006).

11.2.3 Capacitive energy harvesting

Properties and typologies

Capacitive (or electrostatic) generators base their functioning on the relative movement of charged electrodes, separated by a dielectric, under the action of environmental vibrations. When the relative distance between electrodes, or alternatively the facing area of the electrodes, varies the energy stored in the capacitor increases and can serve to charge a separate battery. Three main configurations have been proposed for capacitive harvesters, depending on the kinematics of the electrodes, as represented in Fig. 11.5: in-plane overlap, in-plane gap closing, and out-of-plane. In the first two cases, interdigitated structures (comb drives) are usually used to increase the electrodes' area. The main drawback of this typology of energy harvesters is that a separate voltage source is needed to provide the initial charge of electrodes; the amount of energy required to start the generation

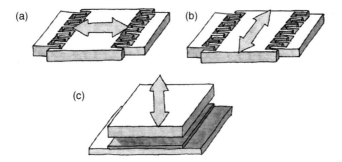

11.5 Kinematic design solutions of electrostatic harvesters: (a) in-plane overlap, (b) in-plane gap closing and (c) out-of-plane.

is proportional to the electrodes' area and travel distance. This limitation leads to the conclusion that the most efficient performance of electrostatic harvesters is limited to the microscale; moreover, the microfabrication processes needed, usually based on silicon material, are well established.

Basics on transduction principle

The basic equations of electrostatic generators that define the capacitance C, the charge Q, and the stored energy E_n are

$$C = \frac{Q}{V} = \varepsilon_{air} \frac{A}{x} \qquad [11.13]$$

$$V = \frac{Qx}{\varepsilon_0 A} \qquad [11.14]$$

$$E_n = \frac{1}{2}QV = \frac{1}{2}\frac{Q^2}{C} = \frac{1}{2}CV^2 \qquad [11.15]$$

where x is the gap between electrodes, A is the area of electrodes, and ε_0 and ε_{air} are the permittivity of free space and air, respectively. According to Equation [11.13], the capacitance varies depending on the gap. Two electrical configurations of the generator can be used to manage the energy increase: constant voltage, or constant charge. In the first case, a separate reservoir is connected to the generator and provides the operative voltage level; when the electrodes move and their gap increases, the capacitance decreases and the surplus of charge moves to the reservoir, representing the output energy of the generator. In the case of constant charge, when the capacitance decreases due to the movement of electrodes, the voltage across them increases and is suitable to charge the separate battery. In both cases, the energy generated is

$$E_n = \frac{1}{2} V_{max} V_0 (C_{max} - C_{min}) \qquad [11.16]$$

where V_{max} is the maximum voltage of the duty cycle and V_0 is the voltage level at the beginning of the duty cycle (in case of constant voltage configuration, $V_0 = V_{max}$); C_{max} and C_{min} are the maximum and minimum capacitances, corresponding to minimum and maximum gap, respectively. Roundy et al. (2003b) provide an expression of the electric damping coefficient affecting capacitive generators:

$$c_e = \lambda \frac{Q^2}{N_g \varepsilon_0 t} \qquad [11.17]$$

where $\lambda = x/4l$ for in-plane gap closing generators, $\lambda = d/2x^2$ for in-plane overlap generators, N_g is the number of gaps among fingers, t is the fingers' thickness, l is the fingers' length, and d is the gap between fingers.

MEMS electret generators

The need for a separate voltage source, as stated before, confines the dimensions of capacitive harvesters in the microscale and leads to high resonance frequencies and low power output. The introduction of electrets can overcome this limitation and offers the possibility to obtain self-charged capacitive generators in the millimetre scale. The electret is a dielectric material with quasi-permanent charge; after its first theorization by Faraday, the term 'electret' was introduced by Oliver Heaviside (1892), in analogy to 'magnet', and the first device was developed by Eguchi (1925). Several methods have been developed to charge electrets, which can be divided into organic (based on polymers) and inorganic (based on SiO_2); a very long-term stability of surface charge of electrets has been demonstrated, in the order of tens of years (Takamatsu, 1991). In capacitive generators, the electret can be used to induce an opposite charge between the electrodes without the need of an external voltage source. Figure 11.6 shows the fundamental configurations of electret generators: the relative motion between the electrodes (where the charge is induced by the electret) or, in the last case, the motion of a high-permittivity insert, causes the current flow in the circuit. A simple equation to calculate the power output of a rotational generator with n poles, a total area A, and rotation frequency f, by neglecting the parasitic capacitance (Boland et al., 2003), is

$$P = \frac{Q^2 t^2 R_{load}}{\left[\varepsilon_0 \varepsilon_{air} R + \frac{1}{nAf}(\varepsilon_{electret} g + \varepsilon_{air} t) \right]^2} \qquad [11.18]$$

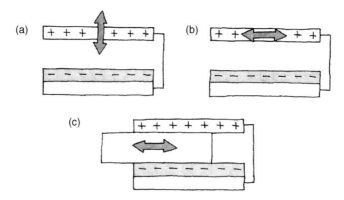

11.6 In MEMS electret generators, the electret (the grey layer) is normally deposited on a ground electrode and is faced to the counter electrode. Design variants include out-of-plane (a) and in-plane (b) motion of the counter electrode, and sliding of a high-permittivity insert (c).

where Q is the charge density, t is the thickness of electret, R_{load} is the load resistance, $\varepsilon_{electret}$ is the relative permittivity of the electret, and g is the gap between the electret and the counter electrode. Suzuki (2011) provides a detailed review of capacitive electret generator devices and technology.

11.2.4 Example devices of kinetic energy harvesters

Table 11.2 summarizes the main advantages and drawbacks of the generators described earlier. Table 11.3 reports the results of experimental characterization of some published prototypes and commercial devices, to compare the operative frequency range and power density of each typology.

Some energy harvesters presented in the literature are reported here as examples. Figure 11.7 shows the piezoelectric harvester built by Elfrink *et al.* (2009), generating 60 µW output power at resonance (572 Hz) at 2 g acceleration; the size of the transducer is $10 \times 10 \times 1$ mm^3. Cheng and Arnold (2010) proposed a particular configuration for the electromagnetic harvester represented in Fig. 11.8: their solution ($54 \times 46 \times 15$ mm^3) includes several coils and magnets organized in two arrays and defining a multi-pole generator able to produce 0.55 mW at 9.25 Hz and 0.8 g. The capacitive generator presented by Chiu and Tseng (2008) includes a proof mass that is made heavier by adding a tungsten ball (4 mm diameter) to reduce its resonance frequency at 120 Hz (Fig. 11.9); the transducer is traditionally based on charged comb fingers and generates 31 µW at 0.23 g. Figure 11.10 (Suzuki *et al.*, 2010) reports an example of capacitive generator with electrets; the mass oscillates in-plane at 63 Hz and 2 g by modifying the facing area of the capacitors situated below the plate; the measured output power is 1 µW.

Table 11.2 Advantages and drawbacks of different energy harvesters typologies

	Advantages	Drawbacks
Piezoelectric	High energy density	High output impedance (low current)
	Response tunability	Low reliability (fatigue)
	High output voltage	Microfabrication issues
Electromagnetic	High output current	Moderate energy density
	High reliability	Limited response tunability
	Performances stability	High velocity required
		Limited integration in microsystems
Capacitive	High integration in microsystems	Electric preload needed
	Consolidated fabrication processes	Almost limited to microscale
		Low output voltage
		High resonance frequencies
Capacitive electret	Passive electric preload	Materials research and processes definition still on-going
	Larger size allowed	Low resonance frequencies

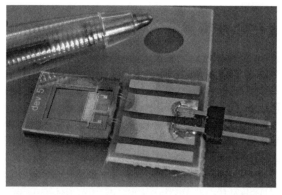

11.7 Piezoelectric generator mounted on a supportive board with electrical connectors (Elfrink *et al.*, 2009). Reproduced with the courtesy of intraocular pressure (IOP).

11.3 Design of kinetic energy harvesters

This section discusses the concepts at the basis of geometry and kinematics definition and material properties selection to design the static and dynamic behaviour of generators. The approaches described are applicable to all the typologies of kinetic harvesters and may be used to compare their performance under different ambient conditions.

Table 11.3 Performances of different typologies of linear energy harvesters

	Resonance/driving frequency (Hz)	Power (µW)	Size (mm³)	Acceleration (g)	Reference
Piezoelectric	80.00	2.10×10^0	1.25×10^2	0.230	Glynne-Jones et al. (2001)
	120.0	3.75×10^2	1.00×10^3	0.250	Roundy and Wright (2004)
	190.0	6.50×10^1	1.20×10^0	7.270	Hong and Moon (2005)
	13900	1.00×10^0	2.70×10^{-2}	5.100	Jeon et al. (2005)
	1495	8.00×10^{-1}	5.00×10^0	2.000	Marzencki et al. (2008)
	60.00	1.50×10^3	9.30×10^4	n.a.	AdaptivEnergy (2009)
	572.0	6.00×10^1	1.00×10^2	2.000	Elfrink et al. (2009)
	100.0	1.00×10^3	4.03×10^4	0.400	Mide Technology Corp. (2011)
	8.560	1.00×10^2	9.62×10^2	0.200	De Pasquale et al. (2011a)
Electromagnetic	4400	3.00×10^{-1}	2.50×10^1	27.30	Williams et al. (2001)
	99.00	4.99×10^3	4.08×10^3	0.700	Glynne-Jones (2001)
	110.0	8.30×10^2	1.00×10^3	9.730	Ching et al. (2002)
	120.0	4.00×10^2	2.45×10^0	0.250	Pérez-Rodríguez et al. (2005)
	52.00	4.60×10^1	1.50×10^2	0.060	Beeby et al. (2007)
	8.000	2.50×10^3	1.27×10^4	0.039	Saha et al. (2008)
	120.0	1.75×10^3	1.30×10^5	0.025	Perpetuum Ltd (2010)
	9.250	5.50×10^2	3.72×10^4	0.800	Cheng and Arnold (2010)
	60.00	1.30×10^3	1.70×10^5	0.050	Ferro Solutions (2011)
	4.300	8.84×10^4	1.42×10^5	0.100	De Pasquale et al. (2011c)
Capacitive	2520	8.00×10^0	1.12×10^0	n.a.	Meninger et al. (2001)
	120.0	3.37×10^{-1}	5.40×10^{-1}	0.230	Roundy et al. (2003a)
	50.00	1.05×10^3	1.80×10^4	1.170	Despesse et al. (2005)
	4300	1.00×10^0	n.a.	372.0	Ma et al. (2005)
	120.0	3.10×10^1	4.00×10^2	0.230	Chiu and Tseng (2008)
	~1400	1.58×10^0	1.50×10^0	13.00	Hoffmann et al. (2009)
Capacitive electret	10.00	6.00×10^0	8.00×10^2	0.400	Arakawa et al. (2004)
	50.00	1.80×10^1	2.70×10^2	58.70	Lo and Tai (2008)
	20.00	7.00×10^2	4.00×10^2	1.930	Sakane et al. (2008)
	30.00	1.00×10^2	1.60×10^3	0.150	Masaki et al. (2010)
	63.00	1.00×10^0	3.05×10^2	2.000	Suzuki et al. (2010)

358   Handbook of MEMS for wireless and mobile applications

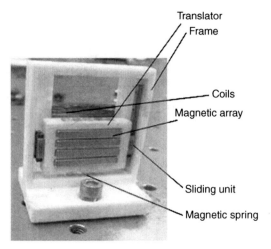

11.8 Four poles electromagnetic generator with magnets mounted on a sliding unit and four coils on the back; the device is 54 mm high and 46 mm wide (Cheng and Arnold, 2010). Reproduced with the courtesy of IOP.

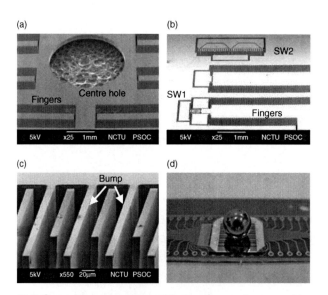

11.9 Capacitive generator with proof mass increased by an external tungsten ball (Chiu and Tseng, 2008): centre hole for positioning the external mass (a), switches (b), comb drive fingers (c) and external mass assembling (d). Reproduced with the courtesy of IOP.

Energy harvesters for powering wireless systems 359

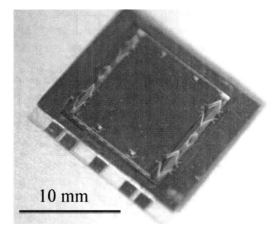

11.10 Capacitive electret generator prototype with suspended mass oscillating in-plane (Suzuki *et al.*, 2010). Reproduced with the courtesy of IOP.

11.3.1 Tools for designing and dimensioning

Static dimensioning

The first goal of the design is to prevent static failure of the structure under a given combination of loads. Static failure is usually induced by the following:

- elastic deformation;
- elastic instability;
- plastic distortion (or ductile fracture);
- fracture.

Elastic deformation is typical of structures that, under the combination of high applied loads and low Young's module of the material, exhibit large deformation in the elastic field; they are accompanied by large displacements, which are not compatible with the confining structures or packages and cause collisions. Elastic instability and buckling effect are associated with long and thin structures loaded with compressive axial forces; in these cases, the expected compressive deformation is no longer respected and another deformation mode is experienced, due to the misalignment between the ends of the structure, which induces a high bending moment. The definition of the plastic distortion threshold is quite arbitrary: conventionally it is associated with a plastic deformation of 0.2% in the stress–strain curve, but in real components the material may experience plastic deformation only in small regions (e.g., surfaces of bended elements) without failure. In general, the propensity to fail under plastic distortion is typical of ductile materials, and the reference parameter identifying this condition is the yield strength σ_y. Fracture is easier to recognize, because it involves the separation of the component; it is the usual failure mode of brittle materials and is identified by the ultimate tensile strength σ_{UTS}.

The actual stress σ induced in the material by the load must be compared with the yield stress (or with the ultimate stress) at every point of the structure; normally, the ratio σ_y/σ must be higher than a specific 'factor of safety' that is properly chosen for the application. If the actual stress has a multiaxial configuration, the comparison is made with an equivalent uniaxial stress that is calculated by one of the many dedicated criteria. In case of complicated geometries, it is important to consider the notch effect in those regions close to strong shape variations (change in section, sharp corners, etc.), where the stress concentration may cause failure although the average stress is much lower. The stress increment can be estimated with the 'stress concentration factor', which is tabulated for many shapes of the notch. A more detailed discussion of the topics introduced is beyond the scope of this work; for additional information the reader is referred to Timoshenko and Goodier (1951) and Collins (1993).

Analytic modelling of the dynamic response

All kinetic energy harvesters are dynamic systems having one or more parts that exhibit a vibration when the environment, to which the harvester is constrained, is vibrating. This common feature allows the introduction of a modelling approach with general validity, which is based on the single degree of freedom (dof) mass–spring–damper dynamic system represented in Fig. 11.11. The general governing equation of kinetic generators has the following form:

$$m(\ddot{x}+\ddot{z})+c\dot{x}+kx = mg + f(t) \qquad [11.19]$$

where x and z are the coordinates in the relative and absolute reference systems, respectively.

The coefficient m usually indicates the proof mass, but it should include also the mass of those portions of suspensions or supports that participate in the oscillation; this mass component is hard to identify, and some empirical assumptions can be used. For instance, a piezoelectric cantilever with mass m_c and proof mass m_p on the tip can be modelled with a global mass of vibrating parts $m = m_p + m_c/3$. The damping coefficient c is the most difficult to determine; it is defined as

$$c = c_m + c_e \qquad [11.20]$$

In Equation [11.20], c_m is the mechanical damping; it refers to the dissipations caused by anchor losses, thermoelastic damping (TED), structural

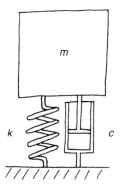

11.11 The mass-spring-damper single-dof dynamic system suitable for a first approximation modelling of kinetic energy harvesters.

dissipations (crystallographic defects), surface effects when the material is subjected to deformation, and viscous dissipations from fluids. For instance, a 400 nm gold coating deposited on a silicon cantilever causes a 50% decrease of the system quality factor because of its high material damping (Sandberg *et al.*, 2008). Depending on the design of the suspensions, mechanical energy may radiate into the environment. Anchor losses can be minimized by placing the suspensions at the natural minima of the modal deformed shape of the structure (De Pasquale *et al.*, 2010). The viscous damping component is associated with the dissipative effects caused by the interactions of the moving structure with fluids, especially air. This damping component can vary considerably depending on geometry, operative frequencies, fluid inertia, fluid compressibility, rarefaction effects, and pressure (Mohite *et al.*, 2008). Viscous dissipation mechanisms are generally divided into 'squeeze film damping' and 'slide film damping', in the case of orthogonal or tangent motion of surfaces, respectively; other typologies are related to fluid flows in perforations and fluid linkages between adjacent surfaces. The component c_e indicates the electric damping and can be estimated with the expression reported in Section 11.2, depending on the transduction principle; a more detailed discussion on damping mechanisms can be found in Priya and Inman (2008). The difficulty of modelling damping mechanisms depends on the strong non-linearities affecting the dissipative processes and on the large number of parameters involved, most of which are device dependent and only predictable through statistical approximation. As a consequence, experimental characterization is often the preferred strategy to quantify the energy losses in the desired range of operation, and it is always recommended that the results predicted by models be validated.

The stiffness coefficient k is usually associated with the properties of the suspensions or the transducer itself (in case of piezoelectric generators).

When small oscillation amplitudes, compared with the device dimensions, are involved, a linear stiffness can be assumed without appreciable errors; this implies considering a linear elastic material for structural suspensions, and negligible second-order effects in the case of other typologies of suspensions (for instance, those based on magnetic levitation). If larger oscillations are present, however, stiffness non-linearities must be considered. The presence of a fluid surrounding the vibrating structure produces viscous forces acting on oscillating components that are represented, in the case of sinusoidal oscillation, by a complex number. In the phase diagram, the force components are 90° shifted, defining in practice a damping force (in phase with the velocity) and a spring force (in phase with the displacement). This means that an additional contribution to the stiffness of the system (k) may appear due to the fluid. Usually, at low frequencies, the fluid damping force is dominant, while at high frequencies the stiffness fluid force prevails. The presence of packages or closed cavities (e.g., in electromagnetic generators with long travel of the magnet) may induce the repetitive compression and expansion of the fluid, with consequent increase of the fluid stiffness contribution.

The term indicating the gravity force (mg) in the governing Equation [11.19] is relevant for large devices, where it is of primary importance to evaluate the static configuration of the system (e.g., long piezoelectric transducers with proof mass on the tip, or large inductors with heavy magnets); on the other hand, it can be neglected to describe the behaviour of generators in the millimetre or micrometre scale. Normally, the force $f(t)$ applied to the proof mass is not present in common designs; however, it is sometimes necessary to modify the response of the system by applying an external force to the oscillating structure. This force can be generated by the transducer itself (e.g., by an electric bias voltage in capacitive harvesters) or by external devices, and it is used to tune the resonance frequency of the harvester on the current vibration frequency of the environment, or to amplify the response bandwidth.

In the case of sinusoidal vibration of the environment, $z(t) = z_0 \sin(\omega t)$, the steady-state solution of the governing Equation [11.19] gives the relative mass displacement $x(t) = x_0 \sin(\omega t + \phi)$, with amplitude and phase angle expressed by

$$|H| = \left|\frac{x_0}{z_0}\right| = \frac{(\omega/\omega_n)^2}{\sqrt{\left[1-(\omega/\omega_n)^2\right]^2 + 2\zeta(\omega/\omega_n)^2}} \qquad [11.21]$$

$$\varphi = \tan^{-1}\left[\frac{2\zeta(\omega/\omega_n)}{1-(\omega/\omega_n)^2}\right] \qquad [11.22]$$

where $\omega_n = \sqrt{k/m}$ is the natural frequency of the undamped system and $\zeta = c/(2m\omega_n)$ is the global damping ratio; Equation [11.21] represents the magnitude of the frequency response function (FRF) of the system, which is plotted in Fig. 11.12a (the phase angle is plotted in Fig. 11.12b). The response curve shows a resonance peak only if $\zeta < 1/\sqrt{2} \cong 0.7$; in this case, the natural frequency of the damped system is

$$\omega_{n,damp} = \omega_n \sqrt{1-2\zeta^2} \qquad [11.23]$$

and the corresponding peak amplitude, also called the 'quality factor', is

$$Q = |H|_{max} = \frac{1}{2\zeta\sqrt{1-\zeta^2}} \qquad [11.24]$$

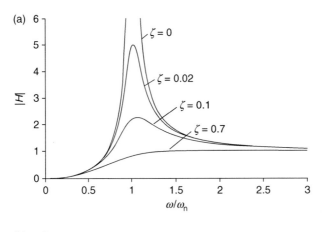

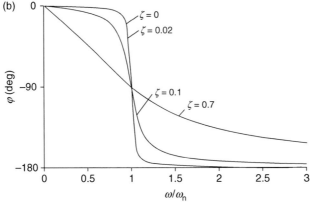

11.12 FRF of the system under sinusoidal excitation and variable damping: (a) amplitude and (b) phase angle.

which is usually approximated with the expression $Q = (2\zeta)^{-1}$ in case of low damping. The 'half power amplitude', situated at approximately −3 dB from the peak, is

$$|H|_{-3dB} = \frac{|H|_{max}}{\sqrt{2}} \qquad [11.25]$$

and the corresponding 'half power points' angular frequencies and 'half power bandwidth' are

$$\omega_{-3dB}^I, \omega_{-3dB}^{II} = \omega_n \sqrt{1 \mp 2\zeta} \qquad [11.26]$$

$$\Delta \omega_{-3dB} = 2\zeta \omega_n \qquad [11.27]$$

The last equation is particularly useful to estimate the damping starting from the experimental measurement of the FRF, where the half power bandwidth and natural frequency are clearly defined.

Reduced order modelling

The solution of the single-dof governing equation provides some basic information about the dynamic response of the system. However, its application is limited by some stringent assumptions: the entire oscillating mass is concentrated in one point; all the dissipative and conservative forces are modelled through the two coefficients c and k that directly act on the single-point mass.

This approach is not sufficiently accurate to evaluate the dynamic behaviour of complicated or flexible structures; additionally, it could be useful to determine the modal deformed shape of the structure and to evaluate the influence of every design parameter (geometry, material properties, etc.) on the dynamic response. The reduced order modelling approach, with the assumption of linear dynamic parameters, can be used for this purpose. The limits introduced by the linearization hypothesis must be verified in relation to the specific transduction principle.

Let us consider, for instance, the double-clamped structure for out-of-plane capacitive generators represented in Fig. 11.13a; the central plate may exhibit a flexural deformation during the vertical oscillation due to its large dimensions. A 3-dof reduced order model of this structure is obtained, as shown in Fig. 11.13b, by separating mass and stiffness properties in some concentrated parameters, depending on shape, kinematics, and constraints. The mass coefficients are defined starting from the total mass of oscillating parts, and the stiffness coefficients are calculated by simple equations based on the beam or plates theory. In the case of additional damping and stiffness

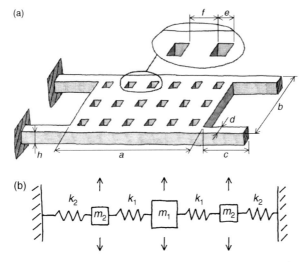

11.13 Basic structure for capacitive generators moving out-of-plane (a) composed by the perforated central electrode and four lateral supporting springs, and its 3-dof compact model (b) built with the concentrated parameters approach. Reported parameters indicate the plate mass splitting (m_1 and m_2), the plate stiffness (k_1) and the suspensions stiffness (k_2).

contributions, they can be added with the same approach. Finally, the structure is described by an eigenfunction having n_{dof} degrees of freedom (where n_{dof} is the number of concentrated masses) that can be solved in the frequency domain, giving the first n_{dof} resonances (from eigenvalues) and modal shapes (from eigenvectors) of the structure. Very practical closed formulas relating the geometry and material properties to the dynamic response can be obtained. In the case considered, the geometrical and material parameters are plate sides (a, b), suspensions sides (c, d), square holes sides (e), holes interspace (f), number of holes ($m \times n$), thickness (h), Young's module (E), and density (ρ). The parameters of the reduced order model can be calculated as follows:

$$m_1 = 0.5M, \ m_2 = 0.25M \quad [11.28]$$

$$k_1 = \frac{2Eh^3 A_{eff}}{a^4}, \ k_2 = \frac{Edh^3}{2c^3} \quad [11.29]$$

where $A_{eff} = ab - mne^2$ is the effective area of the plate and $M = \rho h A_{eff}$ is the mass of the plate. The equilibrium equation of the system is

$$[M]\{\ddot{x}\}+[C]\{\dot{x}\}+[K]\{x\}=\{0\} \quad [11.30]$$

where mass and stiffness matrices are respectively

$$[M] = \begin{bmatrix} m_2 & 0 & 0 \\ 0 & m_1 & 0 \\ 0 & 0 & m_2 \end{bmatrix}, \quad [K] = \begin{bmatrix} k_1+k_2 & -k_1 & 0 \\ -k_1 & 2k_1 & -k_1 \\ 0 & -k_1 & k_1+k_2 \end{bmatrix} \quad [11.31]$$

If the damping coefficients are unknown, the damping matrix can be estimated in first approximation with the Rayleigh formulation:

$$[C] = \alpha[M] + \beta[K] \quad [11.32]$$

By solving the characteristic polynomial associated with Equation [11.30], it is possible to calculate the natural frequencies in the form $\omega_{n,i} = \omega_{n,i}(a,\ldots,f,h,m,n,E,\rho)$ and the modal shapes in the form $\psi_i = \psi_i(a,\ldots,f,h,m,n,E,\rho)$, as described in detail by De Pasquale and Somà (2009), where the linearization hypotheses are also discussed.

Random vibrations

The analytic approaches previously described are based on the stringent assumption of sinusoidal excitation. Unfortunately, energy harvesters are usually applied to randomly vibrating environments, and the reported equations, although very important for the dimensioning stage, are not so useful in calculating the actual device response and power output when it is applied in the field. The most effective procedure to calculate the dynamic response of the system to a random vibration is to decompose the input signal $z(t)$, expressed in the time domain, into the signal $Z(t)$ that is formed by a sum of sinusoids, properly modulated in frequency, amplitude and phase. This can be obtained by applying the Fourier transform to the input displacement:

$$Z(j\omega) = \int_{-\infty}^{\infty} z(t)e^{-j\omega t} dt \quad [11.33]$$

where j is the complex unit. This equation can be applied to the continuous function of the random vibration, which is generally unknown. More frequently, the environmental vibration is measured by sensors (lasers, accelerometers, etc.) with a given sampling frequency that provides a discrete characterization of the displacement (z_n). In this case, it is more practical to apply the discrete Fourier transform (DFT):

$$Z_k = \sum_{n=0}^{N-1} z_n e^{-\frac{2\pi j}{N}kn}, \quad k = 0,\ldots,N-1 \quad [11.34]$$

The sequence of complex samples describing the environmental displacement ($z_0,\ldots,z_{N-1}$) is transformed in a sequence of complex numbers ($Z_0,\ldots,Z_{N-1}$), which represent the amplitude and phase of the different sinusoidal components of the input signal. More precisely, every component has the following magnitude and phase angle:

$$|Z_k| = \sqrt{\text{Re}(Z_k)^2 + \text{Im}(Z_k)^2} \qquad [11.35]$$

$$\varphi_k = \tan^{-1}\left[\frac{\text{Im}(Z_k)}{\text{Re}(Z_k)}\right] \qquad [11.36]$$

The application of the Fourier transform to the random vibration of the environment is usually limited to a small time interval of the function $z(t)$; it is then important to properly select this input range to represent the complete vibration history. This is possible if the environmental vibration is 'stationary', that is, its characteristics remain the same if observed starting from different instants of time, and 'ergodic', that is, the average displacement, its variance, and the value of the autocorrelation function calculated on a single time interval are independent of the interval selected.

When the random input vibration is expressed in terms of a series of sinusoidal vibrations, the system response can be calculated as described in the previous sections for each component of the excitation. In general applications, a large portion of the spectral density of the environmental vibration is concentrated in a small range of frequencies; this implies that a small number of sinusoidal components of the transformed equation include most of the excitation energy. The frequency-domain response of the generator can be expressed in terms of displacement X_k or directly in terms of output power P_k. The components of the response can be combined to obtain the global response of the system or the total output power by using the inverse DFT:

$$x_n = \frac{1}{N}\sum_{k=0}^{N-1} X_k e^{\frac{2\pi j}{N}kn}, \quad n = 0, \ldots, N-1 \qquad [11.37]$$

This last operation may introduce some approximations if large non-linearities affect the system dynamics; the level of approximation should be verified case by case. Figure 11.14 summarizes the procedure described to treat the random excitation. Some strategies to efficiently harvest power from random vibrations, including stochastic resonance, active tuning strategies, and generators with multiple eigenfrequencies, are discussed in Section 11.3.2.

Mechanical fatigue design

Structures subjected to repetitive load cycles may collapse under the effect of mechanical fatigue, although the stress level is considerably lower than

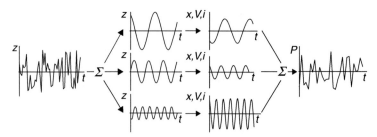

11.14 The random excitation is separated in sinusoidal components with variable frequency, amplitude and phase. For each curve, representing one component of the displacement response, the corresponding electric output can be computed; all the contributions are then combined with the proper phase angle to calculate the dynamic and electric outputs of the generator.

the yield stress. The fatigue mechanism starts with the nucleation of small cracks in correspondence to microscopic defects on the material surface; the alternate loading causes the crack propagation inside the component, orthogonally to the surface, and the actual cross-section of the component is progressively reduced until its catastrophic failure. The studies conducted on fatigue have produced many experimental results, which are usually reported on S–N curves (Fig. 11.15a), demonstrating that the lifetime of components is strongly variable depending on the material, geometry, load characteristics, and environmental parameters. The investigation of fatigue at the microscale is at an early stage, but some results on brittle (Muhlstein *et al.*, 2001; Yoneoka *et al.*, 2010) and ductile (Read, 1998; Somà and De Pasquale, 2009) materials have been presented. The most important parameter to be considered at the fatigue design stage is the 'fatigue limit' σ_L, which identifies the stress level below which the component is not sensitive to fatigue; it is lower than the yield stress for ductile material, but unfortunately it is not possible to identify σ_L for all the materials. Another important result of experiments on fatigue, even at the microscale, is the shortening of lifetime when a non-zero mean stress is added to the cyclic stress applied to the material. The influence of the mean stress on the lifetime is represented by Goodman–Smith diagrams; Fig. 11.15b shows an example for gold samples (De Pasquale and Somà, 2011).

Numerical modelling and FEM simulation

In general, the analytic solution of non-linear differential equations describing the system dynamics is hard to calculate, and this possibility is limited to some specific cases (e.g., in the presence of a non-linear elastic force in levitating suspensions, described in the section on 'Static and dynamic behaviour'). More frequently, it is not possible to get a solution by analytic calculations; numerical integration of the governing equation is needed. Although numerical modelling has an enormous power of calculation, its

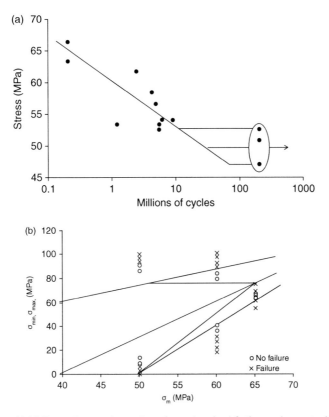

11.15 Experimental results of mechanical fatigue characterization of electroplated gold samples. S–N curve, or Wöhler diagram, under bending and shear alternate load (Somà and De Pasquale, 2009) (a); Goodman-Smith diagram under tensile alternate load with variable mean stress σ_m (De Pasquale and Somà, 2011) (b).

main drawback is the low level of information provided about the influence of design parameters on the system response and about the general comprehension of the system's behaviour.

For the application of numerical integration methods, the governing Equation [11.19] can be written in the form

$$m\ddot{x} + c\dot{x} + kx = -m\ddot{z} + \xi\left\{m_{nl}, c_{nl}, k_{nl}, (\ddot{x})^j, (\dot{x})^k, (x)^w\right\} + mg + f(t) \qquad [11.38]$$

where the function ξ, including all the non-linear terms, is treated as an external force. Unlike Equation [11.38], which has general validity, non-linearities usually interest only damping and elastic forces (i.e., $m_{nl} = 0$ and $j = 0$). In case of explicit integration methods, the equilibrium is written at the time t_i, when the system status is completely defined and non-linear forces ξ can be computed. The finite difference method can be used to calculate the system conditions at the next time step, t_{i+1}, by applying the following expression:

$$x_{i+1} = \frac{1}{(m/(\Delta t)^2)+(c/2\Delta t)} \times \left[\left(\frac{2m}{(\Delta t)^2}-k\right)x_i + \left(\frac{c}{2\Delta t}-\frac{m}{(\Delta t)^2}\right)x_{i-1} - m\ddot{z}_i + \xi_i + mg + f(t_i)\right] \quad [11.39]$$

where Δt is the integration time interval, whose dimension influences the stability of explicit solution methods. Implicit integration methods are numerically stable because the equilibrium is calculated at the time t_{i+1}; the shortening of the time integration interval may improve the accuracy of results. For instance, in the β-Newmark method, a preliminary control on the approximation errors of acceleration (that is arbitrarily assumed for the time t_{i+1}, on the basis of the parameter β that defines its evolution in the time interval) has to be performed by a recursive strategy before proceeding to the following integration step. The solving equation in this case is

$$x_{i+1} = \frac{1}{m+\frac{\Delta t}{2}c+\beta(\Delta t)^2 k}\left\{[2m-(1-2\beta)(\Delta t)^2 k]x_i + \beta(\Delta t)^2\left[F(t_{i+1})+\left(\frac{1}{\beta}-2\right)F(t_i)-F(t_{i-1})\right]\right\} - x_{i-1}$$

$$[11.40]$$

where $F(t)$ indicates all the forces acting on the system.

Methods like these and many others are adopted by commercial software to calculate the response of complicated structures with tens of thousands of degrees of freedom, and more, by means of the finite element method (FEM). This calculation strategy is largely used by designers because of its enormous potential in solving many different kinds of problems. The approach is based on the discretization of the continuous into small parts (finite elements), which are defined by sets of nodes and governing functions (or shape functions for structural problems). The complicated system of differential equations describing the multi-dof model is solved numerically. FEM tools are very important in simulating the behaviour of systems with complicated geometry, of materials' interactions, and of multiphysics problems where many physical domains are involved (e.g., structural, fluidic, electric, magnetic, thermal).

11.3.2 Frequency range of power generation

In common applications, environmental vibrations have small amplitude; this is why energy harvesters are based on resonating systems that are able to amplify the input vibration and improve the efficiency of the transduction device or material. However, the dynamic amplification of vibration has two relevant drawbacks that may greatly limit the generator performance: single working frequency and narrow bandwidth. Because the input vibration has a variable frequency over time, due to the random nature of common excitation sources, several different strategies have been investigated to tune the resonance frequency of the harvester and to widen its bandwidth. Zhu *et al.* (2010) provide a detailed review of the strategies used to increase the operative frequency range of generators.

Resonance tuning

Different tuning strategies can be compared and selected on the basis of a few aspects: the energy consumed with respect to the harvested energy, the frequency range of interest, the frequency resolution needed, and the alterations on the system dynamics (especially on damping and stiffness parameters). Resonance tuning strategies have been effectively divided into 'continuous' and 'intermittent' by Beeby and White (2010), and can be associated with one of the following:

- alteration of dimensions;
- variation of the proof mass centre of gravity;
- application of tuning forces;
- changing of electric load.

Despite the general difficulty in changing the dimensions of a device, it is possible for the free length of vibration, which can be adjusted by modifying the anchoring point; an example is reported in the schematics of Fig. 11.16 (Gieras *et al.*, 2007). The centre of gravity of the proof mass can be moved by acting on translating elements, as shown in Fig. 11.17 (Wu *et al.*, 2008), to modify the resonance frequency of the vibrating system. An external force can be applied to tune the resonance frequency by using different strategies: piezoelectric actuation, electrostatic capacitive bias voltage, magnetic induction, and thermal heating. The application of a tuning force, in general, is responsible for the

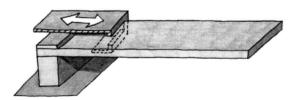

11.16 Resonance tuning strategy based on the variation of the free length of the generator by moving its anchoring point.

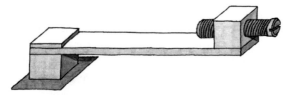

11.17 Tuning strategy of the resonance frequency based on the variation of the gravity centre of the generator by acting on a translating element that moves through the proof mass.

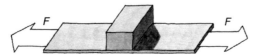

11.18 Application of axial preload to tune the resonance of piezoelectric generators by varying the equivalent structural stiffness.

variation of the elastic properties of the structure; the change of stiffness can be induced directly, for instance, by changing the static equilibrium position, or indirectly, for instance, by applying a compressive or tensile strain to the structure. Some examples are described in Fig. 11.18 (Leland and Wright, 2006), where a variable axial preload is applied to a piezoelectric beam generator; in De Pasquale *et al.* (2009), where a bias voltage is applied to the capacitive harvester to induce an equivalent electric stiffness; and in Fig. 11.19 (Challa *et al.*, 2008), where a magnetic force is used to modify the flexural motion of a piezo harvester. Finally, some experiences on the variation of the electrical damping of piezoelectric generators were reported by adjusting the load and producing the shift of the power spectrum (Wu *et al.*, 2006).

Bandwidth amplification

The simplest way to widen the bandwidth of the dynamic response of the generator is to reduce its quality factor, but this implies increasing the global damping of the system and, consequently, reducing the peak amplitude of the response, making this approach inconvenient in practice. Non-linear suspensions can be used to introduce a dependence of the resonance frequency on the oscillation amplitude, the result being an increase in bandwidth; unfortunately, the real benefits are usually limited to a small range of frequencies and the final bandwidth is dependent on the hardening or softening properties of the suspension. More useful strategies are the following:

- array of structures with different response;
- coupled multi-dof systems;

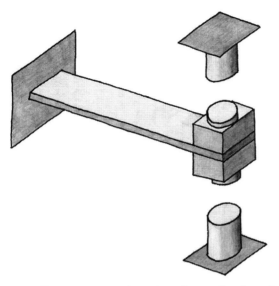

11.19 Tuning strategy based on the application of external forces to the oscillating mass of the generator by means of magnetic interactions.

- bi-stable structures;
- active tuning.

A series of similar harvesting structures can be assembled to form an array: each structure has a different dynamic response, caused by small differences in the structures' geometry and working as a sort of mechanical band-pass filter (Fig. 11.20). The global dynamic response of the generator is the sum of all single contributions, resulting in widened bandwidth frequency content (Shahruz, 2006). Another strategy, related to the previous, is to use a multi-dof design for the energy harvester by introducing multiple proof masses connected to each other with elastic elements; the resulting system response is represented by a broad bandwidth originated by the combination of multiple resonance peaks, each of which is referred to a specific deformation mode. For instance, the capacitive generator introduced by De Pasquale and Wei (2010), composed of three proof masses, associates the first peak with the in-phase oscillation of masses and the other two peaks with out-of-phase oscillation modes (Fig. 11.21). Bi-stable structures are characterized by two stable positions: under the effect of environmental vibration, they repetitively move from one to the other equilibrium configuration. The main advantage of this kinematic strategy is that the movement of the structure can be induced by any excitation frequency, if the acceleration is high enough. As a consequence, bi-stable structures can be used to widen the

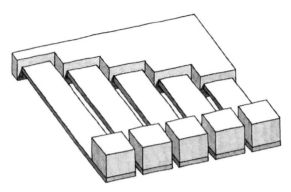

11.20 An array of structures with different response can be used to amplify the bandwidth of the generator; the global response includes the sum of all single contributions.

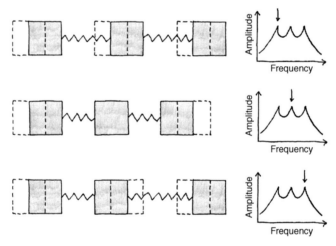

11.21 Working principle of the coupled three-dof generator introduced by De Pasquale and Wei (2010): the proof masses, associated to capacitive comb drives, are connected to each other and provide a multi-peaks response of the generator. The deformation modes reported on the left are referred to the correspondent resonances indicated on the right; the global effect is the widening of the generator bandwidth.

bandwidth of the generator, as well as to harvest power from very low level vibrations, or from highly random excitation sources. The device represented in Fig. 11.22 (Galchev *et al.*, 2010), for instance, has been designed to harvest power from the vibrations of a bridge; it exploits the bi-stable equilibrium of the inertial mass, which excites two membranes connected to lateral inductive generators when snapping from one configuration to the other.

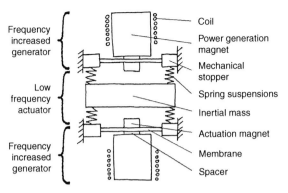

11.22 Example of energy harvester based on the bi-stable structures strategy for the bandwidth amplification. The central proof mass snaps between two stable positions at low frequency and attracts alternatively the two actuation magnets; when one actuation magnet is released, the elastic reaction of the supporting membrane excites the corresponding high-frequency dynamic system that includes the inductive generator. The total volume of the device is 68 cm^3 including the case.

The concept of stochastic resonance applied to bi-stable structures (McInnes *et al.*, 2008) is expected to improve the generated power; it consists in forcing the bi-stable structure with an input force with sinusoidal shape at variable frequency and amplitude depending on the vibration source. The generating structure, for instance a piezoelectric transducer, when excited by the sinusoidal forcing at its stochastic resonance, is induced to switch repetitively between the two stable configurations with significant increasing of travel length and improvement of output power. Although these strategies are theoretically very attractive, they actually belong to the category of active tuning and are affected by its typical drawbacks, in particular the hard practical implementation and the power consumption of control and actuation subsystems. Nevertheless, some real devices based on active tuning, supported by several different approaches, have demonstrated promising performance, such as the piezoelectric harvester by Ahmed Seddik *et al.* (2011), which uses a magnetic clamp to hold and release the seismic mass at every cycle. This allows increasing the oscillation amplitude when the excitation frequency is far from the resonance, making the device an example of active bandwidth amplification.

11.3.3 Magnetic levitation applied to suspensions

This section introduces magnetic levitation as a design approach for suspensions as an alternative to the traditional mechanical springs. The benefits of levitated systems lie in their dynamic response: heavy proof masses are not usable in small-scale harvesters to tune their resonance to low-frequency vibrations, which makes very low stiffness suspensions attractive.

Basic principles

Active magnetic levitation, applied for instance to maglev transports, is allowed by electromagnets; this approach, however, is not indicated for energy harvesting because it consumes power to work. Passive levitation, on the other hand, is powerless and offers several advantages when applied to small-scale generators. There are two main types of passive levitating suspensions, which are based respectively on the repulsive force between magnets and on the diamagnetic force.

The first suspension type is simply made by one or more permanent magnets attached to the frame of the generator and by a magnetic oscillating proof mass (usually represented by another permanent magnet); the polarity orientation of the magnets allows generating the repulsive force between the facing sides. The magnetic force between the magnets representing the suspension can be calculated with compact equations depending on the magnetic properties. For instance, in a suspension composed of one cylindrical fixed magnet and a proof mass with the same shape and having the vectors of magnetization lying on their common axis, the magnetic force is approximated as (Vokoun et al., 2009):

$$F(x) = \frac{\pi \mu_0}{4} M^2 r^4 \left[\frac{1}{x^2} + \frac{1}{(x+2t)^2} - \frac{2}{(x+t)^2} \right] \quad [11.41]$$

where x is the relative distance between magnets, μ_0 is the permeability of free space ($4\pi \cdot 10^{-7}$ N/A²), M is the magnetization, and r and t are the radius and the height of cylinders, respectively.

Diamagnetic levitation is the working principle of the second type of magnetic suspensions. Diamagnetic materials, when situated in a region interested by a magnetic field, can generate a weak field that opposes the external one. The design of the generator may involve a diamagnetic proof mass, connected to the desired transducer (inductive, capacitive, electret, etc.) and placed in a magnetic field. If the configuration is properly studied, the magnetic force acting on the diamagnetic mass may balance the gravitational force and produce levitation; the external magnetic field is generally obtained by some orientated permanent magnets. Unlike other materials, the magnetization of permanent magnets persists even if the external magnetic field intensity $\vec{H}$ is removed; their magnetization can be expressed as

$$\vec{M} = \chi_m \vec{H} \quad [11.42]$$

where χ_m is the magnetic susceptibility. The magnetic field $\vec{B}$ is related to $\vec{H}$ by the equation

$$\vec{H} = \frac{\vec{B}}{\mu_0} - \vec{M} \qquad [11.43]$$

Under the hypothesis of $\chi_m \ll 1$, which is valid for diamagnetic materials, the combination of Equations [11.42] and [11.43] gives the relations

$$\vec{M} \cong \chi_m \frac{\vec{B}}{\mu_0} \qquad [11.44]$$

$$\vec{B} = \mu_0\left(\vec{M} + \vec{H}\right) = \mu_0(1 + \chi_m)\vec{H} = \mu_0\mu_r\vec{H} = \mu\vec{H} \qquad [11.45]$$

where $\mu_r = (1 + \chi_m)$ is the relative magnetic permeability and $\mu = \mu_0\mu_r$ is the magnetic permeability.

Diamagnetic materials are characterized by very small negative susceptibility, which means μ_r is slightly less than 1. The other magnetic materials are divided into paramagnetic (with very small positive χ_m and μ_r slightly higher than 1), which are weakly attracted by magnetic fields, and ferromagnetic (with large positive χ_m and μ_r much larger than 1), which are strongly attracted by magnetic fields. In the case of a diamagnetic levitating proof mass, the magnetic force per unit volume acting on the mass can be calculated by the relation (Barrot, 2008)

$$\vec{f}_m \cong \frac{1}{2\mu_0}\chi_m\nabla\left(\vec{B}^2\right) \qquad [11.46]$$

Solutions for energy harvesters

Magnetic levitation has been successfully applied to inertial sensors to improve their sensitivity to ambient vibrations (Garmire et al., 2007). Krishnamoorthy et al. (2008) estimated the reduction of structural stiffness of the most sensitive MEMS accelerometers from 10 nN/nm to 10 pN/nm, which corresponds to a resolution improvement from 10^{-9} to 10^{-12} g.

The low stiffness of magnetic suspensions can strongly improve the performance of the energy harvesters addressed to low input frequencies. The configuration of inductive generators usually includes a suspended magnet that oscillates inside a coil under the effect of vibrations; by replacing the structural springs with magnetic suspensions, the dynamic response of the generator can be modified. The suspension in this case is simply obtained with one or more additional magnets orientated so as to repulse the proof mass, as represented in Fig. 11.23. The tuning of the stiffness can be simply

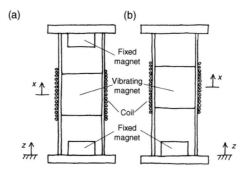

11.23 Layout of inductive generators based on magnetic levitation: symmetric (a) and asymmetric (b) configuration of suspensions.

obtained by varying the distance between magnets. The experimental FRF of a magnetic levitated suspension referred to the configuration of Fig. 11.23b is reported in Fig. 11.24 as an example.

A diamagnetic proof mass associated with capacitive comb drives is the basic structure of a levitated capacitive generator: Fig. 11.25 reports the schematics of this design solution. In this case, a layer of orientated permanent magnets is situated below the proof mass to provide the external magnetic field; the orientation of the magnets is crucial to obtain the configuration of the magnetic field suitable for levitation (Barrot, 2008). The fluctuating armatures of the capacitors can oscillate at very low input frequencies; the direction of oscillation is forced by the constraints introduced by the designer. Figure 11.26 suggests a possible layout for capacitive generators with diamagnetic suspension, and Fig. 11.27 shows alternative kinematic solutions. Figure 11.28 reports the measured FRF of some diamagnetic suspensions made with pyrolytic graphite and NdFeB permanent magnets moving in vertical direction as an example.

Static and dynamic behaviour

The static and dynamic behaviours of levitated generators are generally hard to predict and model because of the complexity of magnetic field distribution and the intrinsic non-linearity of the system. Analytic compact models are rarely applicable. The levitated generator in the configuration of Fig. 11.23a represents one case. Here the symmetric design of the suspension produces a stiffness equation described by an odd function; the governing equation of the system, expressed by

$$m\ddot{x} + c\dot{x} + kx(1 + \eta x^2) = f_0 \sin(\omega t) \qquad [11.47]$$

has the form of the Duffing oscillator (Duffing, 1918) and can be solved for the first harmonic component, getting an accurate approximation of the complete

Energy harvesters for powering wireless systems 379

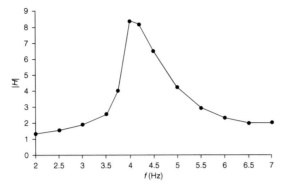

11.24 Experimental FRF of a levitated generator with cylindrical oscillating magnet (10.6 cm³ volume) in the asymmetric configuration of Fig. 11.23b under 2.5 mm imposed oscillation amplitude.

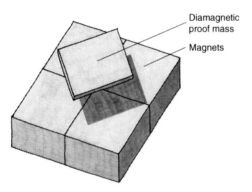

11.25 Schematics of levitating suspension composed by a ground layer with orientated permanent magnets and a levitating proof mass made with diamagnetic material.

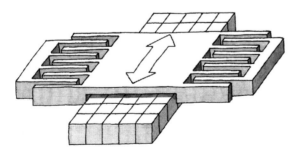

11.26 Possible layout of capacitive generators with diamagnetic suspensions: the diamagnetic proof mass connected to the comb electrodes levitates on a layer of orientated permanent magnets generating the supporting magnetic field.

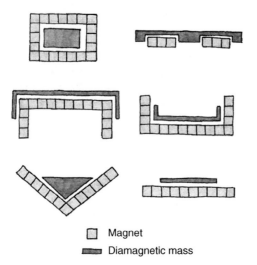

11.27 Design solutions for the layout of generators based on diamagnetic levitating suspensions.

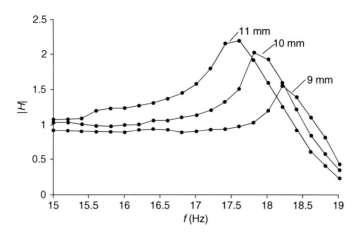

11.28 Experimental FRF of three diamagnetic levitated suspensions made with pyrolytic graphite and NdFeB permanent magnets; the magnetic ground dimensions are 40 × 40 × 3 mm³, the squared levitating masses have thickness 1 mm and the side length is reported near each curve.

solution (the mathematical calculation is reported by Mann and Sims, 2009). The expressions giving the oscillation amplitude and phase angle are

$$\left\{\left[1-(\omega/\omega_n)^2\right]x_0 + \frac{3}{4}\eta x_0^3\right\}^2 + 4x_0^2\zeta^2(\omega/\omega_n)^2 = \left(\frac{f_0}{k}\right)^2 \qquad [11.48]$$

$$\varphi = \arctan\left\{\frac{2\zeta(\omega/\omega_n)}{1-(\omega/\omega_n)^2 + \tfrac{3}{4}\eta x_0^2}\right\} \quad [11.49]$$

where η is the non-linearity coefficient. Previous expressions, when $\eta = 0$, coincide with those describing the behaviour of linear systems (i.e., Equations [11.21] and [11.22]). More generally, numerical models are needed to solve the static and dynamic governing equations of levitating systems; for instance, the response of the harvester (having the configuration of Fig. 11.23b) in the presence of the environmental random vibration input shown in Fig. 11.29 (dashed line) has been calculated with a multibody simulation using commercial software and reported in the same diagram (continuous line). Figure 11.30 also reports the fast Fourier transform (FFT) of the two signals.

A similar approach can be applied to calculating the static levitation curve (represented in Fig. 11.31) of the diamagnetic suspension referred to in the schematics of Fig. 11.25: in this case, a FEM model has been developed to estimate the vertical force acting on each portion of the discretized proof mass (De Pasquale *et al.*, 2011b), by following the meshing approach shown in Fig. 11.32.

11.3.4 Electric power management

The design of the electronic circuit for power management and the dimensioning of its components are crucial for the proper functioning of the energy harvester. The electronic management of the power harvested must

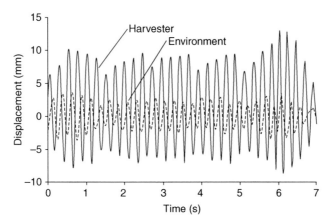

11.29 Simulated time response of a magnetic levitated energy harvester (continuous line) with the configuration of Fig. 11.23b under random excitation (dashed line); both curves have been calculated by a multibody simulation in Simpack 8.6 where the harvester has been placed on a freight train.

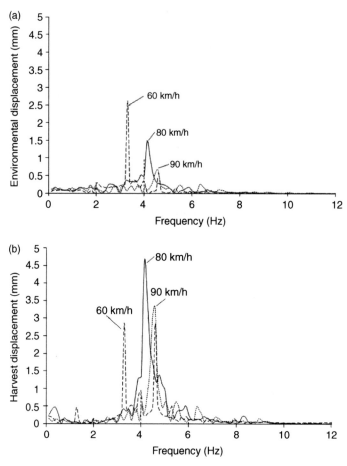

11.30 Multibody simulation of the harvester with asymmetric magnetic suspension (Fig. 11.23b) subjected to a random excitation generated by a freight train travelling at variable velocities: FFT of the environment vibration (a) and of the harvester seismic mass (b).

satisfy some important functions: to control the load impedance, to provide the storage of energy, and to regulate the output voltage.

To achieve the maximum power transfer from the source (i.e., the harvester) to the load, their impedances should be coincident; usually this condition is not verified, and in some applications the impedance of the load can vary depending on the operative conditions. Consequently, an electronic interface connected to the harvester is usually introduced, with the scope to control and match the impedances. The energy storage is represented by one or more batteries, supplied by the generator at a certain voltage that is imposed by the same electronic interface. The function of the battery is

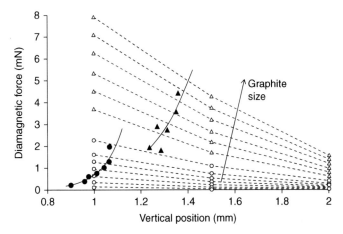

11.31 Numerical estimation (dashed lines) and experimental measurements (black marks) of the diamagnetic force acting on the graphite proof mass in the configuration of Fig. 11.25. The reported curves are referred to increasing sizes of the diamagnetic mass (from 3 to 10 mm) and thicknesses of the magnetic ground (3 mm ○ and 6 mm △).

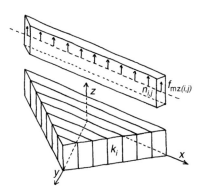

11.32 Finite element model of the levitated suspension for the prediction of the diamagnetic force acting on the proof mass in presence of magnetic field.

to provide a constant power to the load, even if the generation rate of the harvester is not constant, which is a very frequent condition. It is possible to supply the load continuously only if the average power consumed (losses included) in a time interval is lower than the average generated power. The voltage and current needed to supply the load are generally different from the battery output, leading to the introduction of a voltage regulator circuit or component. Figure 11.33 shows the composition of the electric power management for a generic harvester.

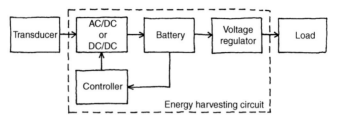

11.33 General composition of the electric power management components for energy harvesters.

The single parts of the configuration described are strongly variable, depending on the typology of transducer and on the design strategy; a detailed description of these variants is beyond the scope of this work, and the reader is referred to the literature for additional information (Ho *et al.*, 2010; Mitcheson and Toh, 2010).

11.4 Other typologies of energy harvesters

After introducing design and modelling strategies of kinetic energy harvesters, this section provides some information about the other most important typologies of energy harvesters.

11.4.1 Kinetic rotating generators

In this type of kinetic harvester the motion of the proof mass is rotational instead of translational. Figure 11.34a shows a very common shape for the mass: thanks to its eccentricity, the mass rotation can be induced either by a rotating or a translating excitation source from the environment. The power conversion is usually electromagnetic: the rotating mass is coupled to a magnetic polar rotor that induces the electric current in a wired coil; some applications include one or more gear stages to increase the rotating velocity of the magnets. Rotating generators are applicable to linear vibration sources with very large oscillation amplitudes, as well as to continuous or alternate rotating environments. The application of elastic and dissipative elements to the rotating mass (Fig. 11.34b) modifies the behaviour of the rotating generator that becomes a resonating system; this architecture is preferred to improve the output power in some excitation conditions. Yeatman (2008) estimates the output power of rotating generators with proof mass m, proof mass radius r, and distance from the axis to the centre of mass r_c in different operative conditions; the maximum power of non-resonant generators, in the case of harmonic rotation input with amplitude Ω_0 and angular frequency ω, is

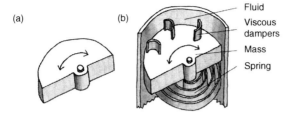

11.34 Typical design solution of kinetic rotating generators. The eccentric shape of the mass allows converting translating or rotating vibrations of the environment to rotation of the mass (a); the output power is generally improved by adjusting the damping and stiffness of the rotating system by dissipative and elastic elements (b).

$$P_{max} = \frac{m\omega^3 \Omega_0^2 r^2}{16} \qquad [11.50]$$

whereas in the case of linear oscillation input with amplitude z_0, it is

$$P_{max} \cong \frac{1}{2} m\omega^3 z_0 r_c \qquad [11.51]$$

For resonant generators, the maximum power is achievable for $c_e = c_m$ (i.e., electric and mechanical damping, respectively) and is given by

$$P_{max} = \frac{I^2 \omega^4 \Omega_0^2}{8 c_m} \qquad [11.52]$$

where $I = mr^2/4$ is the moment of inertia for the half disc. Another example of output power analytic expression for rotating harvesters is reported in Equation [11.18] with reference to electret generators.

Another category of harvesters can be identified as gyroscopic generators. In this case, a rotating proof mass is subjected to the environmental oscillation around an axis orthogonal to its rotation axis; due to the gyroscopic effect, the balance torque induced on the mass is used as a power source. The drawbacks of this solution are related to the complicated architecture, low mechanical quality factor, and above all the input power needed to keep the mass rotation. A similar working principle characterizes the vibrating MEMS gyroscopes, where two planar dof are assigned to the proof mass that oscillates in the driving direction and in the orthogonal one; when an environmental oscillation around the out-of-plane direction takes place, the two motions couple. The strategy described, which is well known for gyroscopic microsensors, may experience future developments in the energy harvesting field. More details on rotating generators and their analytic modelling can be found in the literature (Yeatman, 2008).

11.4.2 Photovoltaic cells

Photovoltaic (or solar) cells are based on semiconductor technology and allow extraction of power from light radiation. They are currently used outdoors and indoors for powering sensor nodes, sensor networks, low-power electronics, and traffic regulators, and for industrial and domestic power generation. The power density available from solar radiation is very large compared with other sources, making this technology very attractive for the future; at present, the main limitations of solar cells are the dimension of surface area needed, the low reliability in harsh environments, and the vulnerability to light intensity variability. Solar cells are obtained by combining an *n-type* semiconductor (doped with donor atoms, such as phosphorus) and a *p-type* semiconductor (doped with acceptor impurities, such as boron) and creating a so-called *p–n junction* between them. In the region close to the junction, defined as the *depletion region*, when the photons are absorbed by the semiconductors, the electrons contained in the n-type material diffuse into the p-type material, determining, respectively, positive and negative charged regions. The photogenerated electrons can produce the flow of a current if a load is connected to the cell, as represented in the schematics of Fig. 11.35.

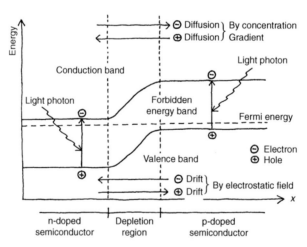

11.35 Band diagram of a photovoltaic cell p–n junction where conduction band, valence band, and forbidden energy band are indicated. Arrows indicate the directions of electrons/holes diffusion (driven by concentration gradient) and electrons/holes drift (driven by electrostatic field).

The output power estimation of a photovoltaic cell placed at a particular site is very complicated due to the strong variability of the natural light source. The light emitted by the sun's surface comes to the earth after a journey through space and the atmosphere, which strongly reduces its power density. Depending on the angle of incidence with the earth's surface, the travel length of light inside the air varies, together with its intensity and spectral distribution due to light scattering; the angle of incidence is influenced by the latitude and by the sun's position in the sky during the day. The presence of clouds increases light diffusion and causes a strong decay of cell performance. The power density of light in the outer atmosphere is referred to the AM0 standard spectrum (1.3661 kW/m^2); for the earth's surface the standard AM1.5 is used (1 kW/m^2). However, the actual values are often fluctuating over time and may be different from the standards; thus, the power estimation of a photovoltaic plant is usually conducted with simulations based on historical data on atmospheric and meteorological conditions for a specific site. For indoor applications with solar light through windows, the same variability of conditions is present, and the average intensity is much lower than outside; in the case of radiation from artificial sources (incandescent bulbs, halogen lamps, fluorescent tubes), the light characteristics are more stable and the cell fabrication can be orientated to maximize the power in the operative conditions. The order of magnitude of the indoor power density of light is 0.005 kW/m^2. From a comparison of solar cell performance based on different technologies from different suppliers, an outdoor efficiency range of 4.3–15.7% and an indoor efficiency range of 3.7–10.5% have been measured (Bagnall and Boden, 2010).

The basic structure of commercial solar cells is composed of several layers (Fig. 11.36): cover glass, front metal contacts, antireflective coating, n-type semiconductor, p-type semiconductor, back metal contact, and glass substrate. Many different solutions have been introduced to improve the efficiency of light conversion starting from the described layout: multijunction cells, layers texturing, etc. Single cells are generally connected in a module

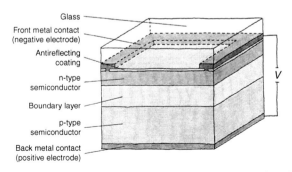

11.36 Basic structure of commercial photovoltaic cells.

to generate higher power levels. Photovoltaic cell properties, loss estimation, experimental measurements, and manufacturing technologies are reported in greater detail in Bagnall and Boden (2010) and Penella-Lopez and Gasulla-Forner (2011).

11.4.3 Radio frequency identification systems

Radio frequency identification systems (RFIDs) are an example of consolidated devices that exploit the RF input signal to generate power and manage information. RF energy harvesters are at a very early stage of development; the basic idea is to convert the energy contained in environmental RF sources (mobile telephony, wireless networks, etc.) to supply small devices or batteries. The estimated power output is influenced by the power density of the RF signal, the characteristics of its polarization and orientation, and, of course, by the distance between the RF source and the harvester.

Figure 11.37 describes the basic layout of RF harvesters. After the antenna, it includes the impedance regulation block that is needed to match the circuit impedance to that of the antenna to maximize the power transmitted; the impedance matching is usually obtained by coils, capacitors in different circuit configurations as transformers, shunt inductors, or LC networks. The filter (eventually followed by another impedance matching block) is used to prevent the high-frequency noise generated by the next rectifier, which comes back to the antenna. Finally, there is the voltage rectifier, which can be represented by a single diode (defining, coupled with the antenna, the so-called rectenna), by a diodes bridge, or by a voltage rectifier multiplier (also called a Dickson charge pump). More information on RF energy harvesters and on the preliminary results of experimental characterizations are reported in the literature (Kocer and Flynn, 2006; Penella-Lopez and Gasulla-Forner, 2011; Singh *et al.*, 2004).

11.4.4 Thermoelectric generators

The interaction between heat and electricity in solids can be used to generate power from temperature gradients by means of thermoelectric effects. The Seebeck effect is at the basis of generators, and it can be explained by

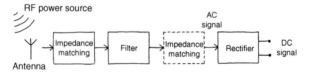

11.37 Schematics of RF harvesters basic layout.

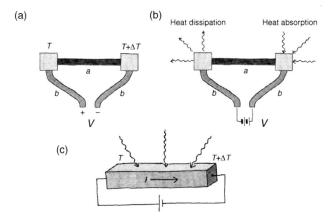

11.38 Thermoelectric effects in solid materials: (a) Seebeck effect, (b) Peltier effect, and (c) Thompson effect.

a circuit made of two different materials (*a* and *b*): when the temperature difference ΔT is applied between the junctions, a voltage difference is generated, as shown in Fig. 11.38a. The output voltage is determined by the relative Seebeck coefficient (α_{ab}) for the two materials:

$$V = \alpha_{ab}\Delta T \qquad [11.53]$$

The highest values of α_{ab} are given by semiconductor materials, in the order of mV/K. Although not directly responsible for power generation, other thermoelectric effects, namely, the Peltier effect and the Thomson effect, are involved in the conversion of heat into electricity. The first is associated with circuits made of two different materials where a voltage difference is applied (Fig. 11.38b); due to the motion of charges, one junction produces heat dissipation and the other heat absorption. The total heat flow between the junctions in the unit of time is

$$\dot{Q} = \pi_{ab} i \qquad [11.54]$$

where i is the electric current passing in the circuit and π_{ab} is the Peltier coefficient. This effect is exploited in heat generators and refrigerators. The Thompson effect is associated with a single material subjected to the temperature difference ΔT and the electric current i, as represented in Fig. 11.38c. In this case, the heat absorbed, or dissipated, by the material is given by

$$\dot{Q} = \beta i \Delta T \qquad [11.55]$$

where β is called the Thompson coefficient.

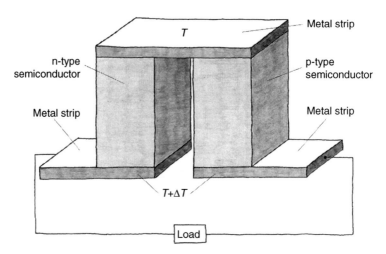

11.39 Basic module of thermoelectric harvesting devices; several modules are connected in series to form the generator.

Although only the Seebeck effect is directly related to power generation and thermoelectric energy harvesting, all the effects are present simultaneously in thermoelectric devices, according to the Kelvin relationships among the three coefficients:

$$\pi_{ab} = \alpha_{ab} T \quad [11.56]$$

$$\frac{d\alpha_{ab}}{dT} = \frac{\beta_a - \beta_b}{T} \quad [11.57]$$

The structure of thermoelectric generators is composed of many modules connected in series; each module is formed by two semiconductor materials (p-type and n-type) connected by a metal strip made of aluminium or copper, as represented in Fig. 11.39. By neglecting the resistance of the metal strip, the internal resistance R is only determined by the semiconductor materials, and, according to the model of Ioffe (1957), the output voltage and current are

$$V = \alpha \Delta T \frac{R_{load}}{R + R_{load}} \quad [11.58]$$

$$i = \frac{\alpha \Delta T}{R + R_{load}} \quad [11.59]$$

where α is the Seebeck coefficient for the two semiconductors and R_{load} is the load resistance. The electrical output power is

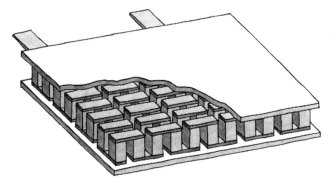

11.40 Thermoelectric generator composed of a matrix of semiconductor modules connected electrically in series by metal strips and thermally in parallel by two ceramic plates.

$$P = \frac{R_{load}}{(R+R_{load})^2}(\alpha\Delta T)^2 \qquad [11.60]$$

and the maximum power of the single block, given by the condition $R = R_{load}$, is

$$P_{max} = \frac{(\alpha\Delta T)^2}{4R} \qquad [11.61]$$

The complete generator is composed of many modules in one single package. The modules are connected electrically in series and thermally in parallel by means of two connecting layers on the opposite sides, as represented in Fig. 11.40. The output power of the device has been formulated (Min, 2006) with a more accurate model that includes the resistances of electric and thermal connections:

$$P_{max} = \frac{AN(\alpha\Delta T)^2}{2\rho(n+l)(1+2rl_c/l)^2} \qquad [11.62]$$

where N is the number of modules in the generator, A and l are the cross-section and length of semiconductor elements, respectively, l_c is the thickness of connecting layers (metal strip and ceramic plate), and $n = 2\rho_c/\rho$, $r = \lambda/\lambda_c$ are the electric and thermal contact parameters, respectively (ρ is the electric resistivity, ρ_c is the electric contact resistivity, λ is the thermal conductivity, and λ_c is the thermal contact conductivity). Typical values of contact parameters are $n \cong 0.1$ mm and $r \cong 0.2$. More information and details on thermoelectric energy harvesters can be found by the reader in the literature (Nolas et al., 2010; Rowe, 1995).

11.5 Conclusion

The purpose of this chapter is to provide the reader with the fundamental principles of energy harvesting strategies and techniques; the contents were organized following an approach of increasing complexity and detail level, to provide some basic tool to the designer. The strategies mentioned include compact analytic calculations and numerical models to solve the static and dynamic governing equations, as well as smart solutions for the improvement of the response, of performance, and of the output power. The critical review of the best in energy harvesting solutions conceived up to now supports the theoretical considerations and may provide useful starting points for new layouts or alternative application fields.

The future development of the energy harvesting discipline is strictly connected to the need to generate electricity somewhere, instead of bringing it by cables or extracting it from a battery. Recently, a lot of potential benefits have been demonstrated by the application of generators to novel fields where this possibility was never investigated. The strongest effort in the development of energy harvesting is probably given by sensorization, as well as by the constant improvement of the sensors' performance in terms of low power consumption and long expected lifetime; the appearance of micrometric devices able to measure environmental parameters is pushing the research to the development of distributed power sources characterized by low intensity and high availability. These properties fit well with the peculiarities of energy harvesting devices that can produce electricity from useless energy, otherwise lost, and store it in a small battery. New technological improvements in the fabrication processes of microdevices, advanced tuning and control strategies, and additional contributions coming from the expertise in more and more application fields will probably lead to an increasing complexity of energy harvesters, accompanied with the fast improvement of their performance in the near future.

11.6 References

AdaptivEnergy, Joule Thief Series (2009), Available from: www.adaptivenergy.com.

Ahmed Seddik, B., Despesse, G., and Defay, E. (2011), 'Increased bandwidth system for mechanical energy harvesting', *Proc. of NSTI Nanotech*, Boston, USA, 1, 751–754.

Arakawa, Y., Suzuki, Y., and Kasagi, N. (2004), 'Micro seismic power generator using electret polymer film', *Proc. of PowerMEMS*, Kyoto, Japan, 187–190.

Bagnall, D. M. and Boden, S.A. (2010), 'Photovoltaic energy harvesting', in Beeby S and White N, *Energy harvesting for autonomous systems*, Boston, Artech House, 45–90.

Barrot, F. (2008), 'Acceleration and inclination sensors based on magnetic levitation. Application in the particular case of structural health monitoring in civil engineering', *PhD Dissertation*, EPFL, Lausanne, Switzerland.

Beeby, S. and White, N. (2010), 'Kinetic energy harvesting', in Beeby S and White N, *Energy harvesting for autonomous systems*, Boston, Artech House, 91–134.

Beeby, S.P., Torah, R.N., Tudor, M.J., Glynne-Jones, P., O'Donnell, T., Saha, C.R., and Roy, S. (2007) 'A micro electromagnetic generator for vibration energy harvesting', *J Micromech Microeng*, **17**, 1257–1265.

Boland, J., Chao, C., Suzuki, Y., and Tai, Y.C. (2003), 'Micro electret power generator', *Proc. of the 16th IEEE Int. Conf. on Micro Electro Mechanical Systems (MEMS)*, Kyoto, Japan, 538–541.

Challa, V.R., Prasad, M.G., Shi, Y., and Fisher, F.T. (2008), 'A vibration energy harvesting device with bidirectional resonance frequency tunability', *Smart Mater Struct*, **17**, 015035.

Cheng, S. and Arnold, D.P. (2010), 'A study of a multi-pole magnetic generator for low-frequency vibrational energy harvesting', *J Micromech Microeng*, **20**, 025015.

Ching, N.N., Wong, H.Y., Li, W.J., Leong, P.H., and Wen, Z. (2002), 'A laser-micromachined multi-modal resonating power transducer for wireless sensing systems', *Sensor Actuator A-Phys*, **97–98**, 685–690.

Chiu, Y. and Tseng, V.F. (2008), 'A capacitive vibration-to-electricity energy converter with integrated mechanical switches', *J Micromech Microeng*, **18**, 104004.

Collins, J.A. (1993), *Failure of materials in mechanical design, analysis, prediction, prevention*, New York, Wiley-Interscience.

De Pasquale, G., Brusa, E., and Somà, A. (2009), 'Capacitive vibration energy harvesting with resonance tuning', *Proc. of Design, Test, Integration and Packaging of MEMS and MOEMS*, Rome, Italy, 280–285.

De Pasquale, G., Iamoni, S., and Somà, A. (2011b), 'Modeling and experimental validation of levitating systems for energy harvesting applications', *Proc. of Design, Test, Integration and Packaging of MEMS and MOEMS*, Aix-en-Provence, France, 97–102.

De Pasquale, G. and Somà, A. (2011), 'MEMS mechanical fatigue: effect of mean stress on gold microbeams', *J Microelectromech S*, **20**, 1054–1063.

De Pasquale, G. and Somà A. (2009), 'Numerical and experimental validation of out-of-plane resonance closed formulas for MEMS suspended plates with square holes', *Microsyst Technol*, **15**, 391–400.

De Pasquale, G., Somà, A., and Fraccarollo, F. (2011a), 'Piezoelectric energy harvesting for autonomous sensors network on safety-improved railway vehicles', *Proc IME C J Mech Eng Sci*, **in press**.

De Pasquale, G., Veijola, T., and Somà, A. (2010), 'Energy dissipation associated with material damping on vibrating MEMS components', *Proc. of Design, Test, Integration and Packaging of MEMS and MOEMS*, Seville, Spain, 99–104.

De Pasquale, G. and Wei, M. (2010), 'Nickel MEMS energy harvester for the self-powering of vehicular sensing systems', *Rom J Inf Sci Tech*, **13**, 3–21.

De Pasquale, G., Zampieri, N., and Somà. A. (2011c), 'Design, simulation and testing of energy harvesters with magnetic suspensions for the conversion of freight trains vibrations into electricity', sub. to *J Comput Nonlin Dyn*.

Despesse, G., Jager, T., Chaillout, J.J., Leger, J.M., and Basrour, S. (2005), 'Design and fabrication of a new energy system for vibration energy harvesting', *Res Microelectron Electron*, **1**, 225–228.

Duffing, G. (1918) *Erzwungene Schwingungen bei veränderlicher Eigenfrequenz und ihre technische Bedeutung*, Braunschweig, Verlag Vieweg.

Eguchi, M. (1925), 'On the permanent electret', *Philos Mag*, **49**, 178.
Elfrink, R., Kamel, T.M., Goedbloed, M., Matova, S., Hohlfeld, D., van Andel, Y., and van Schaijk, R. (2009), 'Vibration energy harvesting with aluminum nitride-based piezoelectric device', *J Micromech Microeng*, **19**, 094005.
Ferro Solutions, VEH-460 (2011), Available from: www.ferrosi.com.
Galchev, T., McCullagh, J., Peterson, R.L., and Najafi, K. (2010), 'A vibration harvesting system for bridge health monitoring applications', *Proc. of PowerMEMS*, Leuven, Belgium, 179–182.
Garmire, D., Choo, H., Kant, R., Govindjee, S., Sequin, C.H., Muller, R.S., and Demmel, J. (2007), 'Diamagnetically levitated MEMS accelerometers', *Proc. of Int. Conf. on Solid-State Sensors, Actuators and Microsystems*, Lyon, France, 1203–1206.
Gieras, J.F., Oh, J.H., Huzmezan, M., and Sane, H.S. (2007). *Electromechanical energy harvesting system*. WO2007070022(A2), WO2007070022(A3).
Glynne-Jones, P. (2001), 'Vibration powered generators for self-powered microsystems', *PhD Dissertation*, Univ. of Southampton, UK.
Glynne-Jones, P., Beeby, S.P., and White, N.M. (2001), 'Towards a piezoelectric vibration powered microgenerator', *IEE Proc Sci Meas Technol*, **148**, 68–72.
El-Hami, M., Glynne-Jones, P., White, N.M., Hill, M., Beeby, S., James, E., Brown, A.D., and Ross, J.N. (2001), 'Design and fabrication of a new vibration-based electromechanical power generator', *Sensor Actuator A-Phys*, **92**, 335–342.
Heaviside, O. (1892) *Electrical papers*, London, Macmillan Publishers.
Ho, C.C., Evans, J.W., and Wright, P.K. (2010), 'Energy storage', in Beeby S and White N, *Energy harvesting for autonomous systems*, Boston, Artech House, 211–251.
Hoffmann, D., Folkmer, B., and Manoli, Y. (2009), 'Fabrication, characterization and modelling of electrostatic micro-generators', *J Micromech Microeng*, **19**, 094001.
Hong, Y.K. and Moon, K.S. (2005), 'Single crystal piezoelectric transducers to harvest vibration energy', *Proc. of SPIE*, **6048**, 60480E-1.
IEEE (1997), 'IEEE standard on piezoelectricity', *ANSI/IEEE Standard*, 176.
Ikeda, T. (1990), *Fundamentals of piezoelectricity*, New York, Oxford University Press.
Ioffe, A.F. (1957), *Semiconductor thermoelements and thermoelectric cooling*, London, Infosearch.
Jaffe, H. and Berlincourt, D.A. (1965), 'Piezoelectric Transducer Materials', *Proc. of the IEEE*, **53**, 1372–1386.
Jeon, Y.B., Sood, R., Jeong, J.H., and Kim, S.G. (2005), 'MEMS power generator with transverse mode thin film PZT', *Sensor Actuator A-Phys*, **122**, 16–22.
Krishnamoorthy, U., Olssson III, R.H., Bogart, G.R., Baker, M.S., Carr, D.W., Swiler, T.P., and Clews, P.J. (2008), 'In-plane MEMS-based nano-g accelerometers with sub-wavelength optical resonant sensor', *Sensor Actuator A-Phys*, **145–146**, 283–290.
Kocer, F. and Flynn, M.P. (2006), 'An RF-powered, wireless CMOS temperature sensor', *IEEE Sens J*, **6**, 557–564.
Leland, E.S. and Wright, P.K. (2006), 'Resonance tuning of piezoelectric vibration energy scavenging generators using compressive axial preload', *Smart Mater Struct*, **15**, 1413–1420.
Lo, H.W. and Tai, Y.C. (2008), 'Parylene-based electret power generators', *J Micromech Microeng*, **18**, 104006.

Ma, W., Wong, M., and Rufer, L. (2005), 'Dynamic simulation of an electrostatic power micro-generator', *Proc. of Design, Test, Integration and Packaging of MEMS and MOEMS*, Montreux, Switzerland, 380–385.

Mann, B.P. and Sims, N.D. (2009), 'Energy harvesting from the nonlinear oscillations of magnetic levitation', *J Sound Vib*, **319**, 515–530.

Marzencki, M., Ammar, Y., and Basrour, S. (2008), 'Integrated power harvesting system including a MEMS generator and a power management circuit', *Sensor Actuator A-Phys*, **145–146**, 363–370.

Masaki, T., Sakurai, K., Yokoyama, T., Ikuta, M., Doi, M., Seki, T., and Oba, M. (2010), 'Power output enhancement of vibration-driven electret generator using concave electrodes', *Proc. of PowerMEMS*, Leuven, Belgium, 57–60.

McInnes, C.R., Gorman, D.G., and Cartmell, M.P. (2008), 'Enhanced vibrational energy harvesting using nonlinear stochastic resonance', *J saSound Vib*, **318**, 655–662.

Meninger, S., Mur-Miranda, J., Amirtharajah R., Chandrakasan, A.P., and Lang, J.H. (2001), 'Vibration-to-electric energy conversion', *IEEE Trans Very Large Scale Integration Syst*, **9**, 64–76.

Mide Technology Corporation, PEH Series (2011), Available from: www.mide.com.

Min, G. (2006), 'TE module design theories', in Rowe D.M. (ed.), *CRC handbook of thermoelectrics: micro to nano*, Boca Raton, CRC Press, 11.1–11.15.

Mitcheson, P.D. and Toh, T.T. (2010), 'Power management electronics', in Beeby S and White N, *Energy harvesting for autonomous systems*, Boston, Artech House, 159–209.

Mohite, S.S., Sonti, V.R., and Pratap, R. (2008), 'A compact squeeze-film model including inertia, compressibility, and rarefaction effects for perforated 3-D MEMS structures', *J Microelectromech S*, **17**, 709–723.

Muhlstein, C.L., Brown, S.B., and Ritchie, R.O. (2001), 'High-cycle fatigue of single-crystal silicon thin films', *J Microelectromech S*, **10**, 593–600.

NASA (1998), 'Properties of PZT-based piezoelectric ceramics between –150 and 250°C', *NASA/CR-1998–208708*, 7.

Nolas, G.S., Sharp, J., and Goldsmid H.J. (2010), *Termo-electrics. Basic principles and new materials developments*, Berlin, Springer.

Penella-Lopez, M.T. and Gasulla-Forner, M. (2011), *Powering autonomous sensors. An integral approach with focus on solar and RF energy harvesting*, Dordrecht, Springer.

Pérez-Rodriguez, A., Serre, C., Fondevilla, N., Morante, J.R., Montserrat, J., and Esteve, J. (2005), 'Electromagnetic inertial generator for vibrational energy scavenging compatible with Si Technology', *Proc. of PowerMEMS*, Tokyo, Japan, 57–60.

Perpetuum Ltd, PMG Series (2010), Available from: www.perpetuum.com.

Priya, S. and Inman, D.J. (2008), *Energy harvesting technologies*, New York, Springer.

Read, D.T. (1998), 'Tension-tension fatigue of copper thin films', *Int J Fatigue*, **20**, 203–209.

Roundy, S. and Wright, P.K. (2004), 'A piezoelectric vibration based generator for wireless electronics', *Smart Mater Struct*, **13**, 1131–1142.

Roundy, S., Wright, P.K., and Rabaey, J.M. (2003a), *Energy Scavenging for Wireless Sensor Networks*, Boston, Kluwer Academic Publishers.

Roundy, S., Wrigth, P.K., and Rabaey, J.M. (2003b), 'A study of low level vibrations as a power source for wireless sensor nodes', *Comput Commun*, **26**, 1131–1144.

Rowe, D.M. (1995), *CRC Handbook of thermoelectric*, Boca Raton, CRC Press.

Saha, C.R., O'Donnell, T., Loder, H., Beeby, S., and Tudor, J. (2006), 'Optimization of an electromagnetic energy harvesting device', *IEEE Trans Magn*, **42**, 3509–3511.

Saha, C.R., O'Donnell, T., Wang, N., and McCloskey, P. (2008), 'Electromagnetic generator for harvesting energy from human motion', *Sensor Actuator A-Phys*, **147**, 248–253.

Sakakibara, T., Izu, H., Kura, T., Shinohara, W., Iwata, H., Kiyama, S., and Tsuda, S. (1994), 'Development of high-voltage photovoltaic micro-devices for an energy supply to micromachines', *Proc. of IEEE 5th Int. Symp. on Micro Machine and Human Science*, Nagoya, Japan, 71–76.

Sakane, Y., Suzuki, Y., and Kasagi, N. (2008), 'The development of a high-performance perfluorinated polymer electret and its application to micro power generation', *J Micromech Microeng*, **18**, 104011.

Sandberg, R., Mølhave, K., Boisen, A., and Svendsen, W. (2008), 'Effect of gold coating on the Q-factor of a resonant cantilever', *J Micromech Microeng*, **15**, 2249–2253.

Shahruz, S.M. (2006), 'Design of mechanical band-pass filters for energy scavenging', *J Sound Vib*, **292**, 987–998.

Singh, P., Xiquan, W., LaFollette, R., and Reisner, D. (2004), 'RF-recharged micro battery for powering miniature sensors', *Proc. of IEEE Sensors*, Vienna, Austria, 1, 349–352.

Somà, A. and De Pasquale, G. (2009), 'MEMS mechanical fatigue: experimental results on gold microbeams', *J Microelectromech S*, **18**, 828–835.

Starner, T. (1996), 'Human-powered wearable computing', *IBM Syst J*, **35**, 618–629.

Stephen, N.G. (2006), 'On energy harvesting from ambient vibration', *J Sound Vib*, **293**, 409–425.

Suzuki, Y. (2011), 'Recent progress in MEMS electret generator for energy harvesting', *IEEJ T Electr Electr*, **6**, 101–111.

Suzuki, Y., Miki, D., and Edamoto, M. (2010), 'A MEMS electret generator with electrostatic levitation for vibration-driven energy harvesting applications', *J Micromech Microeng*, **20**, 104002.

Takamatsu, T. (1991), 'Life time of thermal electrets of carnauba wax, esters, fatty acids and alcohols', *Proc. of 7th Int. Symp. of Electrets*, Berlin, Germany, 106–110.

Timoshenko, S. and Goodier, J.N. (1951), *Theory of elasticity*, 2nd Edition, New York, McGrow-Hill Book Company.

Vokoun, D., Beleggia, M., Heller, L., and Sittner, P. (2009), 'Magnetostatic interactions and forces between cylindrical permanent magnets', *J Magn Magn Mater*, **321**, 3758–3763.

Williams, C.B., Shearwood, C., Harradine M.A., Mellor, P.H., Birch, T.S., and Yates, R.B. (2001), 'Development of an electromagnetic micro-generator', *IEE P-Circ Dev Syst*, **148**, 337–342.

Wu, W.J., Chen, Y.Y., Lee, B.S., He, J.J., and Peng, Y.T. (2006), 'Tunable resonant frequency power harvesting device', *Proc. of SPIE*, **6169**, 55–62.

Wu, X., Lin, J., Kato, S., Zhang, K., Ren, T., and Liu, L. (2008), 'A frequency adjustable vibration energy harvester', *Proc. of PowerMEMS and MicroEMS*, Sendai, Japan, 245–248.

Yeatman, E.M. (2008), 'Energy harvesting from motion using rotating and gyroscopic proof masses', *Proc IME C J Mech Eng Sci*, **222**, 27–36.

Yoneoka, S., Yu, Q.Q., Wang, S., Messana, M.W., Graham, A.B., Salvia, J., Bongsang, K., Melamud, R., Bahl, G., and Kenny, T.W. (2010), 'High-cyclic fatigue experiments of single crystal silicon in an oxygen-free environment', *Proc. of IEEE Micro Electro Mechanical Systems Int. Conf.*, Wanchai, Hong Kong, 224–227.

Zhu, D., Tudor, M.J., and Beeby, S.P. (2010), 'Strategies for increasing the operating frequency range of vibration energy harvesters: a review', *Meas Sci Technol*, **21**, 022001.

11.7 Appendix: list of symbols

A	coil area
	electrodes area
	semiconductor module cross-section
A_{eff}	effective plate area
a	acceleration
	plate length
B	magnetic field
b	plate width
C	electric capacitance
C_{coil}	coil capacitance
C_{load}	load capacitance
C_{max}	maximum capacitance
C_{min}	minimum capacitance
c	damping coefficient
	suspension length
c_e	electric damping coefficient
	electromagnetic damping coefficient
c_m	mechanical damping coefficient
c_{nl}	non-linear damping coefficient
D	charge density
d	piezoelectric charge constant (or strain coefficient)
	gap among fingers
	suspension width
E	Young's module
$\overline{E}$	electric field
E_n	energy
e	hole side
F	force
f	frequency
	holes interspace
	tuning force
f_0	force amplitude

f_m	magnetic force per unit volume
g	acceleration of gravity
	piezoelectric voltage constant
	gap thickness
k	stiffness
	electro-mechanical coupling coefficient
k_{nl}	non-linear stiffness
H	FRF
	magnetic field intensity
$\lvert H \rvert_{-3dB}$	half power amplitude
h	thickness
I	moment of inertia
i	electric current
L_{coil}	coil inductance
l	coil length
	fingers length
	semiconductor module length
l_c	connecting layers thickness
M	plate mass
	magnetization
m	mass
	number of holes rows
m_{nl}	non-linear mass
N	number of turns
	number of thermoelectric modules
N_g	number of gaps among fingers
n	number of poles
	number of holes columns
	electric contact parameter
n_{dof}	number of degrees of freedom
P	output power
P_{max}	maximum output power
Q	quality factor
	electric charge density
	heat
R	electric resistance
R_{coil}	coil resistance
R_{load}	load resistance
$R_{load,opt}$	optimum load resistance
r	magnet radius
	proof mass radius
	thermal contact parameter
r_c	centre mass to axis distance

T_c	Curie temperature
t	piezo layer thickness
	fingers thickness
	electret thickness
	time
	magnet height
V	electric voltage
V_0	initial voltage
V_{max}	maximum voltage
V_{min}	minimum voltage
X	relative displacement Fourier transform
x	relative displacement
	transducer displacement
x_0	relative displacement amplitude
Z	absolute displacement Fourier transform
z	absolute displacement
z_0	absolute displacement amplitude
α	piezoelectric connection parameter
	Rayleigh damping coefficient
α_{ab}	Seebeck coefficient
β	Rayleigh damping coefficient
	Newmark integration parameter
	Thompson coefficient
ΔT	temperature difference
Δt	integration time interval
$\Delta \omega_{-3dB}$	half power bandwidth
ε	strain
ε_0	permittivity of free space
ε_{air}	permittivity of air
$\varepsilon_{electret}$	electret permittivity
ε_p	piezoelectric permittivity (or dielectric constant)
ζ	damping ratio
ζ_e	electric damping ratio
ζ_m	mechanical parasitic damping ratio
η	Duffing oscillator non-linearity
λ	kinematic parameter
	thermal conductivity
λ_c	thermal contact conductivity
μ_0	magnetic permeability of free space
μ_r	relative magnetic permeability
π_{ab}	Peltier coefficient
ρ	density
	electric resistivity

ρ_c	electric contact resistivity
σ	stress
σ_L	fatigue limit
σ_{UTS}	ultimate tensile strength
σ_y	yield strength
ϕ	phase angle
φ	magnetic flux
χ_m	magnetic susceptibility
ψ	modal shape
Ω_0	rotation amplitude
ω	angular frequency
ω_{-3dB}	half power point angular frequency
ω_n	natural frequency of undamped system
$\omega_{n,damp}$	natural frequency of damped system

12
MEMS wireless implantable systems: historical review and perspectives

W. KO and P. X.-L. FENG,
Case Western Reserve University, USA

DOI: 10.1533/9780857098610.2.401

Abstract: We present a historical and perspectival overview of the design and development of wireless implantable microsystems. We first discuss the general considerations for medical implants and telemetry microsystems, where a great number of challenges persist today, even after over 50 years of active and considerable research effort. We then describe and review advances from 1950 to present, with specific examples of design approaches and significant milestones, with an emphasis on implantable and telemetric electronics. We also discuss latest progress and challenges in implant microsystems, and offer insights on future technological trends.

Key words: wireless implantable systems, biocompatibility, telemetry, micropackage, micropower sources.

12.1 Introduction

Implantable systems represent a technique of biomedical instrumentation for sensing body information, or soliciting body reaction, within a living organism from a location outside of the body through a wireless communication link. Exploration inside the body is as exciting as the exploration of outer space. Implantable systems look inward, from body to organs, to tissues, to cells, to sub-cellular molecules including proteins and DNA/RNA. Implantable systems are the tools for our inward exploration, just as spaceships are the tools for exploration of outer space. The science, technology, methodologies and instrumentation for both endeavours are similar, although with great differences terms of scale, size and cost.

The essential building blocks of all implantable systems are shown in Fig. 12.1: the oval is the body, and the rectangular block is the external equipment. The implanted systems, shown schematically in Fig. 12.2, can function as tele-sensing (telemetry) or remote control (tele-actuation), linked together with a closed-loop control system. It may be all electronic, or it may have parts of the implant which are mechanical, chemical or biological. All

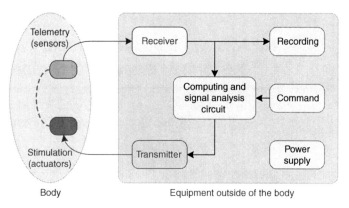

12.1 Conceptual diagram of an implantable system.

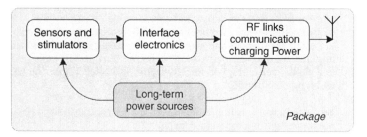

12.2 The essential building blocks of the implantable system for the body.

implantable systems have the same essential building blocks, whether the implant device is for sensing, actuating, or closed-loop control. For implant telemetry systems, the sensors convert the biological parameters into electrical signals that are processed by the interface electronics, then transmitted by radio frequency (RF) (or other wireless means such as ultrasound, optical, etc.) link to an external receiver and recording or processing facilities. For the implant actuation systems, the external command unit sends command signals through the wireless link, which is then processed by the interface electronics to drive the actuators that solicit certain actions in the body. For the implantable electronics system, the common actuators are the electrical stimulators that send currents to the muscles or nerves, through stimulating electrodes that solicit the desired body reactions. For implant control systems, the telemetry unit and the stimulating unit are linked to control specific body function to a desired level, with the telemetric part acting as the feedback unit of conventional control systems. All these systems need to be packaged for biocompatibility before implant insertion (e.g., through surgical operations or ingestion).

The sensor/stimulator, the electronics and the wireless communication link and power supply of an implantable system may be located totally within the body or on the surface layer of the organism. The location may be in the body or intra-cavity (implantable system), within the intestines or mouth (indwelling system), or may be attached on the external surfaces of the body, subcutaneously or on the organ surface (attachable system). The implant electronic systems are valuable instruments for life science research, as well as health care. Telemetry systems are used for monitoring, and diagnosis such as ECG measurement and blood pressure monitoring. Stimulation systems are used for prosthesis, therapy and treatment, such as cochlear implants, heart pacemakers and nerve signal blockage for pain suppression. The closed-loop systems are used for paralysed arm prosthesis, and automated health care and prevention, such as the variable-rate heart pacemaker that can adjust the heart rate according to the oxygenation level in the blood or the activity of the body (Ko and Neuman, 1967).

12.2 Basic considerations and characteristics of wireless MEMS implantable systems

12.2.1 Legal considerations of the radio frequency (RF), field strength and power levels

The wireless operation of implantable systems can be accomplished by modulating a high frequency radiating carrier that can transmit signals through the body to the receiving station nearby or vice versa. The carrier frequency used can be in the range of ultrasound, RF, and infrared (IR). The most commonly used frequencies are in the RF range, from kilohertz (kHz) to megahertz (MHz), to gigahertz (GHz). There are government regulations and international standards to guide the proper use of frequency and radiated carrier power level. These basic considerations are: (1) the carrier signal is non-interfering for other users; and (2) the system is not harmful to the body. In the United States, the regulations are detailed in the electronic Code of Federal Regulations (eCFR) of the Federal Communication Commission (FCC), title 47 Telecommunication, Parts 15, 18, 90, and 95, and IEEE code C-95–2005. These regulations are specific, detailed, and complicated. The following is a greatly simplified sample of the FCC regulations. The designers and the users of implantable systems should seek professional advice on selecting the operation frequency and power level. In many cases, an FCC license would be required.

The IEEE C95-2005 is the IEEE standard for safety levels with respect to human exposure to RF electromagnetic fields from 3 kHz to 300 GHz. It 'provides recommendations to minimize aversive or painful electro-

Table 12.1 ISM frequencies and tolerance

ISM frequency	Tolerance
6.78 MHz	±15.0 kHz
13.56 MHz	±7.0 kHz
27.12 MHz	±163.0 kHz
40.68 MHz	±20.0 kHz
915 MHz	±13.0 MHz
2,450 MHz	±50.0 MHz
5,800 MHz	±75.0 MHz
24,125 MHz	±125.0 MHz
61.25 GHz	±250.0 MHz
122.50 GHz	±500.0 MHz
245.00 GHz	±1.0 GHz

Source: eCFR part 18 § 18.301, 2011.

stimulation in the frequency range of 3 kHz to 5 MHz and to protect against adverse heating in the frequency range of 100 kHz to 300 GHz. In the transition region of 100 kHz to 5 MHz'. Protection against both electro-stimulation and thermal effects is provided through two separate sets of limits. Below 100 kHz only the electro-stimulation limits apply, above 5 MHz only the thermal limits apply, and both sets of limits apply in the transition region. In the transition region, the limits based on electro-stimulation are generally more limiting for low duty cycle exposures, while the thermal-based limits are more limiting for continuous wave fields (IEEE C-95 § 4.1 basic restrictions). The eCFR of the FCC allocates the use of RF frequencies, and regulates RF devices, equipment, and operator licensing.

In the US, implantable systems frequencies may have the following options: (1) the FCC assigned frequency bands for the medical telemetry service (608–614 MHz, 1390–1395 MHz, 1429–1429.5 MHz, 1427–1429 MHz, and 1429.5–1431.5 MHz), as well as the frequency bands for the medical radio-communication service in 401–406 MHz (eCFR title 47 part 95-Subparts H and E); (2) frequency bands assigned to Industry, Science and Medicine (ISM) bands, as listed in Table 12.1 (eCFR, 2011 Title 47, Part 95, Parts 15, and part 18); (3) amateur RF bands; and (4) frequencies satisfying the low-power, non-interference provision.

Operation of the equipment according to the ISM radio bands within the following safety, search and rescue frequency bands is prohibited: 490–510 kHz, 2170–2194 kHz, 8354–8374 kHz, 121.4–121.6 MHz, 156.7–156.9 MHz, and 242.8–243.2 MHz.

The regulation on power level and maximum field strength outside the ISM band are given in IEEE C95. No summary will be given in this chapter. Because the large amount of information contained, and will be updated soon, changes will be made as technology advances and more RF devices are used. Furthermore, the operating power level and the maximum field strength involve personal safety and interference to other's communication. The readers are referred to updated IEEE C 95 or to consult specialists on these topics in selecting operation power level and field strength.

12.2.2 Biocompatibility and protection of the implanted system

The body is a fragile but harsh environment for implantable electronics. The implanted systems should not seriously affect or harm the tissues surrounding the implant, or the body, that is, the device/system has to be biocompatible. At the same time, the implanted system also needs protection from the tissue activity, and damage from corrosive, conducting body fluid. Biocompatibility requires proper design of implantable systems in terms of size, weight, functional electronics and packaging, to minimize electrical, mechanical, thermal and optical interference to the normal activity of surrounding tissues and the body, as well as to eliminate any chemical and biological toxicity and contamination to the tissue and the body.

For physical biocompatibility the size and weight should be small, so that the implant would not affect the normal activity of the body. It is generally accepted that the volume and weight of implantable device or system should not be more than 2% volume and weight of the host organ or body to avoid discomfort or loading stress on the organ or body in normal activity and movement. Besides the small size, the density of the implant should closely match that of the tissues so that, when the body moves, the implant should not cause undue stress to the tissues surrounding the device. For thermal considerations the implant should not have any hot spots that are 2°C higher than the normal temperature of the tissue. The surface of the packaged implant should be smooth, not having any sharp parts that could cause localized stress or irritation to the tissues. Some means to stabilize the position of the implant should be provided, to prevent the implant from migrating from the designated site to other parts of the body (Ko *et al.*, 1969; Ko and Spear, 1983).

When the implantable system is surgically inserted in the body, there will be biological and chemical reactions occurring at the implant location as well as in the body. For biocompatibility the implant should not have any toxic materials leaking out of the package and the package should be designed to minimize biological reaction to the implant and the surgical operation. The small size, the smooth surface, the use of biocompatible packaging materials and techniques, as well as the proper sterilization and surgical operations, can reduce biological reactions to the implant operation. For good implantable systems, inflammatory reactions should be minimized and the thickness of the connecting tissues should be kept thin, in the micrometre range.

For the protection of the implantable device/system, and in order for it to operate properly throughout its designated lifetime, the implant should be designed and packaged to achieve the following: (1) to prevent the electrical damage from the corrosive conducting body fluid to the electronic circuits and devices. The leakage resistance between all parts of the implantable system should be maintained high (with sheet resistance on the order of 100 MΩ/□), to ensure proper operation of the system. This can be achieved by hermetic packaging using compact metal, ceramic and glass boxes and hermetic feed-through; or, alternatively, non-hermetic packaging with polymeric materials and thin film vapour barriers; (2) to protect the system from mechanical damage that may be caused by improper handling during the implant operation and after implantation; (3) to withstand the harsh chemical and biological environment throughout its life time without degradation. Many electronic devices are sensitive to light so some form of shielding would be desirable during the testing or preparatory stages.

In the biocompatibility area there are many unsolved problems related to body reaction and packaging. For example, the correlation between the thickness of the connecting tissue surrounding the implants and the package, as well as the implant processes, are not yet fully understood. Non-hermetic package technology is not fully developed. The understanding and techniques to stabilize and integrate the chronic implant with the surrounding tissue needs further development. The body environment is dynamic besides having a conductive and corrosive body fluid; the body also generates antibodies that attack foreign materials, including implants. The surrounding tissue also may change its properties with time. Sometimes, implants may be rejected by the body. The causes and the processes of implant rejection need to be further studied (Ko et al., 1969; Ko and Spear, 1983).

12.2.3 Characteristics of biological and medical signals

Biological and medical signals have different characteristics when compared with industrial, engineering and scientific signals in requirements for accuracy, sensitivity, reliability and signal bandwidth. When measuring biomedical signals the accuracy may be less important than sensitivity. For biomedical signals, such as blood pressure, heart rate, respiration rate, etc., their normal ranges and useful characteristics may vary between individuals. Even with a single person, the signal may vary a few per cent from time to time, and may be affected by many body and mental activities and health status. The quantitative effects of these personal activities on the biomedical signals are not precisely understood at the present. Therefore, for measurement instruments designed for these signals now, the required accuracy is generally not as high as in other scientific research. Generally, 1% full-scale accuracy is sufficient, although the sensitivity or resolution may need to be very high because the signals are weak. The input electrical signals usually are in the millivolt (mV) to microvolt (μV) to nanovolt (nV) ranges.

Since most biomedical measurement instruments would be used by non-technical personnel under strenuous circumstances, their high reliability, ease of operation, and robust structure may be required beyond the levels set for general instruments used in an engineering laboratory.

Since the biomedical signals are related to molecular manipulations in the body and not to RF processes, the frequency bandwidth required for biomedical signals are generally lower than electronic signals. Generally the bandwidths of biomedical signals are below 10–30 kHz, and many of the clinical instruments would have their signal bandwidths limited to just below 50/60 Hz – the AC power frequency – to avoid the strong interferences of AC power lines. However, the signal amplitude may be in the range from millivolt to microvolt levels for the organ and body signals, and may extend to nanovolts or below for cellular and sub-cellular signals (Ko and Spear, 1983).

12.2.4 Design considerations of MEMS implantable systems

When designing implantable or surface-attached biomedical systems, there are some basic and common considerations related to biocompatibility, reliability, and ease of operation, as discussed before. The fundamental considerations are size and weight, body reaction, and the packaging used to protect the implantable system. When translated to the engineering design of the system, the major considerations are: (1) use micropower components and circuits to reduce the power consumption – including micropower active devices, micropower electronic circuits (use of application specific integrated circuits (ASIC) whenever possible), and micro-sensors and micro-actuators; (2) select the smallest power supply suited to the application – the system may use: (2a) the smallest battery that can last the required life time; (2b) a passive wireless power unit; or (2c) Rechargeable thin battery and wireless charge circuit to charge the battery and to turn off the system when not in use; (2d) Energy scavenging from inside human body; (3). packaging to minimize harmful body reaction and to have adequate protection to the system in the body environment, as well as to minimize volume and weight (Ko and Neuman, 1967). All medical devices or instruments should be designed with *reliability and safety* as their prime consideration, above all cost and technical factors.

On the selection of a power supply unit for the system, there are several developments in high energy density batteries. Among them, the thin film lithium battery is a good candidate. The selection considerations should include (i) the volume and weight per unit stored energy (current × time × voltage), (ii) fast charging time, (iii) small internal resistance or the maximum discharge pulse current, (iv) lifetime recharge cycles, (v) maximum storage and operation temperatures that can withstand steam or other methods of sterilization.

For the passive wireless powered approach, one can use (a) single frequency time sharing for powering and signal transmission with shared antenna; or (b) two frequencies for powering and signal transmission, each having its own antenna. Wireless charging of small batteries is the most popular approach. Here, the wireless charging methods can be: the magnetic field of an RF radiation, low frequency time varying magnetic induction field, and ultrasonic radiation. In all these situations, the surface and tissue power density should be kept below the legal limits for body exposure (for example, the tissue temperature rise should be less than 2°C). When the wireless power source is used to power deep implants, the surface field intensity may be much greater than that at the implantable system site. Wireless charging with on–off control would be the preferred approach whenever possible (Ko and Neuman, 1967).

There are a few interesting design approaches developed for micropower electronics for implantable MEMS systems during the early stages of implantable systems, before the large scale integrated circuit (LSIC) had been developed. They may still be of value even at the present time when we are looking for surface-attached instruments for individualized mobile monitoring and early warning systems. These approaches are: (1) using micropower devices at low-voltage, low-current, such as tunnel diodes and sub-threshold metal oxide semiconductor (MOS) transistors, (2) integrating sensors/actuators with circuits using micropower ASIC, (3) using multi-functional electronic circuits, (4) sharing battery current by cascade electronic circuits, (5) splitting lithium battery voltage to two or three low voltage supplies for the electronic circuits. Some examples will be given in Section 12.3 to explain these approaches.

12.3 Significant research on radio frequency implantable systems from 1955 to 1975

Although radio transmission of analogue signals has been known since 1844 (Prescott, 1884) and frequency-modulation radio links were used to transmit pneumograms in 1948 (Fuller and Gorden, 1948), extensive development of biomedical implant electronic techniques did not really get started until the transistor was discovered in 1948 and made available after 1954.

The comparatively small size and power consumption of this new device made possible the construction of practical telemetry transmitters for implant measurement. Since then, the advances in solid-state devices and microelectronics have further enhanced the development of implant telemetry and stimulation into a field of research in instrumentation. In the late 1950s and early 1960s Mackay, Noller, Wolff, Zworykin, and others developed active radio-telemetry units for use in the gastrointestinal tract and other cavities of the body (Mackay, 1959). Subcutaneous and deep-body implantation of telemetry units were initiated by Essler, Ko, Mackay Cole, Young, and others to measure physiological information in animals as well in humans (Ko and Neuman, 1967). For a historical review of these and other areas of biomedical telemetry, see: Ko and Neuman (1967); Caceres (1967); Slater's (1963, 1966) surveys. See also references: Amlaner and MacDonald (1986) and Hambrecht and Reswick (1977).

The earliest telemetric electronic circuits are shown in Fig. 12.3. Figure 12.3a shows Mackay's blocking oscillator circuit, used to telemeter body temperature or other narrow bandwidth body signals sensed by the sensors R or C1. It is simple, robust and requires very low power. This circuit was modified and improved for use extensively in animal tracking research (Mackay, 1959). A collection of biotelemetric works for radio tracking up to 1975 is given in (Amlaner and MacDonald, 1986). Figure 12.3b is Ko's tunnel diode telemetry circuit with bridge sensor input. The transistor and the tunnel diode share the same supply current (Ko, 1960).

Historically, the development of implantable systems started with telemetry, then stimulation, then closed-loop control. In the period from 1960 to 1975, all design approaches were studied and all biomedical applications were explored. However, due to the limitations of microelectronics and packaging technologies, only the radio tracking was fully developed for animal tracking and monitoring in biology field (Amlaner and MacDonald,

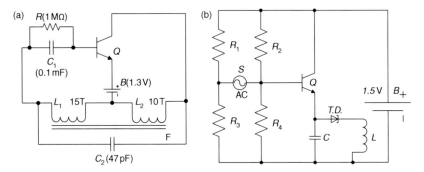

12.3 Examples of implant telemetry circuits of the early 1960 era. (a) Blocking oscillator (Mackay, 1959) and (b) tunnel diode telemetry (Ko, 1960).

1986). In the medical field, several demonstration projects were completed, including: pain blocking by nerve stimulation; indwelling capsules for measurement of pH and motion in the small intestine; hearing and vision prosthetics using skin and brain electrodes; closed-loop electromyography (EMG) control of motions of arms and feet; brain control of machines and body motions through muscle EMG, and the use of brain stimulation to control the emotional status of monkeys. However, none of these reached the stage of being useful products, except for the cardiac pacemaker. A few examples of applications explored and designs from the author's team are shown below.

12.3.1 Implantable telemetry devices

Miniaturized low-power, low-bandwidth telemetric transmitters were developed and packaged with Hysol^R Epoxy and medical grade silicone as short-term implants; flat-pack boxes made of metal and Macor^R (a machinable ceramic), and glass capsule were used for packaging of longer term implants. The sizes are in the range of several cm^3, and the power levels are from milliwatts to microwatts. They are intended for biomedical monitoring and diagnosis, including: (i) physiological research using small animal models; (ii) system biology study; (iii) patient monitoring in the hospital; (iv) response and progress of medical treatment; and (v) monitoring vital signs of patients for preventive care and early warning. Figure 12.4 shows two examples of the telemetric transmitters that were used for many of these applications from 1961 to 1975 (Ko, 1960, 1961, 1962, and 1965). The world first pocket-size mobile microphone was demonstrated in 1964 with a PZT microphone and a MR312 mercury battery (Ko, 1960).

12.3.2 Implant stimulation devices

The peripheral and central nervous system (CNS) in the body can be stimulated by small electrical currents to generate electrical signals, or to block signal transmission, thus inhibiting related functions, such as pain blocking; the tissues also can be stimulated to contract and to generate EMG signals. The theory and applications of *functional electrical stimulation* were developed at the Engineering Design Center, Case Institute of Technology in 1960–70 (Hambrecht and Reswick, 1977). Many research groups tried various applications of the functional stimulation. Examples are: (i) cardiac pacemaker and defibrillation devices; (ii) electrical pain suppressor; (iii) implantable middle ear and cochlear hearing aids; (iv) visual prosthesis (with multi-electrodes attached on the forehead or on the visual cortex surface); (v) diaphragm pacing for respiration; (vi) epileptic seizure control; (vii) hand

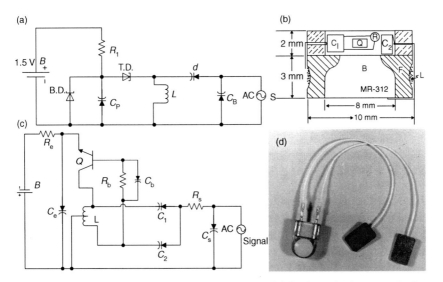

12.4 (a) K-5 tunnel diode telemetry unit. (b) Packaged telemetry device. (c) Circuit and (d) package for K-6 implantable FM telemetry transmitter for voice, EKG and EMK (the world's smallest telemetry unit in 1965; each weights 1.5 g, packaged, including battery and sensors).

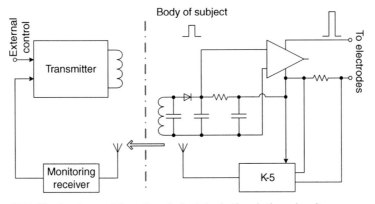

12.5 Single-channel functional electrical stimulation circuit.

and aim control with spinal cord injury, (viii) leg and foot control for walking; and (ix) brain stimulation for emotional control of monkeys and other animal models (Peckham *et al.*, 1981 and 1993).

A typical single-channel electrical stimulation circuit is shown in Fig. 12.5. Here the 'K-5' unit is a feedback circuit used to check on feedback the magnitude of the electrode current being delivered to the body. Multiple-channel stimulation units were developed for hand-control applications for tetraplegic patients (Lin *et al.*, 1972; Peckham, 1993). In the literature, there are hundreds of papers on functional electrical stimulation. Functional stimulation has had many applications, including hearing, vision, respiration, limb motion, pain blockage, and some organ function prosthesis and brain-to-machine interfaces. Much progress has been made. However, use of long-term implanted electrodes for brain recording and stimulation that have a large number of flexible leads connected from the integrated circuit chip to the wide area of brain electrode sites, still presents an interesting challenge and difficult problems to be studied.

12.3.3 Implantable electronic control systems

Many implant control systems have been studied by adding a feedback telemetry circuit to monitor the response of the stimulation for adjusting the strength of command to reach a desired level of body action. Examples include the on-demand pacemaker with heart-rate monitor feedback, and the EMG controlled hand prosthesis that telemeters back the level of muscle response to the command unit to adjust the stimulation level for desired consciously controlled motion. In the early stage of implantable systems many control systems were studied. Examples include:

- paralysed limb control for upper and lower extremities (Crago *et al.*, 1980);
- drug infusion control;
- organ function regulation, such as heart pacing and lung pacing;
- biological research;
- pain suppression, and
- drop foot and other muscle-control systems.

Demonstration projects have been tried, but the practical use of these systems took many years of development work. Figure 12.6 illustrates the arm aid system proposed in 1960 at the Electronics Design Center (EDC), Case Institute of Technology. Only recently has the Case Arm Aid System been approved by Food and Drug Administration (FDA) for patients to gain some use of the hand for daily activity (Peckham, 1993). Figure 12.7 is a photo showing the first demonstration of EMG controlled limb movement, where a K-6 telemetry unit was implanted under the skin on the shoulder of Dr Lojze Vodovnik (Miklavčič *et al.*, 2003), an outstanding visiting scholar of EDC at Case Institute of Technology in the 1960s. The EMG signal of his shoulder muscle was sent to a FM receiver nearby as the command signal. Also, an electrical stimulation unit was implanted in a dog's rear leg muscle. The EMG signal of Dr Vodovnik was then used to control the up and down movement of the dog's leg. Similar experiments have been performed to use EMG signals to control the speed of a motor. These early experiments demonstrated the feasibility of brain-controlled machines, or a brain-controlled environment (Grotz *et al.*, 1964; Lorig *et al.*, 1967).

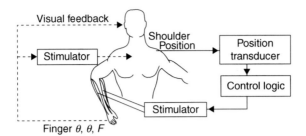

12.6 Illustration of the conceptual arm aid system of 1970 (Hambrecht and Reswick, 1977). In this system, the brain generates the commands and controls through the shoulder muscles; the implanted or surface-mounted telemetry unit on the shoulder sends signals to the external control unit, which in turn generates stimulation signal that controls the arm muscles that actuate the forearm and the fingers; the visual feedback signal closes the control loop.

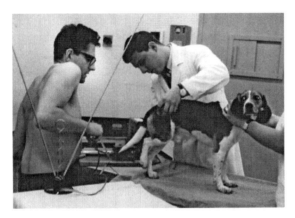

12.7 Human EMG implant device controls leg motion of a dog.

12.3.4 Design approaches and samples of implant electronic devices

As discussed in Sections 12.2.3 and 12.2.4, the implant system design has different considerations from other RF MEMS systems. The implantable systems are operating in a very harsh environment. Body fluids are highly conductive and corrosive. All foreign objects in the body are attacked by antibodies and other biochemical reactions in the body. At the same time, the implant, as a foreign material, may cause inflammation and other toxic reactions in the tissue around the implant and some organs. Therefore, the material used for the implant should be non-toxic and properly packaged to protect the tissue, the implant, and the host body from any harmful reactions.

Implant operations are expensive and time consuming. The implant device takes a long time to reach stable operation after it is implanted. Therefore, when designing implantable systems, reliability and safety are more important than many other quality factors, such as broad-band response, high accuracy, etc.

Biological rhythms generally repeat in fractions of a second to many seconds per cycle. Therefore, the bandwidths of biomedical signals are usually in the range from 0.01 Hz to 10 kHz.

For a long-term implant, with a lifetime from months to years, the basic requirements are: (i) the volume and weight of the packaged implant device should be small and light, so that the device will not affect the normal activity of the host – it is generally agreed that 2% of the host body size and weight are the upper limits; (ii) the biocompatibility – the implant should not contain any toxic or harmful materials, and the package should be able to protect the body and the implant from any harm; and (iii) the implant system – implant and the external unit – should be safe, reliable, and easy to operate by non-technical biomedical personnel.

In the design of long-lifetime implant electronic systems, to meet the size, weight and other requirements all the building blocks in Fig. 12.1 need to be considered. The largest and heaviest blocks are the chronic power supply and the biocompatible package. They have been the most difficult problems, from the early stages of the field to the present.

With the advances of LSICs and MEMS/NEMS the interface electronics and the RF link can be designed to achieve minimal size and weight. Several approaches were developed in the early periods that may still be of interest today. A few examples are given below:

- The use of low-power electronic devices, such as tunnel diodes and low current transistors in Fig. 12.3 (Ko *et al.*, 1970).
- The integration of the sensors with all the signal processing circuits into a single chip.
- The low duty cycle pulse frequency or pulse position modulated RF approach will greatly reduce the power consumption by a factor equal to the duty cycle, which can be of the order of 10^{-2}–10^{-6} (Ko *et al.*, 1970).
- Split power supply voltage, to share the same current for several devices/circuits, such as using two tunnel diodes to share the same battery current with a low voltage transistor, as shown in Fig. 12.8, where the 1.35 V battery is shared by a transistor and two tunnel diodes (as subcarrier oscillators). The two-channel telemetry unit used one sub-milliwatt power (Ko and Neuman, 1967).
- Multiple function of a single active device. Figure 12.9 shows the single-antenna, two-frequency (one for RF powering and one for signal

MEMS wireless implantable systems 415

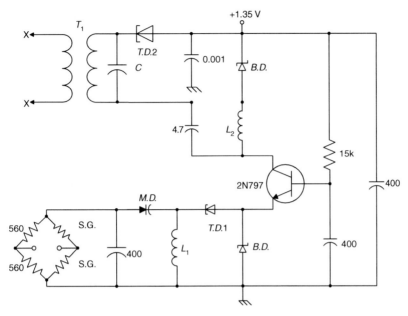

12.8 Two tunnel diodes are in series with a transistor to share the 1.35 V battery current.

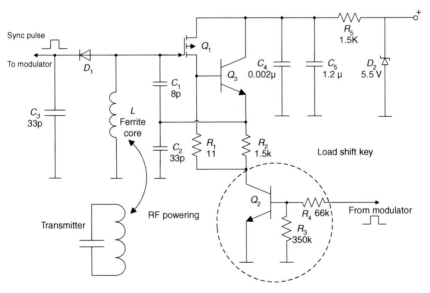

12.9 The single-antenna, two-frequency RF-link circuit (Hynecek and Ko, 1975).

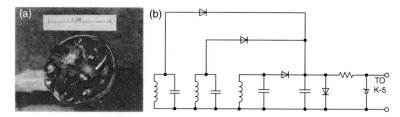

12.10 The three-dimensional RF power receiving coil structure and circuit diagram. (a) Structure of a 3-D RF power unit. (b) Circuit diagram of the RF power unit.

transmission) circuit. Normally Q2 and Q3 are off, and the Q1 field-effect transistor (FET) functions as a diode to rectify the RF power at the frequency tuned by L and (C1, C2); when there is a transmitting signal from the device Q2, Q3 are on, and Q1 and Q3 function as an oscillator and RF transmitter at the frequency of L and C2, respectively (Hynecek and Ko, 1975).

- The three-dimensional RF power receiving coil is shown in Fig. 12.10. High efficiency high power RF powering is achieved by using an external ferrite core to focus the external powering magnetic field to maintain alignment with one of the implant receiving coils as the body moves around (Ko and Neuman, 1967).

12.4 Progress of implantable systems from 1980 to 2010

The great advances of the last three decades in the manufacturing of very large scale integrated circuits (VLSI) and ASIC, and the miniaturization of physical, chemical and biological transducers (sensors, actuators, and electrodes), especially MEMS and NEMS, have cleared many barriers for practicable implantable microsystems in medical care and life-sciences research. The pioneering techniques of short-range MEMS wireless remote monitoring and control have advanced from biomedical research and aerospace applications to preventive care, industrial, environmental, and social communication fields (Haubrich, 2006). Short range RF links (powering and signal transmission) are everywhere in our daily life now. The literature in this field is vast. For instance, a comprehensive literature review can be found in (IEEE Spectrum Webcast, 2006; Receveur *et al.*, 2007). Therefore, no detailed and focused review on implantable MEMS systems from 1980 to the present is included in this chapter. A sample list of implantable systems developed from 1980 to 2010, which have made considerable impacts, are briefly summarized on the next page:

- Implantable electronic devices: telemetry, stimulation and control systems.
  - Limb prostheses: hand, arm, and leg motion control, drop foot stimulator.
  - Sensory prostheses: middle ear and cochlear hearing aids, visual prostheses, touch sensors, artificial taste and smell devices.
  - Assistive/artificial organs: such as cardiovascular assistive devices, heart pacemakers, respiratory pacers, urinary control systems, artificial vocal cords, etc.
  - Drug infusion devices: insulin release devices, cancer treatment drug infusion devices, pain release drug infusion devices, etc.
- Indwelling devices: systems that indwell in the digestive channel or other body cavities. These include ingestive capsules, devices implanted in bladders, oral cavities, and ear channels.
- CNS, for example, brain–machine interface research: With a large electrode array implanted in the brain or on the dural surface for telemetry and stimulation, in order to treat certain diseases and to establish communication links with the brain to develop CNS and computer communication network.
- Surface-attached devices for mobile base line monitoring and early warning of patients' vital signs.
- Body energy harvesting and various wireless powering and distribution techniques.

12.5 Challenges of implantable/attached electronics

The major challenges of implantable, indwelling and surface-attached electronic systems are the same at present as they were 50 years ago. The only difference is the level of sophistication. They have minimum size and weight, long-lifetime power supply, micropackaging, and new and better transducers (sensor and actuator – the large scale stimulator electrode array) integrated with signal processing circuits. As electronic and VLSI technologies progress, the major challenges remaining are the chronic power supply and the packaging.

12.5.1 Long-term power supply

The challenge is to combine a small battery with low internal resistance/impedance for fast recharge and large output transient currents. The supercapacitors and the long-lifetime rechargeable lithium thin film battery developed recently may partially satisfy the present needs for energy storage. The high efficiency wireless charging techniques are challenges. How to transfer microwatts to milliwatts of power though a wireless link to mm-sized receiving coils or plates in the body over a distance of 10–20 cm with reasonable efficiency (0.01–1%) *safely* is a great challenge. Wireless charging can be accomplished by RF magnetic radiation field, ultrasound, infrared light, and low frequency magnetic field, as well as by body energy harvesting. The implantable body energy harvesting and distribution of harvested energy throughout the body are interesting fields of research and challenge. The safe long-term nuclear power source also would be of interest to explore (Ko and Hynecek, 1974).

12.5.2 Micropackage of MEMS/NEMS implantable systems

The function of packaging implantable systems is to protect both the host body and the implant device from harm throughout the system's planted life time. In order to protect the host body: (i) the implant unit should not have any toxic material and should be sterile; (ii) the structure and the surface of the implant should be biocompatible, so that the implant will not irritate surrounding tissues and the body after the wound is healed; (iii) the implant surface temperature should be close to the tissue temperature ($<2°C$ difference); (iv) the specific gravity of the implant should be close to that of the surrounding tissue, so that when the body moves there will be no abnormal stress applied to the tissues (Ko and Spear, 1983); and (v) there should be means to stabilize the implant's position in the body. A good package should have thin flexible layer of tissue layer grown over the implant over the lifetime. Good packaging should prevent the rejection of chronic implant units (Ko, 1995).

In order to protect the implant device the package should: (i) protect the implant from water vapour and ionic chemicals that cause current leakages, and low resistance paths between leads leading to the degradation of the operation of the implant system; (ii) protect the implant from mechanical damage during the implant operation and in the body, and (iii) ensure the proper functioning of the implant over the desired lifetime.

Conventional hermetic packages use hermetically sealed boxes made of non-toxic metal, ceramic and glass with biocompatible outer coating. They can have very long life times, but generally are large, heavy, and costly to make, and have a large amount of wasted space in the box. Presently, the volume and weight of hermetic packages are much larger than the unpackaged MEMS implantable systems with MEMS sensors/actuators and ASIC (Nichols, 1994). Furthermore, the sensors that need to communicate with body environment cannot be boxed. The feed-through and the interconnecting lead are not reliable. New micropackage technology needs to be developed for the micro-implant systems. The package technology has been intensively studied recently (Wong, 1998; Lachhman *et al.*, 2011, 2012). Non-hermetic packages using polymeric materials, such as epoxy, silicone, parylene and ceramic thin films as coating materials, are interesting. Research on non-hermetic packaging of MEMS implant systems with implant lifetimes from several months to several years is being actively studied. When properly developed, the package could be made with low volume and weight and could be made quickly at low cost, but the life time is expected to be shorter, ranging from several months (Bu *et al.*, 2009), up to 2–5 years (Lachhman *et al.*, 2011, 2012). However, the theory and technology need to be developed, and practical tools and processes with proven reliability need to be demonstrated, before they can be used for implantable systems. The development of micropackage technology to have package volume and weight much less than the unpackaged device and have an implant life time up to 10–20 years is challenging.

12.5.3 Microwatt and nanowatt electronic circuits and transducers

Although MEMS/NEMS transducers and integrated circuit technologies have reduced the size and power consumption of sensory and electronic systems by orders of magnitude since 1990, the integration of transducer and integrated circuits (IC) to further reduce the size, weight and power consumption of implant systems are real challenges now. The power consumption per telemetry channel for 1 kHz bandwidth is about 1–5 microwatts for the advanced implantable systems at present (Narasimhan *et al.*, 2011). If the MEMS/NEMS technology could be developed to reduce the per telemetry channel power by two orders of magnitude, to the 10 nanowatt level, and to use electronic devices that require supply voltage in the range of 0.2–1.0 V, then the energy storage component and the implantable systems package could have their volume reduced from larger than 1000 mm^3 now, to 10 mm^3. Many future applications of injected implant systems on or in body organs would then be possible.

12.6 Conclusion and future trends

From 1960 to 2010, implantable electronics systems have made tremendous progress, thanks to the relentless miniaturization of transducers and electronics. The pioneering techniques of short-range MEMS wireless remote monitoring and control have propagated from biomedical research and aerospace applications to clinical health care, industrial, environmental, and social communication fields. Short-range RF links (powering and signal transmission) are everywhere in our daily life now. Implanted or indwelling microsystems will continue to advance to meet human desires and healthcare needs. Based on our experience and understanding of the challenges in implantable systems for biomedical research and health care, we suggest that the trends of implantable, indwelling and attachable systems for biomedical applications may include the following:

- Nanoscale transducers and electronics that can further miniaturize the system volume and weight, and enable minimally invasive, higher-performance implantable systems, for research on organs, tissues, and cells.
- Individualized medical health care – where normal baseline health information can be recorded and monitored through RF links to healthcare institutions while the person assumes normal activities at home or in the office. Deviations from the individualized norm would initiate preventive actions to avoid serious medical problems from developing. The system needs to be reliable, easy and comfortable to use, and available at low cost.
- Home and on line (mobile) monitor and treatment system – when trend A and B are accomplished, the personalized monitoring and warning system can be extended to mobile locations, such as during travel or away from the office. Medical information collection and remotely controlled treatment can be accomplished through cell phone or other mobile communication systems.
- On-organ monitoring and therapeutic devices – when the implantable device is small and reliable, on-organ monitoring and therapeutic devices would be developed, such as a cardiac pacemaker and defibrillator on the heart, and powered by the energy harvested from the heart's motion (Feng and Ko, 2010; Zhang et al., 2011). Similarly, on the liver, on the kidney, on the bladder, on the brain, and other on-organ function monitoring and therapeutic devices would be developed by implant system engineers teaming up with biomedical healthcare researchers.
- Larger scale multiple-channel (1000 and up) brain–machine interconnected network for biology and physiology research, medical diagnosis, prosthesis and treatment of body malfunctions would be developed.
- Artificial organs. such as: artificial heart, lung, kidney, liver, pancreas and others would be developed by multidisciplinary teams including engineers, biomedical, and clinical researchers.
- Large scale multichannel monitoring and control systems as well as brain–computer interfaced RF MEMS networks for biomedical as well as for engineering, industrial, social, environmental, and energy operation and research would be studied.

12.7 Acknowledgements

The authors are grateful for the support from the Advanced Platform Technology (APT) Center, Louis Stokes Cleveland VA Medical Center, Department of Veterans Affairs, and the NIH grant #REB014442A on 'Micropackage Technology for Implantable Biomedical Microsystems'. The editorial assistance of Dr Robert C. Roberts and Dr Linda Ko-Ferrigno are gratefully acknowledged.

12.8 References

Amlaner, C.G. and MacDonald, D.M. Eds (1986) *A Handbook on Biotelemetry and Radio Tracking*, Pergamum Press, Oxford and New York.

Bu, L.P., Cong, P., Kuo, H.-I., Ye, X.S., and Ko W.H. (2009) 'Micro package of short term wireless implantable microfabricated systems', *IEEE EMBC annual Conf.*, Minneapolis, MN, **31**(1); 6395–6399.

Caceres, C.A. Ed. (1967) *Bio-Medical Telemetry*, Academic Press, New York.

Crago, P.E., Mortimer, J.T., and Peckham, P.H. (1980) 'Closed-loop control of force during electrical stimulation of muscle', *IEEE Transactions on Biomedical Engineering*, **27**(6); 306–312.

eCFR (2011) *'Electronic Code of Federal Regulations part 15, part 18, part 90 and part 95'*. Federal Communication Commission.

Feng, P.X.-L. and Ko, W.H. (2010) 'Bioimplantable piezoelectric microsystems for heart health monitoring and self-powered cardiac arrhythmia management', *Pending Disclosure Patent Application*.

Fuller, L. and Gordon, T.M. (1948) 'The radio inductograph – a device for recording physiological activity in unrestrained animal', *Science*, Appleton, New York, **85**, 108, p. 287.

Grotz, R.C., Yon, E.T., Long, C., and Ko, W.H. (1964) 'Intramuscular FM radio transmitter of muscle potential', *42 Congress of Physical Medicine and Rehabilitation*, Chicago, IL.

Hambrecht, F.T. and Reswick, J.B. Eds (1977) *Functional Electrical Stimulation: Applications in Neural Prostheses*, Marcel Dekker, New York.

Haubrich, G. (2006) 'Wireless applications in healthcare: wireless telemetry for active implantable medical device (AIMD) systems', *IEEE Spectrum Webcast*, November 30.

Hynecek, J. and Ko, W.H. (1975) 'Single frequency RF powered telemetry system', *28th Ann. Conf. on Eng. in Med. and Biol.*, p.97, New Orleans, LO.

IEEE C 95 (2005) 'IEEE standard for safety levels with respect to human exposure to radio frequency electromagnetic fields 3 kHz to 300 GHz', *IEEE Standards*.

IEEE Spectrum Webcast (9/13/2006), 'Health monitoring'. Available from: http://www.cse.nd.edu/~cpoellab/teaching/cse40816/Lecture6.pdf

Ko, W.H. (1960) 'Tunnel diode FM wireless microphone', *Electronics*, November 8.

Ko, W.H. (1961) 'Designing tunnel diode oscillators', *Electronics*, February 10.

Ko, W.H. (1962) 'Tunnel diode oscillator delivers RF and audio', *Electronics*, **35**(41): 56.

Ko, W.H. (1965) 'Progress in miniaturized telemetry', *Bioscience*, **15–2**: 118–120.

Ko, W.H. (1995) 'Packaging of microfabricated devices and systems', *Materials Chemistry and Physics*, **42**: 169–175.

Ko, W.H and Neuman, M.R. (1967) 'Implant biotelemetry and microelectronics', *Science*, **156**(773): 351–360.

Ko, W.H., Neuman, M.R., and Lin, K.Y. (1969) 'Body reaction of implant packaging materials', in Stuart L. Ed., *Materials*, Plenum Press, New York, **10**: 55–65.

Ko, W.H., Yon, E.T., and Hynecek, J. (1970) 'Micropower pulse modulated telemetry transmitter', *23nd Ann. Conf. Eng. in Med. and Biol.* p.119, Washington, D.C.

Ko, W.H. and Hynecek, J. (1974) 'Implant evaluation of a nuclear power source-beta-cel battery', *IEEE Transactions on BME*, **21**(3): 238–241.

Ko, W.H. and Spear, T.M. (1983) 'Packaging materials and techniques for implantable instruments', *Engineering in Medicine and Biology*, **2** :24–38.

Lachhman, S. (2011) 'Evaluation and accelerated lifetime studies of medical grade poly-dimethylsiloxane as an encapsulation material', MS Thesis, EECS Department, Case Western Reserve University, Cleveland, Ohio, USA.

Lachhman, S., Zorman, C.A. and Ko, W.H. (2012) 'Multi-layered poly-dimethylsiloxane as a non-hermetic packaging material for medical MEMS', *34th Ann. Int. Conf. of IEEE Eng. Med. Biol. Soc.*, San Diego, CA.

Lin, W.C., Ruffing, F., and Ko, W.H. (1972) 'Feasibility study of engineering problems in multi-electrode visual cortex stimulation system', *Medical and Biological Engineering*, **10**: 365–375.

Lorig, R.J., Vodovnik, L., Reswick, J., Bei et al. (1967) 'An implantable system for the myo-electric stimulation of skeletal muscle using radio frequency links', *20th Ann. Conf. on Eng. in Med. and Biol.* Section 28.6, Boston, MA.

Mackay, R.S. (1959) 'Radio telemetry from within the human body', *IRE Inst. Transactions on Medical Electronics*, ME-6, 100–105.

Miklavčič, D., Kotnik, T., and Serša, G. Eds. (2003) *Lojze Vodovnik – Zbrana Dela (Collected Works)*, University of Ljubljana, Imprint International d.o.o.

Narasimhan, S., Chiel, H.J., and Bhunia, S.K. (2011) 'Ultra low-power and robust digital signal processing hardware for implantable neural interface microsystems', *IEEE Transactions on Biomedical Circuits and Systems (TBioCAS)*, **5**(2), 169–178.

Nichols, M.F. (1994) 'The challenges for hermetic encapsulation of implanted devices – a review', *Biomedical Engineering*, **22**(1): 39–67.

Peckham, P.H., Poon, C.W., Ko, W.H., Marsolais, E.B. and Rosen, J.J. (1981) 'Multichannel implantable stimulator for control of paralyzed muscle', *IEEE Transactions on Biomedical Engineering*, BME-**28**(7): 530–536.

Peckham, P.H., Keith, M. and Kilgore, K. (1993), 'Restoration of upper extremity function in tetraplegia', *IEEE Rehabilitation Engineering*, **1**(1): 8–11.

Prescott, G.B. (1884) *'Bell's electric speaking telephone: its invention, construction, application'*, D. Appleton Co. New York, Reprinted as a Google ebook, ASIN: B0021A0150.

Receveur, R.A.M., Lindemans, F.W. and de Rooij, N.F. (2007) 'Microsystem technologies for implantable applications', *Journal of Micromechanics and Microengineering*, **17**: R50–R80.

Slater, L. Ed. (1963) *Bio-Telemetry*, Pergamon, New York.

Slater, L. (1966) *Survey on Implant Biotelemetry*, BIAC Publ. (Amer. Inst. Biol. Sci.).

Wong, C.P. (1998) 'Polymers for encapsulation: materials processes and reliability', *Chip Scale Review*, **2**(1), 30.

Zhang, R., Chen, Y., Ko, W.H., Rosenbaum, D.S., Yu, X., and Feng, P.X.-L. (2011) '*Ex vivo* monitoring of rat heart wall motion using piezoelectric cantilevers', *Proceedings of the 5th Joint Conference of the 65th IEEE International Frequency Control Symposium (IFCS 2011) and the 25th European Frequency and Time Forum (EFTF 2011)*, San Francisco, CA, USA, 1–5 May 2011, pp. 868–873.

13
Wireless considerations in ocular implants based on microsystems

W. LI, Michigan State University, USA

DOI: 10.1533/9780857098610.2.424

Abstract: Artificial ocular implants have provided effective diagnostic and therapeutic techniques to individuals suffering from neural diseases and injuries of optic nerve and peripheral retinal neurons. Advanced developments in radio-frequency (RF) microelectromechanical systems (MEMS) technology have been widely employed in ocular implants to enable wireless power and data transmission between implanted devices and external units for chronic implants. This chapter provides an insightful overview to state-of-the-art developments and applications of wireless microsystems in ocular implants, with emphasis on wireless microsensors for glaucoma management and artificial retinal prostheses for vision restoration in age-related macular degeneration (AMD) and retinitis pigmentosa (RP) diseases.

Key words: wireless telemetry, RF MEMS, ocular implant, glaucoma, age-related macular degeneration, retinitis pigmentosa, intraocular pressure sensors, subretinal prosthesis, epiretinal prosthesis.

Note: This chapter is a revised and updated version of 'MEMS as ocular implants' by W. Li from the book *MEMS for biomedical applications* edited by S. Bhansali and A. Vasudev, Woodhead Publishing Limited, 2012, ISBN: 978-0-85709-129-1.

13.1 Introduction

Microelectromechanical systems (MEMS), also called micromachines (in Japan) or microsystems technology (MST) (in Europe), are microfabricated systems comprising both electrical and mechanical components. Typical dimensions of such systems range from hundreds of nanometers to millimeters. Over the past few decades, much attention has been drawn to the application of MEMS devices as biomedical implants. In addition to device development, advanced processing technologies and materials are continually evolving, driven by the demand for making biomedical devices that are less expensive and invasive, more biocompatible, and long-term reliable.

Among various implantable devices and systems, artificial ocular implants, which aim at rapid, effective, low-cost diagnosis and treatment of incurable eye diseases, have been developed by many research groups worldwide and are beginning to enter into clinical practice. Despite significant research developments and encouraging clinical results, one of the main challenges behind artificial ocular implants is power and data transmission between an implanted device and components outside of the eye in chronic implant. Conventional implantable systems involve either batteries placed inside the body or wires penetrating through skins and tissues, which are not suitable for long-term implantation for several reasons. Batteries often have a short lifetime of less than 10 years and require surgical procedures for replacement. In addition, physical connections by wires can result in ocular infection and inflammation at the location of implantation. Finally, hermetic sealing of batteries or wires in the sensitive eye environment remains a challenge.

Alternative power sources such as visible light, infrared, piezoelectric, or thermal sources have been investigated. However, they either have limited transfer efficiency or heavily depend on environmental conditions (light intensity, temperatures, etc.). Therefore, wireless power and data telemetry emerges as a critical enabling technology for advanced ocular implant applications. In particular, inductive coupling is considered as the most commonly used technique because of its many favorable properties such as miniaturized size, relatively high energy coupling efficiency, and low cost. Inductive coupling transfers electrical energy and signal using inductively coupled coils (or inductors) through near-field electromagnetic radiation. It has been employed in many ocular microsystems for sensing, diagnosis, and treatment. In this chapter, of particular interest is the management and therapy of chronic eye diseases including glaucoma, age-related macular degeneration (AMD), and retinitis pigmentosa (RP).

Here is a map of this chapter. First, the challenges of wireless ocular implants including device, system, and material constraints are outlined in Section 13.2. Then Section 13.3 discusses the design considerations of ocular microsystems from the perspectives of MEMS coils and inductive telemetric links. Next, a variety of wireless microsystems for applications in glaucoma management and AMD and RP therapy are reviewed and their important characteristics are highlighted in Section 13.4. Finally, the challenges and future research directions of these wireless ocular microsystems are envisioned in Section 13.5.

13.2 Challenges of wireless ocular implants

The human eye has limited volume (<1 cm^3) and is a corrosive environment for electronics. These factors impose multiple constraints on the hardware implementation of wireless ocular implants, pertaining to device size, power, and bandwidth of telemetric link, communication range, and biocompatibility. The following sections will discuss several main challenges from device design, system specifications, and material biocompatibility perspectives.

13.2.1 Device constraints

Typically an inductive link is formed by a pair of loosely coupled coils placed in a coaxial arrangement. In ocular implants, the coupling efficiency is greatly hindered by the presence of air, skin, tissue, and eye fluid between the two coils. In order to enhance the coupling efficiency, a secondary or implanted coil with high inductance and quality factor is required. However, intraocular coils usually suffer from low self-inductances and inevitable parasitic effects, namely parasitic resistances and capacitances, due to their small physical dimensions. Coupling strength of the inductive link is also affected by coil placement including coaxial alignment, angular alignment, and separation. Furthermore, inductive coupling in biomedical implants often occurs at a low frequency, which limits the quality factor of the implanted device. Therefore, it is critical to understand the functional properties of the intraocular coil with respect to its geometric design as well as the relationship between coil dimension and the transfer efficiency of the system, the essential elements of which will be covered in Section 13.3.1.

13.2.2 System constraints

It is important to consider the operating frequency and associated health risks when designing wireless telemetric links for biomedical applications. The most commonly used frequency band is 402–405 MHz Medical Implant Communication Service (MICS) band, regulated by the U.S. Federal Communication Commission (FCC) and the European Radiocommunications Committee (ERC). A comprehensive review of the regulatory standards for implantable medical devices can be found in Savci et al. (2005).

For power transfer via inductive telemetry in the vulnerable areas such as the eyes, the resulting RF heating of the tissue is a primary safety concern because of the relative lack of available blood flow to dissipate the excessive heat load. It is reported that microwave radiation at frequencies above 800 MHz can cause injury to the eye (Kachanov, 1986). In general, temperature increases in the eye must be kept to less than 3°C to avoid tissue damage and microwave-induced cataract formation (Hirata et al., 2000). Safety levels of human exposure to RF electromagnetic fields for frequencies between 3 kHz and 300 GHz are recommended by IEEE Standard C95.1-2005, in terms of the maximum permission exposures (MPEs) and the specific absorption rate (SAR) (2006). In particular, SAR is the quantity used to measure how much energy is actually absorbed in the human body under electromagnetic exposure. It is defined as the power absorbed per mass of the tissue and can be expressed as $SAR = \sigma E^2 / \rho$, where σ is the electrical conductivity of the tissue (in S/m), E is the root-mean-square (RMS) electric field strength in the tissue (in V/m), and ρ is the density of the tissue (in kg/m^3) (Bashirullah, 2010). In the case of whole-body exposure, a maximum SAR can be detected when RF radiation is in the range of about 80 and 100 MHz. Therefore, a whole-body average SAR of 0.4 W/kg has been set as the restriction at these frequencies, which is within the acceptable tolerance range for biological tissue (1998).

13.2.3 Material biocompatibility constraints

Careful selection of materials is critical for making biomedical devices that are intended for chronic implantation. For intraocular implants, complete hermeticity and superior biocompatibility are needed to preserve patient safety and prevent rejection of the implant, while maintaining normal functionality of devices. Presently, gold is considered as the most favorable conductive material for making implantable coils because its relatively high conductivity yields low parasitic resistance for the implantable coil. In addition, gold is highly resistant to chemical corrosion, which prolongs the lifetime of the coil in long-term implantation.

Several factors must be considered when selecting insulation materials for wireless implants, including:

- High permittivity and low loss-tangent values of materials in order to confine the near-field electromagnetic coupling inside a low-loss encapsulation layer for mitigating power loss.
- Hermetic insulation layer to avoid the permeation of the eye fluid and protect electrical components from corrosive environment.
- Biocompatibility and mechanical compatibility to allow intimate contact between implantable devices and biological environment, while minimizing physical damage to the tissue.
- Small encapsulation in order to fit in the limited space inside the eye.

Commonly used packaging approaches based on hard materials (e.g., titanium, glass, and ceramic) provide hermetic sealing of implants. However, they are usually too bulky and require a larger implant space. Other complications, such as surgical difficulty and high-cost manufacturing, are also challenges. As another promising approach, polymer-based packaging provides many advantages over conventional hard material packaging, such as mechanical flexibility, biocompatibility, low-profile encapsulation, and low cost. For example, poly(dimethylsiloxane) (PDMS) has been widely used in the fabrication of biomedical devices because of its biocompatibility approved by the Food and Drug Administration (FDA) and low manufacturing cost. PDMS-based epiretinal electrode arrays have been reported by Humayun *et al.* (2009) and Majji *et al.* (1999). Upon implantation, no retinal detachment, infection, or uncontrolled intraocular bleeding occurred. PDMS did not undergo fibrous encapsulation, discoloration, or structural changes. However, the fabrication of PDMS relies on soft-lithography, which is not compatible with conventional microfabrication techniques. PDMS also has a low Young's module, which makes it very floppy and difficult to handle during surgical operation. Polyimide is another commonly used polymeric material in intraocular implants, but it provides neither the required hermeticity nor satisfactory biocompatibility. It has been reported that polyimide can cause retinal disorganization, retinal pigment endothelium disruption, glial tissue adhesion, and pigment migration in the retina (Montezuma *et al.*, 2006).

Several research groups (Li *et al.*, 2010a; Meng and Gutierrez, 2009; Rodger *et al.*, 2008) have proposed to use parylene C as the structural and packaging material, because of its many unique properties, such as flexibility (Young's modulus ~4 GPa), chemical inertness, United States Pharmacopoeia (USP) Class VI biocompatibility, and lower water permeability compared with other commonly used polymers (e.g., PDMS and polyimide) (Licari and Hughes, 1990). *In vivo* intraocular implantation in two rabbits for six months was performed, during which parylene C did not generate detectable immune response affecting their retinas (Li *et al.*, 2006). Long-term stability of parylene packages has also been studied and preliminary results have suggested that the lifetime of parylene-coated metal at body temperature (37°C) could be more than 60 years (Li *et al.*, 2010a).

Besides the abovementioned methods, other polymer-based packaging efforts include poly(ethylene glycol)-based hydrogels, fibrin, and poly(ethylene glycol) block copolymers (Scholz, 2007). Despite the significant development of polymer packaging approaches, polymers typically do not provide complete hermeticity, and thus additional hermetic coatings are necessary. Several candidates include amorphous aluminum oxide (Henry *et al.*, 1999; Yamada-Takamura *et al.*, 2002) and diamond-like carbon (Fedel *et al.*, 2009; Roy and Lee, 2007; Sweitzer *et al.*, 2006). Detailed reviews of material aspects for biomedical implants can be found in Ghodssi *et al.* (2011) and Scholz (2007).

13.3 Considerations of ocular microsystems

Owing to the abovementioned challenges of the wireless ocular implants, specific consideration should be given to the design and fabrication of RF microcoils and telemetric links, as discussed in the following section.

13.3.1 RF MEMS coil design and microfabrication

One of the key and critical components in the inductive link is the implanted coil, which enables bidirectional communication with the external control and data acquisition units (Fig. 13.1). During the operation, a portion of alternating electromagnetic flux, generated from the primary or the external coil (L_1), is coupled to the secondary or the implanted coil (L_2). The change of flux linkage results in a voltage across the secondary coil, which is proportional to the rate of change of the electromagnetic flux and the turn number of the secondary coil. According to Faraday's law, this induced voltage (V_2) can be expressed as $V_2 = n \partial \psi_m / \partial t$, where n is the number of turns and ψ_m is the magnetic flux linkage.

For the design of the intraocular receiver coil, the competing requirements include small physical geometry, high coupling efficiency, biocompatibility, and long-term mechanical stability. In order to achieve the maximum coupling strength of the inductive link, the intraocular coil is usually implanted in the anterior chamber of the eyes so as to reduce the distance between two coils. Early developed systems mainly use thick and stiff hand-wound coils as the receiver coils, which can cause notable degradation in the implant region. Compared with conventional hand-wound coils, microfabricated coils have miniaturized dimensions more suitable for implantation in the limited space of the anterior chamber. Modern microfabrication technologies are well-established, which enables mass production, high yield, and low cost of the microcoils. Despite their many advantages, microcoils have inherent parasitic effects (e.g., parasitic resistance and capacitance), which lead to a low quality factor and coupling efficiency. To better understand the electrical properties and parasitic effects in the microcoil, several analytical models are studied, where the coil's self-inductance, effective series resistance (ESR), and parasitic capacitance can be modeled with respect to the geometric parameters of the coil.

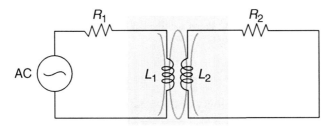

13.1 Concept of inductive coupling through alternating electromagnetic field.

Self-inductance

The self-inductance (L_s) of a planar circular coil can be expressed as (Islam, 2011; Lee, 1998):

$$L_s = \frac{\mu_0 d n^2 c_1}{2}\left[\ln\left(\frac{c_2}{\rho}\right) + c_3\rho + c_4\rho^2 + \cdots\right], \quad [13.1]$$

where μ_0 is permeability of free space, d (in cm) is the mean diameter of the coil, n is the total number of turns, c_n is function of geometry given in Islam (2011), and ρ is the filling factor defined as $\rho = (d_{out} - d_{in})/(d_{out} + d_{in})$. In the case where polygon is used as an approximation, the inductance can be calculated as:

$$L_s = \frac{\mu_0 d n^2 A_{out}}{\pi d_{out}^2}\left[\ln\left(\frac{2.46 - 1.56/N}{\rho}\right) + \left(0.2 - \frac{1.12}{N^2}\rho^2\right)\right], \quad [13.2]$$

where A_{out} is the area computed with the outer dimensions and N is the number of sides of the polygon.

Effective series resistance

ESR (R_s) is commonly used to estimate resistive loss of a microcoil, which plays an important role in designing a power efficient inductive link. The ESR can be divided into two parts: DC resistance and frequency-dependent resistance. Generally the DC resistance can be calculated using Ohm's law as given in (3),

$$R = \rho\frac{L}{A}, \quad [13.3]$$

where ρ is the resistivity (in $\Omega\cdot m$), L is the total length of conductive wire (in m), and A is the cross-section area of the wire (in m²). The frequency-dependent component is attributed to the skin effect and the proximity effect, which can change the current distribution and increase the AC resistance of the conductor. In particular, the skin effect can be evaluated using a frequency-dependent factor, the so-called skip depth δ, as given by:

$$\delta = \sqrt{\frac{2\rho}{\omega\mu}}, \quad [13.4]$$

where ρ is the electrical resistivity of the conductor (in $\Omega\cdot m$), ω is the angular frequency (in rad/s), and μ is the permeability of metal (in H/m). The proximity effect is caused by a time-varying magnetic field induced by an AC current flowing through a conductor. This alternating magnetic field can further induce eddy currents in adjacent conductors, resulting in the change of current distribution in those conductors. Mathematical approaches to model the proximity effect have been reported in several papers (Ferreira, 1994; Huan-Shang et al., 1997; Huo et al., 2006; Xi and Sullivan, 2003).

Parasitic capacitance

Parasitic capacitance (C_s) limits the self-resonant frequency of the coil, above which the coil will not behave as an inductor any more. In a first-order approximation, the parasitic capacitance of a planar coil usually has two major components: the capacitance between turns and the capacitance between layers. A distributed model has been developed to estimate the equivalent parasitic capacitance, as discussed elsewhere (Wu, 2003; Zolfaghari et al., 2001). In this approach, a planar coil is decomposed into equal sections by assuming consistent thickness and width of conductive traces everywhere. The voltage profile is obtained by averaging the beginning and ending potential across the coil structure. With known voltage variations between the correlated sections of adjacent turns and layers, the total capacitive energy stored in the coil structure can be calculated from the distributed capacitance of each segment, which can be derived using the ideal double plate capacitor formula.

Equations [13.5], [13.6], and [13.7] show the analytical formulas for calculating parasitic capacitance, where C_{ii} (in F) denotes the capacitance per unit length between adjacent metal turns, $C_{m,m-1}$ (in F) is the capacitance per unit area between the m-th and $(m-1)$-th metal layer, A_k (in m²) is the trace occupied area of the k-th turn on each layer, and $d(k) = h_1 + h_2 + \cdots + h_k$, in which h_k is defined as the ratio of the wire length of the k-th turn (l_k) to the total wire length (l_{tot}). This simplified model neglects the second order parasitic capacitances between non-adjacent turns and layers, which are much less than the first-order capacitances.

$$C_{\text{eq-turn}} = \sum_{k=1}^{n-1} \frac{1}{4} C_{ii} l_k [d(k+1) - d(k-1)]^2 \qquad [13.5]$$

$$C_{\text{eq-layer}} = \frac{1}{4} \sum_{k=1}^{N} (C_{m,m-1} + C_{m-2,m-3} + \cdots) \frac{A_k}{m^2} [4 - 2d(k-1) - 2d(k)]^2$$

$$+ \frac{1}{4} \sum_{k=1}^{N} (C_{m-1,m-2} + C_{m-3,m-4} + \cdots) \frac{A_k}{m^2} [2d(k-1) + 2d(k)]^2 \qquad [13.6]$$

$$C_{\text{eq-total}} = C_{\text{eq-turns}} + C_{\text{eq-layers}} \qquad [13.7]$$

Quality factor

Quality factor (Q factor) is an important metric for evaluating the efficiency of the microcoil, which is theoretically defined as the ratio of total stored energy to dissipated energy per cycle in a resonating system. With known L_s, R_s, and C_s, the Q factor of the coil can be derived from $Q \approx \omega L_s / R_s = \sqrt{L_s/C_s} R_s$, where the resonant angular frequency ω can be expressed as

$$\omega = \sqrt{\frac{1}{L_s C_s} - \frac{R_s^2}{L_s^2}} \approx \sqrt{\frac{1}{L_s C_s}} \text{ when } R_s \ll \sqrt{\frac{L_s}{C_s}}.$$

For an intraocular coil, the Q factor must be enhanced in order to minimize the power loss in the device as well as to maximize the transfer efficiency of power telemetric link. The enhancement of the Q factor can be achieved by increasing the number of turns (n) and the thickness of the conductive layer. Considerable research efforts have been directed to maximize the coupling efficiency of the three-dimensional (3-D) coils (Fig. 13.2). For example, electroplating is often used to create a thick conductive layer, which can effectively reduce the parasitic resistance (Mokwa *et al.*, 2008). A multilayer polymer–metal thin-film technique has also been developed in order to increase the number of turns, while maintaining the device flexibility. Based on this technique, a variety of flexible polymer-based intraocular MEMS coils have been built (Li *et al.*, 2005, 2006). To minimize the fabrication complication, Li *et al.* proposed a fold-and-bond 3-D coil configuration, which significantly improves the quality factor of microcoils by increasing the number of stacked layers (Chen *et al.*, 2008a). Recently, a microfabricated foil coil with a 17-strand planar Litz design was invented in order to reduce the AC parasitic resistance at high frequencies (Zhao *et al.*, 2012). Future research aims to optimize the design and fabrication of the microcoil and maximize the efficiency of inductive coupling.

13.3.2 Wireless telemetry link for power and data transmission

Inductive coupling is an established field and extensive research has been performed to analyze and optimize the operation of inductive links for biomedical applications (Kendir *et al.*, 2005a; Kim and Wise, 1996; Hamici *et al.*,

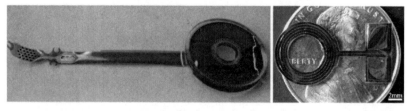

13.2 (Left) An electroplated microcoil developed by EPI-RET. (Image reprinted from Mokwa *et al.* (2008) with permission of IEEE). (Right) A flexible parylene-based microcoil developed by Li *et al.* (2005).

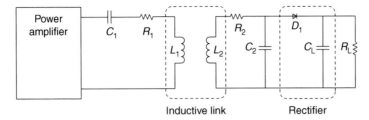

13.3 System overview of an inductive power link for biomedical applications. The secondary stage is modeled as a nonlinear circuit.

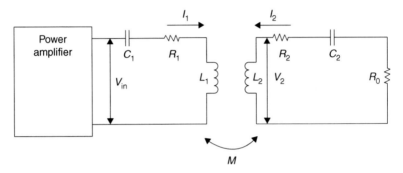

13.4 The secondary stage is simplified with an approximated linear model.

1996; Ziaie *et al.*, 1997). Typically, an inductive link for biomedical applications involves both power and data telemetries to transfer electrical power from an external unit to an internal unit and exchange data between the external and internal units.

Power telemetry

Power telemetry through two coaxially aligned coils is a commonly used configuration for biomedical implantation. A basic inductive power link can be modeled using a nonlinear circuit, as depicted in Fig. 13.3. In this model, the load of the implanted electronics to which power is delivered is represented by R_L. The rectifier is modeled with a diode (D_1) and a capacitor (C_L). The lossy transmitter coil is modeled with an ideal inductance (L_1) and an ESR (R_1). Similarly, the receiver coil is modeled with L_2 and R_2. The parasitic capacitors of the coils and the tuning capacitors are combined together as C_1 and C_2. To maximize coupling efficiency, the primary and secondary stages are both tuned to the same resonant frequency $\omega = 1/\sqrt{L_1 C_1} = 1/\sqrt{L_2 C_2}$.

However, analysis of this model is not trivial due to the nonlinearity of the rectifier. To reduce the complication, this nonlinear circuit can be converted into a linear circuit by transferring the DC load into an AC equivalent load (Fig. 13.4), following the approach in Ko *et al.* (1977b). In this case, the AC linear load can be calculated as $R_0 = 1/(\omega^2 C_2^2 R_L / 2) = 2\omega^2 L_2^2 / R_L$, to maintain a power dissipation equivalent to the DC power. The mutual inductance is associated with L_1 and L_2 by coupling coefficient and defined as $M = k\sqrt{L_1 L_2}$. The coupling coefficient, denoted by k, is a function of coil geometry and alignment, and can be obtained from Ko et al. (1977b).

Based on the equivalent linear circuit, the overall voltage gain of the inductive link can be calculated by keeping the same power consumption between the AC load and DC load, as given by:

$$G_v = \frac{V_{out}}{V_{in}} = \frac{V_0}{V_{in}} \sqrt{\frac{R_L}{R_0}} = \frac{j\sqrt{2}\omega^2 M L_2}{\frac{2\omega^2 L_2^2}{R_L} R_1 + R_2 R_1 + \omega^2 M^2}. \quad [13.8]$$

The total power-transfer efficiency of the inductive link, defined as the ratio between the power delivered to the load and the output power from the power amplifier, is expressed as:

$$\eta = \frac{P_{out}}{P_{in}} = \frac{\frac{1}{2}|V_0 I_0|}{\frac{1}{2}|V_{in} I_1|} = \frac{\omega^2 M^2 R_0}{R_1(R_2 + R_0)^2 + \omega^2 M^2 (R_2 + R_0)}. \quad [13.9]$$

The power lost in the receiver coil is determined by the ratio of P_{R1} over P_{in}:

$$\eta_{lost} = \frac{P_{R1}}{P_{in}} = \left|\frac{I_2^2 R_2}{V_2 I_2}\right| = \frac{\omega^2 M^2 R_2}{R_1(R_2 + R_0)^2 + \omega^2 M^2 (R_2 + R_0)}. \quad [13.10]$$

From the theoretical analysis, it can be seen that the performance of the power telemetry link is affected by several factors. First, the voltage gain and the power-transfer efficiency are functions of the self- and the mutual-inductances of the receiver and transmitter coils, which are dependent on the sizes and the number of turns of the coils (Heetderks, 1988). For implantable systems, the limits on the size of the receiver coil are usually more stringent than those of the transmitter coil. Second, the alignment and spacing between coils can significantly affect the coupling coefficient. Two typical types of misalignment, including lateral misalignment and angular misalignment, can significantly reduce the coupling efficiency (Soma et al., 1987). It is also reported that, when the receiver coil is placed within the circumference of the transmitter coil, the coupling is comparable or even better than that with an exact coaxial alignment (Heetderks, 1988). Third, reasonably high Q factors are desired in order to achieve satisfactory power transfer (Ko et al., 1977a; Vandevoorde and Puers, 2001). The output voltage becomes sensitive to load change if the Q factor is low. Therefore, the frequency of operation should be carefully designed in order to enhance the Q factor, while maintaining the tissue absorption of electromagnetic energy within an acceptable safe range. Finally, low-loss switching amplifiers are desired to drive the transmitter coil. The drive transistor should consume minimum power in order to achieve a power efficient system. Most commonly used circuit topologies reported are class-C (Ko *et al.*, 1977a; Van Schuylenbergh and Puers, 1996b), class-E (Guoxing *et al.*, 2005; Kendir *et al.*, 2005b; Piedade *et al.*, 2005; Puers *et al.*, 2000a; Sokal and Sokal, 1975, Sauer *et al.*, 2005), class-D (Donaldson and Perkins, 1983; Galbraith *et al.*, 1987), and class-C–E (Vandevoorde and Puers, 2001).

Data telemetry

Wireless transmission of data is critical for real-time monitoring and diagnosis. Closed-loop data telemetry involves data transmission from transmitter to power receiver (forward telemetry) and data transmission from receiver to transmitter (backward telemetry). For an inductively powered system, the wireless transmission of the data signal can be conducted through either the power link coils or a separate pair of coils. Several modulation schemes, such as amplitude-shift keying (ASK), frequency-shift keying (FSK), or load-shift keying (LSK), have been explored to achieve high energy efficiency, by taking the benefits of low data rate and short distance communication associated with biomedical telemetry (Ghovanloo and Najafi, 2004; Sacristan-Riquelme *et al.*, 2008; Tang *et al.*, 1995).

Date telemetry for biomedical applications should not interfere with existing communication systems. Therefore, medical devices tend to use industrial, scientific, and medical (ISM) frequency bands with low data rate operation. For example, pacemakers, cardiac defibrillators and analog cochlear processors typically use data bandwidths of around 8 kbps (Sarpeshkar *et al.*, 2005; Wise *et al.*, 2004; Wong *et al.*, 2004); neural recording often uses 800 kbps (Wise *et al.*, 2004); and retinal stimulators use 40 kbps data rate (Weiland *et al.*, 2005).

13.4 Applications of wireless microsystems in ocular implants

This section discusses representative applications of wireless microsystems in intraocular implants, including intraocular pressure (IOP) monitoring devices and wireless retinal prosthetic systems.

13.4.1 Wireless intraocular pressure sensors for glaucoma management

Overview of glaucoma disease

Glaucoma is a group of debilitating eye diseases, and the second leading cause of blindness in the world after cataracts. Worldwide, it is estimated that approximately 66.8 million people have developed visual impairment from glaucoma, with nearly 6.7 million suffering from bilateral blindness (American Health Assistance Foundation (2011a)). It is predicted that the number of glaucoma patients will increase to 79.6 million by 2020 (Quigley and Broman, 2006). Pathological studies reveal that visual impairment and blindness in glaucomatous eyes can be attributed to optic nerve damage, which is characterized by the progression of optic disc cupping (Chauhan et al., 2001). The initial site of injury is the optic nerve head, where retinal ganglion cell axons exit the eye and form the optic nerve. A focal point of axon injury then travels along the optic nerve in both directions, resulting in retrograde degeneration of ganglion cells within the retina and anterograde degeneration of their target neurons in the visual thalamus (Weber et al., 2008).

In many glaucomatous cases, abnormal elevation and fluctuation of IOP are considered as the major risk factors for structural changes in the eye, optical nerve damage, and a progressive loss of vision. In the normal eye, a positive pressure (about 10–15 mmHg), the so-called IOP, is created and maintained by continuous aqueous humor flow. Aqueous humor is produced from the ciliary body, then flows into anterior chamber though the pupil, and finally drains from the eye through a drainage pathway presented by trabecular meshwork and Schlemm's canal between the cornea and iris (Ethier et al., 2004). Among different types of glaucoma diseases, primary open-angle glaucoma is known to be the most common and the most referenced type. In such cases, while the production of aqueous humor remains unaffected, the drainage pathway is often blocked, leading to ocular fluid buildup and elevated IOP (≥ 22 mmHg). Elevated IOP can then result in shearing and compressive forces that damage the nerve fibers by affecting the vasculature that sustains them. Other types of glaucoma, such as angle-closure, low-tension (normal-tension, where no abnormal IOP elevation occurs), congenital, and secondary glaucoma, are not always associated with IOP elevation, but they are not as common as the open-angle form.

Glaucoma diseases often have no pain or significant symptoms until the irreversible and incurable optical nerve damage occurs. Therefore, accurate real-time IOP monitoring and prompt treatments at the early stages of glaucoma development are critical for successful glaucoma management. At present, tonometry is still the gold standard for clinical IOP measurement, in which the IOP is calculated by measuring an external counter force/pressure that balances the internal pressure of the cornea over a pre-determined area. Goldmann applanation tonometry (GAT), dynamic contour tonometer, and pneumotonometry are a few examples based on this technique (Debry et al., 2003; Ducrey et al., 1975; Moses, 1958). Although tonometry provides a simple and non-invasive solution for monitoring IOP, the achievable accuracy of the measurement strongly depends on many factors, such as corneal thickness, corneal curvature, and ocular mechanical rigidity (Chihara, 2008; Elsheikh *et al.*, 2011; Francis *et al.*, 2007; Tonnu *et al.*, 2005). In addition, measurement procedures usually require operation from specialists and cooperation from patients, which are not suitable for continuous monitoring of pressure fluctuations. A direct, convenient, real-time, and reliable sensing technology is necessary for prompt diagnosis and monitoring of the IOP in glaucoma.

MEMS-based IOP sensing devices have received much attention in recent years, by leveraging advanced MEMS technology to realize miniaturized, highly-sensitive, accurate systems for IOP measurement. A number of continuous IOP monitoring devices have been developed, which can be categorized into two types: wired sensors and wireless sensors. Typically, wired IOP sensors are designed based on a non-invasive pressure-sensing technique proposed by Gillman and Greene in 1974, which placed a soft contact lens with embedded strain gauge over cornea to monitor IOP by sensing the deformation of the meridional angle at the corneoscleral junction (Greene and Gilman, 1974). Gauge wires were connected to an external Wheatstone bridge circuit through the temporal canthus. The pressure variation was recorded by balancing the bridge manually. Leonardi *et al.* improved the device by integrating a soft contact lens with microfabricated platinum–titanium strain gauges (Leonardi *et al.*, 2004). The gauges had a built-in Wheatstone bridge configuration and were shaped to match the corneal curvature. The devices were tested in porcine eyes with a sensitivity of 8.36 V/mmHg. Initial clinical trials of such devices in patients with open-angle glaucoma recently have been reported, indicating adequate safety and functionality to monitor IOP fluctuations over 24 h (Mansouri and Shaarawy, 2011). While the wired IOP sensors allow for non-invasive continuous IOP monitoring and eliminate potential surgeical complications, the accuracy of the pressure measurement is still affected by tissue-wall thickness, corneal rigidity, eye size, and other factors, such as eye movement and lid pressure. Unlike wired sensors, wireless IOP sensors permit fully intraocular implantation and thus minimize potential interference from cornea and environment.

Wireless intraocular pressure sensors

Modern wireless IOP sensors can be classified into two categories: passive sensors and active sensors, which will be discussed in the following sections.

Passive wireless IOP sensors: Passive telemetric sensing has been developed for decades as a viable method for continuous and accurate non-contact IOP measurement. The system usually consists of a reader unit mounted on a pair of glasses and a sensing unit implanted in the eye, as illustrated in Fig. 13.5. The implanted sensing unit is designed in an inductor

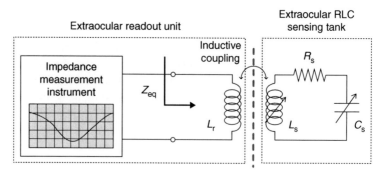

13.5 Conceptual illustration of the passive wireless IOP sensor.

(L)-capacitor (C) resonant configuration, which uses a variable capacitor, or variable inductor, or both as pressure sensitivity elements. The resonant frequency of this LC tank (f_s) can be represented as:

$$f_s = \frac{1}{2\pi}\sqrt{\frac{1}{L_s C_s} - \frac{R_s^2}{L_s^2}} \approx \sqrt{\frac{1}{L_s C_s}}, \quad \text{if } R_s \ll \sqrt{\frac{L_s}{C_s}}. \quad [13.11]$$

When the device operates in sensing mode, the relative frequency variation of the LC circuit is directly related to the variations of inductance and/or capacitance that have resulted from IOP changes, as expressed:

$$\frac{\Delta f_s}{f_s} \sim -\frac{1}{2}\frac{\Delta L_s}{L_s} - \frac{1}{2}\frac{\Delta C_s}{C_s}. \quad [13.12]$$

This frequency shift can be interrogated with the external reader coil by sweeping either impedance magnitude or phase in the frequency domain.

The earliest passive wireless sensor was reported by Collins in 1967 (Collins, 1967). The device contained a gas bubble encapsulated in a glass cylindrical container ranging in size from 2 to 6 mm, with flexible polyester diaphragms to seal the ends of the container. A pair of parallel, coaxial, spiral coils was attached to the inner surfaces of the diaphragms as an inductive link. As IOP rose, the distance between the diaphragms decreased, resulting in the increase of mutual inductance and finally the decrease of the resonant frequency. Based on this concept, Rosengren et al. (1992, 1994) introduced silicon microfabrication technologies into the fabrication of a passive pressure sensor for device miniaturization. In their approach, a micromachined thin membrane and a substrate acted as capacitor plates, which were bonded together using silicon fusion bonding. A hand-wound coil made of 6–12 turns of 50 μm diameter gold wire was attached to the capacitor plates to form a resonant circuit. Silicone encapsulation with overall dimensions of $3 \times 3 \times 1$ mm³ was used to ensure device biocompatiblity and ease of surgery. This sensor was tested in both *in vitro* and *in vivo* (in the anterior chamber of a rabbit eye) experiments, showing an *in vitro* sensitivity of 4 mV/mmHg.

Recently, the rapid growth of MEMS technology has generated tremendous opportunities for the development of IOP sensors. As one of the most significant innovations, MEMS RF coils are adapted to replace bulky hand-wound coils in order to facilitate monolithic integration and packaging of LC elements with a high degree of miniaturization. The first reported MEMS coiled passive sensor involved a plannar coil patterned on capacitor electrodes (Van Schuylenbergh and Puers, 1996a). Further improvements include: the application of electroplating technique to achieve high Q factor of coils (Puers *et al.*, 2000b); the introduction of a ferrite core to enhance telemetric coupling effeciency (Baldi *et al.*, 2003); and the development of inovative integration/packaging techniques (e.g., glass–silicon bonding, flip-chip interconnect, and surface macromachining) (Akar *et al.*, 2001; Dehennis and Wise, 2002; Katuri *et al.*, 2010). These devices, however, are all made of hard materials, such as glass or silicon. Material biocompatibility and long-term reliability still remain as the main challenges.

As an alternative option, polymer-based MEMS techniques have become very attractive, because of their excellent biocompatibility and flexibility compared to conventional semiconductor materials. Forseca *et al.* (2006) reported two types of flexible passive IOP sensor, in which microcoils were fabricated from laminated sheets of copper–clad liquid–crystal polymer (LCP) and polytetrafluoroethylene (PTFE) and bonded with PTFE/ceramic capacitor chambers. The sensors had overall dimensions of ~11 mm in outer diameter and ~0.3 mm in total thickness. The device was very flexible and could be rolled into a catheter with an internal dimater of less than 4 mm. The devices were tested in canine models for over 30 days with a total sensitivity of 5.76 kHz/mmHg and a resonant frequency of 35.677 MHz respectively, indicating the possibility for long-term implant. Similar devices have been monolithically microfabricated by utilizing parylene C (poly-chloropxylylene) as a structural and packaging material to improve the hermeticity of packaging, while maintaining device flexibility and biocompatibility (Chen *et al.*, 2008b, 2010).

Examples of several reported wireless passive IOP sensors are given in Fig. 13.6. Despite the numerous benefits of passive IOP sensors, they often suffer from low inductive coupling efficiency due to the size constraints of microcoils (Katuri *et al.*, 2008). Consequently, such passive sensors are limited in detectable distance, and require perfect alignment between the implant and the external data acquisition unit. In addtion, inevitable dielectric losses in the eye fluid can further impair coil coupling, resulting in malfunction of passive devices in chronic applications.

Active wireless IOP sensors: As the implanted coil becomes smaller and smaller, active telemetry provides a suitable solution to transmitting power

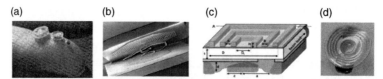

13.6 Examples of several reported wireless passive IOP sensors (a) image reprinted from Collins (1967) with permission of IEEE, (b) image reprinted from Puers *et al.* (2000b) with permission of IOP Publishing Ltd, (c) image reprinted from Dehennis and Wise (2002) with permission of IEEE, (d) image reprinted from Chen *et al.* (2010) with permission of IEEE.

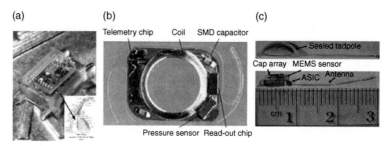

13.7 Examples of several reported wireless active IOP sensors: (a) image reprinted from Chen *et al.* (2011) with permission of IEEE, (b) image reprinted from Eggers *et al.* (2000) with permission of IEEE, (c) image reprinted from Chow *et al.* (2010) with permission of IEEE. The inset figure in panel (a) represents the location of the implanted device in the eye.

and data efficiently and effectively over a larger separation. Capacitive transducers are usually used in active devices as pressure-sensing elements to ensure low power consumption, low noise, high sensitivity, low temperature drift, and good long-term stability. In addition, active sensing systems often contain on-chip circuitry and memory for data analysis and storage and thus do not constantly require an external data acquisition unit. In contrast to passive sensing that has relatively flexible design considerations, the telemetric link design of active sensing has critical concerns such as power/data transmission, coil dimension, and signal-to-noise ratio.

There are many active IOP sensing devices in the research-and-development phase from several leading groups (Fig. 13.7). For example, Eggers *et al.* (2000) reported a flip-chip mounted multichip module (MCM) with overall dimensions of 6.5 mm × 9 mm. The MCM consisted of a capacitive absolute pressure sensor for IOP monitoring, a readout circuitry for data conversion, a telemetric chip for data reduction, and a coil for data transmission. The system operated at a resonant frequency of 125 Hz with a sampling rate of 30 samples per second and a current consumption of less than 85 μA at a supply voltage of 3.5 V. Later on, Stangel *et al.* (2001) made significant improvements by integrating a micromechanical pressure-sensor array, a temperature sensor, readout and calibration electronics, a µC-based digital control unit, and an RF transponder on a single complementary metal oxide semiconductor (CMOS) chip. Pressure independent reference capacitors were incorporated to reduce possible parasitic effects. The sensing unit was mounted to an artificial intraocular lens with a diameter of ~10 mm (Mokwa, 2007). The telemetric link was implemented at an operation frequency of 13.56 MHz. The power consumption of the data readout and calibration electronics was measured to be less than 210 µW. However, these active devices still use inductive coupling for power transmission and thus have a limited operation range. In addition, the devices are mounted on the intraocular lens, resulting in relatively large sizes. The constant requirement of an external data acquisition unit also limits its flexibility for use in continues monitoring.

To address these challenges, Chow *et al.* (2010) proposed a low-power active sensing system for IOP monitoring. The sensor consisted of a MEMS sensor, a microscale antenna, an on-chip memory, a capacitive powering array, and an application-specific integrated circuit (ASIC) assembled on a liquid-crystal polymer-based tadpole-shaped package. The sensor operated at 2.4 GHz, allowing for orientation independent transfer of power and data over a 50-cm telemetric distance. The on-chip FeRAM memory permitted continuous data recording every 5 min over a 24 h monitoring period. At the end of each period, wireless data transmission and power capacitor recharging were performed simultaneously through an external unit. The average power consumption of the entire system over one monitoring period was measured to be ~675.67 pW. A similar system has been reported by Chen and his colleagues at the University of Michigan (Chen *et al.*, 2011). In their approach, a 0.07 mm^2 solar cell and Cymbet thin-film lithium battery were assembled in a 1.5 mm^3 biocompatible transparent housing, along with other system components (e.g., data converter, MEMS sensor, telemetry circuitry, microprocessor, and memory). This system had a large transmission distance of 50 cm in saline. Given the average power consumption of 5.3 nW, it is estimated that this device could be used for 28 days without energy harvesting. The integrated solar cell can convert light energy into electric energy, which can potentially extend the operating lifetime of the implanted device.

Whereas active wireless IOP sensors have shown better performance in transmission distance and data management, such device designs are more complex compared with passive devices. In addition, the fabrication complication makes active devices more expensive and less reliable, and thus batch manufacturing techniques are necessary to improve device productivity and reliability. The device biocompatibility and long-term use in a biological environment will need further investigation. Besides the abovementioned wireless sensing techniques, IOP sensors based on other techniques, such as the mechanical Bourdon tube, have been reported in Chen *et al.* (2007). A comprehensive review of IOP sensing techniques can be found in Katuri *et al.* (2008).

13.4.2 Wireless retinal prosthetic systems

Retinal prosthesis is also a very rapidly moving field of wireless MEMS systems. Whereas the previous section described microsystems that could prevent blindness of individuals by continuous IOP monitoring, this section will concentrate on implantable electronic devices designed to replicate the function of the retina for patients with loss of vision due to AMD and RP.

Overview of age-related macular degeneration and retinitis pigmentosa

AMD and RP are two of the most common outer retinal degenerative diseases that result in the vision impairment and blindness of millions of people worldwide. AMD primarily affects the central vision regions in people age 60 and older. It cannot be easily diagnosed until its advanced stages, because the brain will compensate for central dark patches during its early stages. According to the World Health Organization (WHO), AMD has become the third leading cause of blindness on global scale, and ranks first in developed countries (2008). RP is a genetic eye disease, in which visual deterioration develops gradually and progressively, starting from defective dark adaptation, followed by the reduction of peripheral vision (known as tunnel vision), and, sometimes, a complete vision loss in the advanced stage. It is estimated that RP has affected more than 500,000 people in the United States, among which 20,000 are legally blind (Artificial Retina Project, 2011b).

Although the mechanisms of these diseases have not been fully understood, histopathological studies reveal that they are mainly restricted to the outer retinal region and are associated with damage to the photoreceptor cells (Berson, 1993; Curcio *et al.*, 1996; Green and Enger, 1993; Verhoeff, 1931). The photoreceptor cells (rods and cones) are situated in a deep retinal layer, and they, along with bipolar, ganglion, horizontal, and amacrine cells, perform significant visual processing and communication tasks in normal vision. In a healthy visual pathway, the photoreceptors initiate neural responses to incoming light by converting light into chemical and electrical signals. The bipolar and ganglion cells in the inner retina then pass the visual signals to the optic nerve. Along the way, the horizontal and amacrine cells provide lateral interaction between neighboring cells.

Presently, blindness due to outer retinal degenerative diseases remains incurable. Current clinical interventions include gene replacement therapy, pharmaceutical therapy, nutritional therapy, and dietary measures to slow down the progressive development of retinal degeneration (Bennett *et al.*, 1996; Berson *et al.*, 1993). Whereas photoreceptor and stem cell transplantations can be possible solutions to cure these diseases by replacing the damaged retinal cells (Maclaren *et al.*, 2006; Tropepe *et al.*, 2000), they are still in the early stages of development, and not yet ready for clinical practice. Other concerns, such as high costs and ethical issues, also limit the use of such techniques in neural therapy.

Alternative approaches, known as bioelectronic visual prostheses, have been developed, which utilize electrical stimulation to partially restore the lost vision function of patients, bypassing the damaged photoreceptor cells. Early work toward visual prostheses started from electrical stimulation of visual cortex (Brindley and Lewin, 1968; Dobelle, 2000; Dobelle and Mladejovsky, 1974). This technique provides good protection for implanted devices and enables treatments of various types of blindness due to both optic nerve and retina damages. However, visual cortex usually has complex spatial organization so that patterned electrical stimulations may not produce the same perceptional patterns. Other challenges include surgical complexity, long-term reliability, limited resolution, and local heating. Optic nerve prosthetic devices have also been developed to directly stimulate the optic nerve to treat both retinal degenerative and non-retinal degenerative blindness (Veraart *et al.*, 1998; Yagi *et al.*, 1999). However, several inevitable problems associated with this approach are: (1) difficulties with high-density stimulation and detail perception due to the high density of the axons; (2) surgical complexity and possible harmful side effects after implantation; and (3) the difficulty of implementing a complete intraocular system.

In the 1990s, Humayun *et al.* conducted morphometric analysis of RP patients' retinas and found that, although their photoreceptors are defective, the optic nerves and bipolar and ganglion cells, to which the photoreceptors synapse, still remain largely functional (Humayun *et al.*, 1999). Similar results were discovered later in AMD patients (Kim *et al.*, 2002). These profound results created the possibility of using retinal prostheses to treat AMD and RP patients. To date, many high-quality techniques have been developed and some of them have been utilized in clinical trials. In particular, microscale retinal implants provide many advantages, such as the possibility of high-density stimulation, better heat dissipation through aqueous humor flow, miniaturized overall device dimension, and lower stimulating threshold. Furthermore, the applications of RF microtechnologies in the retinal prosthetic system enable wireless power delivery and data communication between the implanted devices and external units to achieve truly intraocular implants. Depending on the layer of retina receiving the implanted device, there are two main categories of ocular prostheses currently being studied by several groups: subretinal and epiretinal prostheses.

Wireless subretinal prostheses

Subretinal prosthesis is performed behind the retina between the bipolar cell layer and the retinal pigment epithelium by replacing the degenerated photoreceptors with electronic devices. The first form of wireless subretinal implants, known as artificial silicon retinas, was developed based on optical transmission by Chow and his colleagues in the 1990s (Chow, 1993, Chow *et al.*, 2001, 2004). This device contained 5000 integrated microphotodiodes on a disk with thickness of around 50–100 μm and diameter of 2–3 mm. Upon implantation into the subretinal space, these light-sensitive microphotodiodes can be activated by 500–1100 nm incident light through the transparent retina and the resulting electric stimulation pattern is projected onto the retina to excite adjacent sensory neurons in the remaining retinal network. Based on this concept, similar wireless systems have also been investigated with various modifications by: (1) combining amplification circuitry with photovoltaic pixels to improve power efficiency (Loudin *et al.*, 2007; Palanker *et al.*, 2005); (2) incorporating laser diodes to increase image brightness (Asher *et al.*, 2007); (3) improving power consumption and chip resolution (Mazza *et al.*, 2005, Rothermel *et al.*, 2009); and (4) applying an extraocular wired unit as energy sources of photodiodes (Zrenner *et al.*, 2011). The efficacy and safety of these devices have been proven in animal tests and clinical trials (Chow *et al.*, 2004; Zrenner *et al.*, 1997, 1999).

To improve the stimulation efficiency for clinical applications, a subretinal approach based on inductive telemetry (Fig. 13.8) has been investigated by the Boston Retinal Implant Project. In this case, the stimulation current was directly transmitted from an extraocular data acquisition unit through telemetric coupling of a pair of coils (Rizzo, 2011). The external unit consisted of a small camera for collecting visual images and an RF transmitter coil to transfer power and signals to a receiver coil located around the limbus. A stimulation electrode array, with more than 200 individually controlled electrodes, was the only component implanted in the subretinal space. This system allowed independent control and adjustment of the stimulation parameters to individual electrodes based on the feedback of patients. The electrodes integrated on the flexible substrate can bend to match the ocular contours and minimize the disruption of the eye anatomy. Current efforts primarily focus on clinical trials to assess the long-term functionality and biocompatibility of this system. However, similar to the abovementioned subretinal implants, the electrode array introduces a barrier between the outer retina and the choroid, resulting in disruption to the nutritional supply of the retina derived from the choroid. Furthermore, subretinal fluid, which is initially released as the response to subretinal foreign bodies, may disrupt the contact between the retina and the electrode array.

Other wireless approaches, based on optogenetics, have also been explored, which eliminate the need for surgical implant and allow for individual

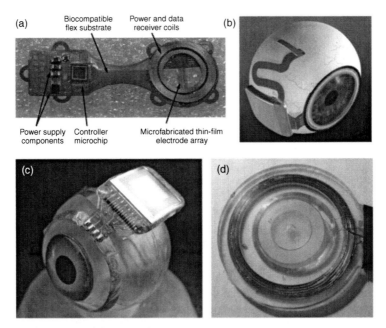

13.8 Images of the first-generation and the second-generation subretinal prosthetic devices developed by the Boston Retinal Implant Project. (a) First generation retinal prosthetic device. (b) Conceptual schematic of the hermetic implant concept. (c) A prototype of the hermetic retinal prosthetic device attached to a plastic model eye. The power and data secondary coils are formed on a sphere to match the eye's curvature. (d) The primary coils are potted in a PDMS mold. (Image reprinted from Kelly *et al.* (2011) with permission of IEEE.)

access to target receptive fields and cells. For example, a biochemical-based photostimulation approach was proposed in which non-light-sensitive retinal ganglion cells (RGCs) and/or bipolar cells were biochemically re-engineered to become light sensitive using a protein (Channelrhodopsin-2) as phototransduction mechanism (Nikolic *et al.*, 2006). However, the effectiveness of subretinal prosthesis could be limited if the inner retinal layers had been damaged following photoreceptor degeneration (Matthaei *et al.*, 2011). Therefore, many researchers are interested in using epiretinal prosthetic devices to directly stimulate ganglion cells with localized stimulator electrodes, bypassing the normal visual pathway.

Wireless epiretinal prostheses

In the epiretinal approach, an array of electrodes must be introduced into the vitreous space in contact with the ganglion cell layer. These electrodes stimulate the remaining neural cells to partially restore vision upon the

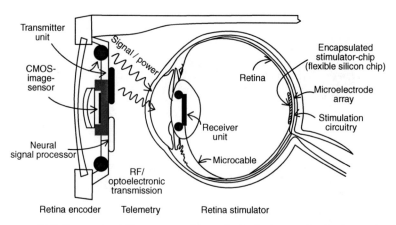

13.9 Conceptual illustration of a typical wireless epiretinal prosthetic system. (Images reprinted from Trieu *et al.* (1998) with permission of IEEE.)

reception of signals through data transmission and processing units. A number of engineering approaches have been developed by several leading groups in the United States, Germany, Australia, and Korea. As shown in Fig. 13.9, these wireless epiretinal prosthetic systems all have similar system configurations, which consist of:

- an electrode array implanted on the surface of the inner retina between the vitreous and internal limiting membrane;
- a data acquisition system located outside of the body for capturing images from the surroundings and converting analog information into patterns of electrical signals;
- a power and data transmission unit through a telemetric link.

As early as 1994, Humayun *et al.* reported that stimulation of the vertebrate inner retinal layers can elicit a localized light perception (Humayun *et al.*, 1994). Since then, his team at the Doheny Eye Institute at the University of Southern California (USC), collaborating with a group of researchers and industrial partners, has developed a series of extraocular retinal prosthesis techniques. The implanted unit of the first generation model consisted of an intraocular part (an electrode array) and an extraocular part (an electronic box including a receiving coil). A 16 platinum microelectrode array on a 5 mm × 5 mm area made by Second Sight Medical Products, Inc (Sylmar, CA, USA) was positioned to the fovea and attached to the inner retinal surface using a retinal tack. A hand-made coil was hung outside of the eye, in the temporal skull, to transfer power and data through inductive coupling. After demonstrating the device functionality in animal models and short-term human studies, clinical trials have started since 2002 to verify the long-term feasibility of this 16-electrode implant (Argus-I). Six human subjects with minimal or no light perception could distinguish motion and locate objects (plate, cup, and knife) after receiving the implants (Weiland *et al.*, 2005). Recently, this research has progressed into its second phase, in which a 60-electrode device (Argus-II) has succeeded in *in vivo* animal studies and is currently being tested in 17 human subjects (Fig. 13.10). It is reported that these patients have shown 86% and 73% improvements in door finding and line tracking 6 months post-operatively (Humayun *et al.*, 2009).

Clinical trials of similar epiretinal implants have also been performed by two German epiretinal prosthesis teams. The first, Intelligent Medical Implants AG, reported the implantation of an intraocular stimulation array with 49 platinum electrodes in human subjects. Patients with such implants were able to see phosphenes and crude shapes correlating to the applied stimuli (Weiland and Humayun, 2008). The second German group, EPI-RET GmbH, has also successfully implanted a 25-electrode array (EPIRET3) into six patients with RP and blindness for a period of 4 weeks (Fig. 13.11).

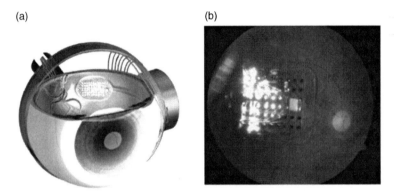

13.10 (a) Schematic view of the Argus™ II system and (b) photograph of the Argus™ II electrode array located on a degenerated retina. (Image reprinted from Mokwa (2011) with permission of IEEE.)

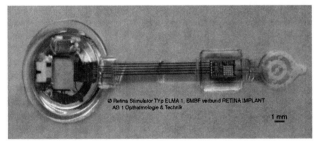

13.11 Epiretinal implant developed by German EPI-RET team. The system is encapsulated with parylene C and silicone rubber. (Image reprinted from Stieglitz (2009) with permission of IOP Publishing Ltd.)

The results show that this wireless implant was well tolerated with temporary moderate postoperative inflammation, and the position of the implants remained stable until removal (Klauke *et al.*, 2011; Walter *et al.*, 2009). Several other groups have also designed varied configurations of epiretinal implants based on the concept of Second Sight. The Australian Vision Prosthesis Group (AVPG) has implemented an epiretinal implant system that features a unique hexagonal electrode array and wireless power/data telemetric link (Wong *et al.*, 2007). The device has been tested in animal models (Kerdraon *et al.*, 2002) and is entering into acute human testing (Dowling, 2008).

Table 13.1 Summary on several date telemetric links for wireless retinal prostheses

Application	Modulation type	Data rate carrier	Reference
Epiretinal prosthesis	ASK	300 kbps 402–405 MHz	David *et al.* (2009)
Epiretinal prosthesis	FSK	~2 Mbps, 20 MHz	Jung *et al.* (2007)
Epiretinal prosthesis	LSK-PWM	3.3 kbps, 1 MHz	Guoxing *et al.* (2005)
Epiretinal prosthesis	ASK	N/A, 200 kHz	Schwarz *et al.* (2000)
Epiretinal prosthesis	ASK–PWM*	25–250 kbps 1–10 MHz	Liu *et al.* (2000)
Subretinal prosthesis	ASK	100 kbps, 13.56 MHz	Theogarajan (2008)
Subretinal prosthesis	ASK	100 kbps 15 MHz	Shire *et al.* (2009)

*PWM: Pulse-Width Modulation

Table 13.2 Summary on several power telemetric links for wireless retinal prostheses

Application	Power transfer	Frequency	Coil type	Reference
Epiretinal prosthesis	45 mW	1–10 MHz	N/A	David *et al.* (2009)
Epiretinal prosthesis	250 mW	1 MHz	Litz wire	Kendir *et al.* (2005b)
Epiretinal prosthesis	N/A	2.5 MHz	Copper wire	Suaning and Lovell (2001)
Epiretinal prosthesis	6 mW	13.56 MHz	Wire	Schwarz *et al.* (1999)
Subretinal prosthesis	2 mW	500 kHz	Gold magnet wire	Rizzo *et al.* (2011)
Subretinal prosthesis	N/A	125 kHz	Wire	Shire *et al.* (2009)

The data and power telemetric links used in several representative epiretinal microsystems are summarized in Tables 13.1 and 13.2, respectively. Extensive reviews on artificial retinal implants can be found in Dowling (2008), Lovell et al. (2010), Ng et al. (2009), Tombran-Tink et al. (2007), and Weiland et al. (2005).

13.5 Necessary improvements in wireless ocular implants

The wireless ocular implants summarized in this chapter, although varying in detail, all rely on inductive coupling for power and/or data transmission between the extraocular and intraocular units. Power telemetry in particular is a major performance-limiting factor for intraocular prostheses, because of several biological constraints including small intraocular space, eye motion, and lossy fluidic environment. In addition, advanced development of high-density retinal interfaces to achieve large-print reading and adequate face-recognition vision requires the delivery of more power to the intraocular system through the telemetric link (Chader et al., 2009). Intensive efforts have been undertaken in recent years to optimize the power-transfer efficiency of the inductive link. For example, Ghovanloo and his group have studied the power telemetric links with 3-coil or 4-coil configurations, both theoretically and experimentally (Kiani et al., 2011, Kiani and Ghovanloo, 2012). The 3-coil inductive link was demonstrated to achieve higher power-transfer efficiency, as well as power delivered to the load, as compared with the conventional 2-coil configuration and the 4-coil design. In addition to the development of innovative inductive telemetry circuits, there is critical need for the improvement of coil design and manufacturing techniques. Advanced surgical tools and operation procedures should also be investigated to optimize the spatial alignment between the intraocular coil and the external transmitter coil, while minimizing the disturbance of biological environment.

System integration plays an important role in the implementation of a fully implantable intraocular system. Techniques should be developed to enable high lead-count interconnects, large-scale integration, high yield, low cost, and system biocompatibility. Traditional packaging technologies such as wire-bonding, flip chip, and tape automated bonding do not meet these requirements, due to their low reliability, non-biocompatibility, and high fabrication costs. A MicroFlex interconnection (MFI) technique has been developed based on a rivet-like approach, utilizing gold ball studs with thermosonic bonding (Meyer et al., 2001). This method can enable high-density electrical and mechanical interconnections between the pads on a flexible polyimide carrier and individual chips or electronic components. Center-to-center bond-pad distances of less than 100 μm have been

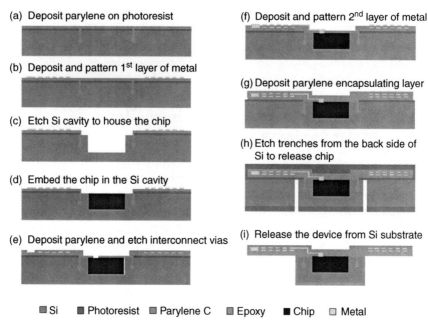

13.12 (a–i) Process flow of the CL-I² technique and an integrated radio-frequency identification (RFID) chip with a flexible MEMS coil (Li et al., 2010b).

achieved. Specifically for epiretinal implant, a chip-level integrated interconnect (CL-I²) packaging technology has been reported based on the bulk-micromachining technology, allowing for direct integration of CMOS IC chips with prosthetic electrodes and microcoil on a single parylene platform to achieve high-level system functionality (Li et al., 2010b; Rodger et al., 2005) (Fig. 13.12). In this approach, individual prefabricated chips and passive components were embedded in a carrier silicon wafer and protected with parylene. Planar MEMS structures, such as electrode arrays and RF coils, were constructed subsequently on the same platform. All interconnections between MEMS devices and chips were processed simultaneously, using standard photolithography and metal patterning method. Although both of these integration techniques are promising for achieving high-density interconnections, their biocompatibility and long-term reliability have not been fully proven in *in vivo* tests and thus require further investigation.

13.6 Conclusion

Advanced RF MEMS technology is a powerful enabling tool for realizing miniaturized, long-term reliable, safe, and complex microsystems for neural prostheses and medical diagnosis and therapy. Of particular interest is the application of wireless microsystems in ocular implants. This chapter has reviewed various types of retinal prosthetic systems that utilize inductive telemetry for power and data transmission. Other innovative wireless microsensors for IOP monitoring in glaucoma have also been discussed. While these research efforts are primarily being conducted at universities and research institutes, an increasing number of companies are being formed based on the initial developments from the academic laboratories. Some devices are currently entering into clinical practice and are being commercialized by existing companies, such as Second Sight, Intelligent Medical Implants, and Boston Retinal Implant, to name just a few. Given the level of technology development and innovation, it is anticipated that within the next few decades these implantable devices will profoundly impact the diagnosis and therapy of incurable eye diseases.

13.7 References

(1998). International commission on non-ionizing radiation protection: Guidelines for limiting exposure to time-varying electric, magnetic, and electromagnetic fields (up to 300 GHz). International commission on non-ionizing radiation protection, *Health Physics*, Vol. **74** (4), pp: 4940–4522.

(2006). Ieee standard for safety levels with respect to human exposure to radio frequency electromagnetic fields, 3 kHz to 300 GHz, *IEEE C95.1-2005*.

Akar, O., Akin, T., and Najafi, K. (2001). A wireless batch sealed absolute capacitive pressure sensor, *Sensors and Actuators A: Physical*, Vol. **95**, No. 1, pp: 29–38.

American Health Assistance Foundation (2011a) *Facts on glaucoma*, 2011, http://www.ahaf.org/glaucoma/about/understanding/facts.html.

Artificial Retina Project (2011b) *Retinal diseases: Age-related macular degeneration and retinitis pigmentosa*, 2011, http://artificialretina.energy.gov/diseases.shtml.

Asher, A., Segal, W. A., Baccus, S. A., Yaroslavsky, L. P., and Palanker, D. V. (2007). Image processing for a high-resolution optoelectronic retinal prosthesis, *Biomedical Engineering, IEEE Transactions on*, Vol. **54**, No. 6, pp: 993–1004.

Baldi, A., Choi, W., and Ziaie, B. (2003). A self-resonant frequency-modulated micromachined passive pressure transensor, *Sensors Journal, IEEE*, Vol. **3**, No. 6, pp: 728–733.

Bashirullah, R. (2010). Wireless implants, *Microwave Magazine, IEEE*, Vol. **11**, No. 7, pp: S14–S23, Doi: 10.1109/mmm.2010.938579.

Bennett, J., Tanabe, T., Sun, D. X., Zeng, Y., Kjeldbye, H., Gouras, P., and Maguire, A. M. (1996). Photoreceptor cell rescue in retinal degeneration (rd) mice by in vivo gene therapy, *Nature Medicine*, Vol. **2**, No. 6, pp: 649–654, Doi: 10.1038/nm0696-649.

Berson, E. L. (1993). Retinitis-pigmentosa – the friedenwald lecture, *Investigative Ophthalmology and Visual Science*, Vol. **34**, No. 5, pp: 1659–1676.

Berson, E. L., Rosner, B., Sandberg, M. A., Hayes, K. C., Nicholson, B. W., Weigeldifranco, C., and Willett, W. (1993). A randomized trial of vitamin-a and vitamin-e supplementation for retinitis-pigmentosa, *Archives of Ophthalmology*, Vol. **111**, No. 6, pp: 761–772.

Brindley, G. S. and Lewin, W. S. (1968). The sensations produced by electrical stimulation of the visual cortex, *The Journal of Physiology*, Vol. **196**, No. 2, pp: 479–493.

Chader, G. J., Weiland, J. W., and Humayun, M. S. (2009). Artificial vision: Needs, functioning, and testing of a retinal electronic prosthesis, *Neurotherapy: Progress in Restorative Neuroscience and Neurology*, Vol. **175**, pp: 317.

Chauhan, B. C., Mccormick, T. A., Nicolela, M. T., and Leblanc, R. P. (2001). Optic disc and visual field changes in a prospective longitudinal study of patients with glaucoma: Comparison of scanning laser tomography with conventional perimetry and optic disc photography, *Arch Ophthalmol*, Vol. **119**, No. 10, pp: 1492–1499, Doi: 10.1001/archopht.119.10.1492.

Chen, G., Ghaed, H., Haque, R., Wieckowski, M., Yejoong, K., Gyouho, K., Fick, D., Daeyeon, K., Mingoo, S., Wise, K., Blaauw, D., and Sylvester, D. (2011). A cubic-millimeter energy-autonomous wireless intraocular pressure monitor, *Solid-State Circuits Conference Digest of Technical Papers (ISSCC), 2011 IEEE International*, pp: 310–312, 20–24 Feb. 2011.

Chen, P. J., Kuo, W. C., Li, W., and Tai, Y. C. (2008a). Q-enhanced fold-and-bond mems inductors, *IEEE NEMS 2008 Conference*, Sanya, Hainan Island, China.

Chen, P. J., Rodger, D. C., Agrawal, R., Saati, S., Meng, E., Varma, R., Humayun, M. S., and Tai, Y. C. (2007). Implantable micromechanical parylene-based pressure sensors for unpowered intraocular pressure sensing, *Journal of Micromechanics and Microengineering*, Vol. **17**, No. 10, pp: 1931–1938, Doi: Doi 10.1088/0960-1317/17/10/002.

Chen, P. J., Rodger, D. C., Saati, S., Humayun, M. S., and Tai, Y. C. (2008b). Microfabricated implantable parylene-based wireless passive intraocular pressure sensors, *Journal of Microelectromechanical Systems*, Vol. **17**, No. 6, pp: 1342–1351, Doi: Doi 10.1109/Jmems.2008.2004945.

Chen, P. J., Saati, S., Varma, R., Humayun, M. S., and Tai, Y. C. (2010). Wireless intraocular pressure sensing using microfabricated minimally invasive flexible-coiled lc sensor implant, *Journal of Microelectromechanical Systems*, Vol. **19**, No. 4, pp: 721–734, Doi:10.1109/Jmems.2010.2049825.

Chihara, E. (2008). Assessment of true intraocular pressure: The gap between theory and practical data, *Survey of Ophthalmology*, Vol. **53**, No. 3, pp: 203–218, Doi: 10.1016/j.survophthal.2008.02.005.

Chow, A. Y. (1993). Electrical-stimulation of the rabbit retina with subretinal electrodes and high-density microphotodiode array implants, *Investigative Ophthalmology and Visual Science*, Vol. **34**, No. 4, pp: 835–835.

Chow, A. Y., Chow, V. Y., Packo, K. H., Pollack, J. S., Peyman, G. A., and Schuchard, R. (2004). The artificial silicon retina microchip for the treatment of vision-loss from retinitis pigmentosa, *Archives of Ophthalmology*, Vol. **122**, No. 4, pp: 460–469.

Chow, A. Y., Pardue, M. T., Chow, V. Y., Peyman, G. A., Liang, C. P., Perlman, J. I., and Peachey, N. S. (2001). Implantation of silicon chip microphotodiode arrays into the cat subretinal space, *IEEE Transactions on Neural Systems and Rehabilitation Engineering*, Vol. **9**, No. 1, pp: 86–95.

Chow, E. Y., Chlebowski, A. L., and Irazoqui, P. P. (2010). A miniature-implantable rf-wireless active glaucoma intraocular pressure monitor, *IEEE Transactions* on *Biomedical Circuits and Systems*, Vol. **4**, No. 6, pp: 340–349, Doi: Doi 10.1109/Tbcas.2010.2081364.

Collins, C. C. (1967). Miniature passive pressure transensor for implanting in the eye, *Biomedical Engineering, IEEE Transactions on*, Vol. BME-14, No. 2, pp: 74–83.

Curcio, C. A., Medeiros, N. E., and Millican, C. L. (1996). Photoreceptor loss in age-related macular degeneration, *Investigative Ophthalmology and Visual Science*, Vol. **37**, No. 7, pp: 1236–1249.

David, C. N., Shun, B., Jiawei, Y., Nhan, T., and Efstratios, S. (2009). Wireless technologies for closed-loop retinal prostheses, *Journal of Neural Engineering*, Vol. **6**, No. 6, pp: 065004.

Debry, P. W., Krishna, R., and Willoughby, T. L. (2003). Comparison of intraocular pressure measurement by dynamic contour tonometry and goldmann applanation tonometry, *Investigative Ophthalmology & Visual Science*, Vol. **44**, pp: U372–U372.

Dehennis, A. and Wise, K. D. (2002). A double-sided single-chip wireless pressure sensor, *Micro Electro Mechanical Systems, 2002. The Fifteenth IEEE International Conference on*, pp: 252–255, 2002.

Dobelle, W. H. (2000). Artificial vision for the blind by connecting a television camera to the visual cortex, *ASAIO Journal*, Vol. **46**, No. 1, pp: 3–9.

Dobelle, W. H. and Mladejovsky, M. G. (1974). Phosphenes produced by electrical stimulation of human occipital cortex, and their application to the development of a prosthesis for the blind, *The Journal of Physiology*, Vol. **243**, No. 2, pp: 553–576.

Donaldson, N. and Perkins, T. (1983). Analysis of resonant coupled coils in the design of radio frequency transcutaneous links, *Medical and Biological Engineering and Computing*, Vol. **21**, No. 5, pp: 612–627, Doi: 10.1007/bf02442388.

Dowling, J. (2008). Current and future prospects for optoelectronic retinal prostheses, *Eye*, Vol. **23**, No. 10, pp: 1999–2005.

Ducrey, N., Geinoz, J., and Faggioni, R. (1975). Non-contact applanation tonometry, *Ophthalmologica*, Vol. **170**, No. 5, pp: 446–449.

Eggers, T., Draeger, J., Hille, K., Marschner, C., Stegmaier, P., Binder, J., and Laur, R. (2000). Wireless intra-ocular pressure monitoring system integrated into an artificial lens, *Microtechnologies in Medicine and Biology, 1st Annual International, Conference On. 2000*, pp: 466–469.

Elsheikh, A., Alhasso, D., Gunvant, P., and Garway-Heath, D. (2011). Multiparameter correction equation for goldmann applanation tonometry, *Optometry and Vision Science*, Vol. **88**, No. 1, pp: E102–E112, Doi: 10.1097/Opx.0b013e3181fc3453

Ethier, C. R., Johnson, M., and Ruberti, J. (2004). Ocular biomechanics and biotransport, *Annual Review of Biomedical Engineering*, Vol. **6**, pp: 249–273, Doi: DOI 10.1146/annurev.bioeng.6.040803.140055.

Fedel, M., Motta, A., Maniglio, D., and Migliaresi, C. (2009). Surface properties and blood compatibility of commercially available diamond-like carbon coatings for cardiovascular devices, *Journal of Biomedical Materials Research Part B: Applied Biomaterials*, Vol. **90B**, No. 1, pp: 338–349, Doi: 10.1002/jbm.b.31291.

Ferreira, J. A. (1994). Improved analytical modeling of conductive losses in magnetic components, *Power Electronics, IEEE Transactions on*, Vol. **9**, No. 1, pp: 127–131, Doi: 10.1109/63.285503.

Fonseca, M. A., Allen, M. G., Kroh, J., and Whit, J. (2006). Flexible wireless passive pressure sensors for biomedical applicatons, *Solid-State Sensors, Actuators, and Microsystems Workshop*, Hilton Head Island, South Carolina, June 4–8, 2006.

Francis, B. A., Hsieh, A., Lai, M. Y., Chopra, V., Pena, F., Azen, S., Varma, R., and Grp, L. A. L. E. S. (2007). Effects of corneal thickness, corneal curvature, and intraocular pressure level on goldmann applanation tonometry and dynamic contour tonomet, *Ophthalmology*, Vol. **114**, No. 1, pp: 20–26, Doi: 10.1016/j.ophtha.2006.06.047.

Galbraith, D. C., Soma, M., and White, R. L. (1987). A wide-band efficient inductive transdennal power and data link with coupling insensitive gain, *Biomedical Engineering, IEEE Transactions on*, Vol. **BME-34**, No. 4, pp: 265–275, Doi: 10.1109/tbme.1987.326076.

Ghodssi, R., Lin, P., Meng, E., Zhang, X., and Benard, W. (2011). Additive processes for polymeric materials, In *MEMS materials and processes handbook*, pp: 193–271, Springer US, Doi: 10.1007/978-0-387-47318-5_4.

Ghovanloo, M. and Najafi, K. (2004). A wideband frequency-shift keying wireless link for inductively powered biomedical implants, *Circuits and Systems I: Regular Papers, IEEE Transactions on*, Vol. **51**, No. 12, pp: 2374–2383, Doi: 10.1109/tcsi.2004.838144.

Green, W. R. and Enger, C. (1993). Age-related macular degeneration histopathologic studies – the 1992 zimmerman,lorenz,e lecture, *Ophthalmology*, Vol. **100**, No. 10, pp: 1519–1535.

Greene, M. E. and Gilman, B. G. (1974). Intraocular pressure measurement with instrumented contact lenses, *Investigative Ophthalmology and Visual Science*, Vol. **13**, No. 4, pp: 299–302.

Guoxing, W., Wentai, L., Sivaprakasam, M., and Kendir, G. A. (2005). Design and analysis of an adaptive transcutaneous power telemetry for biomedical implants, *Circuits and Systems I: Regular Papers, IEEE Transactions on*, Vol. **52**, No. 10, pp: 2109–2117, Doi: 10.1109/tcsi.2005.852923.

Hamici, Z., Itti, R., and Champier, J. (1996). A high-efficiency power and data transmission system for biomedical implanted electronic devices, *Measurement Science and Technology*, Vol. **7**, pp: 192–201.

Heetderks, W. J. (1988). Rf powering of millimeter- and submillimeter-sized neural prosthetic implants, *Biomedical Engineering, IEEE Transactions on*, Vol. **35**, No. 5, pp: 323–327, Doi: 10.1109/10.1388.

Henry, B. M., Dinelli, F., Zhao, K. Y., Grovenor, C. R. M., Kolosov, O. V., Briggs, G. A. D., Roberts, A. P., Kumar, R. S., and Howson, R. P. (1999). A microstructural study of transparent metal oxide gas barrier films, *Thin Solid Films*, Vol. **355–356**, pp: 500–505.

Hirata, A., Matsuyama, S. I., and Shiozawa, T. (2000). Temperature rises in the human eye exposed to em waves in the frequency range 0.6–6 Ghz, *Electromagnetic Compatibility, IEEE Transactions on*, Vol. **42**, No. 4, pp: 386–393, Doi: 10.1109/15.902308.

Huan-Shang, T., Jenshan, L., Frye, R. C., Tai, K. L., Lau, M. Y., Kossives, D., Hrycenko, F., and Young-Kai, C. (1997). Investigation of current crowding effect on spiral inductors, *Wireless Applications Digest, 1997, IEEE MTT-S Symposium on Technologies for*, pp: 139–142, 23–26 Feb 1997, Doi: 10.1109/mttwa.1997.595129.

Humayun, M., Propst, R., De Juan, E., Jr, Mccormick, K., and Hickingbotham, D. (1994). Bipolar surface electrical stimulation of the vertebrate retina, *Archives of Ophthalmology*, Vol. **112**, No. 1, pp: 110–116, Doi: 10.1001/archopht.1994.01090130120028.

Humayun, M. S., De Juan Jr, E., Weiland, J. D., Dagnelie, G., Katona, S., Greenberg, R., and Suzuki, S. (1999). Pattern electrical stimulation of the human retina, *Vision Research*, Vol. **39**, No. 15, pp: 2569–2576.

Humayun, M. S., Dorn, J. D., Ahuja, A. K., Caspi, A., Filley, E., Dagnelie, G., Salzmann, J., Santos, A., Duncan, J., Dacruz, L., Mohand-Said, S., Eliott, D., Mcmahon, M. J., and Greenberg, R. J. (2009). Preliminary 6 month results from the argus™ II epiretinal prosthesis feasibility study, *Engineering in Medicine and Biology Society, 2009. EMBC 2009. Annual International Conference of the IEEE*, pp: 4566–4568, 3–6 Sept. 2009.

Huo, X., Philip, C. H. C., Kevin, J. C., and Howard, C. L. (2006). A physical model for on-chip spiral inductors with accurate substrate modeling, *Electron Devices, IEEE Transactions on*, Vol. **53**, No. 12, pp: 2942–2949, Doi: 10.1109/ted.2006.885091.

Islam, A. B. (2011) Design of wireless power transfer and data telemetry system for biomedical applications.

Jung, L. H., Byrnes-Preston, P., Hessler, R., Lehmann, T., Suaning, G. J., and Lovell, N. H. (2007). A dual band wireless power and fsk data telemetry for biomedical implants, *Engineering in Medicine and Biology Society, 2007. EMBS 2007. 29th Annual International Conference of the IEEE*, pp: 6596–6599, 22–26 Aug. 2007, Doi: 10.1109/iembs.2007.4353871.

Kachanov, L. (1986). *Introduction to continuum damage mechanics (mechanics of elastic stability)*, Springer.

Katuri, K. C., Asrani, S., and Ramasubramanian, M. K. (2008). Intraocular pressure monitoring sensors, *Sensors Journal, IEEE*, Vol. **8**, No. 1, pp: 12–19.

Katuri, K. C., Ramasubramanian, M. K., and Asrani, S. (2010). A surface micromachined capacitive pressure sensor for intraocular pressure measurement, *Mechatronics and Embedded Systems and Applications (MESA), 2010 IEEE/ASME International Conference on*, pp: 149–154, 15–17 July 2010.

Kendir, G. A., Liu, W., Wang, G., Sivaprakasam, M., Bashirullah, R., Humayun, M. S., and Weiland, J. D. (2005a). An optimal design methodology for inductive power link with class-e amplifier, *IEEE Transactions on Circuits and Systems—I: Regular Papers*, Vol. **52**, No. 5, pp: 857–866.

Kendir, G. A., Wentai, L., Guoxing, W., Sivaprakasam, M., Bashirullah, R., Humayun, M. S., and Weiland, J. D. (2005b). An optimal design methodology for inductive power link with class-e amplifier, *Circuits and Systems I: Regular Papers, IEEE Transactions on*, Vol. **52**, No. 5, pp: 857–866, Doi: 10.1109/tcsi.2005.846208.

Kelly, S. K., Shire, D. B., Chen, J., Doyle, P., Gingerich, M. D., Cogan, S. F., Drohan, W. A., Behan, S., Theogarajan, L., Wyatt, J. L., and Rizzo, J. F. (2011). A hermetic wireless subretinal neurostimulator for vision prostheses, *Biomedical Engineering, IEEE Transactions on*, Vol. **58**, No. 11, pp: 3197–3205, Doi: 10.1109/tbme.2011.2165713.

Kerdraon, Y. A., Downie, J. A., Suaning, G. J., Capon, M. R., Coroneo, M. T., and Lovell, N. H. (2002). Development and surgical implantation of a vision prosthesis model into the ovine eye, *Clinical and Experimental Ophthalmology*, Vol. **30**, No. 1, pp: 36–40, Doi: 10.1046/j.1442-9071.2002.00485.x.

Kiani, M. and Ghovanloo, M. (2012). The circuit theory behind coupled-mode magnetic resonance-based wireless power transmission, *Circuits and Systems I: Regular Papers, IEEE Transactions on*, Vol. **59**, No. 9, pp: 2065–2074, Doi: 10.1109/tcsi.2011.2180446.

Kiani, M., Uei-Ming, J., and Ghovanloo, M. (2011). Design and optimization of a 3-coil inductive link for efficient wireless power transmission, *Biomedical Circuits and Systems, IEEE Transactions on*, Vol. **5**, No. 6, pp: 579–591, Doi: 10.1109/tbcas.2011.2158431.

Kim, C. and Wise, K. (1996). A 64-site multishank cmos low-profile neural stimulating probe, *IEEE Journal of Solid-State Circuits*, Vol. **31**, pp: 1230–1238.

Kim, S. Y., Sadda, S., Pearlman, J., Humayun, M. S., De Juan, E. J., Melia, B. M., and Green, W. R. (2002). Morphometric analysis of the macula in eyes with disciform age-related macular degeneration, *RETINA*, Vol. **22**, No. 4, pp: 471–477.

Klauke, S., Goertz, M., Rein, S., Hoehl, D., Thomas, U., Eckhorn, R., Bremmer, F., and Wachtler, T. (2011). Stimulation with a wireless intraocular epiretinal implant elicits visual percepts in blind humans, *Investigative Ophthalmology and Visual Science*, Vol. **52**, No. 1, pp: 449–455, Doi: 10.1167/iovs.09-4410.

Ko, W., Liang, S., and Fung, C. (1977a). Design of radio-frequency powered coils for implant instruments, *Medical and Biological Engineering and Computing*, Vol. **15**, No. 6, pp: 634–640, Doi: 10.1007/bf02457921.

Ko, W. H., Liang, S. P., and Fung, C. D. F. (1977b). Design of radio-frequency powered coils for implant instruments, *Medical and Biological Engineering and Computing*, Vol. **15**, pp: 634–640.

Lee, T. H. (1998). *The design of cmos radio-frequency integrated circuits*, Cambridge University Press.

Leonardi, M., Leuenberger, P., Bertrand, D., Bertsch, A., and Renaud, P. (2004). First steps toward noninvasive intraocular pressure monitoring with a sensing contact lens, *Investigative Ophthalmology and Visual Science*, Vol. **45**, No. 9, pp: 3113–3117, Doi: Doi 10.1167/Iovs.04-0015.

Li, W., Rodger, D. C., Meng, E., Weiland, J. D., Humayun, M. S., and Tai, Y. C. (2006). Flexible parylene packaged intraocular coil for retinal prostheses, *4th Int. IEEE-EMBS Special Topic Conf. on Microtechnologies in Medicine and Biology*, Okinawa, Japan.

Li, W., Rodger, D. C., Meng, E., Weiland, J. D., Humayun, M. S., and Tai, Y.-C. (2010a). Wafer-level parylene packaging with integrated RF electronics for wireless retinal prostheses, *IEEE/ASME Journal of Microelectromechanical Systems (in press)*.

Li, W., Rodger, D. C., Meng, E., Weiland, J. D., Humayun, M. S., and Tai, Y.-C. (2010b). Wafer-level parylene packaging with integrated RF electronics for wireless retinal prostheses, *Microelectromechanical Systems, Journal of*, Vol. **19**, No. 4, pp: 735–742.

Li, W., Rodger, D. C., Weiland, J. D., Humayun, M. S., and Tai, Y. C. (2005). Integrated flexible ocular coil for power and data transfer in retinal prostheses, *Proc. IEEE-EMBS 2005*, Shanghai, China.

Licari, J. J. and Hughes, L. A. (1990). *Handbook of polymer coating for electronics: Chemistry, technology, and applications*, (2nd), Noyes Publications, N.J.

Liu, W., Vichienchom, K., Clements, M., Demarco, S. C., Hughes, C., Mcgucken, E., Humayun, M. S., De Juan, E., Weiland, J. D., and Greenberg, R. (2000).

A neuro-stimulus chip with telemetry unit for retinal prosthetic device, *Solid-State Circuits, IEEE Journal of*, Vol. **35**, No. 10, pp: 1487–1497, Doi: 10.1109/4.871327.

Loudin, J. D., Simanovskii, D. M., Vijayraghavan, K., Sramek, C. K., Butterwick, A. F., Huie, P., Mclean, G. Y., and Palanker, D. V. (2007). Optoelectronic retinal prosthesis: System design and performance, *Journal of Neural Engineering*, Vol. **4**, No. 1, p. S72.

Lovell, N. H., Morley, J. W., Chen, S. C., Hallum, L. E., and Suaning, G. J. (2010). Biological-machine systems integration: Engineering the neural interface, *Proceedings of the IEEE*, Vol. **98**, No. 3, pp: 418–431, Doi: 10.1109/Jproc.2009.2039030.

Maclaren, R. E., Pearson, R. A., Macneil, A., Douglas, R. H., Salt, T. E., Akimoto, M., Swaroop, A., Sowden, J. C., and Ali, R. R. (2006). Retinal repair by transplantation of photoreceptor precursors, *Nature*, Vol. **444**, No. 7116, pp: 203–207, Doi: 10.1038/nature05161.

Majji, A. B., Humayun, M. S., Weiland, J. D., Suzuki, S., D'Anna, S. A., and De Juan, E. (1999). Long-term histological and electrophysiological results of an inactive epiretinal electrode array implantation in dogs, *Investigative Ophthalmology and Visual Science*, Vol. **40**, No. 9, pp: 2073–2081.

Mansouri, K. and Shaarawy, T. (2011). Continuous intraocular pressure monitoring with a wireless ocular telemetry sensor: Initial clinical experience in patients with open angle glaucoma, *British Journal of Ophthalmology*, Vol. **95**, No. 5, pp: 627–629, Doi: DOI 10.1136/bjo.2010.192922.

Matthaei, M., Zeitz, O., Keseru, M., Wagenfeld, L., Hornig, R., Post, N., and Richard, G. (2011). Progress in the development of vision prostheses, *Ophthalmologica*, Vol. **225**, No. 4, pp: 187–192, Doi: Doi 10.1159/000318042.

Mazza, M., Renaud, P., Bertrand, D. C., and Ionescu, A. M. (2005). Cmos pixels for subretinal implantable prothesis, *IEEE Sensors Journal*, Vol. **5**, No. 1, pp: 32–37, Doi: Doi 10.1109/Jsen.2004.839895.

Meng, E. and Gutierrez, C. (2009). Parylene-based encapsulated fluid mems sensors, *31st Annual International Conference of the IEEE EMBS*, Minneapolis, Minnesota, USA, 2–6 September.

Meyer, J. U., Stieglitz, T., Scholz, O., Haberer, W., and Beutel, H. (2001). High density interconnects and flexible hybrid assemblies for active biomedical implants, *Advanced Packaging, IEEE Transactions on*, Vol. **24**, No. 3, pp: 366–374.

Mokwa, W. (2007). Medical implants based on microsystems, *Measurement Science and Technology*, Vol. **18**, No. 5, pp: R47.

Mokwa, W. (2011). Retinal implants to restore vision in blind people, *Solid-State Sensors, Actuators and Microsystems Conference (TRANSDUCERS), 2011 16th International*, pp: 2825–2830, 5–9 June 2011, Doi: 10.1109/transducers.2011.5969883

Mokwa, W., Goertz, M., Koch, C., Krisch, I., Trieu, H. K., and Walter, P. (2008). Intraocular epiretinal prosthesis to restore vision in blind humans, *Engineering in Medicine and Biology Society, 2008. EMBS 2008. 30th Annual International Conference of the IEEE*, pp: 5790–5793, 20–25 Aug. 2008.

Montezuma, S. R., Loewenstein, J., Scholz, C., and Rizzo, J. F. (2006). Biocompatibility of materials implanted into the subretinal space of yucatan pigs, *Investigative*

Ophthalmology and Visual Science, Vol. **47**, No. 8, pp: 3514–3522, Doi: 10.1167/iovs.06-0106.

Moses, R. A. (1958). The goldmann applanation tonometer, *American Journal of Ophthalmology*, Vol. **46**, No. 6, pp: 865–869.

Ng, D. C., Bai, S., Yang, J., Tran, N., and Skafidas, E. (2009). Wireless technologies for closed-loop retinal prostheses, *Journal of Neural Engineering*, Vol. **6**, No. 6, pp: 065004.

Nikolic, K., Degenaar, P., and Toumazou, C. (2006). Modeling and engineering aspects of channelrhodopsin2 system for neural photostimulation, *Engineering in Medicine and Biology Society, 2006. EMBS '06. 28th Annual International Conference of the IEEE*, pp: 1626–1629, 30 Aug. 2006–3 Sept. 2006.

Palanker, D., Vankov, A., Huie, P., and Baccus, S. (2005). Design of a high-resolution optoelectronic retinal prosthesis, *Journal of Neural Engineering*, Vol. **2**, No. 1, p. S105.

Piedade, M., Gerald, J., Sousa, L. A., Tavares, G., and Tomas, P. (2005). Visual neuroprosthesis: A non invasive system for stimulating the cortex, *Circuits and Systems I: Regular Papers, IEEE Transactions on*, Vol. **52**, No. 12, pp: 2648–2662, Doi: 10.1109/tcsi.2005.857923.

Puers, R., Catrysse, M., Vandevoorde, G., Collier, R. J., Louridas, E., Burny, F., Donkerwolcke, M., and Moulart, F. (2000a). A telemetry system for the detection of hip prosthesis loosening by vibration analysis, *Sensors and Actuators A: Physical*, Vol. **85**, No. 1–3, pp: 42–47.

Puers, R., Vandevoorde, G., Bruyker, D. D., Puers, R., and Vandevoorde, G. (2000b). Electrodeposited copper inductors for intraocular pressure telemetry, *Journal of Micromechanics and Microengineering*, Vol. **10**, No. 2, p. 124.

Quigley, H. A. and Broman, A. T. (2006). The number of people with glaucoma worldwide in 2010 and 2020, *British Journal of Ophthalmology*, Vol. **90**, No. 3, pp: 262–267, Doi: DOI 10.1136/bjo.2005.081224.

Rizzo, J. F. (2011). Update on retinal prosthetic research: The boston retinal implant project, *Journal of Neuro-Ophthalmology*, Vol. **31**, No. 2, pp: 160–168, Doi: Doi 10.1097/Wno.0b013e31821eb79e.

Rizzo, J. F., Shire, D. B., Kelly, S. K., Troyk, P., Gingerich, M., Mckee, B., Priplata, A., Chen, J., Drohan, W., Doyle, P., Mendoza, O., Theogarajan, L., Cogan, S., and Wyatt, J. L. (2011). Development of the boston retinal prosthesis, *33rd Annual International Conference of the IEEE EMBS*, Boston, Massachusetts USA, August 30–September 3.

Rodger, D. C., Fong, A. J., Li, W., Ameri, H., Ahuja, A. K., Gutierrez, C., Lavrov, I., Zhong, H., Menon, P. R., Meng, E., Burdick, J. W., Roy, R. R., Edgerton, V. R., Weiland, J. D., Humayun, M. S., and Tai, Y. C. (2008). Flexible parylene-based multielectrode array technology for high-density neural stimulation and recording, *Sensors and Actuators B: Chemical*, Vol. **132**, pp: 449–460.

Rodger, D. C., Weiland, J. D., Humayun, M. S., and Yu-Chong, T. (2005). Scalable flexible chip-level parylene package for high lead count retinal prostheses, *Solid-State Sensors, Actuators and Microsystems, 2005. Digest of Technical Papers. TRANSDUCERS '05. The 13th International Conference on*, Vol. 2, pp: 1973–1976 Vol. 1972, 5–9 June 2005.

Rosengren, L., Backlundt, V., Sjostromt, T., Hokt, B., and Svedbergh, B. (1992). A system for wireless intra-ocular pressure measurements using a silicon micromachined sensor, *Journal of Micromechanics and Microengineering*, Vol. **2**, No. 3, pp: 202.

Rosengren, L., Rangsten, P., Bäcklund, Y., Hök, B., Svedbergh, B., and Selén, G. (1994). A system for passive implantable pressure sensors, *Sensors and Actuators A: Physical*, Vol. **43**, No. 1–3, pp: 55–58.

Rothermel, A., Liu, L., Aryan, N. P., Fischer, M., Wuenschmann, J., Kibbel, S., and Harscher, A. (2009). A cmos chip with active pixel array and specific test features for subretinal implantation, *IEEE Journal of Solid-State Circuits*, Vol. **44**, No. 1, pp: 290–300, Doi: Doi 10.1109/Jssc.2008.2007436.

Roy, R. K. and Lee, K.-R. (2007). Biomedical applications of diamond-like carbon coatings: A review, *Journal of Biomedical Materials Research Part B: Applied Biomaterials*, Vol. **83B**, No. 1, pp: 72–84, Doi: 10.1002/jbm.b.30768.

Sacristan-Riquelme, J., Segura, F., and Oses, M. T. (2008). Simple and efficient inductive telemetry system with data and power transmission, *Microelectronics Journal*, Vol. **39**, No. 1, pp: 103–111.

Sarpeshkar, R., Salthouse, C., Ji-Jon, S., Baker, M. W., Zhak, S. M., Lu, T. K. T., Turicchia, L., and Balster, S. (2005). An ultra-low-power programmable analog bionic ear processor, *Biomedical Engineering, IEEE Transactions on*, Vol. **52**, No. 4, pp: 711–727, Doi: 10.1109/tbme.2005.844043.

Sauer, C., Stanacevic, M., Cauwenberghs, G., and Thakor, N. (2005). Power harvesting and telemetry in cmos for implanted devices, *Circuits and Systems I: Regular Papers, IEEE Transactions on*, Vol. **52**, No. 12, pp: 2605–2613, Doi: 10.1109/tcsi.2005.858183.

Savci, H. S., Sula, A., Wang, Z., Dogan, N. S., and Arvas, E. (2005). Mics transceivers: Regulatory standards and applications [medical implant communications service], *SoutheastCon, 2005. Proceedings. IEEE*, pp: 179–182, 8–10 April 2005, Doi: 10.1109/secon.2005.1423241.

Scholz, C. (2007). Perspectives on: Materials aspects for retinal prostheses, *Journal of Bioactive and Compatible Polymers*, Vol. **22**, No. 5, pp: 539–568, Doi: Doi 10.1177/0883911507082160.

Schwarz, M., Ewe, L., Hijazi, N., Hosticka, B. J., Huppertz, J., Kolnsberg, S., Mokwa, W., and Trieu, H. K. (2000). Micro implantable visual prostheses, *Microtechnologies in Medicine and Biology, 1st Annual International, Conference On. 2000*, pp: 461–465, 2000, Doi: 10.1109/mmb.2000.893826.

Schwarz, M., Hauschild, R., Hosticka, B. J., Huppertz, J., Kneip, T., Kolnsberg, S., Ewe, L., and Hoc Khiem, T. (1999). Single-chip cmos image sensors for a retina implant system, *Circuits and Systems II: Analog and Digital Signal Processing, IEEE Transactions on*, Vol. **46**, No. 7, pp: 870–877, Doi: 10.1109/82.775382.

Shire, D. B., Kelly, S. K., Jinghua, C., Doyle, P., Gingerich, M. D., Cogan, S. F., Drohan, W. A., Mendoza, O., Theogarajan, L., Wyatt, J. L., and Rizzo, J. F. (2009). Development and implantation of a minimally invasive wireless subretinal neurostimulator, *Biomedical Engineering, IEEE Transactions on*, Vol. **56**, No. 10, pp: 2502–2511, Doi: 10.1109/tbme.2009.2021401.

Sokal, N. O. and Sokal, A. D. (1975). Class e-a new class of high-efficiency tuned single-ended switching power amplifiers, *Solid-State Circuits, IEEE Journal of*, Vol. **10**, No. 3, pp: 168–176, Doi: 10.1109/jssc.1975.1050582.

Soma, M., Galbraith, D. C., and White, R. L. (1987). Radio-frequency coils in implantable devices: Misalignment analysis and design procedure, *Biomedical*

Engineering, *IEEE Transactions on*, Vol. **BME-34**, No. 4, pp: 276–282, Doi: 10.1109/tbme.1987.326088.

Stangel, K., Kolnsberg, S., Hammerschmidt, D., Hosticka, B. J., Trieu, H. K., and Mokwa, W. (2001). A programmable intraocular CMOS pressure sensor system implant, *Solid-State Circuits, IEEE Journal of*, Vol. **36**, No. 7, pp: 1094–1100.

Stieglitz, T. (2009). Development of a micromachined epiretinal vision prosthesis, *Journal of Neural Engineering*, Vol. **6**, No. 6, pp: 065005.

Suaning, G. J. and Lovell, N. H. (2001). CMOS neurostimulation ASIC with 100 channels, scaleable output, and bidirectional radio-frequency telemetry, *Biomedical Engineering, IEEE Transactions on*, Vol. **48**, No. 2, pp: 248–260, Doi: 10.1109/10.909646.

Sweitzer, R., Scholz, C., Montezuma, S., and Rizzo, J. F. (2006). Evaluation of subretinal implants coated with amorphous aluminum oxide and diamond-like carbon, *Journal of Bioactive and Compatible Polymers*, Vol. **21**, No. 1, pp: 5–22, Doi: 10.1177/0883911506060202.

Tang, Z., Smith, B., Schild, J. H., and Peckham, P. H. (1995). Data transmission from an implantable biotelemeter by load-shift keying using circuit configuration modulator, *Biomedical Engineering, IEEE Transactions on*, Vol. **42**, No. 5, pp: 524–528, Doi: 10.1109/10.376158.

Theogarajan, L. S. (2008). A low-power fully implantable 15-channel retinal stimulator chip, *Solid-State Circuits, IEEE Journal of*, Vol. **43**, No. 10, pp: 2322–2337, Doi: 10.1109/jssc.2008.2004331.

Tombran-Tink, J., Barnstable, C. J., Rizzo, J. F., Liu, W., Sivaprakasam, M., Wang, G., Zhou, M., Weiland, J. D., and Humayun, M. S. (2007). Development of an intraocular retinal prosthesis to benefit the visually impaired, In *Visual prosthesis and ophthalmic devices*, Tombran-Tink, J. and Barnstable, C. J., pp: 55–69, Humana Press, Doi: 10.1007/978-1-59745-449-0_5.

Tonnu, P. A., Ho, T., Newson, T., El Sheikh, A., Sharma, K., White, E., Bunce, C., and Garway-Heath, D. (2005). The influence of central corneal thickness and age on intraocular pressure measured by pneumotonometry, noncontact tonometry, the tono-pen xl, and goldmann applanation tonometry, *British Journal of Ophthalmology*, Vol. **89**, No. 7, pp: 851–854, Doi: 10.1136/bjo.2004.056622.

Trieu, H. K., Ewe, L., Mokwa, W., Schwarz, M., and Hosticka, B. J. (1998). Flexible silicon structures for a retina implant, *Micro Electro Mechanical Systems, 1998. MEMS 98. Proceedings., The Eleventh Annual International Workshop on*, pp: 515–519, 25–29 Jan 1998, Doi: 10.1109/memsys.1998.659811.

Tropepe, V., Coles, B. L. K., Chiasson, B. J., Horsford, D. J., Elia, A. J., Mcinnes, R. R., and Van Der Kooy, D. (2000). Retinal stem cells in the adult mammalian eye, *Science*, Vol. **287**, No. 5460, pp: 2032–2036, Doi: 10.1126/science.287.5460.2032.

Van Schuylenbergh, K. and Puers, R. (1996a). Passive telemetry by harmonics detection, *Engineering in Medicine and Biology Society, 1996. Bridging Disciplines for Biomedicine. Proceedings of the 18th Annual International Conference of the IEEE*, Vol. 1, pp: 299–300 vol.291, 31 Oct.–3 Nov. 1996.

Van Schuylenbergh, K. and Puers, R. (1996b). Self-tuning inductive powering for implantable telemetric monitoring systems, *Sensors and Actuators A: Physical*, Vol. **52**, No. 1, pp: 1–7.

Vandevoorde, G. and Puers, R. (2001). Wireless energy transfer for stand-alone systems: A comparison between low and high power applicability, *Sensors and Actuators A: Physical*, Vol. **92**, No. 1, pp: 305–311.

Veraart, C., Raftopoulos, C., Mortimer, J. T., Delbeke, J., Pins, D., Michaux, G., Vanlierde, A., Parrini, S., and Wanet-Defalque, M.-C. (1998). Visual sensations produced by optic nerve stimulation using an implanted self-sizing spiral cuff electrode, *Brain Research*, Vol. **813**, No. 1, pp: 181–186.

Verhoeff, F. H. (1931). Microscopic observations in a case of retinitis pigmentosa, *Archives of Ophthalmology*, Vol. **5**, No. 3, pp: 392–407, Doi: 10.1001/archopht.1931.00820030076007.

Walter, P., Roessler, G., Laube, T., Brockmann, C., Kirschkamp, T., Mazinani, B., Goertz, M., Koch, C., Krisch, I., Sellhaus, B., Trieu, H. K., Weis, J., Bornfeld, N., Rothgen, H., Messner, A., and Mokwa, W. (2009). Implantation and explantation of a wireless epiretinal retina implant device: Observations during the epiret3 prospective clinical trial, *Investigative Ophthalmology and Visual Science*, Vol. **50**, No. 6, pp: 3003–3008, Doi: 10.1167/iovs.08-2752.

Weber, A. J., Harman, C. D., and Viswanathan, S. (2008). Effects of optic nerve injury, glaucoma, and neuroprotection on the survival, structure, and function of ganglion cells in the mammalian retina, *The Journal of Physiology*, Vol. **586**, No. 18, pp: 4393–4400, Doi: 10.1113/jphysiol.2008.156729.

Weiland, J. D. and Humayun, M. S. (2008). Visual prosthesis, *Proceedings of the IEEE*, Vol. **96**, No. 7, pp: 1076–1084.

Weiland, J. D., Liu, W., and Humayun, M. S. (2005). Retinal prosthesis, *Annual Review of Biomedical Engineering*, Vol. **7**, No. 1, pp: 361–401, Doi: doi:10.1146/annurev.bioeng.7.060804.100435.

Wise, K. D., Anderson, D. J., Hetke, J. F., Kipke, D. R., and Najafi, K. (2004). Wireless implantable microsystems: High-density electronic interfaces to the nervous system, *Proceedings of the IEEE*, Vol. **92**, No. 1, pp: 76–97, Doi: 10.1109/jproc.2003.820544.

Wong, L. S. Y., Hossain, S., Ta, A., Edvinsson, J., Rivas, D. H., and Naas, H. (2004). A very low-power cmos mixed-signal ic for implantable pacemaker applications, *Solid-State Circuits, IEEE Journal of*, Vol. **39**, No. 12, pp: 2446–2456, Doi: 10.1109/jssc.2004.837027.

Wong, Y. T., Dommel, N., Preston, P., Hallum, L. E., Lehmann, T., Lovell, N. H., and Suaning, G. J. (2007). Retinal neurostimulator for a multifocal vision prosthesis, *Neural Systems and Rehabilitation Engineering, IEEE Transactions on*, Vol. **15**, No. 3, pp: 425–434.

World Health Organization (2008) *Magnitude and causes of visual impairment*, http://www.who.int/mediacentre/factsheets/fs282/en/

Wu, J. J. (2003). Inductive links with integrated receiving coils for MEMS and implantable applications, Electrical Engineering, Doctor of Philosophy, 231.

Xi, N. and Sullivan, C. R. (2003). An improved calculation of proximity-effect loss in high-frequency windings of round conductors, *Power Electronics Specialist Conference, 2003. PESC '03. 2003 IEEE 34th Annual*, Vol. **2**, pp: 853–860 vol. 852, 15–19 June 2003, Doi: 10.1109/pesc.2003.1218168.

Yagi, T., Ito, Y., Kanda, H., Tanaka, S., Watanabe, M., and Uchikawa, Y. (1999). Hybrid retinal implant: Fusion of engineering and neuroscience, *Systems, Man, and Cybernetics, 1999. IEEE SMC '99 Conference Proceedings. 1999 IEEE International Conference on,* Vol. 4, pp: 382–385 vol.384, 1999.

Yamada-Takamura, Y., Koch, F., Maier, H., and Bolt, H. (2002). Hydrogen permeation barrier performance characterization of vapor deposited amorphous aluminum oxide films using coloration of tungsten oxide, *Surface and Coatings Technology*, Vol. **153**, No. 2–3, pp: 114–118.

Zhao, Y., Nandra, M., Yu, C., and Tai, Y. (2012). Reduction of ac resistance in mems intraocular foil coils using microfabricated planar litz structure, *Nano/Micro Engineered and Molecular Systems (NEMS), 2012 7th IEEE International Conference on*, pp: 234–237, 5–8 March 2012, Doi: 10.1109/nems.2012.6196764.

Ziaie, B., Nardin, M., Coghlan, A., and Najafi, K. (1997). A single-channel implantable microstimulator for functional neuromuscular stimulation, *IEEE Transactions on Biomedical Engineering*, Vol. **44**, pp: 909–920.

Zolfaghari, A., Chan, A., and Razavi, B. (2001). Stacked inductors and transformers in cmos technology, *IEEE Journal of Solid-State Circuits,* Vol. **36**, pp: 620–628.

Zrenner, E., Bartz-Schmidt, K. U., Benav, H., Besch, D., Bruckmann, A., Gabel, V. P., Gekeler, F., Greppmaier, U., Harscher, A., Kibbel, S., Koch, J., Kusnyerik, A., Peters, T., Stingl, K., Sachs, H., Stett, A., Szurman, P., Wilhelm, B., and Wilke, R. (2011). Subretinal electronic chips allow blind patients to read letters and combine them to words, *Proceedings of the Royal Society B-Biological Sciences*, Vol. **278**, No. 1711, pp: 1489–1497, Doi: DOI 10.1098/rspb.2010.1747.

Zrenner, E., Miliczek, K. D., Gabel, V. P., Graf, H. G., Guenther, E., Haemmerle, H., Hoefflinger, B., Kohler, K., Nisch, W., Schubert, M., Stett, A., and Weiss, S. (1997). The development of subretinal microphotodiodes for replacement of degenerated photoreceptors, *Ophthalmic Research*, Vol. **29**, No. 5, pp. 269–280.

Zrenner, E., Stett, A., Weiss, S., Aramant, R. B., Guenther, E., Kohler, K., Miliczek, K. D., Seiler, M. J., and Haemmerle, H. (1999). Can subretinal microphotodiodes successfully replace degenerated photoreceptors?, *Vision Research*, Vol. **39**, No. 15, pp. 2555–2567.

14
MEMS-based wireless intraocular pressure sensors

R. BLUE and D. UTTAMCHANDANI,
University of Strathclyde, UK

DOI: 10.1533/9780857098610.2.463

Abstract: Glaucoma is an eye disease resulting from excess intraocular pressure (IOP) and affects millions worldwide; moreover, it gives very little warning sign, until vision is affected. A reliable technique for continuous monitoring of IOP has been long sought after. However, it took the advent of microelectromechanical systems (MEMS) technology to introduce a step change in the possibilities of miniaturization to truly open the door to such a possibility. This chapter tracks the major developments of the interdisciplinary effort to miniaturize the necessary components, such as low-power electronics, energy harvesting, wireless telemetry, and biocompatible materials to realize a fully autonomous IOP system.

Key words: glaucoma, intraocular pressure, MEMS sensor, wireless sensors, microsensors.

14.1 Introduction

Glaucoma is an eye disease that results from blockage of the drainage pathway from the eye for aqueous humour, leading to an increase of intraocular pressure (IOP) and subsequent injury to the optic nerve and even blindness. Presently, almost 70 million people in the world suffer from glaucoma, and it is the second most common cause of blindness around the world. Often there are no visible warning signs to its onset until visual impairment occurs. The elevation of IOP occurs slowly without pain and the first symptoms may be vision reduction itself. Timely intervention via surgery or topically applied drugs to lower the IOP has demonstrated that damage to a patient's vision can be significantly reduced (Fang *et al.*, 2008).

It is therefore highly desirable that the value of IOP in a patient with suspected glaucoma should be regularly or (preferably) continuously monitored. The standard method to measure IOP is Goldmann applanation tonometry (Sarkisian, 2006). During this process, the patient visits a clinic and a skilled operator uses the instrument to measure the force required to flatten an area of the external cornea, and from the measurement infers the fluid pressure inside the eye. For tonometry, a local anaesthetic is used to desensitize the cornea, since the instrument touches the cornea and can be an irritant for the patient. The pressure is usually quoted in millimetres of mercury (mmHg). Millimetres of mercury are manometric units routinely used in medicine and physiology. One mmHg is defined as the pressure exerted at the base of a column of mercury exactly 1 mm high, and 760 mmHg is equal to one atmosphere (101.325 kPa or 760 Torr). Normal eye pressure is in the range 10–20 mmHg above atmospheric pressure, and 21 mmHg is regarded as the onset of glaucoma. The standard tonometric test has a resolution of 1 mmHg. A single measurement of IOP is insufficient since the pressure can vary significantly throughout the day depending on patient activity (Liu et al., 2003).

Rapid spikes in IOP are believed to damage the optic nerve (Asrani et al., 2000) and non-continuous tests are likely to miss the spikes if the IOP peaks are outside the testing hours of a clinic. Using a conventional tonometer for continuous monitoring would require the subject to undertake at least daily visits to a clinic (which is very inconvenient) or even a hospital stay for overnight measurements. In addition, some studies have shown that people with ocular hypertension have thicker corneas than those without, resulting in an applanation measurement from the thicker cornea above that due to an elevated IOP. Hence, a more accurate internal IOP measurement technique is highly desirable to give the most reliable results. (Bron et al., 1999; Copt et al., 1999; Whitacre and Stein, 1993). Therefore, the development of a technique or system for continuous measurement of IOP to an accuracy of 1 mmHg or better by a miniature sensor implanted within the eye would be a revolutionary step, and the desire for such technology has been around for some time.

14.2 Passive miniature implants for intraocular pressure (IOP) sensing

The concept of a wirelessly (inductively) linked implant for IOP measurements can be traced back to when Collins (1967) published his seminal paper on a pressure sensor as small as 2 mm in diameter that could be implanted within the anterior chamber of an animal eye and the pressure accessed via a telemetric link. The device consisted of two separated flat spiral coils encapsulated in glass tubing with polyethylene diaphragms at each end adjacent to the coils (Fig. 14.1). External pressure changes deformed the diaphragms and altered the coil separation (essentially forming a bubble tonometer).

A grid-dip type oscillator supplied electromagnetic energy, which was absorbed by the coils, and the resonant frequency of the circuit varied with high sensitivity to the coil spacing. The resonant frequency is given by:

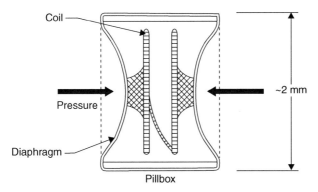

14.1 Illustration of the pressure sensor created by Carter Collins in 1967. External pressure deforms a pair of diaphragms on a small pillbox and the metallic coils are moved closer together, which causes the observed resonant frequency on a grid-dip oscillator to move to a lower value (redrawn with permissions from Collins, 1967).

$$f = \frac{1}{2\pi\sqrt{LC}} \quad\quad [14.1]$$

where L is the mutual inductance and C is the capacitance, which both vary as the coil separation varies, and thus the value of resonant frequency changes as the surrounding pressure deforms the capsule. The dip in the frequency spectrum corresponds to the highest absorbed power at its resonance frequency (RF). After pressure calibration, the device could be repeatedly scanned over a frequency range, and changes in resonant frequency (due to changing surrounding pressure) could be monitored continuously.

The wonderful simplicity of the device (requiring no batteries) facilitated miniaturization and demonstrated a possible methodology towards smaller implants that could remain *in vivo* for an extended period of time and be monitored periodically with external equipment (as illustrated in Fig. 14.2). This demonstration opened up the possibility of continuous monitoring of IOP, as desired for better patient treatment. However, it was not until the early 1990s, with the adoption of microelectromechanical systems (MEMS) processes, that further miniaturization of transducers was enabled, when the next significant miniature IOP device was reported by Uppsala University.

The passive sensing ethos was essentially that which was demonstrated by Collins, but the fabrication of the next generation of passive IOP sensors now took advantage of the material processing capabilities of MEMS to micromachine to at sub-mm dimensions and to fabricate a thin silicon membrane to act as the sensing element in the capacitor device (Backlund *et al.*, 1990). An inductively coupled sensor was made from two silicon wafers (Rosengren *et al.*, 1992). A thin rim 100 μm wide enclosing a 10 μm

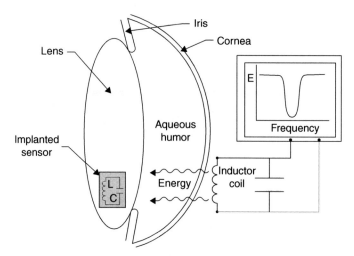

14.2 A passive pressure sensor implanted into the eye can be addressed by electromagnetic energy supplied by an external oscillator.

deep cavity was etched into the top wafer before being inverted and set upon the bottom wafer (Fig. 14.3). A silicon fusion bonding process was used to hermetically seal the wafers together, which has the benefit of reducing the detrimental effects of differential thermal expansion and long-term sensor drift. The bonding requires hydration of the silicon surfaces by boiling in nitric acid then pressing them together at 1000°C in wet oxygen for one hour. A 20 μm thick and 1800 μm wide membrane was then etched into the top wafer to form the pressure-sensitive element of a parallel-plate capacitor. A ten-turn gold wire coil was incorporated into the sensor to form an induction coil for remote detection (up to a maximum distance of 22 mm) of the RF via a grid-dip swept frequency oscillator. This limited distance is due to the small dimensions of the antenna and can thus be regarded as a near-field situation whose magnetic flux density will vary as:

$$B = \frac{\mu I N r^2}{2d^3} \qquad [14.2]$$

where μ is the permeability of the core, I is the loop current, N is the number of turns in the coil, r is the radius of the antenna, and d is separation distance (Hoskins *et al.*, 2009). The sensors demonstrated by Uppsala had good linearity over the range 0 to 100 mmHg, but the device suffered from stray capacitance and a low Q-factor of 5.5, due to inherent series resistance in the bottom wafer.

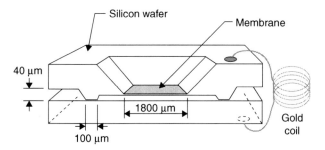

14.3 Schematic of a passive IOP sensor micromachined in silicon with gold induction coil (redrawn from Rosengren *et al.*, 1992).

14.3 Introduction of active MEMS systems for IOP implants

Around the year 2000, Eggers *et al.* (2000) made full use of the advances in micromachining to create an active miniature integrated IOP sensing system comprising a capacitive sensor, a 0.7 μm complementary metal oxide semiconductor (CMOS) readout circuitry, and a telemetry chip. A sensing and a reference capacitor side by side were fabricated on a chip in an eight-mask metal oxide semiconductor (MOS) and micromachining process with overall chip dimensions of 0.8 mm × 2 mm.

The current consumption of the readout circuitry was less than 85 μA for a supply voltage of 3.5 volts and the dimensions of this application-specific integrated circuit (ASIC) was again 0.8 mm × 2 mm × 0.5 mm. The telemetry chip (0.9 mm × 2.9 mm) supplied a rectified 3.5 V to power the system via an inductive transmission on a 125 kHz link. For this prototype, the antenna coil consisted of several hundred turns of 31 μm wire.

The individual chips were assembled using flip-chip technology and encapsulated in poly-methyl-meta-acrylate (PMMA) to form a system of size 6.5 mm × 9 mm that could be located on the edge of a modified intraocular lens implanted during cataract operations. During experimental evaluation using calibration, the IOP system measured to an accuracy ±2 mmHg, thus demonstrating the necessary accuracy and resolution required for implantation.

Also in the year 2000, a group of German researchers comprising RWTH Aachen, Fraunhofer Institute of Microelectronic Circuits and Systems (IMS), and Cologne University discussed and investigated the concept of embedding an IOP sensor in an artificial polydimethylsiloxane ((PDMS), a non-toxic inert silicon-based polymer) lens implanted into the eye and interrogated by a dedicated external reader (Mokwa and Schnakenberg, 2001; Schnakenberg *et al.*, 2000). The micromachined silicon capacitive pressure sensor (plus a reference sensor for drift compensation) sat alongside other

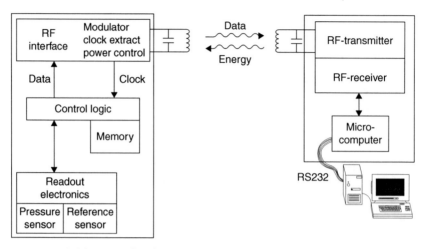

14.4 Layout of active circuitry implant powered remotely for IOP sensing (redrawn with permissions from Schnakenberg *et al.*, 2000).

monolithic components (data conversion, signal conditioning, and wireless modules) and this integrated unit could be wholly implanted into a soft artificial eye during cataract surgery replacing the lens at the front of the anterior chamber. The components were fabricated using a 1.2 μm CMOS process and then subsequent micromachining was applied.

Figure 14.4 illustrates a schematic layout of the sensing scheme. Energy was sent by an RF field to power up the implanted sensor, so again no battery was required. The integrated sensor took a measurement of both pressure and temperature and returned this to the external reader, together with sensor identification and checksum for validation. The algorithm uses sensor-specific calibration data in the external reader's memory for making the calculations of pressure.

In this proof-of-concept, non-optimized telemetric components were positioned on a printed circuit board (PCB) and then encapsulated in PDMS (to give a device of total diameter of 15 mm) and this system was placed into a pressure chamber for testing. The resultant measurements were offset compared to a non-encapsulated sensor, but they showed a good linear correlation and thus the effect could be calibrated out.

The micromachined system was then tested *in vivo* in rabbit eyes for performance under flowing intraocular fluids. At the same time, conventional applanation tonometry was also applied to the same eyes and infusion pressure was varied to directly compare the performance of the intraocular sensor with the external conventional counterpart. Figure 14.5 shows the very good agreement between the traditional measurement system accepted by the ophthalmic industry and the newly developed wireless implant.

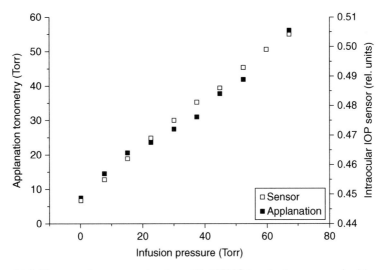

14.5 Measured pressure *in vivo* with MEMS implant compared with a simultaneous external tonometry measurement (reproduced with permission from Schnakenberg *et al.*, 2000).

The IMS continued this area of research to produce a micromechanical pressure sensor containing a non-volatile memory (40-bit EEPROM), a microcontroller, and signal electronics (Stangel *et al.*, 2001). Again a wireless data and power link was established via an antenna coil (flip-chip bonded) and the non-volatile memory could be programmed externally to calibrate the sensor. Data were sent to external electronic modules using an RF carrier operating in the Industrial, Scientific and Medical (ISM) band at 13.6 MHz. The capacitive pressure sensor was formed with deflectable polysilicon diaphragm upon a wafer with a vacuum gap inside the capacitor. Similarly, a reference sensor was fabricated beside the pressure sensor but with an oxide passivation layer upon its diaphragm to increase the rigidity, thereby stopping it flexing with increased pressure. The size of this integrated prototype was 6.8 mm^2, dissipated 210 mW for a power supply voltage of 3 volts. The small footprint of this system gave it the potential for implantation on the edge of an artificial lens and to still have the normal optical transmission path into the eye unhindered.

However, implanting an IOP into an artificial lens has the disadvantage of restricting the possible size of device, thus forcing miniaturization of the RF telemetry, therefore requiring on-chip processing and amplification, which leads to increased manufacturing cost and reduced uptake. In 2008, a group from Flinders University, Australia took a different approach and opted for combining a commercial MEMS capacitive pressure sensor (E1.3N from Microfab Bremen, Germany) together with a planar inductor (formed from copper spiral tracks printed directly onto a polyimide PCB) in order to form a simple parallel resonant circuit that would reduce the complexity of the implanted system and thus the cost (Kakaday et al., 2008).

The researchers also decided to mount this miniature system onto the plate of a glaucoma drainage implant (GDI), which is a medical device implanted below the conjunctiva and connected via a tube to the anterior chamber to allow pressure reduction inside the eye for patients with severe glaucoma. Compared to an artificial lens, the GDI plate can accommodate a larger diameter antenna and sensor, so that passive telemetry can be used with its reduced cost. A frequency-swept external spectrum analyser monitored the RF of the implant. Experiments were conducted with the GDI connected via tubing to the anterior chamber of an explanted sheep's eye, and the infusion pressure varied from 5 to 50 mmHg. Results showed that the pressure at the sensor implant rapidly followed the variation in the anterior chamber. However, the resolution of the sensor implant in the IOP range was reported as 10 mmHg (believed to be due to the low Q-factor of the capacitive sensor), but even this resolution can still be useful for indicating an elevated level of IOP. The non-intraocular lens implant allowed larger diameter antenna coils (4–32.5 mm) to be tested and signals from the sensor implant were detected through 4 mm of PDMS, as well as through sheep corneal and scleral tissue. This demonstrates that a low-cost implant selectively located may find applications for patient use.

14.4 Flexible parylene platforms for long-term MEMS implants

Also in 2008, researchers at Caltech and the University of Southern California fabricated a novel micromachined wireless passive IOP sensor encapsulated in biocompatible parylene C (poly-chloro-p-xylylene) to allow the freedom to locate the implant other than in an artificial lens, thus minimizing surgical complexity (Chen et al., 2008). The US Food and Drug Administration (FDA) has approved the parylene with a Class VI biocompatibility rating suitable for human implantable devices (United States Pharmacopeia Class VI grade and ISO 10993). In fact, in parallel research at Caltech it was found that a 10 μm thick layer of parylene C was sufficient for safe encapsulation of microelectrodes for use in saline (whilst retaining very good flexibility of the platform) and subsequent accelerated ageing experiments predicted that parylene C can stay viable for retinal implants in excess of 60 years (Li, 2009).

Parylene could also be used to fabricate the diaphragm of the capacitor sensor due its ability to form large micromachined areas at room temperature and its inherent flexibility (Wolgemuth, 2000). The encapsulated package was designed with smooth edges to reduce irritation due to the implant,

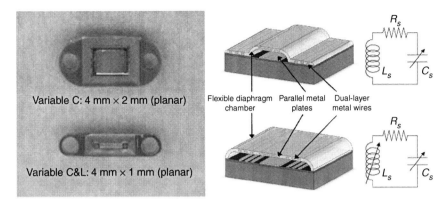

14.6 Designs and dimensions of variable capacitor and variable inductor/capacitor IOP sensors encapsulated in biocompatible parylene for surgical implant (reproduced with permission from Chen *et al.*, 2008).

and the overall size was less than 4 mm × 2 mm × 1 mm. For this prototype device the researchers investigated two sensor configurations, namely that of a variable capacitor with fixed surrounding inductor and that of a variable capacitor and variable inductor as shown in Fig. 14.6. As the diaphragm flexes with pressure, the capacitance changes and also the mutual inductance, which may lead to an improved sensitivity. Experimentally the researchers found that a combined variable capacitor/inductor format gave the same performance as a single capacitor sensor but with a smaller footprint.

The sensors were surgically implanted into an animal, and a six month trial of the implanted sensor demonstrated the *in vivo* compatibility without complications. *Ex vivo* experiments demonstrated successful pressure measurements of an implant; however, the measurement data was noisy, believed to be due to the short wireless transmission distance of this particular sensor through the surrounding fluid and tissue.

The researchers sought to modify the sensing platform to improve upon the sensing distance for an implanted sensor and came up with an alternative geometry. They also exploited the excellent flexibility shown by parylene to create a foldable structure (Fig. 14.7) that would minimize surgical opening required to implant the device (Chen *et al.*, 2010). The sensor was fixed to the iris within the anterior chamber of a rabbit and the surgical implant procedure took less than 15 min and required a corneal incision under 2 mm in length.

The sealed circular capacitor sensor is at the centre of the platform with a circular gold/titanium antenna coil (4 mm diameter), all encapsulated in parylene. Gold layer thicknesses were varied from approximately 3 to 7 μm

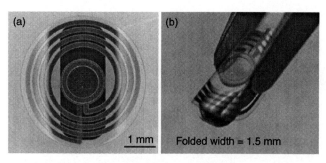

14.7 (a) Unfolded geometry of 4 mm diameter wireless IOP sensor. (b) Reduced width designed for minimizing surgical incision length (reproduced with permission from Chen *et al.*, 2010).

between sensors, which varied the bench test Q-factor from 30 to 45. These bench tests also revealed the strong influence of the surrounding media on the RF and Q-factor. The resonance dip of the sensor changed from 350 to 275 MHz when going from air to water (dielectric constant changing from 1 to 80) as the capacitance of the medium increases, whilst the Q-factor remain unchanged around 45 in each case. However, moving from water to 0.9% saline caused the quality factor to fall dramatically to six, due to this medium being more lossy. The conclusion of this is that the electromagnetic energy reduces faster with distance in the anterior chamber. Bench top tests with a pressure chamber using a minimum signal-to-noise ratio (SNR) of 10 (to achieve an anticipated pressure resolution of 1 mmHg) revealed a maximum sensing distance of 2.5 cm in water, dropping to 1.5 cm in saline solution, thus showing the detrimental influence of the medium around a sensor.

Next the researchers decided to take an alternative approach to placement of the implant for passive IOP sensing as a method for increasing the sensing distance to an external reader. This required a modification of the sensor platform and fabrication procedure (Lin *et al.*, 2012). The fabrication process is shown in Fig. 14.8.

After spin coating a wafer with a sacrificial layer of photoresist, a 5 μm layer of parylene was deposited, followed by a patterned 3 μm Ti/Au layer, and then a second photoresist layer, which was patterned to give a 10 μm thick localized section that would eventually be removed to form the cavity of the capacitor sensor. Another layer of parylene was added to encapsulate the gold tracks already deposited, and a second deposition of 0.5 μm Ti/Au then took place. A last layer of parylene was then deposited and patterned with oxygen plasma to form the final sensing capacitor section. The photoresist between the capacitor plates was removed with acetone, as was

MEMS-based wireless intraocular pressure sensors

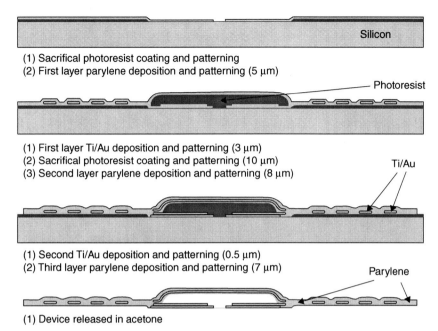

14.8 Summary of processing steps for creating flexible parylene encapsulated IOP sensor (reproduced with permission from Lin *et al.*, 2012).

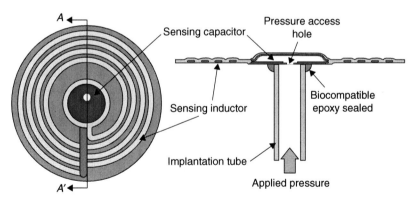

14.9 Illustration of pressure sensor for penetration through the eye wall. Left image is top view showing spiral inductor and right image is side view with added implantation tube (reproduced with permission from Lin *et al.*, 2012).

the underlying silicon substrate. An access hole of 180 μm diameter into the capacitor cavity was created by oxygen plasma, and a tube of inner diameter 320 μm, outer diameter 450 μm, was fixed over the hole using a biocompatible epoxy (Fig. 14.9).

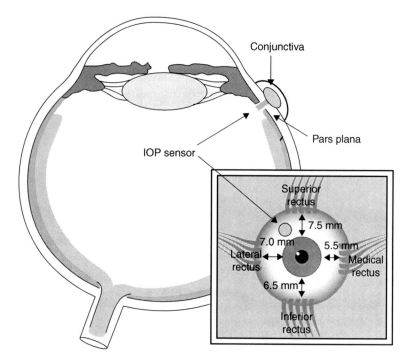

14.10 Intended location of new IOP sensor with implantation tube reaching through the eye wall to measure interior pressure (reproduced with permission from Lin *et al.*, 2012).

The unusual configuration of this sensor was purposely designed to allow the option of implanting the sensor beneath the conjunctiva whilst the tube penetrates the choroid of the eye at pars plana (Fig. 14.10), and thus the IOP modulates the capacitance of the sensing platform.

Furthermore, bench top tests demonstrated that increasing the thickness of parylene (to around 35 µm) upon the sensor could more adequately contain the electric field generated by the coils, and thus it was possible to increase the Q-factor, when immersed in saline, close to that measured in air. This passivation layer finding was useful because, even though the sensor is outside the anterior chamber it is still beneath human tissue that will absorb the electromagnetic energy, and by optimizing the parylene around the sensor, the Q-factor can be maintained at a high value.

14.5 Design of custom ultra-low-power autonomous IOP sensors

In 2010 at the Center for Implantable Devices, Purdue University (Indiana), Chow and co-workers reported the design of a custom circuit

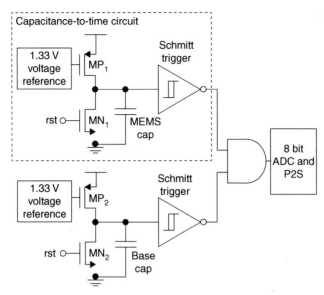

14.11 Ultra-low-power dual capacitance (sensing and reference) to time conversion circuit for autonomous IOP implant (reproduced with permission from Chow *et al.*, 2010).

to allow ultra-low-power operation of an implanted MEMS capacitance sensor using a 1 nanoamp current to charge a capacitor (Chow *et al.*, 2010). The circuit (Fig. 14.11) incorporated a pressure measurement capacitor and a reference capacitor, and the charging time was directly proportional to the capacitance of each. Pulses of different widths proportional to the charging time were digitized and stored in memory. To further facilitate a stand-alone independent measuring system, a non-volatile memory was included, of ferroelectric RAM (FeRAM) type since it has benefits of relatively lower power operation. Data was stored using a sleep–wake cycle that stores capacitance data every 5 min in the FeRAM.

The limited space within the eye limits the suitability of conventional battery technologies as a power source; hence, an array of miniature ceramic capacitors (52 in total) was created as a power-storage unit that was capable of supplying the IOP monitoring system for 24 h.

A liquid-crystal polymer (LCP) (Wang *et al.*, 2003), which is a material found to outperform other biocompatible materials, was employed to create a housing for the IOP measuring system and was shaped into a 'tadpole' geometry (Fig. 14.12). The tail of the tadpole housed an antenna for 2.4 GHz transmitter data transfer and remote powering via a RF rectifier, whilst the head of the tadpole contained the MEMS capacitor sensor, power supply, and customised ASIC. In total, the ASIC had dimensions 700 μm × 700 μm and was fabricated through a Texas Instruments 130 nm CMOS process. The

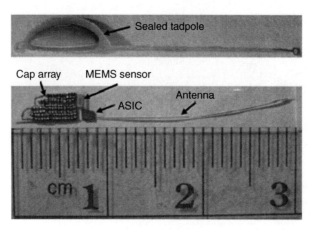

14.12 Tadpole geometry of LCP encapsulated IOP sensor incorporating a long antenna and ultra-low-power circuitry and power-storage unit (reproduced with permission from Chow *et al.*, 2010).

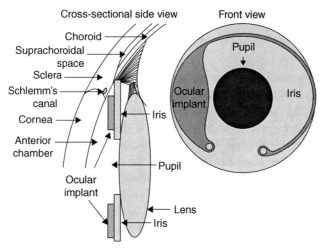

14.13 Recommended implant position of 'tadpole' shaped IOP sensor to allow unobstructed vision (reproduced with permission from Chow *et al.*, 2010).

tadpole geometry (with a 3 × 6 × 0.3 mm head and a 27 mm tail) was also useful, as it was able to follow the curvature of the anterior chamber, and it was suggested that it was best located in front of the of the iris and the natural lens, thereby leaving the natural lens intact and vision unimpeded (Fig. 14.13).

The authors made a comparative evaluation of the power consumption of their developed system (in the wake cycle) with previous implantable

Table 14.1 Comparison of the power consumption of the implant developed by the Centre for Implantable Devices (Indiana) with those reported by previous researchers

Authors	System description	Year	CMOS process node	Supply voltage	Current
Chow et al. (2010)	IOP monitor 5 min sampling with FeRAM and wireless powering and transmission	2009	130 nm	1.5 V	676 pW
Eggers et al. (2000)	IOP SC-relaxation oscillator	2000	700 nm	3.5 V	297 µW
Stangel et al. (2001)	Programmable IOP sensor with EEPROM and RF transponder	2001	1.2 µm	3.0 V	210 µW
Mokwa and Schnakenberg (2001)	IOP sensor and RF transponder	2001	1.2 µm	3.0 V	150 µW

Source: Reproduced with permission from Chow et al. (2010).

IOP devices reported earlier, which revealed that this IOP sensor consumed approximately 200 000 times less power, which alone demonstrates the dramatic progress made in only a few years (see Table 14.1).

The long tail of the tadpole is convenient for increasing the antenna length, and thus the transmission distance. *In vivo* the system had bit error rate (BER) around 10E–4 over a distance of 50 cm operating at 8 Mb/s, whereas this BER was reduced to 7.5 × 10E–5 in free space for the same distance. This sizeable transmission distance is viewed as a significant step forward compared to previous IOP systems, but in addition the telemetry performance was found to be largely independent of orientation, a problem that also plagued previous devices.

After a measurement run that could last for up to 24 h, an external reader could be used to download the data whilst simultaneously supplying power and recharging the capacitor array. The measurement data were sent from the reader via USB for storage on a PC. During evaluation tests of the developed sensor within a pressure chamber (Fig. 14.14) the measurement system demonstrated an average sensitivity of 6.64 fF/mmHg over the IOP range, transmitting this data to a reader situated outside the chamber.

With a similar philosophy of making more autonomous implants, Turner and Naber in the same year (Turner and Naber, 2010) introduced their initial configuration for a commercial capacitive sensor combined with a radio-frequency identification (RFID)-based operating system (operating

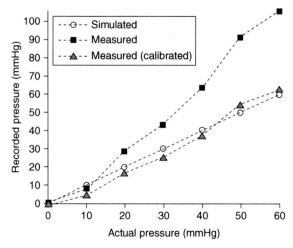

14.14 Experimental evaluation of IOP sensor within a pressure-regulated chamber demonstrating similar trends with and without a calibration factor (reproduced with permission from Chow *et al.*, 2010).

at 13.6 MHz) with on-chip FeRAM. The use of RFID was motivated to reduce the complexity of previous wireless interfaces. A custom ASIC (manufactured using a 0.5 µm CMOS process) sampled the IOP at 10 min intervals and stored the data for later download by an external reader using custom Wireless Serial Peripheral Interface (SPI) to link to external SPI-enabled modules. A super-capacitor power-module was charged externally and allowed the implant to operate independently for 24 h. Power consumption was estimated at 30 µA during wireless transmission. However, the range of the implant was limited to a few centimetres. In the following year (2011), they reported a new prototype system operating at 915 MHz that extended the range up to 100 cm (Faul *et al.*, 2011).

Also that year Haque and Wise at the University of Michigan reported on some fabrication aspects of a project that was developing an autonomous IOP sensor incorporating a capacitive pressure sensor, an ultralow power ASIC, a custom power supply, and wireless components, all of which were hermetically sealed within a glass package and encapsulated in parylene (Haque and Wise, 2010). Micromachining of glass is problematic and therefore a new glass-in-silicon wafer process was developed to form the glass topology, which also allowed electrical connections to be made through the glass to the capacitor thereby keeping these components within the sealed implant. In the fabrication process DRIE was used to form a mould by etching 250 µm deep channels into a silicon wafer substrate, and a 500 µm thick glass wafer was then bonded upon this. These two materials were heated together above 750°C for a period of eight hours, which caused the glass

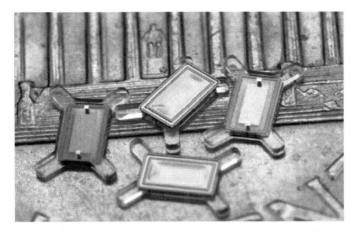

14.15 Capacitive pressure sensors made from a glass reflow process in silicon upon a U.S. penny (reproduced with permission from Wise, 2010).

to flow into the moulded wafer. The silicon was then lapped away until the glass was exposed.

This hybrid structure could then be used with conventional micromachining fabrication techniques to form the final capacitive pressure sensor. The glass-in-silicon wafer serves as the substrate to which the silicon pressure sensing diaphragm (0.85 mm × 1.65 mm) rim is bonded, and an example device is shown in Fig. 14.15 with the vacuum-sealed silicon diaphragm on the front. The capacitance sensors were tested in a pressure-regulated chamber and showed a sensitivity of 26 fF/mmHg, resolving better than 1 mmHg over the IOP range. The second generation of sensor design (Haque and Wise, 2011) using the glass-in-silicon process employed a two-step DRIE process to create additional cavities for an ASIC, and a miniature battery (Fig. 14.16).

In the following year, the University of Michigan team developing an ultralow power IOP implant sensor reported their progress to date (Chen et al., 2011). In the system described in their paper, the researchers have addressed each of the issues to create possibly the most advanced active IOP implant yet, that may make a long-term autonomous implant a real possibility. One significant component of the implant is an energy harvesting technique. A custom rechargeable 1 μAh thin-film lithium battery (EnerChip™) was manufactured by Cymbet™ Corp (Minnesota, USA). With no recharging these batteries can last up to 28 days. However, a miniature photovoltaic diode (of dimensions 0.7 mm^2) is integrated into the system and this converts light entering through the cornea into electrical charge that is stored in

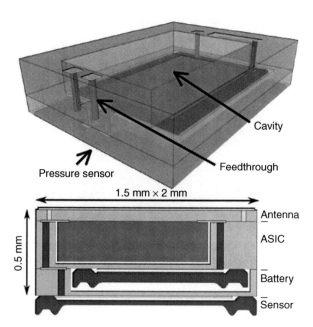

14.16 Multi-layered enclosure fabricated with a novel glass-in-silicon wafer process containing gold interconnects between cavities that will house dedicated circuitry and components for a future IOP sensor. Dimensions given are anticipated following fabrication (reproduced with permission from Haque and Wise, 2011).

the battery. Being rechargeable extends the life of the implant, with possibly as little as 1.5 h of sunlight daily being enough to recharge it.

The implant is fabricated in 0.18 µm CMOS and incorporates a MEMS capacitive pressure sensor, a 7 µW capacitance to digital converter (CDC), 90 nW microcontroller, 4 kb static RAM, and wireless (UWB) transceiver. The standard operation of the implant is waking up and taking a measurement of IOP every 15 min, storing this data and going back to sleep. Using the 10-bit data format means that after 24 h around 1 kb of memory has already been used and therefore there is an option to wirelessly reprogram the microcontroller to compress the memory data so that data logging can be extended to more than one week.

Power consumption is µWs during IOP measurements and rises to mWs for wireless data transmissions. However, these events are periodic and short-lived, and overall average power consumption is kept below 10 nW, which allows the implant to be autonomous. This is facilitated by the processor power being 30 pW when on standby. The integrated circuits and components are wire-bonded together and stacked vertically in four layers (Fig. 14.17) within a biocompatible glass housing formed by the glass reflow

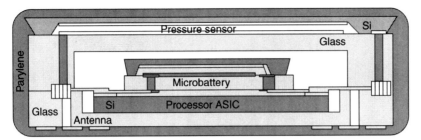

14.17 Final stacked components layout within parylene encapsulated housing (reproduced with permission from Wise, 2010).

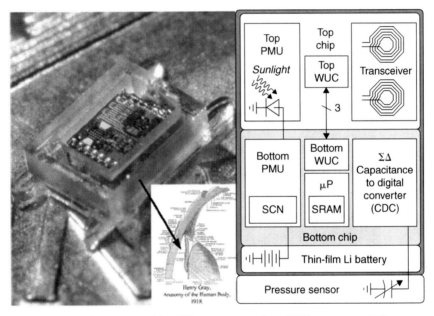

14.18 Final one cubic millimetre operational IOP sensor on U.S. penny (reproduced with permission from Chen *et al.*, 2011).

process developed by Haque and Wise. This glass housing is itself encapsulated inside parylene to give an implant of approximately 1 mm^3 in size (Fig. 14.18).

The recommended implant location is upon the iris (Fig. 14.19) so that the maximum amount of light coming through the transparent cornea can be used to recharge the battery. The researchers have also addressed the surgical aspects of the implantation by including glass fasteners (haptics) on the micromachined platform (Fig. 14.20) that fix the implant with the help of the natural elasticity of the iris. This negates initial tissue damage via tacking but also reduces damage if the implant needs to be removed later.

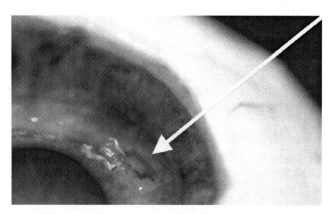

14.19 Demonstrating the implant (minus circuitry) in a human cadaver eye (see arrow) using haptics to negate the need for tacking. Position of implant indicated by white arrow (reproduced with permission from Haque and Wise, 2011).

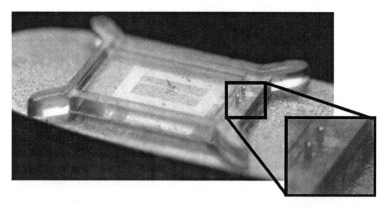

14.20 Close up of glass haptics used to secure IOP sensor (reproduced with permission from Haque and Wise, 2011).

In addition, the IOP sensor resolution of 0.5 mmHg betters the typical 1 mmHg of external tonometric measurement systems. After a desired period of IOP measurements within the eye of the patient, the stored data can be transmitted to an external device using 400 and 900 MHz frequencies to increase the distance. The implant was demonstrated as having a BER less than 10E–6 after passing through 5 mm of saline and then through 10 cm of air. As yet, human testing of the implant is still a few years away but the biocompatibility of the components has been demonstrated previously over extended periods and thus an autonomous long-term implant for IOP monitoring is now a very real possibility.

14.6 Active and passive MEMS contact lenses for IOP monitoring

In 2003 Leonardi et al. (2003) introduced a novel method for the continuous measurement of IOP using an external technique that if successful would alleviate the need for implant and removal surgery, and perhaps lower the cost of IOP sensors, thus promoting their uptake globally. The methodology is to measure changes in the external curvature of the cornea and relate this to internal IOP variations.

Research during the 1990s on human volunteers revealed a direct link between a step change in IOP and changes in radius of corneal curvature (Lam and Douthwaite, 1997) as well as a detailed *in vitro* investigation correlating corneal biomechanics with incremental IOP changes confirming this association (Hjortdal and Jensen, 1995).

Therefore, to try to access these corneal changes, Leonardi and co-workers created microfabricated strain gauges encapsulated in a soft (silicone) contact lens that would measure the changing curvature of the cornea via changes in the measured strain of the gauges. In total, four platinum–titanium strain gauges (two for corneal curvature measurements and two for temperature compensation) were configured in a Wheatstone bridge format. The gauges were composed of 200 nm platinum with 20 nm of titanium encapsulated in insulating polyimide (PI 2611, Dupont), creating a sensor approximately 6 μm thick. The final contact lens was made from silicone (NuSil MED-6015) by several cast moulding steps, which allowed the sensors, microprocessor and antenna to be embedded within the lens. Silicone was used for its known low water absorption and thus the sensor would be less affected by changing atmospheric moisture. In the initial proof-of-concept design a 3 cm connection wire ran from the contact lens to the measuring electronics.

Theoretical analysis revealed that the Wheatstone bridge voltage (V) can be related to the change in IOP (Δp) by the expression

$$\Delta p = \frac{2bV}{\alpha GIR} \qquad [14.3]$$

where I is the applied current, R is the inherent resistance of the gauges, G is a gauge factor, b is a proportionality constant, and α is the initial angle of a point on the contact lens. Thus a change in IOP can be directly related to the Wheatstone bridge voltage.

Initial experiments conducted on model eyes revealed encouraging results yielding a reproducibility of about 2 mmHg for this novel IOP sensor for pressure variations applied to the eye. This research laid the foundation for the company Sensimed AG (Switzerland) in 2003 to commercialize

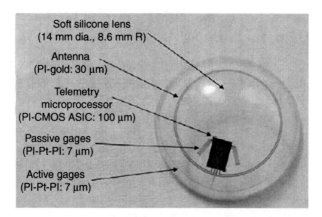

14.21 Soft contact lens technology developed by Sensimed AG for continuous monitoring of IOP (© Sensimed AG-2012).

this non-invasive technology for continuous monitoring of IOP. Subsequent improvements in contact lens design included the removal of the connection wire and replacement with a 50 μm thick ASIC for wireless data transfer to a portable reader operating in the ISM band at 27 MHz. Power is sent externally from either a pair of glasses or an eye patch to a 10 mm diameter, 30 μm thick gold antenna in the contact lens (Fig. 14.21). Antenna and gauges are connected to the ASIC via conductive glue.

In 2009, Leonardi *et al.* reported on *in vitro* experiments using the developed contact lens sensor with ten enucleated pig eyes fed with saline through a cannula and sitting vertically upright. By varying the saline pressure, the IOP could be varied and data from the contact lens sensor was wirelessly transmitted to a computer for analysis. Even though the contact lens was designed for the dimensions of a human eye rather than a pig eye, the results demonstrated that the contact lens sensor followed the variation in IOP between 20 and 30 mmHg very well and in a linear fashion, to a reproducibility of ±0.2 mmHg under these simplified conditions (no blinking or lens movement).

The system developed by Sensimed AG was given the commercial name Triggerfish™ and in early 2009 received its CE-mark paving the way for human clinical trials (Fig. 14.22). One disadvantage of using silicone is that it is naturally hydrophobic and before clinical use the lens has to be oxygen-plasma treated to render a hydrophilic surface between the lens and the cornea. However, if the lens is removed the surface becomes hydrophobic again and thus CE-mark compliance required each lens was for single use up to 24 h.

In 2010, a 24-h study on the continuous monitoring of IOP with the contact lens (Sensimed AG whitepaper, 2010) was conducted on healthy volunteers,

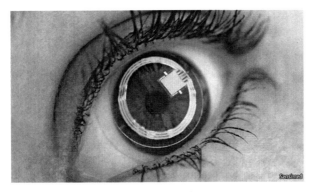

14.22 Approval of European CE-mark has led to human clinic trials of Sensimed AG soft contact lens IOP sensor (© Sensimed AG-2012).

which revealed that the sensor performed well on the subject's eyes (no tolerability issues) and the use of the sensor to monitor peaks and troughs of IOP can support decision making regarding treatment (e.g. effectiveness of medications to lower IOP). However, reproducibility and validation of the results still need to be confirmed at this stage. Another trial more recently in August 2012 (Mansouri *et al.*, 2012) on 40 patients, with and without glaucoma, also revealed good tolerability and concluded that the IOP sensor showed fairly good reproducibility.

Particular issues that arise when using the contact lens on humans are the frequent blinking and eye movements, which can lead to signal fluctuations and deviations of the sensor. The repetitive blink actions are likely to cause short-lived spikes in the sensor trace and can thus be filtered out. The contact lens will also repeatedly move across the cornea during blinking and eye movements, but overall it is expected to return to the same position, thus averaging out errors. Other physiological parameters regarding the living cornea (such as thickness, rigidity and diversity amongst subjects) may affect the calibrated sensor over time and need more research and trials.

A recently established company called Ophtimalia (France) have recently reported initial investigations of a passive contact lens with an embedded coil that uses a mutual inductance system with a secondary external coil to sense changes in resonant frequency in the embedded coil as the curvature of the cornea changes (Auvray *et al.*, 2012). By appropriate modelling of the complete system, the sensor response can be correlated to changes of IOP that can be detected by an external reader built into a spectacle frame. The philosophy behind this methodology is for the contact lenses to be disposable and the complex electronic signal processing to be done externally. If the technology can be sufficiently low cost then this approach may one day allow the technology to be used globally.

14.7 Conclusion

In just two decades microelectronics and MEMS technology and processes, combined with wireless data transfer, have provided the tools to create novel devices that were once the realm of science fiction. For the successful treatment of glaucoma, ophthalmologists have long sought continuous monitoring of IOP whilst allowing the patient to carry on with their daily lives. The steady progress in the field of MEMS and microelectronics in creating ever smaller features and functions, lower power-consuming circuitry, and autonomous self-powering systems, has delivered for the first time technology that can be implanted into the eye, or worn on the eye, to monitor the internal pressure bringing hope that glaucoma can be detected early enough to prevent total blindness. Already several companies, such as AcuMEMS Inc (Menlo Park, California), Implandata Ophthalmic Products GmbH (Hanover, Germany), and LaunchPoint Technolgies Inc (Goleta, California), are developing and commercializing implantable MEMS sensors that collect continuous IOP measurements inside the anterior chamber of the eye and transmit the data to an external device worn by the patient. Other companies, such as Sensimed AG (Switzerland) and Ophtimalia (France), are developing contact-lens-based technologies to be worn for a short time externally, collect a set of IOP measurements, and then be removed. Each approach has its advantages and disadvantages, issues and concerns, but it is always advantageous to have different cross-disciplinary teams addressing a problem from different angles, finding new and unexpected ways to use MEMS to make a meaningful difference in the lives of people. Extrapolating from the progress we have witnessed over the last twenty years, in the next twenty years implanted MEMS IOP sensors may well be integrated with automated MEMS relief valves and a MEMS drug delivery system to lower the IOP to provide a long-term closed-loop monitoring and treatment system.

14.8 References

Asrani, S., Zeimer, R., Wilensky, J., Gieser, D., Vitale, S., and Lindenmuth, K. (2000) 'Large diurnal fluctuations in intraocular pressure are an independent risk factor in patients with glaucoma', *J. Glaucoma*, **9**, 134–142.

Auvray, P., Rousseau, L., Lissorgues, G., Soulier, F., Potin, O., Bernard, S., Dieuleveult, F., Scorsone, E., Bergonzo, P., Chicaud, L., Picaud, S., and Sahel, J. A. (2012) 'A passive pressure sensor for continuously measuring the intraocular pressure in glaucomatous patients', *IRBM*, **33**, 117–122.

Backlund, Y., Rosengren, L., and Hok, B. (1990) 'Passive silicon transensor intended for biomedical, remote pressure monitoring', *Sensors and Actuators*, **A21–A23**, 58–61.

Bron, A. M., Creuzot-Garcher, C., Goudeau-Boutillon, S., and d'Athis, P. (1999) 'Falsely elevated intraocular pressure due to increased central corneal thickness', *Graefes Arch. Clin. Exp. Ophthalmol.*, **237**, 220–224.

Chen, G., Ghaed, H., Haque, R., Wieckowski, M., Kim, Y., Kim, G., Fick, D., Kim, D., Seok, M., Wise, K., Blaauw, D., and Sylvester, D. (2011) 'A cubic-millimeter energy-autonomous wireless intraocular pressure monitor', *IEEE Int. Solid-State Circuits Conference*, 310–312.

Chen, P. J., Rodger, D. C., Saati, S., Humayun, M. S., and Tai, Y. C. (2008) 'Microfabricated implantable parylene-based wireless passive intraocular pressure sensors', *J. MEMS*, **17**, 1342–1351.

Chen, P. J., Saati, S., Varma, R., Humayun, M. S., and Tai, Y. C. (2010) 'Wireless Intraocular pressure sensing using microfabricated minimally invasive flexible-coiled LC sensor implant', *J. MEMS*, **19**, 721–734.

Chow, E. Y., Chlebowski, A. L., and Irazoqui, P. P. (2010) 'A miniature-implantable RF-wireless active glaucoma intraocular pressure monitor', *IEEE Trans. Biomed. Circ. and Sys.*, **4**, 340–349.

Collins, C. C. (1967) 'Miniature passive pressure transensor for implanting in the Eye', *IEEE Trans. Bio-Medical Engineering*, BME-**14**, 74–83.

Copt, R. P., Thomas, R., and Mermoud, A. (1999) 'Corneal thickness in ocular hypertension, primary open-angle glaucoma, and normal tension glaucoma', *Arch. Ophthalmol.*, **117**, 14–16.

Eggers, T., Draeger, J., Hille, K., Marschner, C., Stegmaier, P., Binder, J., and Laur, R. (2000) 'Wireless intra-ocular pressure monitoring system integrated into an artificial lens': In 1st Annual International IEEE-EMBS Special Topic Conference on Microtechnologies in Medicine and Biology, 466–469.

Fang, E. N., Law, S. K., Walt, J. G., Chiang, T. H., and Williams, E. N. (2008) 'The prevalence of glaucomatous risk factors in patients from a managed care setting: A pilot evaluation', *Am. J. Manag. Care*, **14**, S28–S36.

Faul, A., Turner, M., and Naber, J. (2011) 'Implantable wireless microsystems for the measurement of intraocular pressure', *IEEE MWSCAS* **2011**, 1–4.

Haque, R. M. and Wise, K. D. (2010) 'An intraocular pressure sensor based on a glass reflow process', *Solid-State Sensors, Actuators, and Microsystems Workshop*, 49–52.

Haque, R. M. and Wise, K. D. (2011) 'A 3D implantable microsystem for intraocular pressure monitoring using a glass-in-silicon reflow process', *MEMS* **2011**, 995–998.

Hjortdal, J. and Jensen, P. K. (1995) '*In vitro* measurement of corneal strain, thickness, and curvature using digital image processing', *Acta Ophthalmol Scand.*, **73**, 5–11.

Hoskins, S., Sobering, T., Andresen, D., and Warren, S. (2009) 'Near-field wireless magnetic link for an ingestible cattle health monitoring pill', *IEEE EMBC* **2009**, 5401–5404.

Kakaday, T., Plunkett, M., McInnes, S., Jimmy Li, J. S., Voelcker, N. H., and Craig, J. E. (2008) 'Development of a wireless intra-ocular pressure monitoring system for incorporation into a therapeutic glaucoma drainage implant', *SPIE* **7270**, 72700.

Lam, A. K. C. and Douthwaite, W. A. (1997) 'The effect of an artificially elevated intraocular pressure on the central corneal curvature', *Ophthal. Physiol. Opt.*, **17**, 18–24.

Leonardi, M., Leuenberger, P., Batrand, D., Bertsch, A., and Renaud, P. (2003) 'A soft contact lens with a MEMS strain gage embedded for intraocular pressure monitoring', in: Transducers '03, The 12th International Conference on Solid Slate Sensors, Actuators and Microsystems, Boston, 1043–1046.

Leonardi, M., Pitchon, E. M., Bertsch, A., Renaud, P., and Mermoud, A. (2009) 'Wireless contact lens sensor for intraocular pressure monitoring: assessment on enucleated pig eyes', *Acta Ophthalmol.*, **87**, 433–437.

Li, W. (2009) *Integrated Retinal Implants*, Thesis, California Institute of Technology.

Lin, J. C. H., Zhao, Y., Chen, P. J., Humayun, M., and Tai, Y. C. (2012) 'Feeling the pressure A parylene-based intraocular pressure sensor', IEEE Nanotechnology Magazine, September, 8–16.

Liu, J. H. K., Zhang, X., Kripke, D. F. and Weinreb, R. N. (2003) 'Twenty-four hour intraocular pressure pattern associated with early glaucomatous changes', *Invest. Ophthalmol. Vis. Sci.*, **44**, 1586–1590.

Mansouri, K., Medeiros, F. A., Tafreshi, A., and Weinreb, R. N. (2012) 'Continuous 24-hour monitoring of intraocular pressure patterns with a contact lens sensor – safety, tolerability, and reproducibility in patients with glaucoma', *Arch Ophthalmol.* August, 1–6. Available from: http://www.sensimed.ch/images/pdf/2012-08-15_mansouri_safety_tolerability_reproducibility.pdf (accessed October 2012).

Mokwa, W. and Schnakenberg, U. (2001) 'Micro-transponder systems for medical applications', *IEEE Trans. Instrum. Meas.*, **50**, 1551–1555.

Rosengren, L., Backlund, V., Sjostrom, T., Hok, B., and Svedbergh, B. (1992) 'A system for wireless intra-ocular pressure measurements using a silicon micromachined sensor', *J. Micromech. Microeng.*, **2**, 202–204.

Sarkisian, S. R., Jr. (2006) 'An update on tonometry', *Glaucoma Today*, **31**, 31–36.

Schnakenberg, U., Walter, P., vom Bogel, G., Kruger, C., Ludtke-Handjery, H. C., Richter, H. A., Specht, W., Ruokonen, P., and Mokwa, W. (2000) 'Initial investigations on systems for measuring intraocular pressure', *Sens. and Actua.*, **85**, 287–291.

Sensimed AG whitepaper (2010). Available from: http://www.sensimed.ch/images/pdf/white_paper_safety_tolerability.pdf (accessed October 2012).

Stangel, K., Kolnsberg, S., Hammerschmidt, D., Hosticka, B. J., Trieu, H. K., and Mokwa, W. (2001) 'A programmable intraocular CMOS pressure sensor system implant', *IEEE J. Solid-State Circ.*, **36**, 1094–1100.

Turner, M. and Naber, J. (2010) 'The development of a RFID based mixed signal ASIC for the wireless measurement of intraocular pressure', *Micro/Nano Symposium (UGIM)*, 1–4.

Wang, X., Engel, J., and Liu, C. (2003) 'Liquid crystal polymer (LCP) for MEMS: Process and applications', *J. Micromech. Microeng.*, **13**, 628–633.

Whitacre, M. M. and Stein, R. (1993) 'Sources of error with use of Goldmann type tonometers', *Surv. Ophthalmol.*, **38**, 1–30.

Wise, K. D. (2010) 'Microelectronics in the "More than Moore" era', Device Research Conference (DRC), 3–4.

Wolgemuth, L. (2000) 'Assessing the performance and suitability of parylene coating', *Med. Device Diagn. Indust.*, **22**, 42–49.

15
Drug delivery using wireless MEMS

R. SHEYBANI, S. M. SCHOBER and E. MENG,
University of Southern California, USA

DOI: 10.1533/9780857098610.2.489

Abstract: Drug delivery is essential for the treatment of chronic conditions. Implantable site-specific drug delivery devices offer direct delivery to the site of therapy, improving treatment outcomes while reducing side effects and overall associated healthcare costs. Microelectromechanical systems (MEMS) miniaturize infusion pumps such that they are implantable; wirelessly-powered to eliminate the use of bulky, limited lifetime batteries; and volume efficient. Wireless communication allows remote monitoring of device status and performance, and remotely initiated changes to the drug regimen for patient tailored therapy. Requirements for a MEMS drug delivery device with wireless powering and data communication are presented along with an example of such a device.

Key words: implantable site-specific drug delivery device, micro infusion pump, MEMS wireless communication, wireless power and data transmission.

15.1 Introduction

Drug therapy is critical for the management of chronic diseases, such as cardiovascular disease, cancer, diabetes, arthritis, and respiratory disease. Together, these conditions are projected to affect an estimated 50% of Americans by 2030. The management of chronic conditions contributes to an estimated 83% of total healthcare costs today (The Council of State Governments, 2006). The average annual healthcare coverage cost for individuals suffering from a chronic condition is $6032, which is five times higher than for healthy individuals (Menehan, 2006). Therefore, effective drug therapy is a critical healthcare need.

Conventional pharmacological therapies rely on oral, topical, or parenteral drug administration. Parenteral drug injection uses conventional needles and catheters, and requires repeated time- and labor-intensive procedures for chronic treatment. These are associated with frequent clinical visits, lost productivity at the work place or in the field, low patient compliance, and elevated risk of infection. Many drugs are delivered systemically (throughout the entire body directly through circulation, or via the skin or the gastrointestinal route) which requires high doses for efficacy and results in significant waste of expensive drugs and serious unintended side effects.

External infusion pumps are used extensively in hospitals for post-surgery pain management. Most systems currently used, such as Hospira's Symbiq® Infusion System (Hospira Inc., 2011) and the Carefusion Alaris® System (CareFusion Corporation, 2011), are computer-controlled syringe pumps that provide considerable improvement in safety and accuracy over old-fashioned drip-chamber and roller-clamp systems (Fig. 15.1a). Modern infusion pumps provide the desired flow rate to the patient's intravenous line, and include safety features to ensure failures are promptly reported (Maxim, 2010). Recent designs, such as Baxter's Spectrum Infusion System (Fig. 15.1b), include a bi-directional wireless communication system. Wireless pumps reduce the number of cables that tether the patient to the equipment and allow for the freedom of patient movement beyond the hospital bed (Baxter, 2011). However, all these systems deliver the drug systemically, a route which is associated with such side effects as constipation, dizziness, drowsiness, headache, and nausea (Drugs.com, 2000–2011), for which additional medical intervention may be required. Also, the large dose of drug associated with systemic delivery could lead in the case of pain medications to patient dependency.

Site-specific drug delivery systems allow for the precise amount of drug to be delivered in the therapeutic range directly to the site of therapy. Localized delivery lowers the amount of drug required to reach therapeutic concentrations in the body, and enables the use of more potent drugs (Tang et al., 2008). These systems can reduce the cost of healthcare and the number of doctor visits, and improve patient compliance. Furthermore, the use of automated and implantable drug delivery systems for the management of chronic conditions will maximize drug efficacy, reduce side effects, and improve treatment outcomes (Fiering et al., 2009).

In this chapter, we discuss the motivation for wireless drug delivery devices and the advantages of a MEMS approach for implantable infusion pumps. Design requirements for wireless powering and wireless data communication, including biological and security concerns, are reviewed. Finally, we explore a case study of an implantable MEMS drug delivery system.

15.2 Wireless power and data for drug delivery applications

Drug delivery devices that are tetherless are highly desirable. Eliminating the use of wires and catheters would lead to a higher patient mobility range, and allow for drug administration to take place outside of clinical settings. Despite advances in battery technologies on their miniaturization,

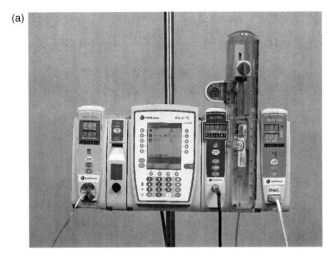

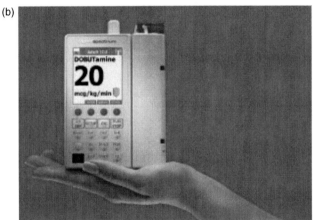

15.1 (a) Carefusion Alaris® System (CareFusion Corporation 2011, used with permission), and (b) Baxter's Spectrum Infusion System (Baxter, 2011, used with permission).

batteries are still large in comparison to MEMS devices and can significantly increase the overall device size and weight. Also, batteries have a limited lifetime and may pose risk to the patient if leakage or malfunctions occur (Si *et al.*, 2007). Wireless powering of drug delivery devices can eliminate the battery and considerably reduce the size of the device. The system lifetime is also improved.

There are two levels of data transfer relevant to medical implants. The first is short-range communication with the device, to monitor device status and performance and send commands to adjust operation. Changes in dosing tailor the therapeutic regimen to each patient's needs during the course

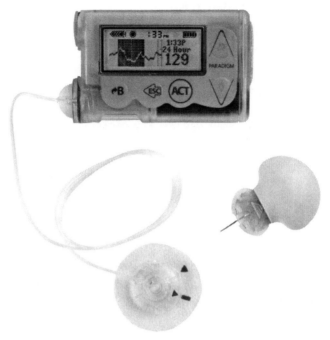

15.2 Medtronic's MiniMed Paradigm® REAL-Time Revel™ System (Medtronic Inc., 2011, Manufactured by the Diabetes business unit of Medtronic, Inc., used with permission).

of therapy. The second is remote monitoring, through data transfer between the device and an internet-based network. Remote monitoring of clinical events and symptoms reduces the frequency of routine follow-up visits. This in turn reduces staff time and costs, while improving the patient's quality of life (Panescu, 2008).

Medtronic's MiniMed Paradigm REAL-Time Revel System (Fig. 15.2) is an example of wireless communication used to inform the drug regimen in the treatment of diabetes. The device combines a wireless glucose sensor with an insulin infusion pump that is worn externally. A catheter delivers insulin through the skin. The sensor wirelessly updates the glucose reading every five minutes. Wireless communication is also used to monitor device activity. The externally worn receiver stores data for up to 30 days, after which it can be downloaded to a computer (Medtronic Inc., 2011). Medtronic has also set up the Medtronic CareLink Pro® Network to provide an internet-based implant monitoring system (Medtronic Inc., 2011).

Many sites cannot be easily accessed through the skin with a simple catheter. For such targets, the diabetes pump format is not suitable. Factors such as discomfort, risk of infection, and the impact on daily activities, may point to the use of a completely implantable pump. MEMS technology can be leveraged to miniaturize drug infusion pumps to meet a form factor that is suitable for implantation.

15.3 A MEMS approach to drug delivery

One of the major concerns for implantable biomedical devices is miniaturization (Albason *et al.*, 2011). Using MEMS technology will allow for complete implantation of miniaturized devices, which reduces patient discomfort, reduces the risk of infection, and eliminates tampering with or damage to the device (Si *et al.*, 2007).

There are two types of MEMS drug delivery systems: passive and active. In passive devices, such as osmotic pumps, the rate of drug delivery is controlled by diffusion and so the flow cannot be modified or stopped after the device is implanted or injected into the targeted area. Such passive devices do not require electrical powering. For active devices, the rate of drug delivery is directly controlled following an external trigger (Smith *et al.*, 2007). Here, we will focus on active devices in which flow of drug can be started or stopped as desired, and the rate can be modified at any time during the course of treatment.

Debiotech's JewelPump® is an example of an insulin micropump for diabetes treatment (Fig. 15.3). The micropump contains a pumping chamber with a flexible membrane, two passive check valves and a pressure sensor. The pressure sensor increases safety by monitoring the performance of the pump during use (Schneeberger *et al.*, 2009). The pump is worn as a patch on the skin and can be wirelessly programmed and monitored using a personal handheld device such as a cellphone. Each disposable reservoir is worn for six days. However, wireless technology is only used for communication, and the device still requires a battery for operation (Debiotech S.A. Switzerland, 2011). Debiotech is in

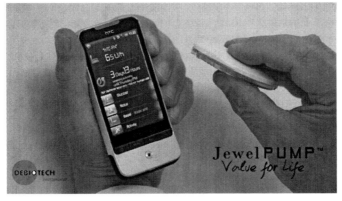

15.3 Debiotech's JewelPump® (Debiotech S.A. Switzerland 2011, used with permission).

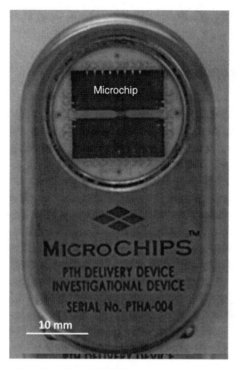

15.4 The MicroCHIPS® micro-reservoir device (Farra *et al.*, 2012, reprinted with permission from AAAS).

the process of further miniaturizing the device so that it can be completely implantable inside the body (Debiotech S.A. Switzerland, 2011).

The MicroCHIPS® micro-reservoir device (Fig. 15.4) is an example where MEMS technology is used to enable an implantable drug delivery system. An array of tiny reservoirs is used to store drug until it is ready to be released in the body. Each individual reservoir is wirelessly actuated to initiate drug release and has the ability to control precisely the dose delivered. Dosing can be terminated without the need for device extraction (Prescott *et al.*, 2006). The devices are compatible with preprogrammed microprocessors, wireless telemetry, and sensor feedback loops, which can be integrated in the future (MicroCHIPS Inc., 2011).

15.3.1 MEMS drug delivery system requirements

A microtechnology-enabled drug delivery system should allow for accurate, efficient, targeted on-demand delivery of drug without the need for patient intervention. The drug pump should be implanted and refillable through the skin, eliminating the need for multiple surgery and catheters. Pumps should be compatible with an assortment of drugs (both conventional and new) to fit the needs of different patients in treating a wide variety of conditions.

From a design standpoint, the pumping mechanism chosen should be small, reliable, and biocompatible, with low power consumption and cost (Laser and Santiago, 2004). Micropumps are categorized into two groups based on the pumping mechanism: mechanical and non-mechanical. A majority of mechanical micropumps (electrostatic, piezoelectric, thermo-pneumatic, bimetallic, shape memory alloy (SMA), and ionic conductive polymer film (ICPF)) operate based on reciprocating displacement, in which a deformable plate with fixed edges does work by periodically applying pressure to the fluid (Amirouche *et al.*, 2009; O'Brien and Santhanam, 1985). Smits introduced the first MEMS-based piezo-electrically actuated peristaltic pump to deliver insulin to diabetic patients in 1984 (Smits, 1989). Since then, there has been a substantial amount of research and development in this field (Amirouche *et al.*, 2009). Electrostatic and piezoelectric micropumps require a high driving voltage and high power, so they are not suitable for wireless applications. SMA micropumps suffer from low flow rate, and are usually not biocompatible. Non-mechanical micropumps utilize the transformation of a certain available non-mechanical energy into kinetic momentum to drive fluid. Generally, non-mechanical micropumps (magnetohydrodynamic (MHD), electrohydrodynamic (EHD), electroosmotic (EO), electrochemical, osmotic, capillary, electrowetting (EW), and diffuser/nozzle) are smaller, simpler in design and easier to fabricate because they do not require physical actuation components; however, their performance with regards to flow rate, response time, and back pressure may be inferior to mechanical micropumps. EHD and MHD micropumps require the working fluid (drug) to be electrically conductive which limits their application (Tsai and Sue, 2007). Electrochemical pumps have low power operation (μW–mW range) making them suitable for wireless applications. Also they generate negligible heat, deliver accurate flow with their large driving force, and can be constructed with biocompatible materials (Sheybani and Meng, 2011).

Case study

An example of an implantable drug delivery system that includes all the requirements mentioned above is being developed at the Biomedical Microsystems Lab at the University of Southern California (Li *et al.*, 2010). The implantable micropump consists of an electrochemical actuator adjacent to, and acting on, a separate drug reservoir, whose outflow leads to a catheter (Fig. 15.5). Constant current applied to an electrode pair in the actuator electrolyzes water, which consequently produces a pressure increase due to gas expansion. This deflects the flexible membrane and drives drug out of the adjacent drug reservoir through the delivery catheter.

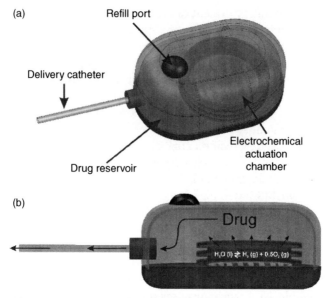

15.5 Implantable MEMS micropump: (a) device schematic and (b) operation principle.

For repeated bolus delivery, the pump is turned on and off by supplying current to the actuator only when dosing is desired. This design allows the catheter to be placed virtually anywhere in the body to target the specific tissue afflicted by the chronic condition. Accurate and reliable dosing is possible by controlling the magnitude of the applied current (to control the flow rate) and its duration (to control of dose). Therefore, the dosing regimen can be altered remotely in an on-demand manner at any point during the treatment. The drug pump is implanted subcutaneously and the reservoir is refillable through the skin, eliminating the need for multiple surgery and daily catheterization. This technology is scalable and compatible with an assortment of drugs (both conventional and new) to enable the treatment of a wide variety of conditions.

15.3.2 Wireless powering requirements for an implantable MEMS drug delivery system

There are four types of wireless power transmission. In practice (through design), only one method is selected as the preferred mode. For transcutaneous powering, inductive transmission is most suitable compared to other forms of wireless powering (radiative, conductive, and capacitive). Due to size restrictions, radiative powering would require the frequency to be in the GHz range for sufficient power reception. This would lead to large power dissipation in biological tissue and attenuation of the transferred power, which are both undesirable. Conductive and capacitive links rely on the electric field. The body acts as a bad conductor and leaky dielectric, which means both these methods would encounter large losses. Inductive powering, however relies on magnetic field coupling and the transmission frequency can be chosen to minimize power dissipation (Lenaerts, 2008). Therefore, we will focus on inductive powering and provide a brief explanation of the design requirements of a simple powering system.

A typical inductive powering system consists of two separate coils, a transmitter (primary) and a receiver (secondary), which, in the case of an implantable device, would be placed inside the body (Albason *et al.*, 2011). An alternating current applied to the transmitting coil can induce a magnetic field, which is then picked up by the receiving coil. The electromotive force that is produced as a result can be converted to a direct current (DC) voltage or current source to drive an attached load (Lenaerts, 2008) (Fig. 15.6).

Transmission efficiency is increased when the coils are tuned to the same resonant frequency. The resonant (e.g. operating) frequency of the device is selected based on the device placement and the resulting attenuation of the magnetic field when traveling through air and biological tissue. At lower carrier frequencies, transmission may be slow and insufficient. However, at higher frequencies (e.g. GHz range), the rate of power attenuation is also higher due to water absorption, and could cause excessive heating that might lead to tissue damage when transmitting a power signal (Albason *et al.*, 2011; Liang *et al.*, 2005). The size of the implant also affects the selected frequency. Generally, higher frequencies would allow for smaller receiver coils sizes; for example, if the frequency is shifted from the MHz to the GHz range, the coil size can be reduced 104 times (Poon *et al.*, 2007). Therefore, the size restrictions and the required transmission power and time should be carefully considered when selecting the operating frequency. It is important

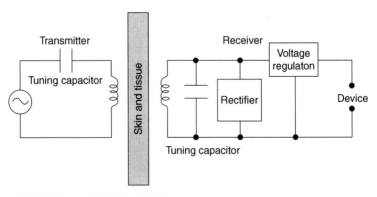

15.6 Wireless powering circuit.

to note that while it is preferable for the receiver coil to be small so that the overall implant size is minimized, within those limits, the largest possible coil is required to maximize pick-up of the transmitter's magnetic flux. Once the size of the receiver and the frequency are decided upon, based on the aforementioned considerations, and the working distance between the coils is finalized, the optimal size for the transmitter can be derived based on a DC finite-element model of the secondary coil explained in Lenaerts (2008).

One of the important quantities defined for inductive coupling is the ratio between mutual inductance and self-inductance of the transmitting and receiving coil, named the coupling coefficient, K. This coefficient is unitless and can be defined as:

$$0 \leq K \equiv \frac{M}{\sqrt{L_1 L_2}} \leq 1$$

where M is the mutual inductance and L_1 and L_2 are the self-inductances of the two coils (Glisson, 2011). K is zero when there is no coupling at all, and equals 1 for perfect coupling. When the geometry is held constant, the value of K is independent of the number of turns of the coils. The coupling coefficient captures the magnitude of the magnetic flux induced by the transmitter that is linked to the receiver (Tang et al., 2008), so it is desirable to maximize the coupling efficiency (Lenaerts, 2008).

Another important coil parameter for each of the coils is the quality factor, Q, which is defined as:

$$Q \equiv \frac{\omega L}{R}$$

where R is the frequency dependent equivalent series resistance of the coil and ω is the transmission frequency (Glisson, 2011). At the selected transmission frequency, a high quality factor (>100) is required to maximize the induced field on the secondary. High Q can be achieved through coil design (Liu et al., 2010; Tesla, 1893) and construction; using multi-wound Litz wire to fabricate the receiver coil will alleviate the shift in resonant frequency caused by winding and ohmic losses; and by increasing self-resonance of the coil due to inherent parasitic capacitances that can be used beneficially (Lenaerts, 2008; Liu et al., 2010). Sullivan uses standard analysis of proximity-effect losses in combination with a power law modeling of insulation thickness to find the optimal stranding of Litz wire when designing coils (Sullivan, 1997). High power transfer efficiency (defined as $\eta = K^2 Q_{transmitter} Q_{receiver} / (1 + K^2 Q_{transmitter} Q_{receiver})^2$ (Schuylenbergh and Puers, 2009)) can be achieved through maximizing Q, or K, or both (Kumar et al.,

2009). However, when maximizing Q and K, it is important to note that these parameters are not independent of each other (Lenaerts, 2008).

Typically, the transmitter circuit is tuned in series to lower load impedance, and the receiver circuit is tuned with a parallel capacitor that cancels the inductive impedance of the coil since this leads to better performance when driving a non-linear rectifier load (Albason *et al.*, 2011). If DC power is required to drive the implant, a rectifier is used to convert alternating current (AC) power to DC power. Even though the transmitted power can be kept constant, the received magnetic field can fluctuate due to coil foveation or changes in distance, with respect to one another or changes in the transmission medium. To limit the voltage supplied to the load, a voltage regulator can be used after the rectifier (Tang *et al.*, 2008). Similarly, if constant current is desired, current regulator circuitry may be utilized. Otherwise the power can be controlled on the transmitter side by detecting changes in the peak to peak AC signal reflected by the receiver circuitry. Donaldson describes the steps required to create the necessary feedback loop to achieve this (Donaldson, 1985).

During the prototyping stage, using surface mount components will reduce size, and negative/positive zero temperature coefficient (NPO) capacitors can reduce power loss due to thermal effects of non-ideal components (Liang *et al.*, 2005). However, once the design of the implantable circuitry is finalized, it is preferable to fabricate the design in customized application specific integrated circuits (ASIC), using complementary metal oxide semiconductor (CMOS) technology. Integrated circuits will increase the reliability and allow for a considerable reduction in device size compared to surface-mounted components. Also, customized chips have reduced power consumption and dissipation which is preferred in order to prevent tissue heating (Albason *et al.*, 2011).

Wireless powering has some limitations, such as short operating range, imperfect transfer efficiency due to frequency tuning, and required alignment between coils (Zhang *et al.*, 2009). When designing a wireless implant, it is assumed that the receiver coil is placed inside a freely moving subject. Depending on the orientation of a single transmitting and receiving coil, if the coils are oriented perpendicularly with regards to each other, then the mutual inductance would be zero and, essentially, no power would be transmitted (Lenaerts, 2008). Therefore, it is important to account for the possible foveation in the design. One solution would be to have multiple transmitting or multiple receiving coils. When using multiple transmitting coils, at least three coils should be used that are linearly independent. In this configuration, feedback from the receiver is used to determine the transmitter coil with the best coupling, and that coil is used for powering while the other two coils are turned off (Fig. 15.7). The second approach would be to use multiple receiving coils with one transmitter. Once again, three coils with perpendicular winding axes are sufficient. With three series resonant

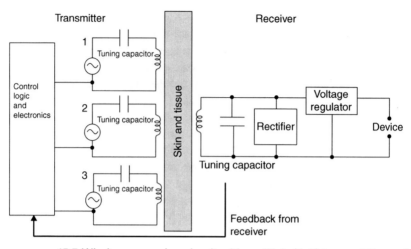

15.7 Wireless powering circuit with multiple (1–3) transmitting coils.

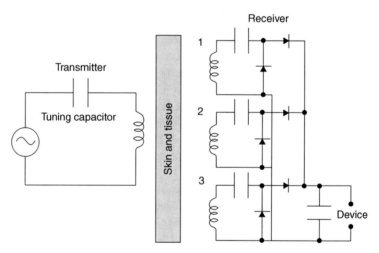

15.8 Wireless powering circuit with multiple (1–3) receiving coils.

secondary tanks, and three parallel rectifiers, the power received from all three coils can be combined in a common filter capacitor (Fig. 15.8). This approach does not require feedback (Lenaerts, 2008).

15.3.3 Wireless data transfer requirements for a MEMS drug delivery system

If designed appropriately, it is possible for the wireless powering inductive link to also support data flow from the transmitter to the receiver and vice versa. For transfer towards the receiver, the current driving the transmitter is manipulated, usually through amplitude modulation. The rectifier on the receiving circuit can be used to demodulate the data signal (Lenaerts, 2008). For data transfer from the receiver to the transmitter, passive absorption modulation can be used, in which a switch is manipulated by the data signal to short the resonant tank, affecting the current passing through the receiver coil. Since the coils are coupled, the modulation is reflected in the transmitter. A separate coil decoupled from the transmitter could be used to better decipher the magnetic field of the receiver (Lenaerts, 2008). Another approach would be to use 'sub-carrier modulation' (Finkenzeller, 2003), in which logic gates are used to multiply the data stream by a subharmonic f/m (f is frequency and m is an integer) obtained using a digital counter (Coosemans and Puers, 2005). After transmission, a band-selective filter is used to filter the power signal and obtain the data stream (Lenaerts, 2008).

Bi-directional data transmission can also be achieved by combining both methods mentioned above, that is, amplitude shift keying (ASK) used for sending commands and data to the receiver, and load shift keying (LSK) or 'reflectance modulation' as a backward transmission method (Fig. 15.9) (Albason *et al.*, 2011).

For wireless communication of data between the transmitter and an internet-based external device, protocols such as Bluetooth and ultra-wide band (UWB) are often used (Chow *et al.*, 2009; Panescu, 2008). Other communication protocols that are specifically designed to work in the Industrial, Scientific, and Medical (ISM) bands, which show promise in the medical device monitoring area, but require a custom integrated circuit (IC) kit to connect to internet-based devices, include the WiseNet sensor network and the IEEE 802.15.4 'ZigBee' wireless standard (El-Hoiydi *et al.*, 2006; IEEE, 2007). The advantage of using Wisenet and ZigBee is that these small

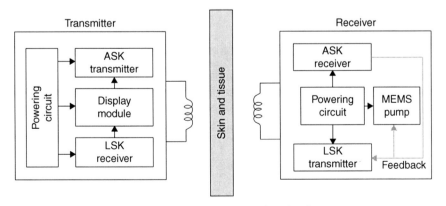

15.9 Bi-directional wireless data transfer circuit.

device communication protocols are much lower power and simpler than Bluetooth and UWB. Attenuation in the data signal due to water in tissue severely limits data transfer for implanted devices in the GHz range; therefore, it is important to consider the data communication protocol operating frequency.

The GHz frequency range can be utilized for data communication to achieve faster data transfer without concerns over high attenuation since higher bandwidths are available (Lenaerts, 2008). However, while faster transfer rates are desirable, faster rates generally require more power and more sophisticated integrated circuit designs, (Panescu, 2008) therefore a careful balance should be reached.

When designing wireless data transfer, the environment in which the device is primarily used should be considered and the carrier frequency and communication protocol should be carefully chosen, so that other RF sources do not interfere with communication. The U.S. Federal Communications Commission (FCC) has allocated a 14 MHz range (608–614, 1395–1400, and 1427–1432 MHz) as a wireless medical telemetry service (WMTS) spectrum to be used by medical telemetry systems without interference to and from other users of the electromagnetic radio spectrum. Authorized healthcare providers are eligible to use this spectrum without a license as long as their device is registered with FCC's designated frequency coordinator, the American Society for Healthcare Engineering of the American Hospital Association (ASHE/AHA) (Federal Communications Commission, 2010).

Qualcomm Life has recently developed the 2net™ platform, a cloud-based system designed to be universally-interoperable with different medical devices and applications. Access to the platform is via a 'plug-and-play' gateway hub that supports Bluetooth, Bluetooth Low Energy, WiFi, and ANT+ local area radio protocols. Data is acquired from the medical device through the 2net hub™, and then transferred and stored in the cloud. This information can be accessed securely by medical device users and their physicians or caregivers (Qualcomm Life Inc., 2011).

15.4 Biological constraints and requirements

Wireless powering and data communication with an implantable device requires an inductive coupling link through skin and biological tissue. When designing such a system, it is important to consider the effects of the device and inductive coupling on the surrounding tissue and vice versa.

15.4.1 Effects of an inductive field on biological tissue

At frequencies below 100 kHz, direct physiological interaction with the tissue should be considered, in which the field causes particle displacement inside living tissue. Excessive displacement may result in difficult breathing, pain, uncontrolled muscle contractions, and interfere with heart function (Polk and Postow, 1995). At higher frequencies, particles do not move effectively, and instead the dominant issue is tissue heating. To assess the heating effects, specific absorption rate (SAR), which is the amount power absorbed per unit of mass, is used as a metric. The thermo-regulatory system of the body is affected if the overall SAR exceeds 4 W/kg (International Commision on Non-Ionizing Radiation Protection, 1998). It is also advised to limit exposure time to prevent heating. Regardless of the frequency used, a healthy human adult cannot perceive current densities below 10 mA/m^2 (International Commision on Non-Ionizing Radiation Protection, 1998).

International Commission on Non-Ionizing Radiation Protection (ICNIRPs) guidelines (International Commision on Non-Ionizing Radiation Protection, 1998) and IEEE standard levels with respect to human exposure to radio frequency electromagnetic fields (Committee, 1999; Committee, 2002) should be used to limit exposure and prevent damage to biological tissue.

15.4.2 Effects of biological tissue on an inductive field

Electromagnetic fields are affected by biological tissue. Brown describes tissue as a leaky dielectric (Brown, 1999). This could cause losses in transfer efficiency and limit the operating distance between the transmitter and receiver. The effects vary, depending on the location and depth of the implant and also on the composition of the surrounding tissue (Chow *et al.*, 2009), including a fibrous capsule of collagenous tissue that may be created around the implant as a result of the body's natural immune system response (Prescott *et al.*, 2006).

It is essential that medical implant development includes stringent tests and experiments to identify possible harmful effects of the device on the body and the body on the device. Saline and *ex vivo* tissue are good models for first preliminary evaluation. It is important to remember that when using *ex vivo* tissue, additional tissue material should be placed behind the implant to simulate back-scattering and better represent the actual implant conditions (Chow *et al.*, 2009). Several formulas have been proposed to simulate the electrical properties of biological tissue (Chou *et al.*, 1984; Fukunaga *et al.*, 2004; Karacolak *et al.*, 2009; Lazebnik *et al.*, 2005; Stuchly *et al.*, 1987). As an example, Table 15.1 lists simple formulas to simulate the electromagnetic properties of muscle, brain, lung, and bone tissue (Hartsgrove *et al.*, 1987).

15.5 Security concerns for wireless implants

While there are many advantages to wireless powering and data transfer, there are also vulnerabilities that need to be considered. Wireless

Table 15.1 Simple formulas to simulate the electromagnetic properties of muscle, brain, lung, and bone tissue

	Material	Percentage by weight
Muscle tissue	Water	52.4
	NaCl salt	1.4
	Sucrose sugar	45.0
	Hydroxyethyl cellulose (HEC)	1.0
	Bacteriacide (Dowicil 75®)	0.1
Brain tissue	Water	40.4
	NaCl salt	2.5
	Sucrose sugar	56.0
	Hydroxyethyl cellulose (HEC)	1.0
	Bacteriacide (Dowicil 75®)	0.1
Lung tissue	Muscle Material	47
	Hollow silica microspheres (Ø 30–180 μm)	54
Bone tissue	TWEEN	57.0
	n-Amyl alcohol	28.5
	Paraffin oil	9.5
	Water	4.5
	NaCl salt	0.5

Source: Hartsgrove *et al.*, 1987 (reprinted with permission from Wiley Company).

communication between devices opens the device to possibilities of tampering or information theft. Devices triggered by a wireless cue can allow a hacker to cause harm to a patient by sending commands that alter the prescribed drug regimen. For instance, on 4 August 2011, Jerome Radcliffe, a security researcher and diabetic, showed the audience at the Black Hat security conference in Las Vegas, how he could hack into his wireless insulin pump and tamper with the dose regimen (Takahashi, 2011). Data transfer from the device may allow a 'data harvester' or a hacker to steal patient information. Therefore, communication to and from the device should be secure (Malasri and Wang, 2009; Panescu, 2008).

In order to prevent tampering with an implantable device, measures should be taken so the device only responds to requests and commands from an approved external device. Two approaches have been patented:

1. In U.S. Patent 6,880,085 by Balczewski and Lent, a password-based approach was proposed. Before implantation of a device, a specific password is programmed that would be required for all subsequent communication with the device (Balczewski and Lent, 2005). However, as pointed out by Malasari and Wang, the patent does not explain how the password is protected after implantation when it is transmitted between the implant and external device (Malasri and Wang, 2009).

2. In U.S. Patent 7,155,290, von Arx, Koshiol, and Bange present a two-step method to secure wireless communication. First, the external device should send an unlock command to the implant through short-range communication. Then the two devices must share an authentication code before communication can commence (von Arx *et al.*, 2003).

However, the problem with both schemes is that the device needs to be extracted before the password can be reprogrammed after the device security has been compromised (Malasri and Wang, 2009).

Besides intended tampering, there is also the issue of accidental device compromise due to interference from surrounding wireless communication. For this, the European Communication Commission (ECC) has recommended two types of interference avoidance techniques. The first is to 'listen before talk' in which frequency agility is used to adapt to a frequency band with low ambient signals, and the second is to use a decreased transmitted power level with a duty cycle of <0.1% (Panescu, 2008).

It is the responsibility of developers of wireless implantable drug delivery devices to implement security measures to protect the device from tampering by unauthorized users, including the patients themselves.

15.6 Wireless inductive powering and uni-directional data system for a MEMS drug pump

The electrochemical micropump in the aforementioned case study requires constant current to be supplied to a pair of interdigitated electrodes to electrolyze water into hydrogen and oxygen and provide the actuation driving force. Depending on the desired flow rate (0.3–141.9 μL/min), the current is set (0.1–13 mA). Power ranging from 0.6 to 60 mW is required to supply the constant current. The wireless power system should be capable of providing this power, with high transfer efficiency and low heat dissipation in the surrounding tissue. The operating distance is affected by the implant depth. The pump is designed to be placed under the skin to be refilled percutaneously.

15.6.1 Case study

For the first prototype, a simple Class D amplifier wireless powering system (Fig. 15.10) was developed (Sheybani *et al.*, 2011). Class D systems can provide the large current needed to create the magnetic field; however, series-tuning of the primary coil cancels inductance leakage through the coil, lowering the required driving voltage. They are also less dependent on coupling as long as the load stays well above the switch-on resistance (Schuylenbergh and Puers, 2009). These features make Class D systems suitable for simple

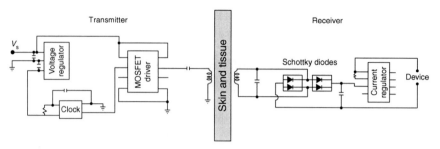

15.10 Class D amplifier wireless powering system (Sheybani and Meng, 2011).

first stage prototyping. The transmitter circuit consisted of a voltage regulator (LM2937IMP-5.OCT-ND, National Semiconductor, Agoura Hills, CA), a metal oxide semiconductor field effect transistor (MOSFET) Class D amplifier (TC4420CPA-ND, Microchip Technology, Chandler, AZ), and a 2MHz clock crystal (CTX755- ND, CTS-Frequency Controls, Albuquerque, NM). The receiver circuit included a full wave rectifier with Schottky diodes (BAS7006ZXCT-ND and BAS7005CT-ND, Diodes Zetex Semiconductors, Oldham, United Kingdom), along with a current regulator (LM334SM, National Semiconductor, Agoura Hills, CA) to control the power being delivered to the electrochemically driven MEMS drug delivery system.

The design was implemented using discrete components. The effects of distance between coils and foveation between the transmitter and receiver were studied (Fig. 15.11) before flow rate testing was performed on the drug delivery device (Table 15.2). Flow rates higher than that of a constant current source (Keithley, 2400 source meter, Cleveland, OH) were measured for the same set current with <2% standard error for each set current. While simple in design, this Class D system using discrete components had several drawbacks. The MOSFET driver chip had large process variations, making it difficult to fine-tune the amplifier. MOSFET switching and the open loop configuration caused the MOSFET driver to heat up and sometimes burn out.

A second receiver device was designed with a low drop-out (LDO) switching regulator (LTC3670EDDB#PBF, Linear Technology, Woodland Hills, CA) with a faster response time and higher linear efficiency compared to the current regulator previously used (Fig. 15.12). In this design, a half-wave rectifier was implemented to reduce the noise level and the number of components needed. A Zener diode (MM3Z4V3CCT-ND, Fairchild Semiconductor, San Jose, CA) was attached in parallel with the circuit to limit the input voltage (4.3 V) to the regulator. This design was first simulated using LTSpice, before being implemented using surface mount components on a flexible printed circuit board (PCB) on a scale that could be integrated to an implantable drug delivery device. Benchtop testing was performed

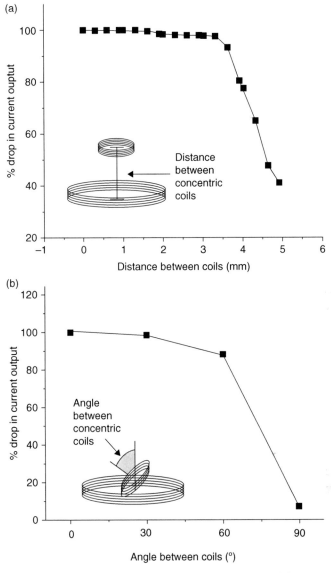

15.11 The effects of (a) distance between coils and (b) foveation between the transmitter and receiver on current output.

using the transmitter described in (Givrad, 2007). Flow rates were comparable to that achieved with (Keithley 2400 source meter, Cleveland, OH). The results of changing distance between coils and foveation between the transmitter and receiver are shown below (Fig. 15.13). The device was then packaged for *in vivo* testing: electronics were encapsulated using epoxy and

Table 15.2 Flow rate results

Current (mA)	Flow rate with constant current source (µL/min)	Flow rate with wireless system (µL/min)
2	14.16 ± 0.34	20.00 ± 0.14
5	46.40 ± 0.32	59.00 ± 1.11
8	82.65 ± 0.38	98.67 ± 0.41
10	106.8 ± 0.72	125.67 ± 1.44

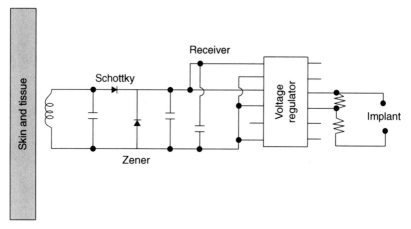

15.12 Second receiver device with a LDO switching regulator.

attached to the drug delivery device. The completely packaged system was covered in medical-grade silicone rubber (MDX-4, Factor II Inc., Lakeside, AZ) before being coated by a 9 µm thick conformal layer of Parylene C to enhance biocompatibility and reduce moisture permeability. A 30 day trial, with the packaged device immersed in a 37°C water bath, showed continued accurate and reliable dosing with <3.7% standard error.

It is important to note that due to the nature of electrolysis and the linear relationship between current and flow rate, a receiver with a constant current output would be more suitable for this application.

The next phase in design was connecting a purchased Bluetooth radio (2.4 GHz) to the transmitter circuitry for wireless control. A Parallax Board of Education USB carrier board kit, a Basic Stamp 2 Module microcontroller, and an Easy Bluetooth Module were purchased (Parallax Inc., Rocklin, CA). The output of the Bluetooth module was used to control a single pole OptoMos relay (LCA 717, Clare, Inc., Beverly, MA), controlling the power to the transmitter circuit. Basic Stamp 2 Editor (v. 2.5.2) was used to program the communication. The program created allowed for the transmitter circuit to be controlled wirelessly via Bluetooth. Figure 15.14 shows a photograph

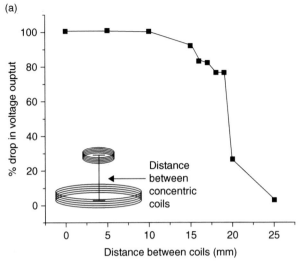

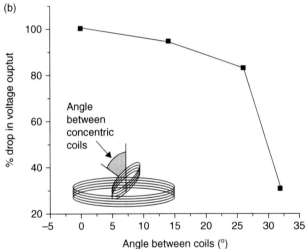

15.13 The effects of (a) distance between coils and (b) foveation between the transmitter and receiver on voltage output.

of the entire setup for wireless powering with wireless Bluetooth control of the transmitter.

15.7 Suggested improvements and future generation device

An improved wireless power and bi-directional control data system composed of new transmitter and receiver will require establishing a new set

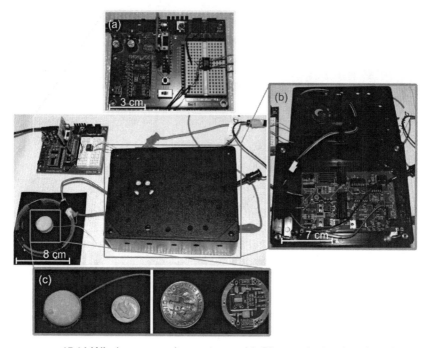

15.14 Wireless powering system with Bluetooth circuitry for wireless control: (a) Parallax Board of Education, Basic Stamp 2 Module microcontroller, and an Easy Bluetooth Module; (b) transmitter circuit; (c) packaged micropump and receiver PCB.

of design goals to improve the wireless power transfer and to include control data transfer at the desired 2 MHz frequency. These include: (1) to design a receiver coil which possesses a higher Q in order to more effectively transfer power to the implanted circuitry; (2) to be able to increase or decrease the transmitted power delivered by the transmitter to accommodate for when changes in distance and/or foveation between the transmitter and receiver coils occur; and (3) to have a method for controlling and monitoring the amount of drug delivered by the drug pump.

In the receiver implanted circuitry, obtaining a high Q in the coil is of prime importance, in order to allow for efficient power transfer and generally a smaller implanted coil. Also, equally important is matching the resonant frequency of the receiver circuitry to the transmitter's transmitted frequency signal to reach maximum power transfer between the two coils, since the coupling coefficient, K, is usually low (i.e. on the order of 0.1–0.3) when transmitting power through tissue (Ghovanloo and Atluri, 2007). A parallel RLC (resistor, inductor, and capacitor) tank circuit can be utilized for matching to the desired resonant frequency of 2 MHz in the receiver. Two techniques to increase the inductor quality factor, Q, and further match the self-resonant frequency, ω, of the receiver parallel tank inductor to the desired 2 MHz signal include: (1) using multi-wound Litz wire; and (2) applying the Tesla bifilar coil structure to the design (Tesla, 1893). These two techniques could potentially allow for the tank's tuning capacitor component to be eliminated, due to the creative utilization of the natural, distributed parasitic parallel capacitances between the wires (in both the Litz and the Tesla bifilar coils).

Improvements could also be made to both the transmitter and receiver circuitry to account for undesired fluctuations in the transmitted power levels, which must be kept in check in order to maintain a constant current delivered to the drug pump. Common circumstances when the power drops lower than desired include the transmitter and receiver coils moving away from the optimal distance (e.g. 1 cm) or when misalignment in the angle between the coils takes place. To remedy this, the transmitter circuitry can be designed so that it is able to sense reflected power off the receiver in a wireless closed loop fashion and adjust the amount of power sent from the transmitter circuitry.

There are a variety of methods on how to approach controlling the amount of drug delivered by the drug pump if given minimal limitations in the areas of power, size, and cost. For example, in the receiver, a microcontroller could be added to the design and programmed with an implantable radio to change the desired current levels (e.g. 8–10–12 mA), thus changing the rate of drug dosage. This receiver design is confined by size, due to the desire for the device to be implantable, and cost. Therefore, tradeoffs must be accounted for and analyzed. The challenges faced with employing a pre-packaged microcontroller and a separate implantable radio include power consumption, complexity, size, cost, and programming effort. Ideally, a microcontroller, inductive powering circuitry, and a low power implantable radio designed on a single custom integrated circuit would be the end-all solution. A different approach that allows for a much simpler, low power system design is to keep the current delivered to the drug pump constant, and to change the duty cycle of the transmitted primary signal to alter the rate of flow of drug dosage.

The future goal for the wireless powering and bi-directional data transfer circuitry is to take the re-design and characterize the transmitter and receiver design for the MEMS drug pump based on the aforementioned requirements, and then to create a custom integrated circuit chip in CMOS technology based on the finalized design. The planned future design includes the wireless control circuitry, a microcontroller, and a custom implanted medical band radio on the same die.

15.8 Conclusion

Management of chronic conditions that require drug therapy contributes to a large portion of healthcare costs. Current methods are inadequate and give rise to large overdoses and associated side effects that adversely affect the patient's quality of life, while further imposing burden on healthcare providers. Wireless implantable site-specific drug delivery systems can alleviate these problems and allow for safe and effective treatment. Several factors need to be carefully considered when designing a wireless system for an implantable device, including power consumption, communication range, data transfer rates, size and cost, security, and the effects of environment on the device and vice versa (Panescu, 2008).

Using MEMS technology will allow for complete implantation of miniaturized devices that reduce patient discomfort, reduce the risk of infection, and eliminate tampering or damage to the device (Si *et al.*, 2007). MEMS micropumps can be divided into active and passive pumps, based on the actuation method they employ, and there are several pumping mechanisms. Depending on the specific application, the appropriate actuation mechanism should be chosen based on the size, power consumption, flow rate, response time, fabrication requirements, reliability, biocompatibility, and cost. This chapter has focused on active MEMS micropumps that could be programmed to release the required amount of drug at a specific time and be tailored to each patient's needs. These pumps need to be powered.

Batteries are often employed to power fully implantable devices. However, despite advances in battery technologies on their miniaturization, batteries are still large in comparison to MEMS devices and can significantly increase the overall device size. Also, batteries have a limited lifetime and may pose risk to the patient if leakage or malfunctions occur (Si *et al.*, 2007; Tang *et al.*, 2008). Wireless powering of drug delivery devices can eliminate the battery and considerably reduce the size of the device.

Of the four types of wireless power transfer, inductive transmission is most suitable for transcutaneous powering. When designing the powering system, several factors considered: transmission frequency should be carefully chosen; Q and K need to be maximized to achieve higher transfer efficiency; and solutions for limited power transfer due to foveation between transmitting and receiving coils, as a result of the subject movement, should be implicated (Lenaerts, 2008).

Wireless data communication allows device status and performance to be monitored remotely, as well as remotely initiated changes to the drug regimen by caregivers throughout the course of treatment to tailor the drug regimen to the individual needs of each patient. There are two levels of data transfer relevant to medical implants. The first is short-range communication with the device to monitor device status and performance and send commands to adjust operation. Changes in dosing tailor the therapeutic regimen to each patient's needs during the course of therapy. The second is remote monitoring through data transfer between the device and internet-based network. Remote monitoring of clinical events and symptoms reduces the frequency of routine follow-up visits. This in turn reduces the staff time and costs, while improving the patient's quality of life (Panescu, 2008).

Wireless powering and data communication with an implantable device requires inductive coupling linkage through skin and biological tissue. When designing such a system, it is important to consider the effects of the device and inductive coupling on the surrounding tissue and vice versa.

Lastly, it is the responsibility of developers of wireless implantable drug delivery devices to implement security measures to protect the device from tampering by unauthorized users, including the patients themselves, as well as interference from other wireless devices the patients may come in contact with through everyday life.

The case study example presented in this chapter introduces a MEMS electrochemically actuated micropump. The pump allows for accurate and reliable dosing, so that the dosing regimen can be altered remotely in an on-demand manner at any point during the treatment. The drug pump is implanted subcutaneously and the reservoir is refillable through the skin when drug is exhausted, eliminating the need for multiple surgeries and daily catheterization. This technology is scalable and compatible with an assortment of drugs (both conventional and new) to enable the treatment of a wide variety of conditions. A Class E wireless powering system is presented, which could be fabricated in a modular fashion apart from the pump. Wireless control of the transmitter is enabled through a commercially available Bluetooth kit and feedback data transfer from the implanted micropump is underway. Suggestions for further improvements are also presented.

15.9 Acknowledgment

This work was supported by Henry M. Jackson Foundation agreement #2267 through the Qualcomm/TATRC Wireless Health Innovation Challenge and National Science Foundation (NSF) IIP-1157852.

15.10 References

Albason, A. C., D. W.-Y. Chung and S.-L. Lou. (2011). 'A 2 MHz wireless CMOS transceiver for implantable biosignal sensing systems'. *Journal of Signal Processing Systems* **62**(3): 263–272.

Amirouche, F., Z. Yu and T. Johnson. (2009). 'Current micropump technologies and their biomedical applications'. *Microsystem Technologies* **15**(5): 647–666.

Balczewski, R. A. and K. Lent (2005). *Security system for implantable medical devices.* U. S. P. Office. United States.

Baxter (2011). 'Baxter's SIGMA spectrum infusion', from http://www.baxter.com/healthcare_professionals/products/sigma_spectrum.html.

Brown, B. H. (1999). *Medical physics and biomedical engineering.* Bristol; Philadelphia, Institute of Physics Pub.

CareFusion Corporation (2011). 'Carefusion alaris system'. from http://www.carefusion.com/medical-products/infusion/alaris-system/index.aspx.

Chou, C. K., G. W. Chen, A. W. Guy and K. H. Luk (1984). 'Formulas for preparing phantom muscle tissue at various radiofrequencies'. *Bioelectromagnetics* **5**(4): 435–441.

Chow, E. Y., B. L. Beier, A. Francino, W. J. Chappell and P. P. Irazoqui (2009). 'Toward an implantable wireless cardiac monitoring platform integrated with an FDA-approved cardiovascular stent'. *Journal of Interventional Cardiology* **22**(5): 479–487.

Committee, I. S. C. (1999). IEEE standard for safety levels with respect to human exposure to radio frequency electromagnetic fields, 3 kHz to 300 GHz. USA, Inst. Electr. and; Electron. Eng., New York, NY, USA. IEEE Std C95.1, 1999 Edition: ix+73.

Committee, I. S. C. (2002). IEEE standard for safety levels with respect to human exposure to electromagnetic fields, 0–3 kHz. USA, Inst. Electr. and Electron. Eng., New York, NY, USA. IEEE Std C95.6-2002: vi+43.

Coosemans, J. and R. Puers (2005). 'An autonomous bladder pressure monitoring system'. *Sensors and Actuators A (Physical)* **123–124**: 155–161.

Debiotech S.A. Switzerland (2011). 'Debiotech jewel pump'. from http://www.jewelpump.com/.

Donaldson, N. D. N. (1985). 'Use of feedback with voltage regulators for implants powered by coupled coils'. *Medical and Biological Engineering and Computing* **23**(3): 291.

Drugs.com (2000–2011). 'Morphine side effects'.

El-Hoiydi, A., C. Arm, R. Caseiro, S. Cserveny, J. D. Decotignie, C. Enz, F. Giroud, S. Gyger, E. Leroux, T. Melly, V. Peiris, F. Pengg, P. D. Pfister, N. Raemy, A. Ribordy, D. Ruffieux and P. Volet (2006). *The ultra low-power WiseNET system.* 2006 Design, Automation and Test in Europe, 6–10 March 2006, Piscataway, NJ, USA, IEEE.

Farra, R., N. F. Sheppard, L. McCabe, R. M. Neer, J. M. Anderson, J. T. Santini, M. J. Cima and R. Langer (2012). 'First-in-human testing of a wirelessly controlled drug delivery microchip'. *Science Translational Medicine* **4**(122): 122ra121.

Federal Communications Commission (2010). Wireless medical telemetry service (WMTS). *Code of federal regulations (CFR), title 47.*

Fiering, J., M. J. Mescher, E. E. Leary Swan, M. E. Holmboe, B. A. Murphy, Z. Chen, M. Peppi, W. F. Sewell, M. J. McKenna, S. G. Kujawa and J. T. Borenstein (2009). 'Local drug delivery with a self-contained, programmable, microfluidic system'. *Biomedical Microdevices* **11**(Compendex): 571–578.

Finkenzeller, K. (2003). *RFID handbook: fundamentals and applications in contactless smart cards and identification.* Chichester, England; Hoboken, N.J., Wiley.

Fukunaga, K., S. Watanabe and Y. Yamanaka (2004). 'Dielectric properties of tissue-equivalent liquids and their effects on specific absorption rate'. *IEEE Transactions on Electromagnetic Compatibility* **46**(1): 126–129.

Ghovanloo, M. and S. Atluri (2007). 'A wide-band power-efficient inductive wireless link for implantable microelectronic devices using multiple carriers'. *IEEE Transactions on Circuits and Systems – I: Fundamental Theory and Applications* **54**(10): 2211–2221.

Givrad, T (2007). Induction power microbolus infusion pump used for functional neuroimaging applications in rodents. J.-M. I. Maarek. United States – California, University of Southern California. University of Southern California.

Glisson, T. H., Jr. (2011). *Introduction to circuit analysis and design*. New York, Springer Science + Business Media.

Hartsgrove, G., A. Kraszewski and A. Surowiec (1987). 'Simulated biological materials for electromagnetic radiation absorption studies'. *Bioelectromagnetics* **8**(1): 29–36.

Hospira Inc. (2011). 'Hospira symbiq infusion system'. from http://www.hospira.com/Products/symbiqinfusionsystem.aspx.

IEEE (2007). 'IEEE standard for information technology – telecommunications and information exchange between systems – local and metropolitan area networks – specific requirements part 15.4: Wireless medium access control (MAC) and physical layer (PHY) specifications f'. IEEE Std 802.15.4a: xiv+187.

International Commision on Non-Ionizing Radiation Protection (1998). 'Guidelines for limiting exposure to time-varying electric, magnetic, and electromagnetic Fields (up to 300GHz)'. *International Commission on Non-Ionizing Radiation Protection, Health Physics Society*.

Karacolak, T., R. Cooper and E. Topsakal (2009). 'Electrical properties of rat skin and design of implantable antennas for medical wireless telemetry'. *IEEE Transactions on Antennas and Propagation* **57**(9): 2806–2812.

Kumar, A., S. Mirabbasi and M. Chiao (26 November 2009–28 November 2009). *Resonance-based wireless power delivery for implantable devices*. 2009 IEEE Biomedical Circuits and Systems Conference, BioCAS 2009, Beijing, China, IEEE Computer Society.

Laser, D. J. and J. G. Santiago (2004). 'A review of micropumps'. *Journal of Micromechanics and Microengineering* **14**(6): 35–64.

Lazebnik, M., E. L. Madsen, G. R. Frank and S. C. Hagness (2005). 'Tissue-mimicking phantom materials for narrowband and ultrawideband microwave applications'. *Physics in Medicine and Biology* **50**(18): 4245–4258.

Lenaerts, B. (2008). *Omnidirectional inductive powering for biomedical implants*. New York, Springer.

Li, P.-Y., R. Sheybani, C. A. Gutierrez, J. T. W. Kuo and E. Meng (2010). 'A parylene bellows electrochemical actuator'. *Journal of Microelectromechanical Systems* **19**(Copyright 2010, The Institution of Engineering and Technology): 215–228.

Liang, C.-K., J. J. J. Chen, C. Cho-Liang, C. Chen-Li, and W. Chua-Chin *et al.* (2005). 'An implantable bi-directional wireless transmission system for transcutaneous biological signal recording'. *Physiological Measurement* **26**(1): 83–97.

Liu, L., X. Shao, F. Wu, X. Huo, W. Li and L. Mo (10 December 2010–12 December 2010). *Design and application research of implantable wireless power transmission micro electro mechanical system*. 4th International Seminar on Modern Cutting and Measurement Engineering, Beijing, China, SPIE.

Malasri, K. and L. Wang (2009). 'Securing wireless implantable devices for healthcare: Ideas and challenges [Accepted from Open Call]'. *IEEE Communications Magazine* **47**(7): 74–80.

Maxim (2010). 'Important considerations for infusion pump and portable medical designs'. *Maxim*.

Medtronic Inc. (2011). 'Medtronic CareLink® Network'.

Medtronic Inc. (2011). 'MiniMed paradigm revel insulin pump'. from http://www.medtronicdiabetes.net/products/paradigmrevelpump.

Menehan, K. (2006). Partnership for solutions: Better lives for people with chronic conditions. *National program report*. M. B. Janet Heroux, Robert Wood Johnson Foundation.

MicroCHIPS Inc. (2011). 'MicroCHIPS platform'. from http://www.mchips.com/technology.html.

O'Brien, R. N. and K. S. V. Santhanam (1985). *Anodic oxidation and deposition of polymer films as electrodes on metals*. Extended Abstracts, Spring Meeting – Electrochemical Society, Toronto, Ont, Can, Electrochemical Soc.

Panescu, D. (2008). 'Wireless communication systems for implantable medical devices'. *IEEE Engineering in Medicine and Biology Magazine* **27**(2): 96–101.

Polk, C. and E. Postow (1995). Interaction of DC and ELF electric fields with biological materials and Systems. *Biological effects of electromagnetic fields*, CRC Press.

Poon, A. S. Y., S. O'Driscoll and T. H. Meng (23–26 August 2007). *Optimal operating frequency in wireless power transmission for implantable devices*. 29th Annual International Conference of IEEE-EMBS, Engineering in Medicine and Biology Society, EMBC'07, Lyon, France, Inst. of Elec. and Elec. Eng. Computer Society.

Prescott, J. H., S. Lipka, S. Baldwin, N. F. Sheppard Jr, J. M. Maloney, J. Coppeta, B. Yomtov, M. A. Staples and J. T. Santini Jr. (2006). 'Chronic, programmed polypeptide delivery from an implanted, multireservoir microchip device'. *Nature Biotechnology* **24**(4): 437–438.

Qualcomm Life Inc. (2011). 'Introducing the 2Net Platform'. from http://www.qualcommlife.com/wireless-health.

Schneeberger, N., R. Allendes, F. Bianchi, E. Chappel, C. Conan, S. Gamper and M. Schlund (2009). 'Drug delivery micropump with built-in monitoring'. *Procedia Chemistry* **1**(1): 1339–1342.

Schuylenbergh, K. V. and R. Puers (2009). *Inductive powering: basic theory and application to biomedical systems*. Dordrecht, Springer.

Sheybani, R., H. Gensler and E. Meng (5–9 June 2011). *Rapid and repeated bolus drug delivery enabled by high efficiency electrochemical bellows actuators*. 2011 16th International Solid-State Sensors, Actuators and Microsystems Conference, Transducers '11 Beijing, China, IEEE.

Sheybani, R. and E. Meng (23 January 2011–27 January 2011). *High efficiency wireless electrochemical actuators: Design, fabrication and characterization by electrochemical impedance spectroscopy*. 24th IEEE International Conference on Micro Electro Mechanical Systems, MEMS '11, Cancun, Mexico, Institute of Electrical and Electronics Engineers Inc.

Si, P., A. P. Hu, J. W. Hsu, M. Chiang, Y. Wang, S. Malpas and D. Budgett (23–25 May 2007). *Wireless power supply for implantable biomedical device based on primary input voltage regulation*. 2007 Second IEEE Conference on Industrial Electronics and Applications, Piscataway, NJ, USA, IEEE.

Smith, S., T. B. Tang, J. G. Terry, J. T. M. Stevenson, B. W. Flynn, H. M. Reekie, A. F. Murray, A. M. Gundlach, D. Renshaw, B. Dhillon, A. Ohtori, Y. Inoue and A. J.

Walton (2007). 'Development of a miniaturised drug delivery system with wireless power transfer and communication'. *IET Nanobiotechnology* **1**(5): 80–86.

Smits, J. G. (12 June 1989–14 June 1989). *Piezoelectric micropump with microvalves*. Proceedings of the Eighth Biennial University/Government/Industry Microelectronics Symposium, Westborough, MA, USA, Publ by IEEE.

Stuchly, M. A., A. Kraszewski, S. S. Stuchly, G. W. Hartsgrove and R. J. Spiegel. (1987). 'RF energy deposition in a heterogeneous model of man: near-field exposures'. *IEEE Transactions on Biomedical Engineering* **BME-34**(12): 944–950.

Sullivan, C. R. (22–27 June 1997). *Optimal choice for number of strands in a litz-wire transformer winding*. PESC97. Record 28th Annual IEEE Power Electronics Specialists Conference. Formerly Power Conditioning Specialists Conference 1970–71. Power Processing and Electronic Specialists Conference 1972, New York, NY, USA, IEEE.

Takahashi, D. (2011) 'Excuse me while I turn off your insulin pump'. *Venture Beat, Interpreting Innovation*. Available at: http://venturebeat.com/2011/08/04/excuse-me-while-i-turn-off-your-insulin-pump/

Tang, T. B., S. Smith, B. W. Flynn, J. T. M. Stevenson, A. M. Gundlach, H. M. Reekie, A. F. Murray, D. Renshaw, B. Dhillon, A. Ohtori, Y. Inoue, J. G. Terry and A. J. Walton (2008). 'Implementation of wireless power transfer and communications for an implantable ocular drug delivery system'. *IET Nanobiotechnology* **2**(3): 72–79.

Tesla, N. (1893). *Coil for electromagnets*. U. S. P. Office.

The Council of State Governments (2006). *Costs of chronic diseases: What are states facing?*

Tsai, N.-C. and C. Y. Sue (2007). 'Review of MEMS-based drug delivery and dosing systems'. *Sensors and Actuators A (Physical)* **134**(2): 555–564.

Von Arx, J. A., A. T. Koshiol and J. E. Bange (2003). *Secure long-range telemetry for implantable medical device*. U. S. P. Office. United States.

Zhang, F., L. Xiaoyu, S. A. Hackworth, R. J. Sclabassi and S. Mingui (2009). *In vitro and in vivo studies on wireless powering of medical sensors and implantable devices*. 2009 IEEE/NIH Life Science Systems and Applications Workshop (LiSSA 2009), Piscataway, NJ, USA, IEEE.

16
RF MEMS for automotive radar

J. OBERHAMMER, N. SOMJIT,
U. SHAH and Z. BAGHCHEHSARAEI,
KTH Royal Institute of Technology, Sweden

DOI: 10.1533/9780857098610.2.518

Abstract: Radio-frequency microelectromechanical systems (RF MEMS) devices and circuits have attracted interest in applications such as car radar systems, particularly in the 76–81 GHz frequency band, due to their near ideal signal performance and compatibility with semiconductor fabrication technology. This chapter gives an introduction to state-of-the-art car radar sensors and architectures, describes the most commonly engaged RF MEMS components and circuits, and gives examples of RF MEMS-based automotive radar prototypes.

Key words: RF, MEMS, car radar, automotive radar, phase shifter.

Note: This chapter is a revised and updated version of Chapter 5 'RF MEMS for automotive radar sensors' by J. Oberhammer, N. Somjit, U. Shah and Z. Baghchehsaraei, originally published in *MEMS for automotive and aerospace applications*, eds M. Kraft and N. M. White, Woodhead Publishing Limited, 2013, ISBN 978-085709-118-5.

16.1 Introduction

Automotive safety is evolving from the use of passive systems, such as airbags and seat belts, to the use of active sensors for collision avoidance. The competing technologies to achieve active vehicular surround sensing functions include radar, lidar, ultrasonic, and video cameras.[1] Automotive radar is one of the leading technologies, owing to its weather independence and high information content, including range and speed detection, when compared to many alternative sensors, especially visual sensors. Additional information from the radar signal, for example angle of targets, can be extracted using advanced techniques. Automotive radar has been under development since the mid-1960s. The first applications using automotive radar were adaptive cruise control and collision warning systems. The collision warning systems were successfully introduced in the United States in the 1990s, with Greyhound installing more than 1600 radar systems in their buses resulting in reduction of accidents by 21%

in 1993 compared to the previous year.[2] Radar based autonomous cruise control (ACC) systems were first introduced in the Mercedes S class series in 1999.[3] Additional safety functions, such as pre-crash sensing and collision mitigation using active brake assist, are also offered in the 77 GHz radar sensor providing much higher braking forces for deceleration when a threat situation arises.[2,3] Frequency regulation is an important aspect of any commercially functioning radar and same is true for automotive radar. The 76–77 GHz band was regulated in the 1990s and now it is allocated for Intelligent Transport Services (ITS) in Europe, North America and Japan.[2] The Federal Communications Commission (FCC) regulated ultra-wide band (UWB) for the North American market in 2002. For the automotive UWB short-range radar systems the FCC allocated the band 22–29 GHz.[2] Because of strong objections from the telecom industry and earth observation institutions, a considerable effort was dedicated to finding a compromise and hence to enabling automotive UWB radar systems. In January 2005 it was decided by the European Commission to allocate the frequency band of 21.625–26.625 GHz for UWB short-range radar (SRR) for automotive applications on a temporary basis from July 2005 to 30 June 2013. It is expected that in eight years work will be done towards the introduction of inexpensive SRR sensors operating at a new frequency, without impairing other commercial, scientific or military systems and services. Hence, in March 2004 the European Commission allocated the frequency range 77–81 GHz for UWB SRR with permitted usage from 2005 onwards. Anticipating the allocation of this band also in Japan and North America, the SRR suppliers will probably shift their UWB developments from 24 to 79 GHz in the medium term.

16.1.1 Sensor types and architecture

Automotive radar sensors can be divided into two categories: short-range radar (SRR), and long-range radar (LRR). The combination of these types of radar provides valuable data for advanced driver assistance systems. The combination of SRR and LRR can be seen in Fig. 16.1, where LRR can track three motorway lanes over a distance of up to 150 m and SRR uses an angle of 80° to monitor the immediate area up to 30 m.[3]

Short-range radar (SRR)

For short-range applications, UWB sensors are preferred because of their low-cost perspective and their high resolution in range. Since these sensors do not require long-range capability, lower frequencies are preferred.[2] The applications of SRR are shown in Fig. 16.2, which include[3]: (1) ACC support with Stop and Go functionality; (2) collision warning; (3) collision

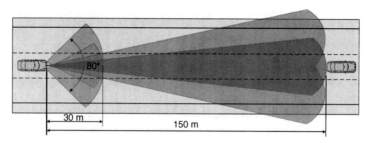

16.1 Combination of LRR and SRR for advanced safety features.[1]

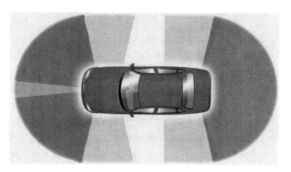

16.2 Applications using SRR.[1]

mitigation; (4) blind spot monitoring; (5) parking aid (forward and reverse); (6) lane change assistant; (7) rear crash collision warning.

Long-range radar (LRR)

The automotive LRR functions at 77 GHz to access blind areas in front of the automobile. This sensor provides information about the traffic situation in front of the vehicle, making it possible to react to altered traffic conditions. This radar is the fundamental part of the ACC with active brake assist. In contrast to the smooth deceleration capability of the ACC, the active brake assist provide much higher braking forces for deceleration.[2] LRRs measure the range, angle and relative radial velocity of multiple targets by using multi-beam antenna systems.

Radar sensors for automotive applications are typically divided into two categories: (1) continuous-wave (CW) radar and (2) pulse radar.

Continuous-wave radar

CW radar transmits and receives at the same time. The transmitter generates a continuous sinusoidal oscillation at frequency f_t which is radiated by the antenna. On reflection by a moving target, the transmitted signal is shifted via the Doppler effect by an amount f_d. It is also possible to measure range using a CW radar system by frequency modulation, or digital modulation techniques such as phase shift keying (PSK). A systematic variation of transmitted frequency or phase places a unique time stamp on the transmitted wave at every instant. By measuring the frequency or phase of the received signal, the time delay between transmission and reception can be measured and therefore the range can be measured.[4]

$$R = c \frac{T}{2} \frac{\Delta f}{f_2 - f_1}$$

where c is the speed of light, Δf is the difference between the transmitted and received signals, f_2 is the maximum transmitted frequency, f_1 is the minimum transmitted frequency and T is the period between f_1 and f_2, and the velocity is given by[4]

$$v = \frac{dR}{dt}$$

Pulse radar

The pulse Doppler-radar has the advantage of being able to detect small amplitude moving target returns against a large amplitude clutter background. Pulse-delay ranging is based on the measurement of the time delay between the transmitted pulse and the received echo.[4]

$$R = c \frac{\Delta T}{2}$$

where c is the speed of light, ΔT is the time difference between transmitted and received pulse and echo. The velocity is related to the Doppler frequency shift between the transmitted pulse and received echo:[4]

$$v = \frac{f_d \lambda_o}{2}$$

where f_d is the Doppler frequency shift and λ_o is the free space wavelength at the centre frequency. Pulse Doppler radars are half duplex, meaning that they either transmit or receive, which results in high isolation between the transmitter and receiver, thus increasing the dynamic range of the receiver and the range detection of the radar. The disadvantage of this system is the existence of a blind zone given by:[4]

$$R_b = c \frac{(\tau_p + t_s)}{2}$$

where τ_p is the pulse width, and t_s is the switching time of the transmit and receive switch, if applicable. Pulse Doppler radar systems are therefore better suited for long-range detection, whereas frequency-modulated continuous wave (FMCW) radar is better suited for short-range detection.[4]

16.1.2 Requirements for car radar sensors

The acquisition parameters for high resolution LRR data are given below:[3]

- Centre frequency 76.5 GHz
- Maximum field of view ±10°
- Azimuthbeamwidth 1°
- Elevation beamwidth 5°
- Range resolution 1 m
- Velocity resolution 1 km/h
- System sensitivity −20 dBm at 150 m

Typical specifications for a 79 GHz SRR sensor are as follows[3]:

- Frequency 79 GHz
- Bandwidth 4000 MHz
- Maximum field of view ±80°
- Range 30 m
- Range Accuracy ±5 cm
- Bearingaccuracy ±5°

16.2 RF MEMS components for automotive radar

This section gives an overview of RF MEMS components suitable for automotive radar, in particular switches, phase shifters, and oscillators.

16.2.1 RF MEMS switches and tunable capacitors

RF MEMS switches and tunable capacitors are the principal components of most RF MEMS circuits and devices, such as phase shifters,[5] reconfigurable antennas and matching circuits,[6,7] and beam-steering applications,[6,8,9] which are suitable for automotive radar applications.

Low insertion loss, high signal linearity, high isolation, near-zero power consumption, large bandwidth of RF MEMS switches, high tuning range, low series resistance and high linearity of mechanically tunable capacitors are the advantages of these components as compared to their semiconductor equivalents. As their semiconductor counterparts, they can be fabricated in large volume parallel processes on semiconductor wafers, resulting in high product uniformity, potentially very low cost, and ease of integration/assembly with semiconductor components and systems. However, they suffer from reliability issues, low switching or actuation speed, low number of cycles corresponding to lifetime, low power handling capabilities and limited hot switching in high power applications; and most of them require complex fabrication and integration processes in non-standardized process flows.[10]

Electrostatic actuation is the most widely used, because of the near-zero actuation power consumption, simple design and fabrication, well-developed theory, maximum force in the contact position, pull-in hysteresis for robustness, and good integration compatibility with IC technology.

In general, RF MEMS switches can be categorized by the nature of the switching mechanism (metal contact or capacitive contact), and the usage on a circuit level (series or shunt configuration). The most commonly used embodiments are electrostatically actuated metal-contact series switches and electrostatically actuated capacitive shunt switches, schematically illustrated in Fig. 16.3, and shortly summarized in the following:

- Electrostatically actuated series switch with metal contacts: a cantilever or membrane with a metal contact bar opens or closes the signal line by a metal-to-metal direct ohmic contact. Switches of this category are normally OFF. The ohmic contact characteristic of this switch type makes it capable of switching direct current (DC) to RF signals of even up to 100 GHz, but they normally suffer from low isolation at high frequencies

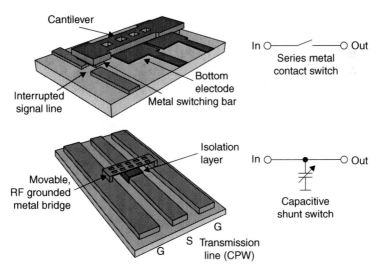

16.3 The two most commonly used electrostatically actuated MEMS switch types.[10]

because of the UP-state capacitance and substrate wave coupling. The metal contact physics is rather complicated and large-force actuators must be employed for high reliability. Lifetime is limited by contact degradation, and these switches typically fail in short-circuit by the metal contacts getting stuck, the most mature designs surviving billions to trillions of switching cycles.
- Electrostatically actuated capacitive shunt switches: these consist of a metal bridge or membrane connected to an RF ground and moving vertically above the signal line which is isolated by a thin dielectric film. The switch is normally in up position (ON-state) where the signal freely propagates. In the DOWN-state, the bridge capacitively short-circuits the signal line to the RF ground (OFF-state). Due to its capacitive nature, this switch type is not suitable for low frequency signals and mostly used in applications above 10 GHz. Its performance is limited by the DOWN-state parasitic inductance. The main reliability factor is the dielectric charging of the isolation layer, which results in non-reproducible actuation, or even in failure of the switch to open the signal line.

As an example, an inline DC-contact microelectromechanical systems (MEMS) series switch,[11] developed for V-band applications (50–75 GHz) is shown in Fig. 16.4. Table 16.1 gives an overview of MEMS switches, mainly designed for W-band (75–110 GHz), thus suitable for 76–81 GHz automotive radar.

Another RF MEMS component of importance is the tunable capacitor. In MEMS-based tuning circuits, either MEMS-switched capacitor banks are used, or electromechanically tunable capacitors. The capacitance can be tuned, either by varying the gap between parallel plates, or by changing the

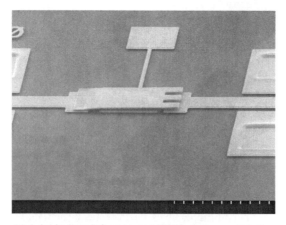

16.4 An in-line DC-contact MEMS series switch.[11]

Table 16.1 Comparison of RF MEMS switches

Device	Frequency band	Actuation voltage (V)	On/off speed (µs)	Insertion loss (dB)	Isolation (dB)	Reference
DC-contact series switch	V-band	80	0.3 and 0.16	1.94 at 60 GHz	14.79 at 60 GHz	Vu et al. (2009)[11]
Capacitive series switch	W-band	–	15	0.3 at 50–100 GHz	17 at 76.5 GHz	Stehle et al. (2008)[12]
T-match capacitive shunt switch	W-band	30	–	0.25 ± 0.1	20 at 80–110 GHz	Rizk et al. (2001)[13]
π-match capacitive shunt switch	W-band	30	–	0.4 ± 0.1 at 90 GHz	30–40 at 75–110 GHz	Rizk et al. (2001)[13]
Longitudinal coplanar shunt switch	W-band	25	–	0.3 at 75–100 GHz	30 at 77–94 GHz	Ulm et al. (2003)[7]
T-match and π-match capacitive shunt switch on quartz substrate	W-band	40	–	0.2–0.5	25 over the W-band	Rizk and Rebeiz (2003)[14]
Metal-to-metal contact shunt switch	DC to 100 GHz	22	0.5 with 40 V bias in g voltage	1 at 75 GHz, 1.4 at 100 GHz	22 at 100 GHz	Mercier et al. (2004)[15]
DC-contact series switch	1–40 GHz and W-band	39	45	0.36 at 77 GHz	17.3 at 77 GHz	Ghodsian et al. (2008)[16]

overlapping area between a fixed and a moving electrode. An example of the latter concept, i.e. area-tuning capacitors, is a comb-drive tunable capacitor which, however, is not suitable for higher-GHz frequencies because of limited Q-factors. Actuators tuning the gap between two parallel plates are built similar to RF MEMS capacitive shunt switches. However, instead of keeping the suspended part either in the DOWN-state or UP-state, it is possible to tune the position of the capacitive membrane in analogue mode, and thus the capacitive loading of the line, which results in very high Q-factors and hence suitability for W-band applications. The limited tuning range and non-linearity effects of analogue tuning, though, have rendered tunable capacitors less suitable for W-band circuits as compared to MEMS-switched capacitive loads.

Examples of a MEMS tunable W-band capacitor for beam-steering applications are demonstrated in.[8,17] The tunable varactors are composed of metal patches suspended with four folded flexures above the fixed electrode. The gap can be tuned gradually from the initial distance of 1.0–0.4 μm with an actuation voltage below 35 V.

16.2.2 MEMS phase shifters

Phase shifters are widely employed in radar systems based on phased antenna arrays. MEMS technology offers much lower insertion loss, higher linearity over a large bandwidth and lower power consumption as compared to solid-state technology. Ferrite-based phase shifters have good performance, but cannot be easily integrated and are more expensive in fabrication as compared to MEMS technology.

Three main types of MEMS phase shifters have been presented in the literature to date: (a) MEMS-switched true-time delay (TTD)-line phase shifter networks;[12] (b) distributed MEMS transmission line (DMTL) phase shifters;[7] and (c) a novel concept based on tuning the loading of a three dimensioned (3D) micromachined transmission line by a dielectric block placed on top of the line, which is vertically moved by MEMS actuators.[18] A discussion of each of these types with examples is provided in the following.

MEMS-switched true-time delay (TTD) phase shifter networks

MEMS-switched TTD-line phase shifters consist of various phase shifter sections in a cascaded arrangement. MEMS switches are employed in different lines to switch the line length of the signal, resulting in different phase shifts. Since RF MEMS switches are used to switch between different paths, this kind of phase shifter inherits all the advantages of RF MEMS switches, resulting in excellent performance. However, they are not suitable for the millimetre-wave frequency, including W-band, because the performance of multiple switches and the necessary lengths of the transmission line degrade the performance.[18]

Stehle et al.[12] describe a phase shifter consisting of a 45° loaded-line phase shifter element, and a 90° as well as a 180° switched-line phase shifter element, resulting in a three-bit RF MEMS phase shifter. For the complete device, return loss was better than −12 dB, and the insertion loss was −5.7 dB at 76.5 GHz.

Design equations for a MEMS-switched TTD phase shifter comprising impedance-matched slow-wave unit cells, with the optimization goal to maximize the figure-of-merit $\Delta\varphi$/dB, are presented by B. Lakshminarayanan et al.[20] To verify the equations, one-bit phase shifters were implemented by cascading numbers of unit cells corresponding to various maximum design frequencies. The phase shifter with maximum frequency of 110 GHz showed insertion loss of about 2.65 dB, measured $\Delta\varphi$/dB of 150°/dB, and return loss below −19 dB.

Distributed MEMS transmission line phase shifters

The second type, DMTL phase shifter, is based on periodically loading the transmission line with capacitive MEMS bridges to vary the line capacitance. Consequently, the propagation coefficient of the line and the signal phase between the input and the output of the phase shifter are altered. Varying the capacitance of the line, in addition to changing the propagation coefficient, changes the line impedance. This effect imposes another limitation on the maximum usable capacitance ratio, in addition to those required by the switch design parameters, according to the acceptable mismatch. The capacitance ratio is reported to be limited to approximately 1.3–1.6 in.[7]

In general, DMTL phase shifters have excellent performance in the millimetre-wave regime, in comparison to TTD phase shifters. However, there are some disadvantages to take into consideration. Capacitive MEMS bridges incorporated in DMTL phase shifters are composed of thin metal bridges that cannot handle large induced current densities at high RF power because of limited heat conductivity to the substrate due to their suspension above the substrate. This results in reliability issues due to buckling (plastic deformation) or even melting of the thin metal layer. Additionally, thin gold bridges, as employed in both types of MEMS phase shifters, are subject to drastically losing their elastic behaviour, at even slightly elevated temperatures of around 80°C, resulting in decreased reliability.[18]

It is also possible to load the transmission line digitally by employing fixed capacitances, which can be switched to load the line. This alternative method provides the capability of increasing the capacitance ratio, which is more suitable in the millimetre-wave regime.[7]

Barker and Rebeiz[5] presented the design and optimization of DMTL phase shifters for U-band and W-band with analogue tuning capability of the bits on quartz substrate. The W-band DMTL phase shifter consisted of 48-bridge DMTL elements with pull-down voltage of just over 26 V and corresponding capacitance ratio of 1.15. Measured phase shift per decibel loss was 70°/dB from 75 to 110 GHz. Average measured insertion loss was −2.5 dB and return loss was −11 dB at 94 GHz.

Hung, Dussopt and Rebeiz[21] demonstrated a low-loss distributed two-bit W-band MEMS phase shifter on glass substrate, as shown in Fig. 16.5. Each unit cell of this phase shifter consisted of a MEMS bridge and the sum of two metal–air–metal (MAM) capacitors, which were fabricated using the crossover between the MEMS bridge and the coplanar waveguide (CPW) ground plane. Since the simulated phase shift of the unit cell was about 1.2° at 80 GHz, a 90° section with eight switches and a 180° degree section with 16 switches were cascaded. Phase shifts of 0°, 89.3°, 180.1°, and 272° were measured at

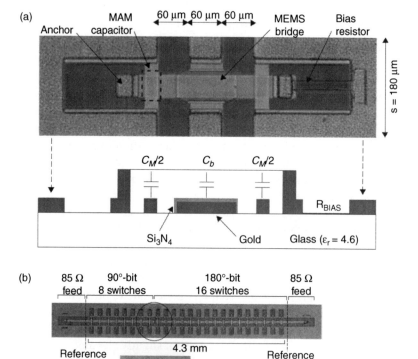

16.5 A low-loss distributed two-bit W-band MEMS DMTL phase shifter: (a) single cell with its corresponding profile; (b) entire two-bit DMTL phase shifter composed of 24 switches.[21]

81 GHz that were close to the designed frequency and phase shifts. Return loss was better than −11 dB, the average insertion loss was −2.2 dB and phase error was equal to ±2°. The worst insertion loss was −2.9 dB at 94 GHz.

MEMS tunable dielectric-block loaded-line phase shifter

The third type of MEMS phase shifter was presented by Somjit et al.,[18] based on tuning the loading of a 3D-micromachined transmission line by a dielectric block placed on top of the line and moved by MEMS actuators, shown in Fig. 16.6. The single cell of this phase shifter consisted of a high-resistivity monocrystalline silicon block placed upon and loading a 3D high-impedance micromachined CPW. The relative phase shift was achieved by vertically moving the dielectric block above the transmission line by electrostatic actuation, which resulted in different propagation constants for the microwave signal depending on the vertical displacement of the dielectric block. Periodic patterns were etched into the dielectric block, and the ratio of the etched to the unetched area made it possible to artificially tune the macroscopically effective dielectric constant of each individual block. By cascading multiple stages of such unit cells a binary coded $15° + 30° + 5 \times 45°$ phase shifter was implemented. At the design frequency of 75 GHz, maximum return and insertion loss were −17 and −3.5 dB, respectively, which was corresponding to a loss of −0.82 dB/bit, and a phase shift efficiency of 71.1°/dB and 490.02°/cm. This phase shifter type was found to be very linear with a third-order intercept point IIP3 of 49.27 dB.[18] Also, as this concept does not employ any thin metallic bridges, which limit the current and thus the power handling of conventional MEMS TTD and DMTL phase shifters, the power handling is effectively only limited by the heat-sink capability of the transmission line itself, i.e. not by the MEMS part. A comparable study found that even at 40 dBm power at 75 GHz, the hottest spot on this phase shifter design has only increased by 30 °C, which is 10–20 times less than for conventional MEMS TTD and DMTL phase shifter designs.[19]

To summarize the section on RF MEMS phase shifters, a comparison among several W-band phase shifters is provided in Table 16.2. Most data are reproduced from Somjit et al.[18] with some additions.

16.2.3 MEMS oscillators

Resonators can be classified into two types; electromagnetic wave resonators, and electromechanical or (electro)acoustic wave resonators, based upon their principles of operation. Since the second type is mostly based on mechanical resonance, it is not usable in high frequency applications. Among various resonators of the first type, cavity and dielectric resonators can be used at millimetre-wave frequencies with Q-factors above 500. Since dielectric resonators

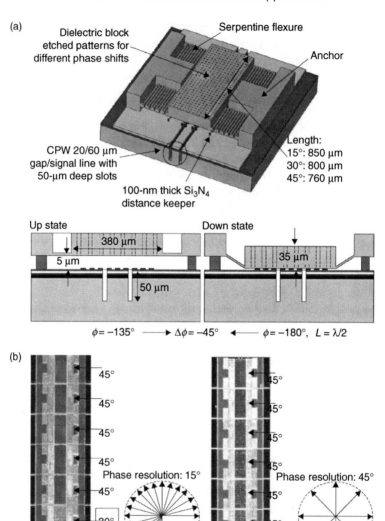

16.6 Binary-coded 4.25-bit W-band monocrystalline-silicon MEMS multistage dielectric-block phase shifters: (a) working principle of a single stage of the phase shifter, (b) microscopic pictures of fabricated seven-stage phase shifters.[18]

Table 16.2 Comparison among several W-band RF MEMS phase shifters

Reference	Stehle et al. (2008)[12]	Rizk and Rebeiz (2003)[14]	Rizk and Rebeiz (2003)[22]	Lakshmi-narayanan and Weller (2007)[20]	Hung et al. (2004)[23]	Barker and Rebeiz (2000)[5]	Hung et al. (2003)[21]	Somjit et al. (2009)[18]
Type	Loaded line and switched line	Switched line	Switched line and reflect line	TTD	DMTL	DMTL	DMTL	Loaded line with dielectric block
Substrate	Si	Quartz	Quartz	Quartz	Glass	Quartz	Glass	Si
Nominal frequency f_n (GHz)	76.5	90	80	110	78	94	81	75
Number of bits	3	1	2	1	3	Analogue	2	4.25
Config. possibilities	8	2	4	2	8	Analogue	4	19
Max. $\Delta\varphi$ of f_n (°)	315	180	282	410	315	170	272	270
Max. IL of f_n (dB)	≥5.8	≥2.5	≥6.1	≥2.65	≥3.2	≥2.5	>2.2	≥3.5
Max. IL/bit of f_n (dB/bit)	−1.93	−2.5	−3.05	−2.65	−1.07	−	−1.1	−0.82
Max. $\Delta\varphi$ loss of (°/dB)	55.26	85.71	70.5	150	95.75	70	−	71.05
Max. $\Delta\varphi$/loss (°/dB)	−	32.85	−	−	83.3	−	−	98.3
Max. RL of f_n (dB)	≤12	≤12	≤9.5	≤19	≤12	≤11	≤11	≤17
Max. IL at W (dB)	≥8	≥6	≥7	−	≥6	≥2.7	≥2.9	≥4.1
Max. RL at W (dB)	≤7.5	≤3	≤9	≤19	≤9	≤10	≤11	≤12

Source: Somjit et al., 2009.

consist of a piece of a high ε_r material, generally their size is smaller by a factor of $\sqrt{\varepsilon_r}$ in comparison to air-filled cavity resonators.[25]

Micromachining (MEMS) technology can be employed to enhance the performance of resonators at higher frequencies, or to add the tuning capability. However, most of the resonators investigated in the literature for the millimetre-wave regime are mainly measured at resonance frequency below 60 GHz,[26,27] and just a few have been demonstrated for W-band.

Dancila et al.[24] presented a variable-sized MEMS-based Faraday cage, used to tune the resonant frequency of a silicon micromachined cavity resonator, as shown in Fig. 16.7. An electrostatically tunable micoelectromechanical cantilever array, which forms a Faraday cage, incorporated in the cavity could change the resonance frequency of the resonator by influencing the electromagnetic field inside the cavity resonator. The dimension of the cavity resonator designed for the resonance frequency of 60 GHz was 3844 μm × 3844 μm × 440 μm. MEMS cantilevers could be actuated gradually from 0 to 30 V. The measured unloaded and loaded quality factors were 55 and 48, respectively, which were rather low because of the reported flaw in the metallization of the cavity resonator.

16.3 Examples of RF MEMS-based automotive radar front-end technology

In this section, concepts, implementations and advantages of two RF MEMS-based radar front-ends for automotive applications are discussed. These MEMS automotive radar front-ends were developed at the University of Michigan (USA),[28,29] and Robert Bosch GmbH (Germany).[7,9]

16.3.1 The University of Michigan 38-GHz RF MEMS car radar front-end

A 38-GHz high-pulse repetition frequency (HPRF) mono-pulse Doppler-radar front-end was developed at the University of Michigan by Caekenberghe et al.[28,29] for a long-range automotive radar application such as pre-crash detection and ACC. The radar front-end is based on an RF MEMS electronically scanned array (ESA) design and low-loss MEMS time-delay units (TDU), which offer cost and performance advantages over the other technologies. A maximum radar range up to 150 m and a resolution of 1.5 m are obtained from this design. The scanning angle resolution for this car radar is ±11° in the azimuth plane with an angular deviation of ±2.5° from an amplitude mono-pulse tracking, as compared to the scanning angle. This front-end was optimized for 38 GHz; however, it can be scaled to 77 GHz to match the ITU-Rs recommendations.[28] The front-end concept of the RF MEMS-based HPRF automotive radar is shown in Fig. 16.8.

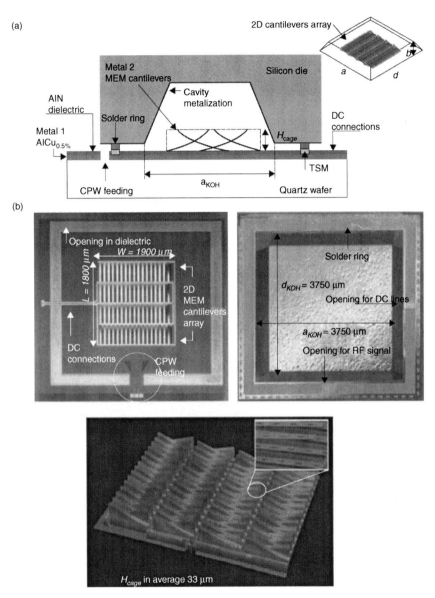

16.7 A MEMS variable Faraday cage as tuning element for integrated silicon micromachined cavity resonators: (a) cross-section of the MEMS tunable cavity resonator, (b) bottom part, top part and plot of the 2-D MEM cantilever array implementing the Faraday cage.[24]

As shown in Fig. 16.8, the radar front-end consists of a T/R module, an intermediate-frequency (IF) impulse processor and two passive sub-arrays which are individually connected to the T/R module. In the transmitting mode, a transmitted signal is fed to the transmitter module via an IF impulse

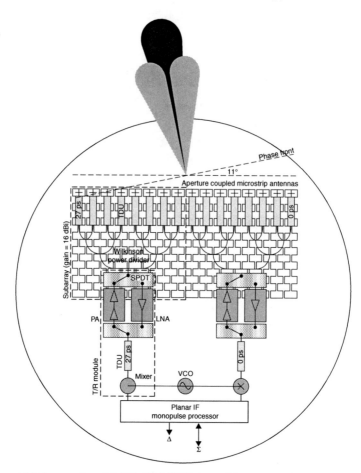

16.8 A complete 38-GHz RF MEMS-based front end of a HPRF monopulse Doppler-radar at the University of Michigan.[28]

processor, while the received signal is separated and fed to the sum and the azimuth-different channels to correct the angular errors. The radiation patterns of the transmitting and receiving modules are shown in Fig. 16.9a and b. Two passive sub-arrays, as the key units, are composed of 16-dB-gain 64 elements of microstrip antennas optimized at 38 GHz. The line antenna arrays fed through a slotted aperture from a microstrip corporate feed a network consisting of Wilkinson power dividers and grounded coplanar waveguide (GCPW) TDUs, which are analogue DMTLs, and each line is loaded with 60 elements of RF MEMS varactor. This design offers a low-loss and wideband device with good power handling capability at 38 GHz.

The front-end module was fabricated on a 6-inch fused silica wafer and a Rogers TMM3 substrate using wafer-scale monolithic tile construction.

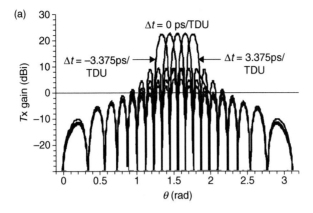

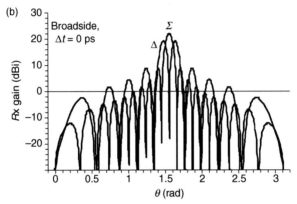

16.9 Radiation characteristic of the transmit (a) and receive (b) mode of the 38-GHz HPRF mono-pulse Doppler-radar.[28, 29]

The fused silica wafer contains two passive sub-arrays which are the MEMS TTD feed networks coupled to microstrip antenna arrays which are fabricated on the Rogers substrate. Apart from the microstrip antenna arrays, the other modules were fabricated in a class-100 cleanroom with a wafer-scale RF MEMS process with SiCr integrated thin-film resistors and high-resistivity bias lines.

16.3.2 Robert Bosch 77-GHz automotive radar front-end

Schoebel *et al.* at Robert Bosch GmbH developed two designs for 77-GHz analogue-beam-forming automotive radar front-end. The first approach was based on a MEMS single-pole–multi-throw switch, which

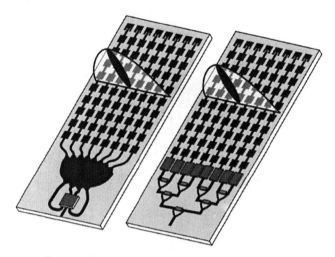

16.10 Two 77-GHz RF MEMS automotive-radar front ends from Robert Bosch GmbH.[9] The designs are based on Rotman lens (left) and MEMS phase shifters (right).

is employed to select one of several beams of a planar Rotman lens and then feeding branches of a patch-antenna array. The second approach was a more conventional patch-antenna array beam-steering concept, whereby RF MEMS phase shifters, fed via a Wilkinson power divider, were used for configuring the phase distribution of the signals of the antenna array.[7,9] These designs offer better performance, ease of design, and low manufacturing costs in comparison to the other millimetre-wave technologies. These two 77-GHz RF MEMS-based automotive radar concepts are shown in Fig. 16.10.

For the first design, an automotive radar front-end implemented with RF MEMS phase shifters, with less than three bits, and a patch-antenna array was investigated. The distance between each antenna element was half-wavelength, as compared to the wavelength in free space. Therefore, fixed scanning beams of 0°, ±14.5°, ±30°, and ±48.6° from the boresight axis are obtained from this design. The beam forming is implemented by constructing three stages of a two-port Wilkinson power divider with the employment of a 20-dB Chebyshev pattern. RF MEMS stub-loaded-line phase shifters employed in this automotive radar design are based on MEMS capacitive shunt switches, offering 90° and 180° phase shift and less than 4° phase tolerance. This phase shifter exhibits a very wide bandwidth, which is very suitable for ultra-wideband (UWB) applications.

The second alternative design consists of a Rotman lens and a single-pole–quadruple-throw (SP4T) switch. This design is very straightforward and offers a completely symmetrical device, exhibiting uniform loss for all

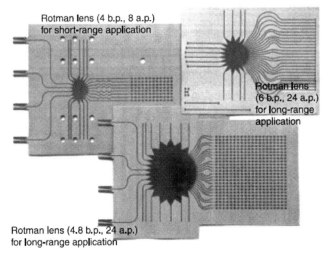

16.11 77-GHz MEMS automotive radar realized by RFMEMS SP4T switch and Rotman lens.[9]

scan beams. The number of scan angles reduces to four, pointing to ±6° and ±18° from boresight axis. The Rotman lens was implemented by microstrip technology, and the body of the lens is designed as a parallel-plate waveguide with microstrip feeding. The Rotman lens with patch-antenna and waveguide interconnects is realized on a 5-mil Ro3003 substrate. The SP4T switch is designed based on the capacitive shunt single-pole–double-throw (SP2T) switch design. The SP2T switch offers an insertion loss of 1.8 dB at 77 GHz. Figure 16.11 shows the fabricated MEMS automotive radar based on the Rotman lens and the SP4T switch. The radiation pattern of the design with the Rotman lens and the antenna array is shown in Fig. 16.12, in comparison to the three-stage Wilkinson power divider and MEMS phase shifters, with the same microstrip antenna array.

16.4 Unconventional MEMS radar beam-steering technologies

This section gives an overview of MEMS components that enable unconventional radar architectures. This includes tunable microwave surfaces, leaky-wave antennas (LWA) and micromechanically reconfigurable antennas.

16.4.1 MEMS tunable reflective microwave surfaces

MEMS tunable high-impedance surface (HIS) has been used by several research teams[8,30–32] for designing low-loss analogue-type phase shifters. HIS

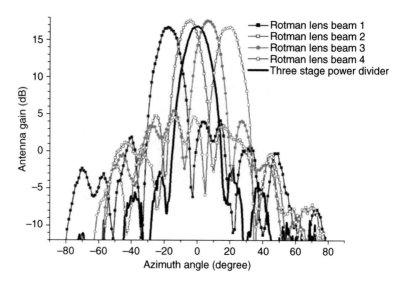

16.12 Radiation characteristics of the 77-GHz MEMS automotive radar based on Rotman lens with microstrip antenna array compared with the alternative design implemented with MEMS phase shifters, three-stage Wilkinson power divider and the microstrip antenna array.[9,7]

consisting of electrically small MEMS varactors placed on a dielectric substrate with a ground plane shown in Fig. 16.13 was used to achieve tunability of the effective surface input impedance. Since the size of the MEMS varactors is much smaller than the wavelength of the field above the structure, its electromagnetic response can be described in terms of the effective surface impedance. The array of MEMS varactors provides a capacitive response to the electromagnetic field above the structure, the grounded dielectric below provides an inductive response. Consequently, as a whole, the structure possesses resonant properties, and at the resonance frequency its impedance becomes very high. When bias voltage is applied to the MEMS varactors, the gap of the varactors decreases, thereby increasing the effective capacitance of the structure and hence changing the effective surface impedance. This affects the phase of the reflection coefficient or propagation constant of the field reflecting from the structure or propagating above it, which can be used in beam-steering and phase shifting applications. Electronic beam steering is achieved by inducing a gradient of the effective surface impedance throughout of the HIS by applying different bias voltages to the different rows of elements of the structure (see Fig. 16.14). Effectively this allows tuning the phase of the reflection coefficient in different sections of the HIS, which affects the direction of the reflecting beam.

Reflection-type analogue phase shifters can be obtained by placing the MEMS tunable HIS as a back-short of the rectangular metal waveguide

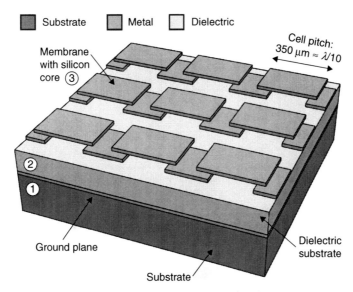

16.13 Periodic high-impedance metamaterial surface, composed of a low-loss dielectric substrate (2) integrated with a silicon substrate (1) and a transferred monocrystalline silicon membrane (3).[8]

in order to control the reflection phase. The fabricated MEMS-based HIS was placed as back-short of the rectangular metal waveguide WR-10 measuring S_{11}. As soon as the MEMS varactors are actuated, the reflection phase decreases, creating an analogue tunable reflection-type phase shifter. Transmission type analogue phase shifters can be obtained by introducing MEMS tunable HIS into waveguide structures in order to affect the phase factor of the propagation constant. The HIS can be placed adjacent to a dielectric rod waveguide (DRW) at a distance d, as shown in Fig. 16.15. Changing the effective impedance of the HIS by applying different bias voltage to all MEMS varactors of the structure dramatically changes the phase at Port 2 of the waveguide, when the operation frequency is close to the resonance frequency. The phase shift is proportional to the length of the HIS.

16.4.2 MEMS steerable leaky-wave antennas

The LWA presented in Reference 33 comprises a right–left-handed transmission line, where a microstrip is used as the right-handed (RH) transmission line and the left-handed loading comprises series reconfigurable MEMS capacitors and shunt narrow strip inductors. Microstrip as an RH transmission line offers two main advantages: ease and low cost of fabrication, and suitability for MEMS implementation. Tunable MEMS capacitors

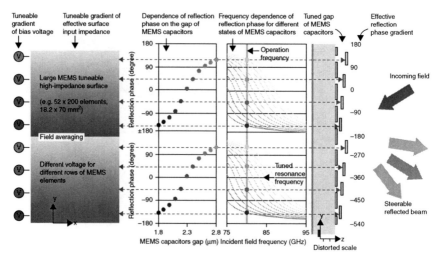

16.14 MEMS-based HIS with induced tunable gradient of the effective surface impedance for electric beam steering.[32]

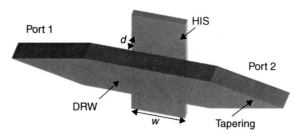

16.15 Phase shifter based on a DRW with an adjacent MEMS tunable HIS of a width, *w*, at a distance, *d*.[31]

are connected in series, and shunt inductors are built, in the initial design, from thin strip lumped inductors, resulting in a transmission line circuit of distributed resonance element along the line. The resulting antenna is built from such cascaded unit cell resonators as is shown in Fig. 16.16. The length of the unit cell is just a fraction of the wavelength, making the transmission line effectively homogenous.

In Fig. 16.17, scattering parameters (obtained from electromagnetic (EM) simulation software) of a single unit cell are shown. It is assumed that the scattering of one unit cell (in the case of a balanced unit cell) is enough to determine the main resonance frequency of the structure composed of such cells.

Figure 16.18 shows a scanning-electron microscopy (SEM) picture of a micromachined tunable LWA comprising 30 sequentially cascaded unit cells.

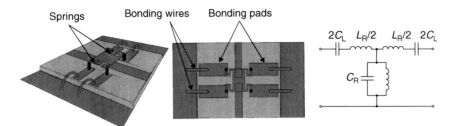

16.16 Unit cell of a MEMS-tunable LWA, and its equivalent lumped element circuit.[33]

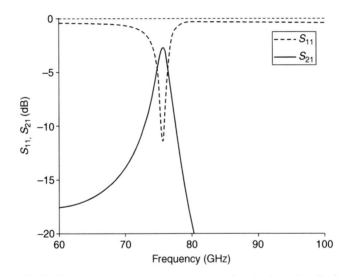

16.17 Simulated scattering parameters of a single unit cell of a LWA.[33]

16.4.3 Mechanically driven antenna platform

A single antenna platform steered by an external magnetic field where a monolithic microwave integrated circuit (MMIC) and capacitors are vertically integrated has been shown by Kim et al.[34] The electrical steering scheme using phase shifters is already mature and shows a fast scan speed. However, it requires a number of phase shifters and power amplifiers to obtain a large scan angle, resulting in bigger and more expensive systems. A mechanical steering antenna can radiate beam directly, and it has a constant RF gain at any scan angle. The absence of multiple phase shifters and amplifiers, even at large scan angles, makes the mechanical beam-steering antenna smaller, and more efficient in terms of RF capability. The required deflection of the antenna in Reference 34 is over 1.3 mm. A schematic of the RF antenna and steering method is shown in Fig. 16.19.

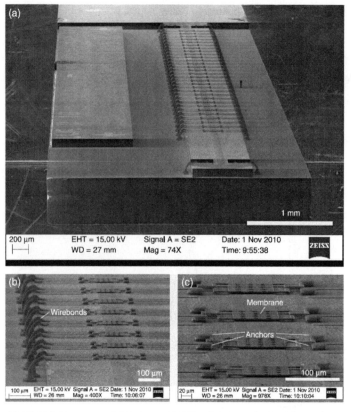

16.18 SEM images of fabricated LWAs: (a) the whole chip with a 30 element array; (b) close-up of the wire bonds connecting the membranes to the ground plane (c) close-up of the membranes with springs and anchors.[33]

The antenna consists of two pairs of mechanical springs made of benzocyclobutene (BCB) with a thickness of 40 μm. Two metal–insulator–metal (MIM) capacitors are implemented by conventional micromachining and are vertically flip chip bonded to the suspended antenna substrate. Currents with the same magnitude and direction flow through a pair of adjacent coils under the movable antenna substrate and generate the driving magnetic force. When the current flows through two pairs of coils, the magnetic field is extended to the nickel underneath the silicon substrate, and the plate rotates. The average tilting angles are 5.4°, 8.2°, 13.4°, and 18.3°, respectively, when the applied currents are 200, 300, 400, and 500 mA in the H-plane. The average tilting angles are 4.7°, 6.8°, 12.1°, and 17.7° in the E-plane. The measured radiation beam patterns and tilting angles are depicted in Fig. 16.20. The beam radiation patterns shifts originating from the rotation at the angles of −14°, 0°, and +18° in the H-plane and the beam patterns at −18°, −12°, 0°, +12°, and +16° in the E-plane are shown in Fig. 16.20.

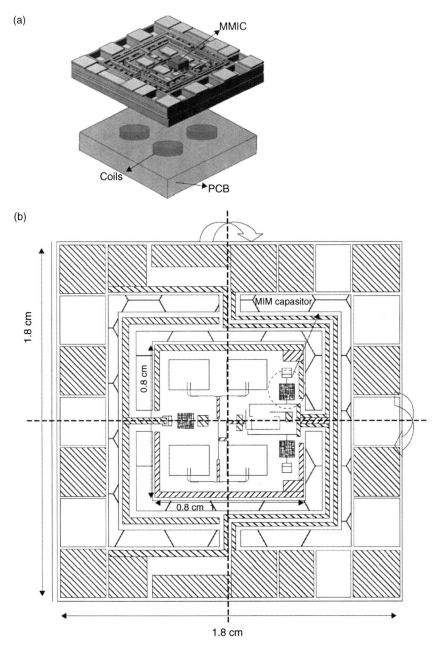

16.19 Micro-mechanically driven antenna platform: (a) schematic view of the proposed RF antenna; (b) design layout.[34]

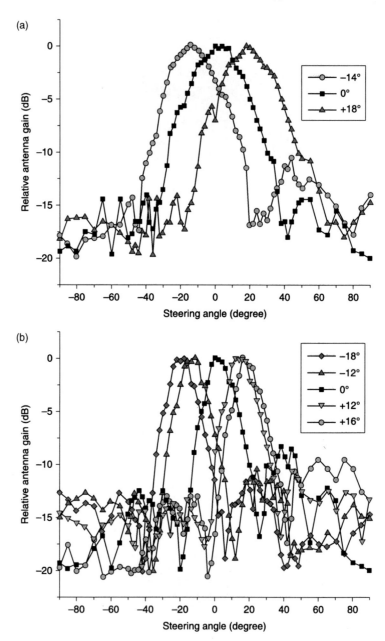

16.20 Radiation beam pattern of the mechanically tilted RF antenna actuated by magnetic field: (a) H-plane; (b) E-plane.[34]

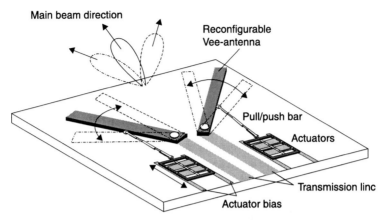

16.21 Concept of micro-mechanically reconfigurable Vee-antenna.[9]

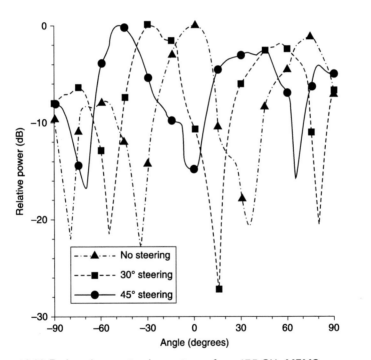

16.22 E-plane beam-steering patterns for a 17.5 GHz MEMS reconfigurable Vee-antenna.[9]

16.4.4 MEMS reconfigurable Vee-antennas

In Reference 35, a planar antenna structure is dynamically reconfigured to steer the radiation beam or change the shape of the beam using electrically-controlled microactuators. Figure 16.21 shows the concept and the cross-section of the reconfigurable Vee-antenna.

The antenna arms of the Vee-antenna are moved through pulling or pushing by microactuators. One end of the antenna arm is held by a fixed rotation hinge locked on the substrate, which allows the arm to rotate with the hinge as the centre of a circle. Both antenna arms were rotated by 30° and 45° in the same direction, while the Vee-angle was kept at 75°. Figure 16.22 shows that the main beams shift by 30° and 48°. It also shows that the first null shifts from 35° to 15° for the 30°-steering and from 35° to 0° for the 45°-steering.

16.5 Conclusion

RF MEMS is a very interesting technology for 76–81 GHz automotive radar, mainly because of the near ideal signal properties of RF MEMS devices, such as switches and phase shifters. Various RF MEMS components and demonstrators for RF MEMS-based automotive radar have been presented, and alternative beam-steering technologies, enabled by microelectromechanical tunable components, are summarized in this chapter. Developing RF MEMS components to market maturity still requires a major effort, especially as it is difficult to overcome such reliability problems as contact stiction and dielectric charging of isolation layers, and to realize low-cost packaging methods that also provide package hermeticity and good RF feed-through. As of 2011, about a handful of companies have succeeded in developing reliable RF MEMS components and circuits, which are fulfilling customer specifications both in electrical performance and in reliability requirements. Switches, for instance, already exceed the lifetime of mechanical RF relays by a factor of 100. For the low power requirements of automotive radar of 1–10 mW, state-of-the-art RF MEMS components are able to fulfil the reliability requirements. Still, as of 2011, no RF MEMS-based car radars are on the market, but various RF MEMS components, mainly switches and circuits, for instance antenna matching networks, have reached maturity and are commercially offered.

16.6 References

1. D.M. Gavrila, M. Kunert, and U. Lages, 'A multi-sensor approach for the protection of vulnerable traffic participants – the PROTECTOR project', *Proc. IEEE Instrumentation and Measurement Technology Conference*, Budapest, Hungary, 21–23 May (2001).

2. M. Schneider, 'Automotive radar – status and trends', *Proc. German Microwave Conference GeMiC*, pp. 144–147, Ulm, Germany, April (2005).
3. J. Wenger, 'Automotive radar – status and perspective', *Compound Semiconductor Integrated Circuits Symposium 2005*, Palm Springs, CA, USA, Oct. (2005).
4. K. A. P. A. Van Caekenberghe, 'RF MEMS technology for millimeter-wave radar sensors', PhD Dissertation, The University of Michigan (2007).
5. N. S. Barker and G. M. Rebeiz, 'Optimization of distributed MEMS transmission-line phase shifters-U-band and W-band designs', *IEEE Transactions on Microwave Theory and Techniques*, vol. **48**, no. 11, pp. 1957–1966, Nov. (2000).
6. E. R. Brown, 'RF-MEMS switches for reconfigurable integrated circuits', *IEEE Transactions on Microwave Theory and Techniques*, vol. **46**, no. 11, pp. 1868–1880, Nov. (1998).
7. M. Ulm, J. Schobel, M. Reimann, T. Buck, J. Dechow, R. Muller-Fiedler, H.-P. Trah, E. Kasper, 'Millimeter-wave microelectromechanical (MEMS) switches for automotive surround sensing systems', *Proc. 2003 Topical Meeting on Silicon Monolithic Integrated Circuits in RF Systems*, pp. 142–149, 9–11 April (2003).
8. M. Sterner, D. Chicherin, A. V. Raisenen, G. Stemme, and J. Oberhammer, 'RF MEMS high-impedance tuneable metamaterials for millimeter-wave beam steering', *Proc. IEEE Micro Electro Mechanical Systems*, Sorrento, Italy, 25–29 Jan. (2009), pp. 896–899.
9. J. Schoebel, T. Buck, M. Reimann, M. Ulm, M. Schneider, A. Jourdain, G. J. Carchon, and H. A. C. Tilmans, 'Design considerations and technology assessment of phased-array antenna systems with RF MEMS for automotive radar applications', *IEEE Transactions on Microwave Theory and Techniques*, vol. **53**, no. 6, pp. 1968–1975, June (2005).
10. J. Oberhammer, 'Novel RF MEMS switches and packaging concepts', Ph.D. dissertation, KTH Royal Institute of Technology, Stockholm, ISBN 91-7283-831-0, (2004).
11. T. M. Vu, G. Prigent, J. Ruan, A. Rumeau, P. Pons, and R. Plana, 'Fabrication and characterization of RF-MEMS switch in V-band', *IEEE Asia-Pacific Microwave Conference*, 7–10 Dec. (2009), pp. 202–205.
12. A. Stehle, G. Georgiev, V. Ziegler, B. Schoenlinner, U. Prechtel, H. Seidel, and U. Schmid, 'RF-MEMS switch and phase shifter optimized for W-band', *IEEE/EuMA European Microwave Conference*, 27–31 Oct. (2008), pp. 104–107.
13. J. Rizk, G.-L. Tan, J. B. Muldavin, and G. M. Rebeiz, 'High-isolation W-band MEMS switches', *IEEE Microwave and Wireless Components Letters*, vol. **11**, no. 1, pp. 10–12, Jan. (2001).
14. J. B. Rizk and G. M. Rebeiz, 'W-band CPW RF MEMS circuits on quartz substrates', *IEEE Transactions on Microwave Theory and Techniques*, vol. **51**, no. 7, pp. 1857–1862, July (2003).
15. D. Mercier, P. L. Charvet, P. Berruye, C. Zancy, L. Lapierre, O. Vendier, J. L. Cazaux, and P. Blondy, 'A DC to 100 GHz high performance ohmic shunt switch', *Proc. IEEE International Microwave Symposium Digest*, vol. **3**, 6–11 June (2004), pp. 1931–1934.
16. B. Ghodsian, P. Bogdanoff, and D. Hyman, 'Wideband DC-contact MEMS series switch', *IET Micro and Nano Letters*, vol. **3**, no. 3, pp. 66–69, Sept. (2008).

17. D. Chicherin, M. Sterner, J. Oberhammer, S. Dudorov, J. Åberg, and A.V. Räisänen, 'Analog type millimeter wave phase shifters based on MEMS tunable high-impedance surface in rectangular metal waveguide', *IEEE International Microwave Symposium 2010*, Anaheim, CA, USA, 23–28 May (2010), pp. 61–64.
18. N. Somjit, G. Stemme, and J. Oberhammer, 'Binary-coded 4.25-bit-band monocrystalline–silicon MEMS multistage dielectric-block phase shifters', *IEEE Transactions on Microwave Theory and Techniques*, vol. **57**, no. 11, pp. 2834–2840, Nov. (2009).
19. N. Somjit, G. Stemme, and J. Oberhammer, 'Power handling analysis of high-power W-band all-silicon MEMS phase shifters', *IEEE Transactions on Electron Devices*, vol. **58**, no. 5, pp. 1584–1555, May (2011).
20. B. Lakshminarayanan and T.M. Weller, 'Optimization and implementation of impedance-matched true-time-delay phase shifters on quartz substrate', *IEEE Transactions on Microwave Theory and Techniques*, vol. **55**, no. 2, pp. 335–342, Feb. (2007).
21. J.-J. Hung, L. Dussopt, and G.M. Rebeiz, 'A low-loss distributed 2-bit W-band MEMS phase shifter', *Proc. IEEE/EuMA Microwave Conference 2003*, Oct. (2003), pp. 983–985.
22. J.B. Rizk and G.A. Rebeiz, 'W-band microstrip RF-MEMS switches and phase shifters', *Proc. IEEE MTT-S International Microwave Symposium*, vol. **3**, 8–13 June (2003), pp. 1485–1488.
23. J.-J. Hung, L. Dussopt, and G.M. Rebeiz, 'Distributed 2- and 3-bit W-band MEMS phase shifters on glass substrates', *IEEE Transactions on Microwave Theory and Techniques*, vol. **52**, no. 2, pp. 600–606, Feb. (2004).
24. D. Dancila, P. Ekkels, X. Rottenberg, I. Huynen, W. De Raedt, and H. A. C. Tilmans, 'A MEMS variable Faraday cage as tuning element for integrated silicon micromachined cavity resonators', *Proc. IEEE Micro Electro Mechanical Systems*, 24–28 Jan. (2010), pp. 723–726.
25. W. De Raedt, E. Beyne, and H.A.C. Tilmans, 'MEMS for wireless communications: "from RF-MEMS components to RF-MEMS-SiP"', *Journal of Micromechanics and Microengineering*, vol. **13**, no. 4 (2003) pp. 139–163.
26. B. Guillon, D. Cros, P. Pons, K. Grenier, T. Parra, J. L. Cazaux, J. C. Lalaurie J. Graffeui, and R. Plana, 'Design and realization of high Q millimeter-wave structures through micromachining techniques', *Proc. IEEE International Microwave Symposium*, vol. **4** (1999), pp. 1519–1522.
27. I. Ocket, B. Nauwelaers, G. Carchon, A. Jourdain, and W. De Raedt, '60 GHz Si micromachined cavity resonator on MCM-D', *Proc. Topical Meeting on Silicon Monolithic Integrated Circuits in RF Systems*, 18–20 Jan. (2006), p. 4.
28. K. Van Caekenberghe and K. Sarabandi, 'Monopulse-Doppler radar front-end concept for automotive applications based on RF MEMS technology', *Proc. IEEE International Conference on Electro/Information Technology* (2006), pp. 1–5.
29. K. Van Caekenberghe, 'RF MEMS technology for radar sensors', *International Radar Conference – Surveillance for a Safer World* (2009), pp. 1–6.
30. M. Sterner, G. Stemme, and J. Oberhammer, 'Wafer counter-bonding for integrating CTE-mismatched substrates and its application to MEMS tuneable metamaterials', *Proc. IEEE TRANSDUCERS 2009*, Denver, CO, USA, 22–25 June (2009), pp. 1722–1725.

31. D. Chicherin, M. Sterner, J. Oberhammer, S. Dudorov, D. Lioubtchenko, A. J. Niskanen, V. Ovchinnikov, and A.V. Räisänen, 'MEMS based high-impedance surface for millimetre wave dielectric rod waveguide phase shifter', *Proc. IEEE European Microwave Conference 2010*, Paris, France, 26 Sept.–1 Oct. (2010), pp. 950–953.
32. D. Chicherin, M. Sterner, J. Oberhammer, S. Dudorov, D. Lioubtchenko, V. Ovchinnikov, and A.V. Räisänen, 'MEMS tunable metamaterials surfaces and their applications', *Proc. IEEE Asia Pacific Microwave Conference 2010*, Yokohama, Japan, 7–10 Dec. (2010), pp. 239–242.
33. T. Zvolensky, D. Chicherin, A. Räisänen, C. Simovski, M. Sterner, J. Oberhammer, and H. Hakojärvi, 'Leaky-wave antenna at 77 GHz', *Proc. IEEE/EuMA European Microwave Conference 2011*, Manchester, UK, 9–14 Oct. (2011), pp. 1039–1042.
34. Y. Kim, N.-G. Kim, J.-M. Kim, S.H. Lee, Y. Kwon, and Y.-K. Kim, '60-GHz full MEMS antenna platform mechanically driven by magnetic actuator', *IEEE Transactions on Industrial Electronics*, vol. **58**, no. 10 (2011), pp. 4830–4836.
35. J.C. Chiao, Y. Fu, J.M. Chio, M. DeLisio, and L.Y. Lin, 'MEMS reconfigurable antenna', in *IEEE MTT-S International Microwave Symposium*, June (1999), pp. 1515–1518.

17
Telecommunications reliability monitoring using wireless MEMS

M. HAUTEFEUILLE,
Universidad Nacional Autónoma de México, Mexico

DOI: 10.1533/9780857098610.2.550

Abstract: Wireless sensor networks (WSNs) technology is becoming a very promising solution to better address reliability in general, thanks to constant, accurate environmental monitoring. After reviewing the current reliability issues of the telecommunications sector, this chapter describes how the integration of multiple microelectromechanical systems (MEMS) sensors on small, low-power, low-cost WSN platforms may help answer the current and future needs of this key industry. Finally, a miniaturized WSN environmental platform is presented as a case study to suggest one possible fabrication methodology for the designer.

Key words: MEMS sensors, reliability, cross-correlation, wireless sensor network (WSN), telecommunications.

17.1 Introduction

Thanks to the recent progress made in modern telecommunication systems in constantly guaranteeing secure, good quality transmissions from nearly any emitting source to any receiver, this industrial sector has converted itself into one of the major economies worldwide. In 2010, the global revenue of telecommunications has been estimated by the Telecommunications Industry Association (TIA) at approximately US$3.1 trillion (TIA, 2010). The actors in this expanding technology are seeking an ever wider distribution of more modern systems available at an increasing transfer rate and decreasing price. The subsequent reliability requirements of telecommunications equipment are thus often compared to those of very demanding and more strategic fields, such as aerospace and military. Indeed, the general procedures to address and improve lifetime quality and reliability of the global telecommunication infrastructures and their performance are often similar to those used in such delicate areas (Jones and Hayes, 1999). Henceforth, although the majority of consumer electronics manufacturers seem to have abandoned their earlier customs that consisted in following strict reliability guidelines provided by military handbooks to lower their costs, it is a trend that the telecommunication industry cannot afford.

WSN is a modern technology that consists of low-cost, low-power, autonomous, modular platforms offering spatially distributed sensor modules with wireless communication capabilities. They are currently being developed to monitor, collect and communicate crucial information about environmental, contextual or behavioural conditions in real-time on an application-specific fashion. WSN technology is particularly beneficial in applications where reliability must be addressed; thanks to a relatively high integration level made possible with the recent progress in electronics miniaturization and especially in WSN, multiple MEMS sensors may be attached directly onboard to enable accurate readings, detection redundancy and cross-sensitivity compensation. This chapter gives a generic overview of the current reliability issues that modern telecommunication systems have to cope with, and goes on to demonstrate how wireless MEMS, combined with WSN technologies, may offer very promising prognostics and point-of-care diagnostics solutions to respond to these current needs. A practical and affordable WSN platform, based on a variety of complementary metal oxide semiconductor (CMOS)-compatible MEMS environmental sensors, is finally presented as a case study to suggest a methodology for the design, development, fabrication and characterization of a possible future commercial solution.

17.2 Typical reliability issues in telecommunication systems

In the past decades, with the breakthrough of computer science and progress in complex modelling, reliability research has been converted from a purely statistical field to a multidisciplinary science. This transformation is now enabling more accurate fatigue, stress and ageing models of sophisticated systems for failure predictions and diagnostics. A better understanding of malfunction and breakdown causes and consequences even allows engineers and developers to foresee the overall performance and lifespan of their manufactured designs, leading to a new discipline called prognostics (Hess, 2001).

Telecommunication systems functionalities are mainly based on electronic components that are likely to fail at some point (Shapiro *et al.*, 2004). The ever increasing level of miniaturization and device integration on complex electronic systems and circuit boards is complicating the task of reliability engineers, as it is becoming less and less evident to apply component-level reliability models to higher levels. In addition to these hierarchical issues, more complex systems also present interdependent architectures and circuits that may influence each other, resulting in greater difficulty in establishing reliability models from empirical observations and determining environmental or behavioural factors that are responsible for possible issues. Finally, the current market-driven consumer electronics trends are discarding the necessity to fabricate and sell reliable components that perform well over a long period of time. This lowers the global quality requirements as well as the quantities of valuable data that would be collected from all different failing parts of a particular piece of equipment to improve the quality of its future generations.

17.2.1 Reliability in electronics and implications in telecommunications

In addition to the obvious practical consequences and constraints that unreliable telecommunication devices may impose on manufacturers and users, the economic implications are the real motives that drive reliability research. In the telecommunication industry as in every successful technological sector, the total life-cycle cost of a device must be carefully addressed to help define the proper methodology that will guarantee the lowest costs possible, from conception to maintenance and disposal (Barringer, 2003). It is thus commonly advised to consider investigating reliability issues as much as, if not more than, replacement and maintainability (SAE, 1995).

There are several parameters that may be considered as critical criteria in the estimation of reliability in telecommunications. No software-specific or computing-reliability issues will be discussed in this chapter, as the vast majority of them may not be remedied using wireless MEMS solutions. However, telecommunication systems in general, and especially modern ones, present deficiencies mainly provoked by malfunctioning, failure or breakdown of electronic components (Salmela, 2005). Most of the time, telecommunication reliability is then directly associated with electronics or microelectronics reliability. Therefore, the methods to characterize, determine and predict failure rates, as well as the factors that affect the normal behaviour of the systems or aggravate their operating conditions, are quite similar.

In the case of complex architectures such as those typically found in modern telecommunication technology, reliability research is based on predictive simulation models built from probability theory. Moreover, the failure rate of the whole system is typically inferred from existing reliability information of all discrete components that constitute the considered platform (EPSMA, 2005). As the failure rate determination process is time-consuming for each component, extensive databases of relevant reliability data are needed and carefully kept up-to-date in published handbooks. However, this information may sometimes be inappropriate, especially if it was obtained under different operating conditions or in different application schemes. Finding specific, pertinent reliability data applicable to the preventive maintenance of complex systems can be particularly tedious, and empirical observations usually differ significantly from predictive models (Vichare et al., 2007). Moreover, when external environmental conditions are responsible for reliability issues, the combination of common prediction methods with application-specific life tests may also be inaccurate or erroneous in some cases, especially when the systems are deployed and operated in different surroundings (EPSMA, 2005).

17.2.2 Monitoring and construction of reliability models

To address reliability, in addition to extensive prototype testing, recent efforts have been made to constantly monitor both the performance and the environmental conditions of operations of various systems in real-time. Important amounts of data may then be recorded at the desired sampling rate and then analysed to help construct more accurate and more specific reliability databases. Indeed, the collection of several key parameters, and the possibility to combine various environmental and behavioural criteria, allow a better understanding of possible failure without limiting the reliability scope to malfunctioning or breakdown caused by ageing. A complete historical panorama of a given system may finally be obtained from constant, correctly defined monitoring data and this should help in acquiring a more detailed knowledge of possible failures, and to construct more accurate reliability models.

Ideal sensors produce repeatable responses which are not influenced by any cross-sensitivity. The type of output signals, sampling frequencies, input power consumption, cost of fabrication, dimensions, and ease of use are amongst examples of sensor specifications that are defined by target applications. Modern technologies have enabled development and deployment of ubiquitous discrete sensors with great sensitivity. Discrete individual sensors are stand-alone components that sense one particular parameter in their vicinity. They usually require adapted circuits to condition their signal and make it readable. It has recently been shown that discrete sensors are currently being investigated to improve the performance of smart sensor systems, thanks to their accurate, reliable response and cost-effective manufacturing (Assaf and Dugan, 2008). The development of such intelligent structures raises new challenges, such as structural integrity, long-term reliability, placement and organization, collection of sensed data, and remote querying (Berger-Wolf et al., 2005). The quantity of discrete sensors can also be a critical issue for the large deployment of sensing systems, and it has been proven that not only redundancy but also collaboration between different sensors is desirable (Rachlin et al., 2005). This communication between individual sensors leads to the concept of sensor networks.

17.2.3 Prognostics solutions

Predictive modelling, based on existing reliability databases and known failure rates of specific components, is quite limited in new systems architectures. Prior warnings are thus almost non-existent or non-detectable. Moreover, reliability research is not always capable of manufacturing more reliable components or of providing accurate data on device quality, especially for large systems. Although some practical solutions, such as component redundancy (where different units function in parallel), have been proposed, most of them are difficult to implement in telecommunication systems.

Prognostics and health management (Engel *et al.*, 2000; Hess, 2001) is a recent reliability method based on constant monitoring that enables the evaluation of complex systems in their actual application conditions. By assessing the impact of measurement uncertainties and extracting irregular time-load data, existing models may be actualized and improved for specific systems. The prognostics approach thus allows the construction of more accurate accumulative damage models and helps identify dominant failure precursors in real-time. It also improves decision-making by constantly addressing remaining lifetime, thanks to adequate feedback-controlled regression algorithms (Feldman *et al.*, 2008). In 2005, the prognostics approach was identified as one of the greatest maintenance requirements for electronics systems in key sectors where functionality and performance must be maintained (Cutter and Thompson, 2005). Reliability monitoring implementation has then become a critical need in telecommunication systems and specific sensors are required to address it.

Until recently, typical prognostics and reliability approaches were based on early warning devices, called canaries and fuses (Ramakrishnan *et al.*, 2000), and built-in test or self-verification devices (Motorola, 2002). For large volume and complex devices, this type of system, however, is prone to false alarms provoking unnecessary costly replacement and inaccurate model construction (Pecht *et al.*, 2001). In order to collect valuable data and better assess health management of complex systems, failure precursor monitoring is thus necessary. It consists in measuring several parameters directly related to failure or damage. Current prognostics techniques are then based on constantly sensing and collecting data correlated to the performance of a system. Precise interpretation of recorded information is also required to build predictive point-of-care models (Pecht *et al.*, 1999).

17.3 Reliability monitoring with wireless MEMS

A low-cost, low-power, easily interrogated solution to current telecommunication systems reliability needs is now possible with the recent use of WSNs. These allow the deployment of both sensing and data-processing remotely:

data-mining and communication to the outside world are organized in coordination with other nodes, enabling the consultation of data off-site, thanks to networking. Each individual device in a WSN has a limited power supply, processing speed, storage capacity, and communication bandwidth although the overall network can offer substantial processing capability. All these assets permit the WSNs to have a broad range of applications nowadays, and their deployment is expected to increase even further (Culler et al., 2004; Mukhopadhyay and Leung, 2010).

Most of the time, the level of sensor integration that environmental monitoring systems offer is too low for a practical use in a large range of applications, from environmental monitoring to quality, reliability and precision control, where low-cost, reliable sensors are demanded. Moreover, in telecommunications reliability monitoring, although the type of sensors is mainly application specific, multiple sensing capabilities are now requested to offer greater flexibility, better quality response and cross-sensitivity assessment via simultaneous readings from multiple sensors. This is seen for example in the aircraft industry, where tyre condition monitoring requires the investigation of multiple parameters at the same time (Tiju et al., 2004). It is also preferable to enable sensing redundancy when possible (Chong and Kumar, 2003).

17.3.1 Existing monitoring solutions

The key in addressing reliability to construct models is in the capability of implementing constant and programmed monitoring during the infrastructure application, on-site. Today, novel sensor networks are promising to merge data sets from different sensor types and to enhance the understanding of larger monitored systems as a whole. The convergence of these sensor platforms with global communication networks makes the chain from raw data to useful information available where needed.

Some environmental monitoring commercial solutions embeddable in larger systems already exist and cover a large range of applications, from the automotive industry to avionics and consumer electronics. Some electronics industry companies have already taken part in the global aim of improving reliability with prognostics solutions. For example, Honeywell, Crossbow, Sensatronics and Dust Networks are already offering a range of environmental monitoring platforms integrating discrete off-the-shelf sensors, such as for light, temperature and humidity. Application-specific solutions already exist as well in different key domains, such as the energy sector where Advanced Energy Industries has recently developed a site-monitoring solution for photovoltaic systems compatible with several energy monitoring software providers. Finally, at the research level, the number of academic projects currently utilizing WSN capabilities and performances is only limited by the number of possible applications and technical surveys reviewing the latest research achievements that have to be updated on a regular basis (Hart and Martinez, 2006).

However, although most of commercial environmental monitoring solutions are often responding to specific needs, they only integrate a limited amount of sensor readings, typically temperature and humidity, in macroscale ranges. The unreliability or high cost of more complex structures integrating several other sensors impedes a different approach with smaller components. However, it is desirable to enhance the sensing capabilities and reduce the overall size of the monitoring modules to offer more flexibility. In order to set a vision for future WSN technologies close interactions between research and development are necessary and adapted approaches are to be sought (Vichare *et al.*, 2007).

17.3.2 Development of reliability monitoring solutions using MEMS technology

Advances in microsensor fabrication, microprocessors, compact memories, batteries and wireless technologies have permitted the implementation of miniature, autonomous platforms and modules that are able to respond the current needs in environmental monitoring, even for remote deployment of the system to be analysed. As power consumption is currently the greatest limiting factor for WSN solutions, low-power devices are needed for life-cycle data collection.

MEMS technology presents advantages for the development of reliability monitoring solutions in general, and telecommunication reliability in particular, where the sensors must be more reliable than the system they have to monitor. Although non-mature MEMS structures may suffer some reliability issues, especially with packaging (Hartley *et al.*, 2002), commercial microsystems developed with a fabrication process linked to high-volume integrated circuits (IC) enable a range of actuation and sensing at a lower cost and increased robustness, even in harsh environments. MEMS sensors thus provide significant advantages in a broad range of applications: batch fabrication and low-power actuation reduce costs, high precision and response speed enable accurate monitoring, micron-sized fabrication and CMOS compatibility enable a higher level of integration, and redundancy is made feasible on a single die for better accuracy and reliability.

Miniaturized, wireless, self-powered, low-power, low-cost, redundant and even self-reconfigurable monitoring platforms are then possible with MEMS technology (Hautefeuille *et al.*, 2011), and MEMS sensors seem to offer the best solution to design environmental monitoring platforms called Health and Usage Monitoring Systems (HUMS). These enable specific, precise multi-mode or multi-function sensor systems that respond well to current reliability needs (Xu et al., 2010). In 2007, a HUMS Service Cluster, comprising more than 30 leading experts, was established. Its goals are to build an extensive reliability information database, achieve on-line test and diagnostics capabilities, and conduct studies on HUMS solutions for constant environmental monitoring (HUMS, 2007).

17.3.3 Advantages of wireless MEMS

Smart sensor nodes are the building blocks of WSN modules. These can sense, measure and collect information from their environment and, based on a user-defined decision process, they can transmit useful data to the outside world. Therefore, the modules are typically equipped with one or more sensors, a processor with necessary signal conditioning circuitry, and a radio-frequency (RF) module for wireless communication. For some specific applications, memory and power supply can be embedded on board as well, even though WSNs typically have little infrastructure for remote sensing application and greater autonomy. In contrast with traditional communication networks, each WSN possesses its own application-specific limitations such as: available energy supply, bandwidth, communication range, processing, storage capabilities, and design constraints. Most of these resource restrictions are addressed at different programming and scheduling levels. However, the design constraints, such as network size, deployment, choice of sensors, and topology are dependent on the environment to monitor and hence on the application. This is why the development of sensor networks may require different research works in various fields of science and technology, including the development of intelligent, miniature scale and low-power sensors.

Indeed, the continued demand for novel WSN modules requires not only software or organization improvements; novel, low-cost, reliable, small sized sensor platforms are greatly needed platform in order to further reduce the size of the node and its power consumption. Indeed, when developing these data-acquisition systems, the information collected by the sensors is the most important parameter, and it is too often limited by existing technology. A higher level of sensor integration is thus required today, and long-term integrity, quality performance, interactivity, cross-sensitivity and minimal power consumption are amongst the most important requirements and specifications that are raised for integration in WSN. Finally, the development of reliable sensors may allow a better correlation of all relevant parameters and even provide a broader understanding of long-term systems performance in different environments.

MEMS technology has already demonstrated its potential to develop mature, commercial sensors. Nowadays, it also permits the integration of

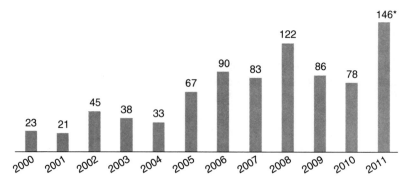

17.1 Timeline of indexed scientific publications in the 'wireless MEMS and reliability' context (*results of an Internet web search conducted on Science Direct at the end of November 2011). (*Source*: Science Direct.)

multiple sensor structures on a single miniaturized platform to enable accurate multi-mode readings and cross-sensitivity compensation, thanks to a combination of simultaneous readings (Hautefeuille *et al.*, 2011). MEMS sensors may then be integrated on specifically-designed circuit boards or existing platforms for the development of prognostics solutions, Health and Usage Monitoring Microsystems (HUMMs) modules and multi-function sensing platforms that are non-intrusive. Real-time communication to the outside world is ensured via RF protocols, and data collection in a serial memory is also made possible for diagnostics applications.

The advantages presented by MEMS technology to build wireless solutions have also permitted the fabrication of many application-specific autonomous MEMS-based WSN modules (Warneke and Pister, 2002). A simple web search conducted in September 2011 and presented in Fig. 17.1 shows that the number of scientific publications where both expressions '*wireless MEMS*' and '*telecommunication reliability*' appear has increased from the early days of WSN modules. The levels achieved in more recent times, however, suggest that less progress has been made in this field lately. This is probably due to the known difficulty in maturing MEMS applications and managing to pass the commercialization barrier (Grace, 2006). In the meantime, additional advanced capabilities, such as self-recalibration, reconfiguration and energy scavenging, are also sought for more flexibility and more autonomy for the wireless MEMS solutions (Kerkhoff, 2009).

To conclude, it may be useful to summarize that WSNs are now arguably on the way to becoming one of the new technological revolutions, able to answer the current needs of reliability research where good quality real-time monitoring systems are required. It has become utterly important to build intelligent, modular platforms with the capability to sense multiple parameters, at a lower cost, and lower scale, even remotely. It has been proven that MEMS technology is a very good solution to consider today, in order to match all these recent requirements. Although an ideal solution does not exist, MEMS-based WSN platforms seem to offer an appropriate flexibility in environmental monitoring.

17.4   Case study: multi-MEMS platform

In the present case study, a MEMS-based environmental platform, developed to address reliability issues due to external stress and ageing, is presented (Hautefeuille et al., 2011). The purpose of this section is to demonstrate that a simple methodology may be used by a MEMS designer to develop a wireless platform with multiple microsensors relatively rapidly, using existing fabrication processes and WSN modules. This approach of fabricating multiple MEMS structures functions on one single substrate has been called multi-MEMS. By combining precise and trustable monitoring multi-MEMS structures with wireless capabilities, important data may then be gathered on field and during operation, thus helping to improve understanding or even prevent failure of telecommunication systems.

An existing CMOS-compatible MEMS fabrication process has been modified and extended to manufacture temperature, relative humidity, corrosion, gas detection, and gas flow velocity sensors on a single silicon substrate and to offer good sensitivity with limited power consumption. All MEMS sensors have been easily simulated prior to their fabrication and designed according to application-specific requirements. Final characterization of each sensor is necessary at different levels after fabrication to prove good agreement with analytical models. They have been tested at a bare-die level and after onboard integration (Hautefeuille et al., 2011). As presented in Fig. 17.2, this type of multi-MEMS fabrication on a single substrate may allow a greater integration level on a package than the multi-chip module approach with different discrete dies that must be attached to it (Fig. 17.2a). As previously mentioned, the presented MEMS sensors are compatible with CMOS technology as the fabrication processes are similar. Monolithic integration of all MEMS sensors on top of their own CMOS signal conditioning circuitry is then possible and presents other important advantages in the global aim to reduce dimensions, costs, interconnect issues and even power consumption. When the fabrication processes are not compatible or concurrent, a hybrid integration where two die are attached to each other is chosen. It is a more common strategy as it is generally easier to achieve.

The choice of sensors is always based on the reliability requirements of high-value telecommunications components during shipping, storage and operation, where monitoring and recording of temperature, humidity,

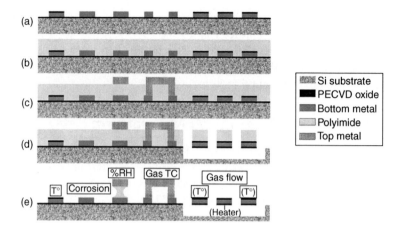

17.2 Multi-MEMS fabrication process on a silicon substrate: (a) selective metal deposition and passivation on PECVD oxide; (b) spin coating of a 3-µm-thick polyimide layer; (c) selective top metal deposition; (d) selective silicon etching; (e) polyimide removal.

corrosion, gas thermal conductivity and gas flow rates are needed. All information gathered from these sensors then needed to be accessible in real-time by wired or wireless communication and logged in a memory for possible further use. However, the choice of the sensor structure is not always straightforward and depends on several factors, such as the fabrication facilities, processes and materials available, application, etc. The technological requirements and limitations of this particular type of project always represent the bottom-line that dictates the specifications of the corresponding MEMS sensors that should be developed. The following gives a rapid, summarized overview of the sensors that have been fabricated for integration on a WSN platform. Although there is no single solution to a particular problem, it is hoped to provide valuable information to MEMS sensors designers.

17.4.1 Temperature sensors

Temperature is a very important parameter to monitor in telecommunication reliability and over a very large range of values. However, it is not particularly important to fabricate very fast sensors or measure its value at a high sampling rate, as it is a relatively slow process. Metal meanders may be fabricated to measure temperature. Their sensing principle is based on a linear dependence of their electrical resistance with temperature. A simple measurement of a resistance change will then be easily translated into a temperature modification, as can be seen in Fig. 17.3. Depending on the meanders total length on the die surface, the sensitivity of the fabricated structures presented in this case study may vary in the mΩ/°C to kΩ/°C

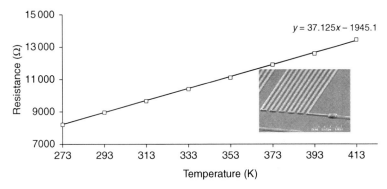

17.3 Typical temperature sensor linear response of a 2 μm wide, 0.5 μm thick and 250 mm long Al/1%Si meander. (Adapted from Hautefeuille et al., 2011.)

range, enabling a precision of approximately 1°C. Moreover, MEMS technology typically allows large temperature operation range of operations. In this case study, the structures have been successfully tested for temperature changes occurring within seconds, which is considered to be in the range of normal electronic components heating and much faster than environmental changes. The full temperature range covered by these structures is between −10°C and 85°C, which is very acceptable for telecommunication reliability applications. Simple Wheatstone bridges or voltage dividers are used for temperature readings when integrating these sensors on a WSN platform.

17.4.2 Humidity sensors

Relative humidity is an even slower process to monitor. Moreover, great precision is not required in this case and typical telecommunication reliability specifications require a precision between 1%RH and 10%RH in the full 0–100%RH range. Many different MEMS humidity sensors solutions exist. In this case, capacitive structures have been designed to offer a 5%RH precision with a sensitivity of a few femtofarad per relative humidity percent (fF per %RH). Figure 17.4 shows the characteristic response of a polyimide-based capacitive sensor with interdigitated electrodes. As mentioned in Hautefeuille et al. (2011) and although it is not commonly addressed, humidity sensors ageing must be characterized to guarantee reliable measurements over a long time. Capacitance-to-voltage circuits are required to utilize this type of capacitive sensor on a WSN module.

17.4.3 Corrosion sensors

The structures consist of interdigitated aluminium triple-track comb patterns, which suffer leakage currents between their inversely biased electrodes due to

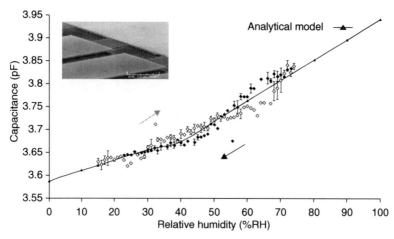

17.4 Response of a polyimide-based capacitive humidity sensor with interdigitated electrodes. Sensor dimensions are: 1.2 mm × 1.2 mm × 3 μm. In the figure, the ◊ represent ascending values and the ♦ represent descending values. (Adapted from Hautefeuille et al., 2011.)

electrolytic migration between metal tracks in the presence of moisture, salts and other impurities that influence metal degradation. This type of miniaturized canary-like structure may be adequately designed to monitor the desired corrosion rates, thanks to direct resistance readings even under low voltage bias. Indeed, as the MEMS corrosion sensor suffers degradation, its electrical resistance increases slowly in a stepwise fashion. As resistive sensors, these early warning corrosion sensors require the same conditioning circuits as the resistive sensors.

17.4.4 Gas sensors

Suspended beam thermal conductivity sensors operate by measuring variations in the thermal conductance of a structure in response to changes in the surrounding gaseous ambient. This type of sensor is heated electrically and may be configured to detect pressure changes in real-time. It may also detect the presence of different gases with a thermal conductivity different to that of air, as shown in Fig. 17.5, although this capability is limited. It is indeed almost impossible to discriminate between gases when the structure is located in a complex mixture of various gases. The determination of the thermal conductance given by the microsensor is possible by calculating it from an electrical resistance measurement when a constant voltage V is applied across the structure. This is practical for its integration on a wireless module. It is, however, critical to limit the input voltage to avoid physical damage of the structure caused by high electrical currents.

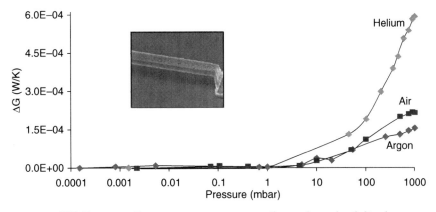

17.5 Free-standing gas sensor response: thermal conductivity change with pressure as a function of ambient gas. (Adapted from Hautefeuille *et al.*, 2011.)

An application-specific programmable alarm may be configured for maximum pressure or dangerous gas detection levels.

17.4.5 Gas flow sensors

There exist many approaches to fabricating MEMS gas flow sensors. The one developed in this case study consists of three similar metallic meander structures that can monitor a flow velocity and its direction: one resistive heater is located in the centre of two temperature sensors. By measuring the temperature difference between the sensors upstream and downstream, it is possible to conclude on air flow direction and velocity with great precision. The final dimensions of the structures depend highly on the reliability specifications and the system to monitor. It is recommended to fabricate several of these structures onboard with different orientations, to be able to detect complex flows on the surface. As the detection principle is also based on resistive measurements, its integration on WSN platforms is quite straightforward.

17.4.6 Results of case study

A dedicated conditioning circuit layer has been built around the fabricated MEMS multisensor die for integration on an existing WSN module with data-processing, memory, communication and power capabilities for flexibility in remote sensing. The design needed to be in agreement with many different onboard limitations of the existing module like: available

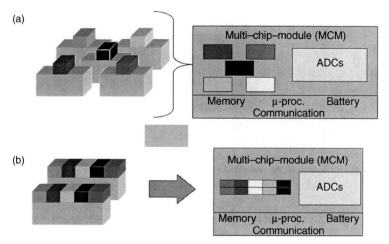

17.6 Different approaches for MEMS sensors integration: (a) multiple discrete sensor chips integrated on a module, (b) optimized integration of a multisensor die fabricated on a single substrate.

real-estate, power, communication packet-size, robustness, etc. The fabrication of multiple MEMS sensors on a single die, however, offers more integration flexibility than multiple discrete dice when attached on existing modules (Fig. 17.6). It also presents the advantage of permitting a completely new design developed around the multi-MEMS structure.

Two of the resulting MEMS-based multisensor chips presented here have finally been attached on a 25 mm × 25 mm *Tyndall25* node used as a data-logging and communications platform (Barton *et al.*, 2006). When compared to the majority of similar current modules, the final MEMS-based WSN solution offers greater simplicity of operation, lower costs of production and a simpler utilization for a reliable data collection from a great number of sensors. Real-time communication of all sensed data to the outside world is ensured via RF protocols, and data collection in a serial memory is also made possible for future use or diagnostics applications.

The combination of simultaneous readings from multiple environmental sensors not only enables redundancy and accurate readings in real-time but also permits cross-sensitivity compensation. The great integration level achieved thanks to MEMS technology and illustrated in Fig. 17.7 has indeed enabled study of the cross-correlation between sensors and minimizing its influence to acquire better quality data from the WSN module (Hautefeuille *et al.*, 2008). Although self-recalibration has not been realized in this case, the first steps towards this capability have been achieved successfully with the multi-MEMS approach: cross-correlation and redundancy are available onboard.

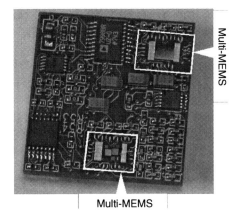

17.7 Top layer of the MEMS-based environmental WSN platform with multiple sensing capabilities. Two 3 mm × 3 mm bare dies have been wire-bonded on a 25 mm × 25 mm circuit board here.

17.5 Conclusion

As previously mentioned, five different sensors required for environmental monitoring have been proposed and developed in order to answer a series of current specifications and requirements of the telecommunication industry. This multi-MEMS approach has enabled the following achievements:

- Multiple sensing capabilities have been integrated on a single silicon substrate and different associations of some or all of temperature, humidity, pressure, gas, gas flow, and corrosion sensors have been integrated on a single 4.5 mm × 3 mm die.
- The dimensions of the different sensors are conditioned by the application and space available onboard. Although these user-defined dimensions will influence the final device performance, the designer has the opportunity to predict this behaviour as good agreement has been found between measured and simulated outputs from all MEMS sensors.
- A specific sensor layer may carefully developed to limit the overall power consumption of the platform thanks to programmable analogue signals and well-designed conditioning circuits.
- Thanks to MEMS technology, redundancy and cross-sensitivity are enabled on such a small space to aid in distinguishing false alarms, correcting faulty structures and building new models by interpreting raw data from multiple sensors.
- An additional memory layer compatible with the existing wireless sensor module has been programmed to record all necessary information that will be communicated to the outside world when desired. The final version of the WSN module developed here then forms a data-logger.

For each sensor, a user-defined sampling rate may be programmed via the processor or microcontroller that constitutes the core of any sensor module. The total memory space utilized for a single sampling of a multisensor output depends on the application and specifications of the platform. Once again, MEMS sensors and multi-MEMS platforms offer flexibility in data collection thanks to their low-power and reliable operation conditions. The fabrication of a number of miniature sensing elements using MEMS technology on 3 mm × 3 mm silicon die helps save manufacturing costs and substrate area for further integration on WSN platforms. A significant limitation to future commercialization has however been identified in this particular case. All multi-MEMS sensor platforms have been attached and wire-bonded in their bare-die form on the WSN module. This results in a very sensitive but fragile sensor layer, located on top of the module. For practical reasons, packaging has not been studied and its potential implications on sensor performance are completely unknown. Although it is a common limitation of MEMS structures in general, it should be carefully addressed in the future.

17.6 Acknowledgements

Most of the material presented here is based on works funded by the Centre for Value-Chain Research (CTVR, Ireland) and achieved when the author was working at the Tyndall National Institute, Lee Maltings, Prospect Row, Cork, Ireland.

17.7 References

Assaf T and Dugan J B (2008), 'Diagnosis based on reliability analysis using monitors and sensors', *Reliability Engineering and System Safety*, **93**, pp. 509–521, doi:10.1016/j.ress.2006.10.024.

Barringer H P (2003), 'A life cycle cost summary', *Proceedings of the International Conference of Maintenance Societies*, ICOMS 2003, p. 10.

Barton J, Hynes G, O'Flynn B, Aherne K, Norman A, and Morrissey A (2006), 'A 25 mm Sensor-Actuator Layer: A miniature, highly adaptable interface layer', *Sensors and Actuators A*, **132**, pp. 362–369, doi:10.1016/j.sna.2006.04.004.

Berger-Wolf T Y, Hart E, and Saia J (2005), 'Discrete sensor placement problems in distribution networks', *Mathematical and Computer Modelling*, **42**(13), pp. 1385–1396.

Chong C Y and Kumar S P (2003), 'Sensor networks: evolution, opportunities and challenges', *Proceedings of the IEEE*, **91**(8), pp. 1247–1256, doi:10.1109/JPROC.2003.814918.

Culler D, Estrin D, and Srivastava M (2004), 'Overview of sensor networks', *IEEE Computer*, **37**(8), pp. 41–49, doi:10.1109/MC.2004.93.

Cutter D and Thompson O (2005), 'Condition-based maintenance plus select program survey', Report LG301T6.

Engel S J, Gilmartin B J, Bongort K, and Hess A (2000), 'Prognostics, the real issues involved with predicting. Life remaining', *IEEE Aerospace Conference* (IEEE 0-7803-5846-5/00).

EPSMA (2005), *Guidelines to Understanding Reliability Prediction*, Report of the European Power Supply Manufacturers Association, p. 29.

Feldman K, Sandborn P, and Jazouli T (2008), 'The analysis of return on investment for PHM applied to electronic systems', *Proceedings of the International Conference on Prognostics and Health Management*, pp. 1–9, doi:10.1109/PHM.2008.4711415.

Grace R H (2006), 'The 2006 report card on the barriers to the commercialization of MEMS and Nanotechnology'. Available online: http://www.rgrace.com/Papers/2006_Report_Card.pdf Accessed on september 29th 2011-

Hart J K and Martinez K (2006), 'Environmental sensor networks: A revolution in the earth system science?', *Earth-Science Reviews*, **78**, pp. 177–191, doi:10.1016/j.earscirev.2006.05.00.

Hartley F T, Arney S, and Sexton F (2002), 'Microsystems reliability, test and metrology', in *MANCEF, Micro Nano roadmap, 1st Edition*, pp. 341–391.

Hautefeuille M, O'Flynn B, Peters F H, and O'Mahony C (2011), 'Development of a MEMS-based multisensor platform for environmental monitoring', *Micromachines* 2011, **2**(4), pp. 410–430, doi:10.3390/mi2040410.

Hautefeuille M, O'Mahony C, O'Flynn B, Khalfi K, and Peters F (2008), 'A MEMS-based wireless multisensor module for environmental monitoring', *Journal of Microelectronics Reliability*, **48**(6), pp. 906–910, doi:10.1016/j.microrel.2008.03.007.

Hess A (2001), 'The joint strike fighter (JSF) prognostics and health management', NDIA Conference.

HUMS Service Cluster (2007), Available online: http://www.mns-minds.org/outputs-and-publications/downloadfile.html?id=58&entryid=55 Accessed on September 29th 2011.

Jones J and Hayes J (1999), 'A comparison of electronic-reliability prediction models', *IEEE Transactions on Reliability*, **48**(2), pp. 127–134, doi:10.1109/24.784270.

Kerkhoff H G (2009), 'Dependable reconfigurable multi-sensor poles for security', *Proceedings of the 15th IEEE Mixed-Signals, Sensors and Systems Test Workshop (IMS3TW'09)*, Scottsdale, AZ, USA, pp. 1–4, doi:10.1109/IMS3TW.2009.5158681.

Motorola (2002), 'Motorola built-in test diagnostic software'. Available online: http://www.bnl.gov/cad/sns/documents/vme/MVME5500.pdf. Accessed in April 2013.

Mukhopadhyay S C and Leung H (2010), *Advances in Wireless Sensors and Sensor Networks*, Springer-Verlag, Berlin, Heidelberg.

Pecht M G, Dube M, Natishan M, and Knowles I (2001), 'An evaluation of built-in test', *IEEE Transactions on Aerospace and Electronics Systems*, **37**(1), pp. 266–272, doi:10.1109/7.913684.

Pecht M G, Radojcic R, and Rao G (1999), *Guidebook for Managing Silicon Chip Reliability*, CRC Press, Boca Raton, FL, USA.

Rachlin Y, Negi R, and Khosla P (2005), 'Sensing capacity for discrete sensor network applications', *Proceedings of the 4th International Symposium on Information Processing in Sensor Networks*, Los Angeles, USA, doi:10.1109/IPSN.2005.1440911.

Ramakrishnan A, Syrus T, and Pecht M G (2000), *Electronic Hardware Reliability*, Avionics Handbook, CRC Press, Boca Raton, FL, USA, pp. 22-1–22-21.

Society of Automotive Engineers (1995), *Reliability, Maintainability and Supportability Guidebook*, 3rd Edition, Warrendale, PA.

Salmela O (2005), 'The effect of introducing increased-reliability risk electronic components into 3rd generation telecommunications systems', *Reliability Engineering and System Safety*, **89**(2), pp. 208–218, doi:10.1016/j.ress.2004.08.020.

Shapiro A A, Ling S X, Ganesan S, Cozy R S, Hunter D J, Schatzel D V, Mojarradi M M, and Kolawa E A (2004), 'Electronic packaging for extended mars surface missions', *Proceedings of IEEE Aerospace Conference*, **4**, pp. 2515–2527, doi:10.1109/AERO.2004.1368046.

Telecommunications Industry Association (2010), *TIA's 2010 Information and Communications Technology Market Review and Forecast*.

Tiju W, Ahanchian A, and Majlis B Y (2004), 'Development of tire condition monitoring system (TCMS) based on MEMS sensors', *Proceedings of ICSE 2004*, Kuala Lumpur, Malaysia, pp. 350–353, doi:10.1109/SMELEC.2004.1620903.

Vichare N, Rodgers P, Eveloy V, and Pecht M (2007), 'Environment and usage monitoring of electronic products for health assessment and product design', *Quality Technology and Quantitative Management*, **4**(2), pp. 235–250.

Warneke B A and Pister K S J (2002), 'MEMS for distributed wireless sensor networks', *Proceedings of the 9th International Conference on Electronics, Circuits and Systems*, pp. 291–294, doi:10.1109/ICECS.2002.1045391.

Xu Z, Koltsov D, Richardson A, Le L, and Begbie M (2010), 'Design and simulation of a multi-function MEMS sensor for health and usage monitoring', *Prognostics and Health Management Conference*, Macao, pp. 1–7, doi:10.1109/PHM.2010.5413415.

18
Optical MEMS for displays in portable systems

W. O. DAVIS, MicroVision, Inc., USA

DOI: 10.1533/9780857098610.2.569

Abstract: This chapter discusses several optical microelectromechanical systems (MEMS) devices that are used as displays for portable wireless systems. Two direct-view MEMS-based displays are summarized; these seek to displace the incumbent liquid-crystal based displays that are widely employed in mobile devices. MEMS picoprojector displays are reviewed, including mirror array-based projection and laser beam scanning (LBS). The further application of MEMS-based LBS to head-up and eyewear displays is discussed.

Key words: optical MEMS, display, picoprojector, laser beam scanning.

18.1 Introduction

In a wireless system requiring a display there will be obvious tradeoffs involved in reconciling portability with the display's usability. Size and power consumption requirements in particular can be expected to force compromises. In the case of size, either the display may be smaller than one would prefer, so that it fits within the allowable system volume, or the mobile system is made larger than desired, so that it can have a usable display. Furthermore, the power consumption for a wireless mobile device display must be low enough to serve its application on a battery charge, and this can be expected to force a limit on the maximum display brightness. Both the size and the power constraints suggest a role for optical MEMS, with recent examples showing the potential to simultaneously address critical size and power limitations. Especially when combined with miniaturized and efficient light sources, optical MEMS may have a large impact on wireless system capabilities.

For directly viewed displays, the substitution of MEMS-based technology for the traditional liquid-crystal displays (LCDs) in current widespread use has been recently demonstrated, including a technology that creates MEMS within the existing LCD manufacturing infrastructure. Another technology forms a color displayed image using ambient light, filtered and reflected, to combat the overwhelming of backlit displays by bright ambient outdoor light. For these direct-view displays, however, the size requirements for the display and the portable system are in their usual tension.

Handheld picoprojectors provide a means of relieving this tension, providing a display much larger than the confines of its mechanical assembly. MEMS technologies that currently address this concept include mirror array-based image plane projection and laser beam scanning (LBS) with a micromirror. These systems can create monitor-sized displays using a projection engine that occupies only a few cubic centimeters, or even widescreen television or movie-screen sized displays when ambient lighting conditions permit. LBS also lends itself well to heads-up displays (HUDs) for automobiles.

The eye itself is the ultimate display surface. Extending the picoprojection concept to wearable 'eyewear' displays overcomes the need to find a convenient projection surface and suitable lighting conditions, and therefore represents a very attractive direction for the MEMS-based technologies. Inherently portable, the eyewear concept can also address a desire for a more immersive and private viewing experience and enables augmented- and virtual-reality technology. Future developments are likely to increase the value of displays for wireless systems by making them more immersive and interactive through three-dimensional (3-D) display and user interface improvements.

18.2 MEMS-based direct-view displays

Direct-view displays can be considered as those comprising a matrix of pixels that emit light directly into the viewer's eye. Wireless systems currently use LCD and organic LED (OLED) technology; however, MEMS devices may have a role to play as well.

18.2.1 Qualcomm™ IMOD™ display

Backlit LCD displays do not perform well in outdoor ambient light, the backlight being overwhelmed by the light incident on the display surface. The mirasol® IMOD™ display by Qualcomm™ seeks to address the need for power-efficient mobile displays under such conditions by using the ambient light itself to illuminate the display. This is accomplished using an array of MEMS membranes to form optical cavities tuned to red, green, and blue (RGB) wavelengths (Qualcomm, 2009a,b).

A display pixel is subdivided into RGB subpixels, each comprising a MEMS device as illustrated in Fig. 18.1. In an open state, an optical cavity is formed that is tuned to reflect the red, green, or blue components of

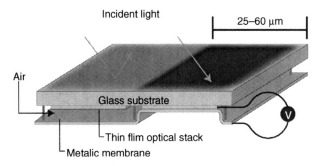

18.1 Illustration of Qualcomm™ IMOD™ MEMS device to form a wavelength-dependent switchable reflector (from Gally (2004)).

the incident light spectrum. The cavity lengths are determined during the MEMS fabrication process by the selective removal of a sacrificial layer. A voltage is applied between the optical cavity surfaces formed by a stationary optical stack of metals and metal oxides such as indium–tin–oxide (ITO) and a moveable metal membrane, the voltage creating an electrostatic attractive force that causes the cavity to collapse. In the collapsed state the cavity reflects light in invisible ultraviolet wavelengths, while the reflectance of visible light drops to near zero and the subpixel appears black (Qualcomm, 2009b). Qualcomm (2009b) reports reflectivity of 60% and a contrast ratio of 10:1, which is comparable to printed text.

The subpixels are further divided into sub-elements that enable 3-bit grayscale within each color, as in Figs 18.2 and 18.3 (Qualcomm, 2009b). Additional grayscale resolution up to 64 gray levels per color can be derived by additional temporal modulation of the subpixels' reflectance state, taking advantage of the MEMS membrane's fast switching time, on the order of tens of microseconds (Qualcomm, 2009b). Being a reflective display, the color balance is not under control without a feedback system using detection of the incident light spectrum. Still, Gally (2004) reports favorable performance in terms of reflectance, color gamut, and contrast ratio compared to reflective and transflective (transmissive when a backlight is in use, reflective when ambient conditions overwhelm the backlight) LCD displays, which face the same color issue.

The IMOD device can be operated in a bistable mode of operation (Miles *et al.*, 2003; Qualcomm, 2009a,b), exploiting the electromechanical pull-in phenomenon that is a common occurrence in electrostatic MEMS devices. At a critical value of the voltage across the optical cavity (illustrated in Fig. 18.1), the electrostatic force overwhelms the ability of the mechanical elastic restoring force to maintain an intermediate equilibrium position. The membrane suddenly pulls into contact with the optical stack and the

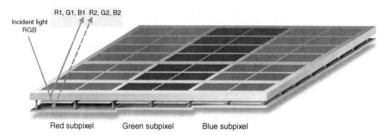

18.2 Color IMOD™ pixel formed by RGB subpixels (from Qualcomm (2009b)).

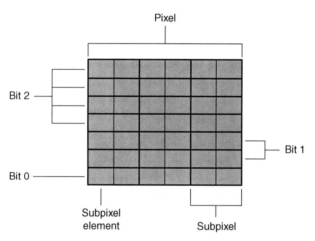

18.3 Subdivision of RGB subpixels into subpixel elements, for three-bit grayscale resolution achieved by spatial dithering (from Qualcomm (2009b)).

reflectance is switched off. Thereafter, the voltage can be reduced somewhat while still maintaining the collapsed pull-in state. Further reduction of the voltage to a second critical value finally enables the elastic forces to overwhelm the electrostatic attraction, and the membrane returns to its original position where the cavity reflects visible light. The hysteresis is used to operate the device with three voltage levels, where an intermediate hold voltage can maintain either the reflective or the black optical states and transient pulses to two other voltage levels can switch the reflective state, as illustrated in Fig. 18.4.

Because of the bistability characteristic, and the fact that the electrical load of the MEMS is capacitive, the IMOD display can be operated in a very low electrical power mode when temporal dithering is not necessary for grayscale resolution and the displayed image content is static or

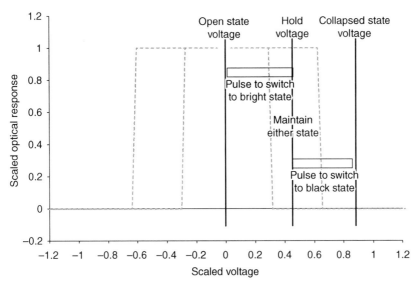

18.4 Bistability of IMOD™ device reflectance enabled by electromechanical hysteresis (from Qualcomm (2009a)).

changing slowly. The only power consumption occurs when the display content changes and, unlike LCD displays, the IMOD does not need to be occasionally refreshed due to degradation over time. In Miles *et al.* (2003), a power consumption of 0.84 µW/in^2 was reported for the IMOD display showing static text, compared to 68 µW/in^2 for a thin film transistor (TFT)–LCD display that has to be refreshed frequently to maintain even the static image. For a battery-powered wireless device such as a smartphone, whose power consumption today is dominated by the LCD display, a factor of 80 reduction in the battery discharge rate for the display of static text using the IMOD device could enable significantly longer use times between charges.

The use of pull-in and contact means that attention must be paid to the prevalent issue of stiction, where surfaces, once in contact, are hard to separate. Stiction would cause the black state of the element to persist when attempts are being made to change to the reflective state. The IMOD device is packaged in a sealed environment with a getter material to absorb moisture, a factor promoting stiction. Floyd *et al.* (2006) report a prediction of lifetime of 10 years based on the dessicant reaching its absorption capacity.

Future adoption will be dependent on certain wireless devices' need for low-power displays in bright ambient lighting, where increasing the brightness of a backlit display carries an unacceptable penalty in power consumption. Reaching the consumer mass market has so far proved difficult: in 2012 Qualcomm announced plans to limit production and instead seek to license the technology (Davies, 2012).

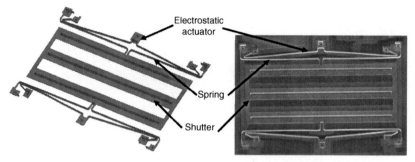

18.5 Pixtronix DMS™ MEMS device (from Brosnihan *et al.* (2010)).

18.2.2 Pixtronix Digital Micro Shutter

Another direct-view display technology using an array of MEMS devices is the Pixtronix PerfectLight™ Display using the Digital Micro Shutter (DMS™). This display uses field sequential color (FSC), such that the entire display is illuminated with RGB light each in their turn, at a fast enough rate that the viewer perceives a color image. An array of MEMS shutters is reconfigured corresponding to the color content of the image. An individual DMS device is shown in Fig. 18.5. This approach multiplexes the subpixels temporally, in contrast to approaches that multiplex spatially such as the IMOD™ device in the previous subsection with subpixels dedicated to a certain color each occupying a unique volume. In 2012 Qualcomm acquired Pixtronix (Clarke, 2012), adding this approach to the company's direct-view MEMS-based display portfolio.

The DMS is formed using the manufacturing infrastructure in use to produce TFT and LCDs. The polarizers and filters that would be part of an LCD display are replaced by FSC illumination and the MEMS shutters. The MEMS is formed on a TFT backplane which forms the shutter driver array, and attached to a backlight panel with an aperture pattern that will be covered or uncovered by the shutters depending on their actuation state. In LCD displays, individual liquid-crystal pixels' states are switched to either transmit or absorb light from the backlight source. The transmission efficiency for light that exits the display through polarizers, filters, and the LCD material is of the order of 10%. The DMS is more optically efficient, since it does not contribute to transmission losses when opened, and because of the light recycling structure designed to give the light only one way out, through the apertures, as shown in Fig. 18.6. Transmission efficiencies of 50–80% have been reported (Brosnihan *et al.*, 2010; Hagood *et al.*, 2007), even though the apertures' area coverage of the display is only in the range of 5–20% (Hagood *et al.*, 2007).

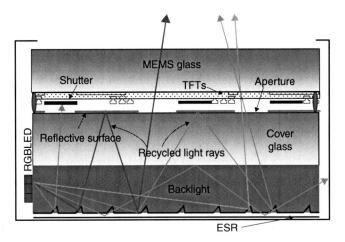

18.6 Illustration of Pixtronix PerfectLight™ display device (from Hagood *et al.* (2008)).

The DMS device is a flexure-suspended shuttle mass, with a gap-closing lateral electrostatic actuator that acts on the suspension beam springs, as shown in Fig. 18.5. As described by Legtenberg *et al.* (1997), the springs are attracted to the actuator under an applied voltage. They come into physical contact at a small voltage, with the contact area increasing with increasing voltage until the full travel range is reached, akin to the joining of two structures with a zipper. The material choices were restricted to those in use in the production of LCD displays in order to take advantage of the scale of existing manufacturing infrastructure. As described by Brosnihan *et al.* (2010), the films in use are not thick enough to create mechanical flexure springs with a thickness-to-width aspect ratio high enough to create the desired in-plane compliance and out-of-plane stiffness. Instead, MEMS structures with the desired mechanical properties were formed by conformal coating of the sidewalls of a layer used as a sacrificial mold (Brosnihan *et al.*, 2010).

Brosnihan *et al.* (2010) reported 10 μm of travel actuated with 20 V, with a shutter switching time of 100 μsec. The fast switching time for opening and closing the shutter is used to create 8-bit per color digitization of the illumination, providing 24-bit color depth with a 60 Hz frame rate. The time-division multiplexed color-sequential approach carries a power penalty associated with more frequent display state changes compared to LCD or IMOD™; however, when combined with the optical efficiency improvement the company claims the net power savings is 60–80% over LCD (Brosnihan *et al.*, 2010). The LED light sources provide excellent color gamut of 150% NTSC over viewing angles from −85° to +85°, compared to 50–80% NTSC for LCD displays not using LED light sources. Reported contrast ratios are greater than 100:1, with one contrast reducing factor being the light leakage around the shutters.

18.3 Handheld picoprojectors

Projection is a familiar technology that inherently decouples the size of a portable system from the size of its display. While image sharing by projection of slide-format prints has fallen out of fashion, it remains in principle an effective way for people to simultaneously view images. In its heyday slide-format print projection required a lot of setup on the part of the projectionist, with significant risk that the viewers' enjoyment could not match the efforts spent on production. Today, digital, miniaturized, and mobile image storage is now taken for granted but sharing is still limited by the tradeoff between portability of the storage device and the size of a direct-view display. The time is ripe for 'picoprojector' technology that enables effortless spontaneous image sharing, using a pocket-sized projector running on battery power. MEMS devices are contributing to this emerging technology, as will by shown by two examples.

18.3.1 Digital Micromirror Device™

One of the most famous MEMS devices is the Digital Micromirror Device™ (DMD™) by Texas Instruments (TI), first conceived in the 1980s (Hornbeck, 1996). It consists of an array of micromirrors, each on the order of 10 μm in width with an individually controllable tilt degree of freedom. It went into commercial production in 1996 as a 640 by 480 pixel VGA array, that is, with 307 200 individual micromirror devices (Hornbeck, 1996). The successful manufacturing of this device is an historic achievement in the MEMS industry, and TI has enjoyed many years of commercial success in projection display for cinema and office environments with its continued production.

The DMD is fabricated by surface micromachining on top of a complementary metal oxide semiconductor (CMOS) memory circuit using a six photomask MEMS process that patterns three aluminum alloy layers, including the reflector itself (Hornbeck, 1996, 2007). A diagram of an individual DMD micromirror is shown in Fig. 18.7 (Hornbeck, 1996). Each micromirror corresponds to a pixel in the display. Its rotation is actuated by the electrostatic force between the mirror and electrodes underneath. The micromirror position is digital, in that it is positioned in one of two states created by rotating the micromirror until it contacts a mechanical stop. In one position the micromirror reflects light into a display pixel, while in the other it sends the light in an unviewed direction. Since the device is an electrostatic pull-in device, it exhibits a hysteretic behavior (Senturia, 2001, p. 541) similar to that already discussed for the IMOD™ MEMS device, where the mirror can be held in a deflected position with a voltage that is less than the pull-in voltage (Hornbeck, 2007). Anti-stiction countermeasures are part of the design: the contact to the mechanical stop is made through contact springs,

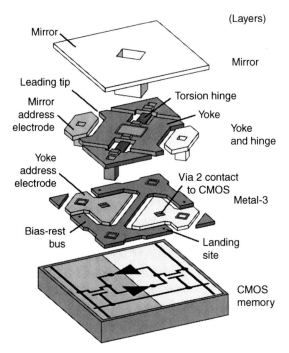

18.7 Exploded diagram of TI DMD™ MEMS device (courtesy of TI).

and when a mirror rotation state change is to be made the mirror is actually briefly pulled closer to the stops so that the contact springs' restoring forces help to release the mirror from any stiction forces (Hornbeck, 2007).

The primary use of the DMD device has been in DLP® projectors, implemented for displays in color-multiplexed forms. In a three-DMD configuration, each DMD array is dedicated to modulating the light intensity corresponding to one of the component colors. This arrangement is in widespread use in office projectors and digital cinema. In a one-DMD color-sequential configuration, the DMD mirror array is FSC illuminated in turn with RGB light (for example), created from LED or laser light sources, or a sequence of colors created using a white lamp and a color wheel. The reduced composite duty cycle of projected multicolor light results in a less bright display compared to that of the three-DMD arrangement.

Displays for highly portable wireless systems will be restricted to single DMD arrangements with FSC using LED or laser light sources, due to size and power consumption limitations. The achievable small size is directly related to the display resolution: when the mirrors can be made at a 10.8 μm pitch, as in (Hornbeck, 2007), then the size of a DMD array will be about 20.7 mm by 11.7 mm for a high-definition 1920 by 1080 pixel display. The need for packaging providing encapsulation, and for projection optics somewhat larger than the DMD array, will add to the size, yet even so the size of the display engine is merely a fraction of what a direct-view display would be for a reasonable projected image size. For example, one commercial pico-projector offering by Optoma using the DMD has a volume of 1.7 cm by 11.2 cm by 6.1 cm, about the size of several smartphones, yet it can project an image the size of a computer monitor or even larger (Optoma, 2011).

18.3.2 Laser beam scanning projection

In marked contrast to approaches using an array of elements, where each one corresponds to a display pixel, is a technique that uses a single high-speed scanning mirror to build up the displayed image pixel-by-pixel. MicroVision has been a pioneer in the commercialization of this type of display engine, using high-speed MEMS scanning mirrors and laser light sources. The LBS method is similar to the cathode-ray tube (CRT) technology, which scans an electron beam onto a phosphor grid; however, for LBS there is no special projection surface needed. To achieve a high pixel count, a scanning mirror deflects a laser spot with a high-speed horizontal scan, as illustrated in Fig. 18.8. Practical implementations require using the mechanical resonance of a MEMS scanning mirror, and the horizontal component of the

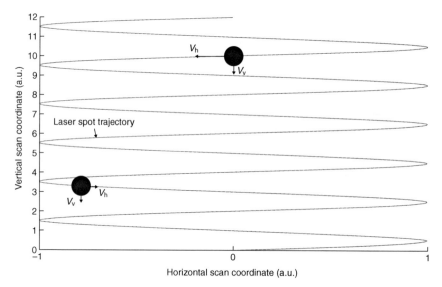

18.8 Laser spot trajectory for LBS projection consisting of a high-speed sinusoidal horizontal scan and a constant-velocity vertical scan. The laser spot's constant vertical velocity and sinusoidal horizontal components V_v and V_h are shown for illustration at two different times within the scanning of a display frame and are not to scale.

spot velocity V_h on the projection surface is sinusoidal under small angle assumptions. The high-speed horizontal scan lines are swept vertically by an orthogonal scanning mirror motion. To achieve uniform pixel placement and the highest quality image, the vertical scan is a sawtooth raster with constant velocity V_v during the active video portion of the scan.

The LBS technology was used by MicroVision in head-mounted retinal scanned display (RSD) systems in the mid-1990s, starting with conventionally machined metallic resonant scanners, and using silicon MEMS scanning mirrors in the early 2000s (Lippert *et al.*, 2000; Tauscher *et al.*, 2010; Urey *et al.*, 2000; Wine *et al.*, 2000). The RSD technology will be further discussed in Section 18.5. More recently, the MEMS-based LBS has been deployed in the PicoP® miniaturized display engine for picoprojection, illustrated in Fig. 18.9. The technology was commercialized in 2009 as the SHOWWX™ handheld projector. Inside the projection engine, RGB laser

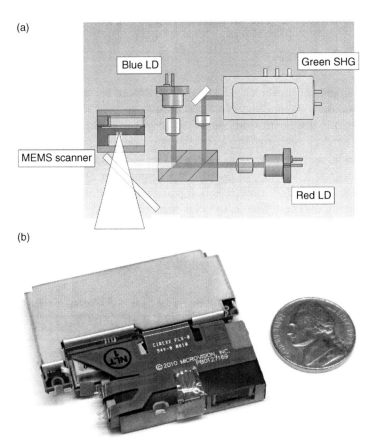

18.9 MicroVision PicoP™ MEMS-based LBS projection engine. (a) Schematic and (b) photograph of actual system.

light is combined into a single beam. A biaxial MEMS scanning mirror scans the combined beam in a two-dimensional 60 Hz frame rate raster pattern. High-speed modulation of the laser light controls the display of individual pixels. The red and blue lasers are available as laser diodes, while the green laser is a device using second-harmonic generation (SHG) to halve the wavelength of an infrared source.

The key component inside the PicoP is the MEMS scanning mirror. Requirements for mirrors that are capable of scanning a modulated laser spot, such that common display resolutions can be achieved with 60 Hz refresh rates, have been derived by Urey *et al.* (1999, 2000) and Urey (2004) and summarized with several examples by Tauscher *et al.* (2010). Consider a scanned projection generated by deflecting a laser spot in a horizontal scan with frequency f, and with a vertical scan providing a given frame rate (e.g. 60 Hz). Briefly, the number of resolvable pixels generated in a frame period is proportional to the mirror scan angle amplitude θ, the scanning mirror's diameter D, and the scanning frequency f:

$$N \propto \theta \cdot D \cdot f \qquad [18.1]$$

Accordingly, the product $\theta \cdot D$ and the high-speed horizontal scan frequency f are standard figures of merit for scanning mirrors, and the requirements for common display resolutions are listed in Table 18.1.

The MEMS device is an electromagnetically actuated single-crystal silicon biaxial scanning mirror as shown in Fig. 18.10. A roughly 1 mm diameter inner mirror is suspended by stiff horizontal scan flexures within a gimbal frame, which has a metallic coil patterned on it as shown in Fig. 18.11. Permanent magnets are assembled around the MEMS die, so that the Lorentz forces generated by the current flowing through the coil provide the actuating torques. The scanning mirror is driven into rotations about two orthogonal axes by the single coil. The target scanning trajectory consists of

Table 18.1 Scanning mirror requirements for common display resolutions

	VGA	WVGA	SVGA	HD720	SXGA	HD1080
Horizontal resolution (pixels)	640	840	800	1280	1280	1920
Vertical resolution (pixels)	480	480	600	720	1024	1080
$\theta \cdot D$ product (deg · mm)	7.0	9.4	8.8	14.1	14.1	21.1
Horizontal scan frequency, f (kHz)	18	18	22.5	27	38.4	40.5

Source: From Urey, 2004; Tauscuer *et al.*, 2010.

Optical MEMS for displays in portable systems 581

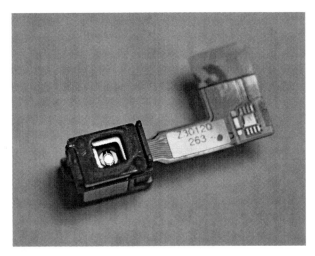

18.10 MicroVision magnetically-actuated MEMS scanning mirror.

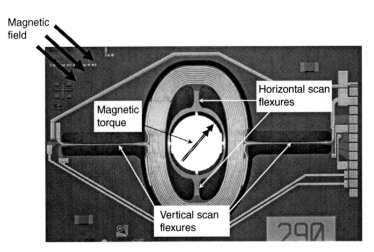

18.11 MicroVision MEMS scanning mirror die.

a 60 Hz sawtooth ramp used for the vertical raster scan, and a high-speed horizontal scan using a resonance of a vibration mode at a frequency in the range of 18–42 kHz for display resolutions from 480 lines (VGA) to 1080 lines (high-definition). The scanning mirror acts as a mechanical filter, in the sense that a 60 Hz drive waveform to the coil mainly generates rotations of the gimbal frame about the vertical scan flexures, while a high-frequency drive waveform only generates a scanning response when the frequency corresponds to a resonant mode of vibration, and so the two drive signals are superimposed and applied simultaneously to the coil (Davis et al., 2008; Yalcinkaya et al., 2006).

The inertial and elastic forces developed in high-speed resonant scanning are large enough to cause deformations of the mirror that could result in a projected laser spot with unacceptable aberrations. These forces will reach their peaks at the extrema of the oscillating rotations, so the resulting dynamic deformations of the mirror can cause the apparent sharpness of a LBS display to be diminished away from the center. As explained by Urey et al. (2000), in order to project an unaberrated laser spot throughout the extents of the scanned field-of-view, the amplitude of the dynamic deformation should be kept to one-tenth of the wavelength: that is, less than 63 nm peak-to-valley mirror deformation for projection of 635 nm laser light. This requirement factors strongly into the scanning mirror design, for example thin-films a few microns thick fabricated by surface micromachining processes would not supply enough structural stiffness to keep a 1 mm diameter mirror sufficiently rigid under high-speed scanning, and so scanning mirrors are commonly fabricated out of thicker single-crystal silicon material.

A discriminating feature of the LBS technique, compared to array-based projection, is that the use of a single scanning mirror as a pixel generator decouples the size of the MEMS pixel generator from the desired number of projected pixels. The projection display resolution can be scaled up with MEMS device changes that preserve the size of the reflective portion of the scanning mirror device and the overall die size. This is illustrated by comparing the sizes of the MEMS devices in Fig. 18.12, where the smallest MEMS die also happens to be the one providing the highest display resolution. By comparison, array-based pixel generators, such as DMD devices, must either grow larger to increase the display resolution, or shrink the size of the pixels and thereby suffer increased diffraction effects. Due to this scalability, LBS picoprojection with MEMS holds much promise for use in portable wireless systems.

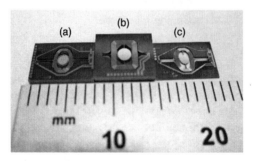

18.12 Comparison of MEMS die sizes for scanning mirrors corresponding to three different projection display resolutions. (a) WVGA; (b) SVGA; (c) HD 720.

The acronym LBS implies the scanning method is married to laser light sources, while array-based display engines such as DMD or LCD can use other light sources such as lamps or LEDs. Some scanned beam displays have been created, however, that use LED light sources (Freeman, 2003). Continued advances in laser technology will produce RGB sources with cost and efficiency that will likely make laser light a compelling choice for any picoprojector. In addition to their efficiency, laser light is attractive due to the wide color gamut spanned by combined RGB sources and the pleasing display produced by deeply saturated colors. A further capability enabled by the use of laser light is the ability to design the optical system such that the output beam divergence creates display pixels that grow proportionally to the projection distance (Brown *et al.*, 2011). This eliminates the need for bulky focusing projection optics and enables projectors to operate 'focus-free,' with every pixel in the projected display in focus for the viewer no matter how it is projected, even on curved or distorted projection surfaces.

Other MEMS devices used to demonstrate the LBS display include electrostatic comb-drive actuated devices, which seek to take advantage of the integration of the scanning mirror actuator with the other etched silicon features, such that no extra fabrication or assembly steps are needed to form the actuator. This is unlike magnetically-actuated MEMS, which require the formation of a magnetic field using permanent or electromagnets. Examples of electrostatic MEMS include those produced by the Fraunhofer Institute of Photonic Microsystems (IPMS). A noteworthy characteristic of these devices is that they operate resonantly on both the horizontal and vertical axes.

Such bi-resonant scanning creates a nonuniform spatial distribution of scan lines because of the Lissajous pattern followed by the projected laser spot. A side effect is the perception by the viewer of display artifacts, such as image break-up under eye *saccade* motion or motion of the projector (Hsu *et al.*, 2008). Consider the Lissajous pattern shown in Fig. 18.13, which represents one period of the scan trajectory that generates one image frame.

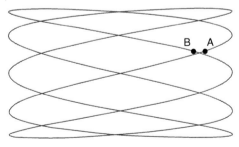

18.13 Illustrative example of a laser spot trajectory following a Lissajous figure from a bi-resonant scanning mirror.

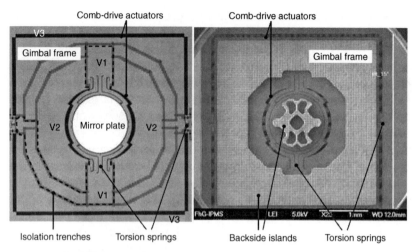

18.14 Electrostatic comb-drive scanning mirror by Fraunhofer IPMS (from Hsu *et al.* (2008)).

A Lissajous trajectory for a high resolution projection display will be far denser; however, this simple version makes a useful illustration. Consider a pixel displayed at position A and its neighbor at position B. In a high-density Lissajous trajectory, these could be two pixels that are nearest neighbors on the same horizontal line in the input image. Mapping the pixels A and B onto the Lissajous scan trajectory results in a separation in time that is nearly a full frame period. Relative motion between the viewer and the projected image that occurs during this time delay will cause a spatial separation, and therefore a break-up of the image. Rapid eye motion (or saccade), such as that occurring from the viewer's changing the focus of his attention from one portion of the image to another, or from involuntary blinking, similarly causes spatio-temporal image artifacts. The effect is somewhat similar to the color break-up or 'rainbow effect' that occurs for FSC displays (Järvenpää, 2004), due to temporal delay in displaying an image's color components. The Lissajous image artifact can be minimized by making the resonant vertical scan have a frequency sufficiently low to approximate a progressive scan. However, it is a major challenge to make a resonant vertical scan that provides a frame rate of 60 Hz using silicon MEMS, which, due to their high stiffness and low inertia, are generally more suited to resonant frequencies on the order of 1 kHz and greater. Fraunhofer IPMS has reported significant progress in this direction, recently having fabricated MEMS devices such as the one shown in Fig. 18.14 with vertical scan resonant frequencies around 100 Hz (Drabe *et al.*, 2012), which help make the artifacts less visible (Hsu *et al.*, 2008).

Btendo (2008) and Mirrorcle Technologies (Milanovic, 2007) are among some who have addressed the sawtooth ramp issue using electrostatic comb drives by adding some complexity to the MEMS fabrication in order to create vertically-offset comb finger structures, which enable the non-resonant quasistatic motion required for a sawtooth ramp scan. Because the electrostatic forces generated in the comb finger structures are still rather weak compared to electromagnetic forces, the comb-drive MEMS devices tend to require rather high voltages. Scanning mirror performance commensurate with VGA display resolution with 60Hz sawtooth frame rate leads to high drive voltages on the order of 150 V for either a horizontal or vertical scan axis (Hsu, 2008; Milanovic et al., 2004). The low power consumption and miniaturization sought by the choice of electrostatic actuation must therefore account for parasitic capacitive loads in the high-frequency (greater than 18 kHz for at least VGA display resolution) horizontal scan drive channel, and for the size, cost, and power consumption of high voltage generation. The parties involved with the MEMS–based LBS technology seem to weigh the tradeoffs rather differently, and there may very well be multiple paths to a competitive solution with acceptable size, power consumption, and cost.

18.4 Automobile head-up display

LBS projection technology is well-suited to automotive head-up display (Auto-HUD) applications. Because it reduces driver inattention and keeps his eyes on the road, AutoHUD is increasingly available as a safety-enhancement. As discussed by Freeman (2011), there are some particular requirements for Auto-HUD that are well-addressed by LBS. For one, laser light produces highly saturated color that helps the viewer distinguish the information displayed by the HUD from the background scene. For another, LBS completely turns off the laser light sources for 'black' pixels; this helps maintain the desired see-through characteristics at very low night-time ambient light levels compared to other technologies, which tend to have some background glow.

It is straightforward to simply position a picoprojector on the driver's side of the windshield for use as an Auto-HUD. Using narrowband laser light is instrumental to satisfying the requirement for a see-through display not obstructing the driver's view of the road, because the projection surface can be engineered to be transmissive across the visible spectrum except for narrowband reflectance corresponding to the laser colors, as illustrated in Fig. 18.15.

Auto-HUD as a safety feature is more effective if the display can be made to appear out in front of the car instead of on the windshield, so that the

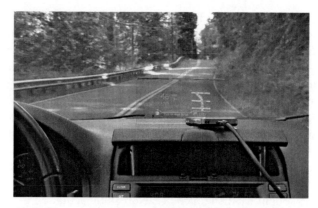

18.15 Direct projection see-through Auto-HUD using a surface with narrowband reflectance corresponding to a picoprojector's laser light sources.

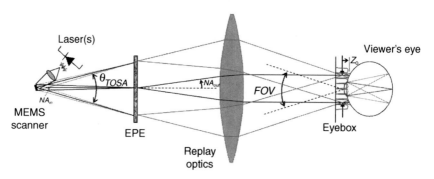

18.16 MicroVision Auto-HUD optical design.

information is better overlaid over the scene that should be the focus of attention anyway. MicroVision's optical design for Auto-HUD that achieves this effect is discussed in Freeman (2011) and is illustrated in Fig. 18.16. An exit-pupil expander (EPE) is positioned at an image plane. Relay optics transmit the image to the viewer's eye, and the role of the EPE is to create copies of the image that occupy a reasonably-sized eyebox so that minor movements of the driver's position do not cause the image to go in and out of view.

A compact implementation of the optical design is shown in Fig. 18.17. The system uses several optical elements that create an optical path length long enough to make the image appear to the viewer to be floating out beyond the windshield. A similar design using PicoP was a part of the Carrozzeria Cyber Navi HUD product released by Pioneer in 2012 and shown in Fig. 18.17.

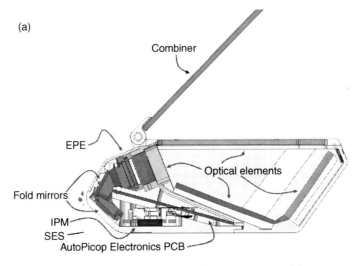

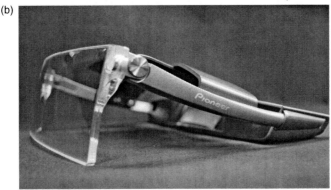

18.17 MicroVision Auto-HUD system, (a) schematic; (b) Carrozzeria Cyber Navi HUD by Pioneer.

18.5 Eyewear displays

The goal for so-called eyewear display is a lightweight and comfortable display that resembles a pair of glasses. The display can be occluded for applications where the viewer's awareness of her surroundings is not important, for example while consuming immersive entertainment. Or, the display can be see-through, which is desirable for augmented reality applications where supplementary information about the surroundings ought to be superimposed on the environment. The eyewear displays that involve MEMS are mainly the work of MicroVision, who applied LBS devices including MEMS to eyewear displays starting in 1997 (Tauscher *et al.*, 2010; Wine *et al.*, 2000).

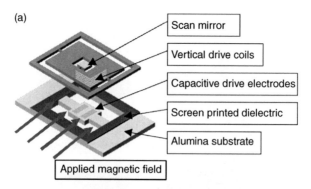

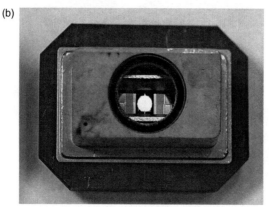

18.18 MEMS scanning mirror by MicroVision, using electrostatic actuation for the fast horizontal scan axis and electromagnetic actuation (permanent magnets not shown) for the sawtooth raster vertical scan. (a) Schematic; (b) vacuum-packaged device.

The optical design for eyewear dubbed RSD or virtual retinal display (VRD) is conceptually the same as that used for Auto-HUD, as shown in Fig. 18.16. The first MEMS scanning mirrors used by MicroVision design used parallel-plate electrostatic actuation for the fast scanning horizontal axis and electromagnetic actuation for the quasistatic, raster-scanning vertical axis. An early version is shown in Fig. 18.18.

Parallel-plate electrostatic actuation was a poor fit for the torsional scanning application: the large motion clearance for mirror rotation mandated a large electrostatic gap, which made for a correspondingly feeble torque dependent on the inverse of this gap-squared (Senturia, 2001, p. 135). The MEMS device required vacuum packaging in order for the weak electrostatic torque to balance the gas drag damping on the resonant scanning mirror, and in spite of this the device still required very high actuation voltages on the order of 200 V (Tauscher *et al.*, 2010). Early devices had

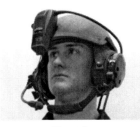 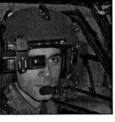 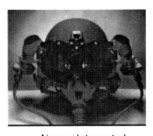

Nomad Spectrum Aircrew Intergrated Common Helmet

18.19 Military eyewear displays by MicroVision, using MEMS scanning mirrors and laser light sources.

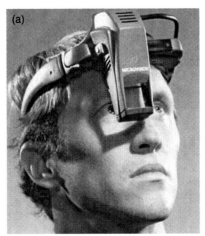 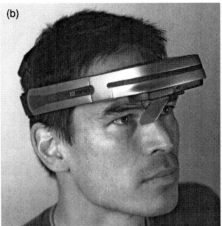

18.20 Commercialized wearable displays by MicroVision. (a) NOMAD I; (b) NOMAD II.

sealed-can vacuum packaging, with subsequent efforts made to minimize the size, including wafer scale vacuum packaging (Tauscher *et al.*, 2010). Several military display prototypes such as that shown in Fig. 18.19 came out of this work (Sainsbury and Clevenger, 2003), as did the general-purpose NOMAD I wearable display shown in Fig. 18.20.

By 2005 MicroVision was using electromagnetic actuation, as shown in Fig. 18.10, for both the resonant horizontal scan and the vertical sawtooth scan, which enabled the abandonment of both the vacuum packaging and the high voltage for MEMS actuation. These developments resulted in the NOMAD II product offering, shown in Fig. 18.20. At the time the only laser diodes suitable for the application were red, so the display was monochrome, and the form factor was still short of the desired eyeglass style, which limited its consumer adoption.

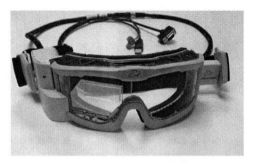

18.21 Eyewear display using LBS display engine.

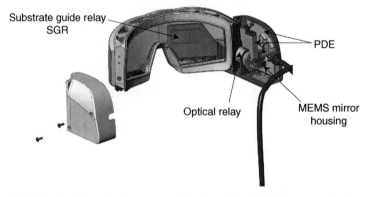

18.22 Optical layout of eyewear display using LBS display engine.

The MEMS design and light sources continued to mature, however, being used in the color LBS picoprojector engine discussed in Section 18.3.2. Progress toward color eyewear with better form factor has recently been made using this PicoP™ engine (DeJong, 2011), resulting in the prototype system shown in Fig. 18.21. In this work, the projection engine was moved from a position hanging out in front of the viewer's forehead to a more comfortable position at the side of the head, as shown in Fig. 18.22. An optical element called a substrate-guide relay (SGR) is introduced to deliver the image to the eye. The scanned beam from the PicoP Display Engine (PDE) is fed into the SGR through an input coupler. It propagates through the SGR by total internal reflection, and is waveguided to the output coupler as in Fig. 18.23, which reflectively turns the image to the viewer's eye. The display provides a WVGA resolution image viewable under any lighting conditions (DeJong, 2011). The use of the SGR is amenable to future miniaturization and eventual eyeglass form factor.

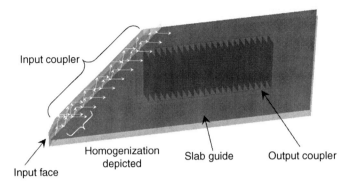

18.23 SGR ('slab guide') schematic.

18.6 Conclusion

We have seen above that MEMS devices can offer several improvements over the state of the art for mobile displays, namely LCDs. Some of the future trends for both direct-view and projection MEMS-based displays will parallel developments in conventional displays, with basic improvements in brightness, image quality, efficiency, and cost, and new features will become available, such as three-dimensional image display. Beyond these developments, the MEMS-based projection technologies in particular can provide some new capabilities that help people interact with their environments. Some thought-provoking demonstrations have been made by the MIT Media Lab's work on the 'Sixth Sense' wearable gesture interface (Maes and Mistry, 2009). Yet there are still intrinsic capabilities that have yet to be fully exploited.

A projection display that is sending light out into a scene simply needs an optical detector to collect reflected light and thereby obtain information about objects in the scene. Any projection system that puts structured light onto an object can use a camera and image processing techniques to obtain accurate three-dimensional information about the object's surface (Brown *et al.*, 2011). However, LBS projection provides additional unique capabilities, since there are inherently available electrical signals representing the two-dimensional mirror orientation. This enables rapid detection of the locations of objects within the projection field, and can be used to create a 'touch' interface capability for picoprojectors with the simple introduction of a photodiode sensor to the projection module. Furthermore, the time-of-flight of a laser pulse with invisible wavelength can be used to measure the three-dimensional position of objects in the projector's field-of-view, the principle behind light detection and ranging (LIDAR). Exploiting the LBS projector's use of light sources with distinct wavelengths brings possibilities for wireless and highly portable object analysis, for example wound analysis of the human skin (Brown et al., 2011). The introduction of optical MEMS displays into wireless systems could therefore simultaneously enable several new interactive capabilities that go well beyond the basic functions of a display.

18.7 References

Brosnihan T, Payne R, Gandhi J, Lewis S, Steyn L, Halfman M, and Hasgood N (2010), 'Pixtronix digital micro shutter display technology – A MEMS display for low power mobile multimedia displays', *Proc. SPIE*, vol. **7594**. DOI:10.1117/12.84834.

Brown M, Valliath G, Masood T, Niesten M, and DeJong D (2011), 'MEMS-based handheld projection systems and a survey of applications', *Proc. SPIE*, vol. **7930**. DOI:10.1117/12.876154.

Btendo (2008), Executive discussion on two uni-axial mirrors vs one bi-axial mirror scanningavailable (whitepaper). Available from: http://btendo.com/tech_papers_minor.html [accessed 30 August 2011].

Clarke P (2012), 'Qualcomm buys MEMS display startup, reportedly for $175M', *EE Times*. Available from http://cdn.eetimes.com/electronics-news/4235298/Qualcomm-buys-MEMS-display-startup [accessed 13 February 2013].

Davies C (2012), 'Mirasol production doused as Qualcomm chases licensing instead', *Slashgear.com*, available at http://www.slashgear.com/mirasol-production-doused-as-qualcomm-chases-licensing-instead-23239751/. [accessed 13 February 2013].

Davis W, Sprague R, and Miller J (2008), 'MEMS-based picoprojector display', *Proc. 2008 IEEE/LEOS Optical MEMS and Nanophotonics*, pp. 31–32. DOI: 10.1109/OMEMS.2008.4607813.

DeJong C D (2011), 'Full-color, see-through, daylight-readable, goggle-mounted display', *Proc. SPIE*, vol. **8041**. DOI:10.1117/12.883488.

Drabe C, Kallweit D, Dreyhaupt A, Grahmann J, Schenk H, and Davis W O (2012), 'Bi-resonant scanning mirror with piezo-resistive position sensor for WVGA laser projection systems', *Proc. SPIE*, vol. **8252**.

Floyd P D, Heald D, Arbuckle B, Lewis A, Kothari M, Gally B J, Cummings B, Natarajan B R, Palmateer L, Bos J, Chang D, Chiang J, Chu D, Wang L-M, Pao E, Su F, Huang V, Lin W-J, Tang W-C, Yeh J-J, Chan C-C, Shu F-A, and Ju Y-D (2006), 'IMOD™ display manufacturing', *SID Symposium Dig. of Tech. Papers*, vol. **37**, pp. 1980–1983. DOI:10.1889/1.2433440.

Freeman M (2011), 'MEMS scanned laser head-up display', *Proc. SPIE*, vol. **7930**. DOI:10.1117/12.879031.

Freeman M (2003), 'Miniature high-fidelity displays using a biaxial MEMS scanning mirror', *Proc. SPIE*, vol. **4985**, pp. 56–62. DOI:10.1117/12.477816.

Gally B J (2004), 'Wide-Gamut color reflective displays using IMOD™ interference technology', *SID Symposium Digest*, **35**. DOI:10.1889/1.1831063.

Hagood N, Barton R, Brosnihan T, Fijol J, Gandhi J, Halfman M, Payne R, and Steyn J L (2007), 'A direct-view MEMS display for mobile applications', *SID Symposium Dig. of Tech. Papers*, vol. **38**, pp. 1278–1281.

Hagood N, Payne R, Steyn L, Fijol J, Gandhi J, Brosnihan T, Lewis S, Fike G, Barton R, and Halfman M (2008), Pixtronix DMS™ display technology: ultra-low power consumption and exceptional video image quality. Available from http://www.pixtronix.com/technology/white-paper.asp [accessed 28 August 2011].

Hornbeck L (1996), 'Digital Light Processing and MEMS: An overview', *Advanced Applications of Lasers in Materials Processing/Broadband Optical Networks/Smart Pixels/Optical MEMs and Their Applications. IEEE/LEOS 1996 Summer Topical Meetings*, pp.7–8. DOI: 10.1109/LEOSST.1996.540770.

Hornbeck L J (2007), 'Combining digital optical MEMS, CMOS and algorithms for unique display solutions', *Proc. Electron Devices Meeting, 2007*, pp. 17–24. DOI: 10.1109/IEDM.2007.4418852.

Hornbeck L J (1998), 'Current status and future applications for DMD-based projection displays', *Proc. Fifth International Display Workshop IDW '98*.

Hsu S-T, Klose T, Drabe C, and Schenk H (2008), 'Two dimensional microscanners with large horizontal-vertical scanning frequency ratio for high resolution laser projectors', *Proc. SPIE*, vol. **6887**. DOI: 10.1117/12.761617.

Järvenpää T (2004), 'Measuring color breakup of stationary images in field-sequential-color displays', *Society of Information Display (SID) Symposium Digest of Technical Papers*, vol. **35**, No. 1, pp. 82–85. DOI:10.1889/1.1811462.

Legtenberg R, Gilbert J, Senturia S, and Elwenspoek M (1997), 'Electrostatic curved electrode actuators', *JMEMS*, vol. **6**, No. 3, pp. 257–265. DOI:10.1109/84.623115.

Lippert T M, Rash C E, and Hauser J (2000), 'A helmet-mounted laser display', *Information Display*, 1 January 2000, pp. 12–16.

Maes P and Mistry P (2009), 'Unveiling the "Sixth Sense," game-changing wearable tech', *TED 2009*. Available from: http://www.ted.com/talks/pattie_maes_demos_the_sixth_sense.html [accessed 30 August 2011].

Milanovic V (2007), 'Improved control of the vertical scan for MEMS projection displays', *Proc. IEEE/LEOS Int. Conf. on Optical MEMS and Nanophotonics*, pp. 89–90. DOI: 10.1109/JSTQE.2004.829205.

Milanovic V, Matus G, and McCormick D T (2004), 'Gimbal-less monolithic silicon actuators for tip-tilt-piston micromirror applications', *IEEE J. of Selected Topics in Quantum Elec.*, vol. **10**, No. 3, pp. 462–471.

Miles M, Larson E, Chui C, Kothari M, Gally B, and Batey J (2003), 'Digital Paper™ for reflective displays', *J. Soc. Inf. Display*, vol. **11**, No. 209. DOI:10.1889/1.1831708.

Optoma Technology Inc. (2011), Pico PK201 datasheet. Available at http://www.optomausa.com/products/detail/Pico-PK201, 2011 [accessed 28 August 2011].

Qualcomm (2009a), Operating principles of the IMOD drive (whitepaper). Available from: http://www.qualcomm.com/documents/mirasol-displays-operating-principles-IMOD-drive, 2009 [accessed 28 August 2011].

Qualcomm (2009b), Technology overview (whitepaper). Available from: http://www.qualcomm.com/documents/mirasol-displays-IMOD-technology-overview, 2209 [accessed 28 August 2011].

Sainsbury R and Clevenger J D (2003), 'High performance, versatile HMDs', *Proc. SPIE*, vol. **5080**. DOI:10.1117/12.500911.

Senturia S D (2001), *Microsystem Design*, Norwell, Massachusetts, Kulwer Academic Publishers. DOI: 10.1007/0-306-47601.

Tauscher J, Davis W O, Brown D, Ellis M, Ma Y, Sherwood M, Bowman D, Helsel M P, Lee S, and Coy J W (2010), 'Evolution of MEMS scanning mirrors for laser projection in compact consumer electronics', *Proc. SPIE*, vol. **7594**, 2010. DOI: 10.1117/12.843095.

Urey H (2004), 'MEMS scanners for display and imaging applications', *Proc. SPIE*, vol. **5604**, pp. 218–229. DOI: 10.1117/12.580450.

Urey H, Wine D, and Lewis J, (1999), 'Scanner design and resolution tradeoffs for miniature scanning displays', *Proc. SPIE*, vol. **3636**. DOI:10.1117/12.344656.

Urey H, Wine D, and Osborn T D (2000), 'Optical performance requirements for MEMS-based microdisplays', *Proc. SPIE*, vol. **4178**. DOI:10.1117/12.396486.

Wine D, Helsel M P, Jenkins L, Urey H, and Osborn T D (2000), 'Performance of a biaxial MEMS-based scanner for microdisplay applications', *Proc. SPIE*, vol. **4178**. 10.1117/12.396487.

Yalcinkaya A D, Urey H, Brown D, Montague T, and Sprague R. (2006), 'Two-axis electromagnetic microscanner for high resolution displays', *JMEMS*, vol. **15**, No. 4, pp. 786–794. DOI: 10.1109/JMEMS.2006.879380.

Index

active magnetic levitation, 376
active MEMS device, 493
active wireless IOP sensors, 439
actuation electrodes, 245
actuation voltage, 14–15
age-related macular degeneration, 442–3
AM0 standard spectrum, 387
amplitude-shift keying (ASK), 435
AMPS standard, 209–10
angular frequency, 384–5
anisotropic wet etching, 244
antenna switches, 213–14
  conventional antenna switch in a cell phone, 214
antennas
  applications, 177–8
  design considerations, 197–201
    biasing network, 198–9
    design flow and simulation, 197–8
    feflect-array cell, 200
    gain analysis for a reconfigurable aperture with lossy switches, 199
    insertion losses, packaging and reliability effects, 199–201
  future trends, 201–2
    circular Yagi-Uda antenna, 202
  reconfigurable antennas, 185–97
  reconfigurable feeding networks, 179–85
  RF MEMS for wireless applications, 176–202
  technology, 178–9
    technological approaches for the combination of RF MEMS, 178
application-specific integrated circuit (ASIC), 407, 441, 467, 475, 499
Argus-II, 447
artificial silicon retinas, 444

Australian Vision Prosthesis Group (AVPG), 448
automatic repeat request (ARQ), 34–5, 38–42
automobile head-up display (Auto-HUD), 585–7
  direct projection see-through Auto-HUD, 586
  MicroVision Auto-HUD optical design, 586
  MicroVision Auto-HUD system, 587
automotive radar
  components of RF MEMS, 522–32
    MEMS oscillators, 529–32
    MEMS phase shifters, 526–9
    switches and tunable capacitors, 522–6
  examples of automotive radar front-end technology, 532–7
    radar front-end consists of a T/R module, 534
    radiation pattern of the design with the Rotman lens and the antenna array, 538
    radiation patterns of the transmitting and receiving modules, 535
    RFMEMS SP4Tswitch and Rotman lens, 537
    Robert Borsch 77-GHz automotiveradar front-end, 535–7
    two 77-GHz RF MEMS automotive-radar front ends, 536
    University of Michigan 38-GHz RF MEMS car radar front-end, 532–5
  RF MEMS, 518–46
    LRR and SRR for advanced AQ1 safety features, 520

595

596   Index

automotive radar (*cont.*)
    requirements for car radar sensors, 522
    sensor types and architecture, 519–22
    unconventional MEMS radar beam-steering technologies, 537–46
    mechanically driven antenna platform, 541–5
    MEMS reconfigurable Vee-antennas, 546
    MEMS steerable leaky-wave antennas, 539–41
    MEMS tunable reflective microwave surfaces, 537–9

β-Newmark method, 370
band select filters, 218–19
    BAW, Bulk Acoustic Filter physical design, 219
    FBAR *vs.* SAW filters, 219
    radio part of a triple band GSM phone, 215
    SAW-filter structure, 215
bandwidth amplification, 372–5
base station controller (BSC), 41
base transceiver stations (BTS), 41
BCB cap packaging, 275–80
benchtop testing, 506–7
benzocyclobutene (BCB), 259, 328, 542
bi-directional data transmission, 501
bias circuitry, 87–8
    MEM switch with integrated germanium resistors and MIM capacitors, 89
    resistive materials, 88
biasing lines, 232, 245
biasing network, 198–9
    coupling mitigation techniques, 198
binary amplitude shift keying (BASK), 45
binary frequency shift keying (BFSK), 46–7, 48
binary phase shift keying (BPSK), 46
bioelectronic visual prostheses, 443
bit error, 46
bit error ratio (BER), 46
Boston Retinal Implant, 444, 451

'bridge' layer, 249
bulk micromachined waveguides, 68

capacitive contact switches, 237–40
    capacitive shunt switch, 237
    capacitive shunt switch in 'boosted' configuration, 241
    isolation parameters of a capacitive shunt switch, 238
capacitive energy harvesting, 352–5
    basic transduction principle, 353–4
    design variants of MEMS electret generators, 355
    kinematic design solutions of electrostatic harvesters, 353
    MEMS electret generators, 354–5
    properties and typologies, 352–3
capacitive powering, 497
capacitive switches, 81–2, 120–6
    CNT doped SiN layer, 83
    dielectric charging, 82
    measured reflection parameter, 124
    measured transmission parameter, 125
    transfer function that RF MEMS microswitches, 122
carbon nanotubes (CNT), 82, 94
Carefusion Alaris, 490
carrier sense multiple access with collision detection (CSMA/CD), 42–3
Carrozzeria Cyber Navi HUD, 586
Case Arm Aid System, 412
charge/discharge transient measurements (C/DCT), 299
charged device model (CDM), 320
chemical mechanical polishing (CMP), 84–5
code division multiple access (CDMA), 54
cognitive radio, 59
complementary metal oxide semiconductor (CMOS), 68, 101, 287, 320, 441, 467, 499
compound reconfiguration, 194–7
    frequency and pattern-reconfigurable pixel antenna, 196
    frequency and radiation pattern-reconfigurable Yagi patch antenna, 195

pixel reconfigurable antenna with planar monopole architecture, 196
techniques, 195
conductive powering, 497
conductive seed layer, 249
continuous-wave radar, 520–1
coplanar waveguide (CPW), 106–7, 140, 182, 232, 258, 297
corrosion, 295
corrosion sensors, 561–2
creep, 294

data-link layer, 38–43
  2G and 3G systems, 41
  medium access control (MAC), 42–3
  probability of bit error vs. E_b/N_0 with and without FECC, 40
data telemetry, 435
DC resistance, 430
deep reactive ion etching (DRIE), 69, 242, 244
depletion region, 386
device under test (DUT), 321
diamagnetic levitation, 376
dielectric breakdown of the air gap, 293
dielectric breakdown of the dielectric, 293
dielectric charging, 13–14, 292, 297
dielectric phase shifter, 158–9
  7-stage dielectric-block phase shifters, 159
  fabricated seven-stage phase shifters, 160
differential encoded phase shift keying (DEPSK), 49
differential phase shift keying (DPSK), 49
Digital Micromirror Device (DMD), 576–8
  schematic diagram, 577
'digital' tuning, 19
direct sequence spread spectrum (DSSS), 53
direct sequence ultra-wideband (DS-UWB), 58
discrete Fourier transform (DFT), 366
display pixel, 571
distributed-line phase shifter, 150–5

analog and digital implementations, 152–4
  circuit model of the MEMS bridges, 154
  DMTL phase shifters with MIM and MAM capacitors, 155
  phase shift and S-parameters vs. frequency of DMTL, 153
  two-units of the DMTL phase shifter, 154
comparison, 154–5
  analogue type DMTL phase shifters, 157
  digital-type DMTL phase shifters, 156
theory, 151–2
  CPW implementation and circuit model, 152
distributed MEMS transmission lines (DMTL), 22, 150–5
DLP projectors, 577
drug delivery
  biological constraints and requirements, 502–3
  effects of an inductive field on biological tissue, 502–3
  effects of biological tissue, 503
  formulas to simulate the electromagnetic properties of tissues, 504
  improvements and future generation device, 509–11
  inductive powering and uni-directional data system, 505–9
  MEMS approach, 493–502
    Debiotech's JewelPump, 493
    drug delivery system requirements, 494–6
    implantable MEMS micropump, 496
    MicroCHIPS micro-reservoir device, 494
    wireless data transfer requirements, 500–2
    wireless powering requirements, 496–500
  security concerns for wireless implants, 503–5
  wireless MEMS, 489–513

598   Index

drug delivery (cont.)
    Carefusion Alaris and Baxter's Spectrum Infusion System, 491
  wireless power and data, 490–3
    MiniMed Paradigm REAL-Time Revel System, 492
dwell time, 336
dynamic contour tonometer, 436
dynamic pull-in, 7–8

effective isotropic radiated power (EIRP), 60
effective series resistance (ESR), 429, 430–1
elastic deformation, 359
  temperature-induced, 294
elastic instability, 359
electret, 354
electric dampling coefficient, 349
electric power management, 381–4
  general composition, 384
electrical lifetime test (ELT), 301
electrical short, 296
electrical voltage overstress (EOS), 321
electro-magnetic switches, 230
electromagnetic actuation, 589
electromagnetic energy harvesting, 350–2
  basics on transduction principle, 351–2
  properties and typologies, 350–1
  schematics of linear electromagnetic generators, 351
electromagnetic fields, 503
electromagnetic mechanism, 110
electromigration, 295
Electronics Design Center (EDC), 412
electrostatic actuation, 523
electrostatic attraction force, 114
electrostatic discharge, 319–23
  damage caused by ESD to MEMS, 322
  DC leakage measurements on unprotected MEMS, 323
  effect on MEMS, 321–7
electrostatic force, 6
electrostatic mechanism, 109
electrostatic MEMS, 584
electrostatically actuated switches, 231

EnerChip, 479
energy harvesters
  design of kinetic energy harvesters, 356–84
  kinetic energy harvesters, 346–56
  other typologies, 384–91
    band diagram of photovoltaic cell p-n junction, 386
    basic module of thermoelectric harvesting devices, 390
    basic structure of commercial photovoltaic cell, 387
    design solution of kinetic rotating generators, 385
    kinetic rotating generators, 384–6
    photovoltaic cells, 386–8
    radio frequency identification systems, 388
    schematics of RF harvesters basic layout, 388
    thermoelectric effects in solid materials, 389
    thermoelectric generator composed of matrix of semiconductor modules, 391
    thermoelectric generators, 388–91
  powering wireless systems, 345–92
EPI-RET GmbH, 447
equivalent surface charge distribution, 314
ESD, 320
European Communication Commission (ECC), 505
European Radiocommunications Committee (ERC), 426
eyewear displays, 587–91
  commercialized wearable displays by MicroVision, 589
  LBS display engine, 590
  MEMS scanning mirror by MicroVision, 588
  military eyewear displays, 589
  optical layout using LBS display engine, 590
  SGR ('slab guide') schematic, 591

Faraday's law, 429
fast Fourier transform (FFT), 381
fatigue, 293

'fatigue limit,' 368
Federal Communication Commission (FCC), 426, 519
FeRAM memory, 441
ferroelectric RAM (FeRAM), 475
field sequential colour (FSC), 574
fieldeffect-transistor (FET), 209
figure of merit (FoM), 138
fine leak testing, 328
finite difference method, 369
finite-differences in the time-domain (FDTD), 197–8
finite element method (FEM), 370
fly-catching effect, 295
focusing ion beam (FIB), 334
forward error correction coding (FECC), 39
fracture, 295–6, 360
frequency bands, 208–9
frequency-dependent resistance, 430
frequency hopping spread spectrum (FHSS), 54
frequency reconfiguration, 186–9
 frequency-tunable MEMS-switched fractal antenna, 187
 frequency-tunable MEMS-switched slot antenna, 186
 frequency-tunable patch antenna based on variable reactive loading, 188
 frequency-tunable patch antenna with MEMS actuated ground plane, 187
 mechanisms, 186
 UWB elliptical monopole with a reconfigurable band notch, 188
frequency response function (FRF), 363
frequency-selective surfaces (FSS), 189
frequency-shift keying (FSK), 435
friction, 295
functional electrical stimulation, 410
fusing, 296

gas sensors, 562–3
 free-standing gas sensor response, 563
General Packet Radio Service (GPRS), 40

glaucoma, 435–7
 wireless intraocular pressure sensors for management, 435–42
glaucoma drainage implant (GDI), 470
global damping ratio, 363
Goldmann applanation tonometry (GAT), 436, 463–4
gross leak testing, 328
gyroscopic generators, 385

half power amplitude, 364
half power bandwidth, 364
half power points, 364
handheld picoprojectors, 570, 576–85
 Digital Micromirror Device, 576–8
 laser beam scanning projection, 578–85
He bomb, 335, 337
Health and Usage Monitoring Systems (HUMS), 556–7, 558
heterodyne receiver, 211–12
 basic principle, 211
 front end with filter to suppress image frequency, 211
high actuation voltage, 14–15
high resistivity silicon (HRS), 107, 284
high speed packet access (HSPA), 42
homodyne receiver, 212–13
 complete RF front end in a handset, 213
 front end, 212
human body model (HBM), 320
human metal model (HMM), 320
humidity sensors, 561
 response of a polyimide-based capacitive humidity sensor, 562
hybrid automatic repeat request (HARQ), 42
hybrid integration, 90–1
 tunable in frequency LNA with MEMS capacitors networks, 91

IEEE C95-2005, 403
IEEE Standard C95.1-2005, 426
impedance matching tuners, 129–30
 schematic diagram, 130
impulse radio (IR), 58
inductive coupling, 425

inductive powering system, 496, 497
    wireless and uni-directional data system, 505–9
        Class D amplifier wireless powering system, 506
        effects of distance between coils and foveation, 507, 509
        flow rate results, 508
        receiver device with LDO switching regulator, 508
        wireless powering system with Bluetooth circuitry, 510
inductors, 116–20, 243–4
    air-suspended inductors, 243
    RF MEMS concept, 117
    RF MEMS suspended square loop, 118
    S11 parameter, 119
insertion losses, 199–201
integrated circuit (IC), 229
Intelligent Medical Implants, 447, 451
inter-symbol interference (ISI), 51
interferometry, 334
International Commission on Non-Ionizing Radiation Protection (ICNIRP), 503
Internet service providers (ISP), 35
intraocular pressure implants
    active MEMS systems, 467–70
        layout of active circuitry implant, 468
        measured pressure *in vivo* with MEMS implant, 469
intraocular pressure (IOP), 435
intraocular pressure sensing
    passive miniature implants, 464–7
        IOP sensor micromachined in silicon with gold induction coil, 467
        passive pressure sensor implanted into the eye, 466
        pressure sensor created by Carter Collins, 465
intraocular pressure sensors
    active and passive MEMS contact lenses for IOP monitoring, 483–7
        Sensimed AG soft contact lens IOP sensor, 485
        soft contact lens technology, 484
    custom ultra-low-power autonomous, design of, 474–82
        capacitive pressure sensors, 479
        experimental evaluation, 478
        final one cubic millimetre operational IOP sensor, 481
        glass haptics used to secure IOP sensor, 482
        implant in human cadaver, 482
        layout of final stacked components, 481
        multi-layered enclosure, 480
        power consumption of the implants, 477
        recommended implant position, 476
        tadpole geometry of LCP encapsulated IOP sensor, 476
        ultra-low-power dual capacitance, 475
IP address, 35–8
IS-95, 10

JewelPump, 493

Karlsuss SB6 bonder, 266
Kelvin probe force microscopy (KPFM), 300
kinetic energy harvesters, 346–56
    capacitive energy harvesting, 352–5
        basic transduction principle, 353–4
        design variants of MEMS electret generators, 355
        kinematic design solutions of electrostatic harvesters, 353
        MEMS electret generators, 354–5
        properties and typologies, 352–3
    design, 356, 359–84
    electric power management, 381–4
        general composition, 384
    electromagnetic energy harvesting, 350–2
        basics on transduction principle, 351–2
        properties and typologies, 350–1
        schematics of linear electromagnetic generators, 351
    example devices, 355–6, 357–9

advantages and drawbacks of different typologies, 356
capacitive electret generator prototype with suspended mass oscillating in-plane, 359
capacitive generator with proof mass increased by an external tungsten ball, 358
four poles electromagnetic generator, 358
performances of different typologies of linear energy harvesters, 357
piezoelectric generator mounted on supportive board with electrical connectors, 356
frequency range of power generation, 370–5
application of axial preload to tune the resonance of piezoelectric generators, 372
bandwidth amplification, 372–5
energy harvester based on bi-stable structures, 375
resonance tuning, 371–2
resonance tuning strategy based on variation of the free length of generator, 371
structures with different response, 374
tuning strategy based on application of external forces to the oscillating mass of the generator, 373
tuning strategy of resonance frequency based on variation of gravity centre of the generator, 372
working principle of coupled three-dof generator, 374
magnetic levitation applied to suspensions, 375–81, 382, 383
basic principles, 376–7
capacitive generators with diamagnetic suspensions, 379
design solutions for the layout of generators based on diamagnetic levitating suspensions, 380

diamagnetic force acting on the graphite proof mass, 383
experimental FRF of levitated generator with cylindrical oscillating magnet, 379
experimental FRF of three diamagnetic levitated suspensions, 380
finite element model of the levitated suspension, 383
layout of inductive generators based on magnetic levitation, 378
multibody simulation of the harvester with asymmetric magnetic suspension, 382
schematics of levitating suspension, 379
simulated time response of magnetic levitated energy harvester, 381
solutions for energy harvesters, 377–8
static and dynamic behaviour, 378–81
piezoelectric energy harvesting, 346–50
basics on transduction principle, 348–50
output power measured on a piezoelectric generator, 349
piezoelectric cantilever for energy harvesting applications, 349
piezoelectric materials operation modes, 347
properties and typologies, 346–8
properties of piezoelectric materials for energy harvesters, 348
tools for designing and dimensioning, 359–70
analytic modelling of dynamic response, 360–4
basic structure for capacitive generators moving out-of-plane, 365
FRF of system under sinusoidal excitation and variable damping, 363

kinetic energy harvesters (*cont.*)
  mass-spring-damper single-dof-dynamic system, 361
  mechanical fatigue characterisation of electroplated gold samples, 369
  mechanical fatigue design, 367–8
  numerical modelling and FEM simulation, 368
  random excitation is separated in sinusoidal components with variable frequency, amplitude and phase, 368
  random vibrations, 366–7
  reduced order modelling, 364–6
  static dimensioning, 359–60
kinetic rotating generators, 384–6

laser beam scanning projection, 578–85
  comparison of MEMS die sizes, 582
  laser spot trajectory for LBS projection, 578
  MicroVision magnetically-actuated MEMS scanning mirror, 581
  MicroVision MEMS scanning mirror die, 581
  scanning mirror requirements for common display resolutions, 580
  schematic diagram of laser spot trajectory, 583
laser Doppler vibrometer, 300, 322, 332
lead zirconate titanate, 348
lead zirconium titanate, 239
leaky-wave antennas (LWA), 539–41
  simulated scattering parameters, 541
  SEM of fabricated LWA, 542
  unit cell of a MEMS-tunable LWA, 541
line-of-site (LOS), 61
linear generators, 350
liquid-crystal polymer (LCP), 475
Lissajous pattern, 583–4
lm bulk acoustic-wave resonators (FBAR), 75
load-shift keying (LSK), 435
loaded-line phase shifter, 142, 144–7
  comparison, 146–8
    phased array module and packaged loaded-line phase shifters, 148
  schematic diagram, 147
  equations, 144
  implementation, 144
  three classes for implementation, 145–6
    class I, II and III, 145
    CPW implementation of Class I phase shifter, 145
    proposed implementation, 146
local area network (LAN), 42
logical link control (LLC), 38
long-range radar (LRR), 520, 522
long-term evolution (LTE), 41
low-noise amplifier (LNA), 90
  band-switchable 56/72 GHz, 17–19
  micrograph, 18
  schematic diagram, 18
low pressure chemical vapour deposition (LPCVD), 69

M-ary phase shift keying (MPSK), 49
M-ary quadrature amplitude modulation (MQAM), 49
machine model (MM), 320
Mackay's blocking oscillator circuit, 409
maximum permission exposures (MPEs), 426
Meandered ribbon inductors, 243
mechanical micropumps, 495
mechanical or acoustic coupling, 296
mechanical parasitic damping ratio, 349
mechanical steering antenna, 541–5
  micro-mechanically driven antenna platform, 543
  radiation beam pattern, 544
Medical Implant Communication Service (MICS) band, 426
medium access control (MAC), 38, 42–3
MEMS oscillators, 529, 532
  MEMS variable Faraday cage, 533
MEMS phase shifters, 526–9
  comparison among several W-band RF MEMS phase shifters, 531
  distributed MEMS transmission line phase shifters, 527–9
  low-loss distributed two-bit W-band MEMS DMTL phase shifter, 528

MEMS-switched true-time delay (TTD) phase shifter networks, 526–7
MEMS tunable dielectric-block loaded-line phase shifter, 529
  binary-coded 4.25-bit W-band monocrystalline-silicon MEMS multistage dielectric-block phase shifters, 530
MEMS scanning mirror, 580
MEMS tunable high-impedance surface (HIS), 537–8
  periodic high-impedance metamaterial surface, 539
  phase shifter based on a DRW, 540
  surface impedance for electric beam steering, 540
MEMS wireless implantable systems
  basic considerations and characteristics, 403–8
    biocompatibility and protection of the implanted system, 405–6
    characteristics of biological and medical signals, 406–7
    design considerations, 407–8
    ISM frequencies and tolerance, 404
    legal considerations of the radio frequency, field strength and power levels, 403–5
  challenges of implantable/attached electronics, 417–19
    long-term power supply, 417–18
    micropackage of MEM/NEMS implantable systems, 418–19
    microwatt and nanowatt electronic circuits and transducers, 419
  conceptual diagram of an implantable system, 402
  essential building blocks of implantable system for the body, 402
  future trends, 419–20
  historical review and perspectives, 401–20
  progress from 1980 to 2010, 416–17
    3-dimension RF power receiving coil structure and circuit diagram, 416
  significant research on radio frequency implantable systems from 1955 to 1975, 408–15
    conceptual arm aid system of 1970, 413
    design approaches and samples of implant electronic devices, 413–15, 416
    human EMG implant device control legs motion of a dog, 413
    implant stimulation devices, 410–12
    implant telemetry circuits of the early 1960 era, 409
    implantable electronic control systems, 412–13
    implantable telemetry devices, 410
    K-5 tunnel diode telemetry unit and packaged telemetry device, 411
    single-antenna, two-frequency RF-link circuit, 415
    single-channel functional electrical stimulation circuit, 411
metal/air/metal (MAM) capacitors, 87–8
metal-insulator-metal (MIM) capacitors, 87–8, 299, 542
methods-of-moments (MoM), 197–8
micro-welding and wear, 294–5
MicroCHIPS, 494
microelectromechanical systems (MEMS)
  data-link layer, 38–43
  network layer mobility, 35–8
  physical layer, 43–59
  physical layer system design, 63–4
  telecommunications reliability monitoring, 550–66
    issues, 551–4
    multi-MEMS platform, 559–65
    reliability monitoring, 554–9
  transport layer, 31–5
  wireless, drug delivery using, 489–513
    biological constraints and requirements, 502–3
    improvements and future generation device, 509–11
    inductive powering and uni-directional data system, 505–9

microelectromechanical systems (MEMS) (cont.)
  MEMS approach to drug delivery, 493–502
  security concerns for wireless implants, 503–5
  wireless power and data, 490–3
  wireless intraocular pressure sensors, 463–86
    active and passive MEMS contact lenses for IOP monitoring, 483–7
    active MEMS systems for IOP implants, 467–70
    design of custom ultra-low-power autonomous IOP sensors, 474–82
    flexible parylene platforms, 470–4
    passive miniature implants for intraocular pressure sensing, 464–7
  wireless link budget, 59–63
  wireless techniques, 30–65
MicroFlex interconnection (MFI) technique, 449
micromachines, 424
microstrip lines, 247
microsystems technology (MST), 424
microwave microelectromechanical systems
  high-performance devices enabled by RF MEMS technology, 250–3
  next-generation wireless communications, 225–53
  RF MEMS complex circuit fabrication, 244–9
  RF MEMS technology, 228–31
  RF MEMS technology for high performance passive components, 231–44
MIL-STD-883H, 335
millimetre-wave impedance tuners, 22–4
  impedance tuner circuit with capacitive tuning, 23
  measured impedance coverage of DMTL impedance tuner, 23
  W-band DMTL impedance tuner, 23
millimetre-wave switches, 17–22
MiniMed Paradigm REAL-Time Revel System, 492

mirasol IMOD, 570
modulation, 45–53
  BER vs. E_b/N_0 for common binary modulation techniques, 50
  BER vs. E_b/N_0 for MPSK and MQAM systems, 52
  BFSK modulation, 46
  constellation for 16-PSK, 64-QAM and QPSK, 51
  correlation coefficient for common binary modulation methods, 49
  OOK (BASK) modulation, 45
  PRK (BPSK) modulation, 45
  spectral vs. power efficiencies of popular modulation schemes, 53
monolithic integration, 91–4
  low frequency noise measurement, 92
  MEMS capacitor with top dielectric and metal layers of CMOS substrate, 94
  post-processing of MEMS structures of CMOS or SiGe-based substrates, 92
  RF communication module, 93
monolithic microwave integrated circuit (MMIC), 287
MOSFET, 506
movable membrane, 86–7
multi-antenna switching, 181–4
  polarisation-reconfigurable antenna, 184
  switched multi-antenna systems composed of three CPW slot-based antennas, 183
  switched multi-antenna systems composed of two printed Yagi antennas, 182
  switched multi-antenna systems providing frequency reconfiguration, 183
multi-band integrated circuits, 17–22
multi-band orthogonal frequency division multiplexing (MB-OFDM), 58
multi-carrier ultra-wideband (MC-UWB), 58
multi-input multi-output (MIMO), 178, 222–3

array of transmitters and receivers and resulting transfer matrix H, 223
multi-MEMS platform, 559–65
　case study results, 563–5
　　approaches for MEMS sensors integration, 564
　　top layer of the MEMS-based environmental WSN platform, 565
　　corrosion sensors, 561–2
　　fabrication process, 560
　　gas flow sensors, 563
　　gas sensors, 562–3
　　humidity sensors, 561
　　temperature sensors, 560–1
multi-port switching, 181–4
multichip module (MCM), 440

n-type semiconductor, 386
nanoelectromechanical systems (NEMS), 94
neodymium iron boron (NdFeB), 351
network layer mobility, 35–8
　node mobility, 37
network mobility (NEMO), 38
NMT-450 analogue networks, 210
noise-budget, 62
non-mechanical micropumps, 495
non-semiconducting 'all-MEMS' system, 24
notching, 71

ocular implants
　challenges wireless ocular implants, 425–8
　　device constraints, 426
　　material biocompatibility constraints, 427–8
　　system constraints, 426–7
　considerations of ocular microsystems, 428–35
　　inductive power link for biomedical applications, 433
　　secondary stage simplified with an approximated linear model, 433
　necessary improvements in wireless ocular implants, 449–50
　　process flow of the CL-I^2 technique and an integrated RFID chip with flexible MEMS coil, 450
　RF MEMS coil design and microfabrication, 429–32
　　effective series resistance, 430–1
　　electroplated microcoil developed by EPI-RET, 432
　　inductive coupling through alternating electromagnetic field, 429
　　parasitic capacitance, 431
　　quality factor, 431–2
　　self-inductance, 430
　wireless considerations based on microsystems, 424–51
　wireless intraocular pressure sensors for glaucoma management, 435–42
　　conceptual illustration of the passive wireless IOP sensor, 438
　　overview of glaucoma disease, 435–7
　　wireless active IOP sensors, 440
　　wireless intraocular pressure sensors, 437–42
　　wireless passive IOP sensors, 440
　wireless microsystems applications, 435–49
　wireless retinal prosthetic systems, 442–9
　　age-related macular degeneration and retinitis pigmentosa, 442–3
　　Argus II system, 447
　　conceptual illustration of epiretinal prosthetic system, 446
　　epiretinal implant by German EPI-RET team, 447
　　first-generation and second-generation subretinal prosthetic devices, 445
　　several date telemetric links for wireless retinal prostheses, 448
　　several power telemetric links for wireless retinal prostheses, 448
　　wireless epiretinal prostheses, 445–9
　　wireless subretinal prostheses, 444–5

ocular implants (*cont.*)
  wireless telemetry link for power and data transmission, 432–5
    data telemetry, 435
    power telemetry, 433–5
ohmic metal to metal contact switches, 234–7
  electrostatic actuated ohmic switch, 235
  electrostatically actuated cantilever ohmic switch, 236
ohmic switch, 87, 120–6
  clamped-clamped RF MEMS series, 121
  lumped element network, 126
  measured reflection parameter, 122
  measured transmission parameter, 123
  transfer function that RF MEMS microswitches, 122
Ohm's law, 430
on-off keying (OOK), 44, 47, 48
open system interconnection (OSI), 38
optical interferometry, 300
optical microelectromechanical systems (MEMS)
  displays in portable system, 569–92
    automobile head-up display, 585–7
    eyewear displays, 587–91
    handheld picoprojectors, 576–85
    MEMS-based direct-view displays, 570–5
orthogonal frequency division multiplexing access (OFDMA), 59
orthogonal frequency division multiplexing (OFDM), 55–7
  adjacent (unmodulated) carriers, 56
  transmitter conceptual representation, 56
outgassing, 328
outgassing and adsorption, 296

p-n junction, 386
p-type semiconductor, 386
packaging, 199–201
parallel-plate movement, 5
parasitic capacitance, 429, 431

parylene C
  flexible platforms for long-term MEMS implants, 470–4
    designs and dimensions of variable capacitor and inductor/capacitor IOP sensors, 471
    foldable structure, 472
    illustration of pressure sensor, 473
    intended location of new IOP sensor, 474
    summary of processing steps, 473
passive absorption modulation, 501
passive components
  applications, 102–5
    fabrication technology platform, 102–3
    radar system employing electronically steerable beam antennae, 105
    super-heterodyne radio receiver, 104
    super-heterodyne radio receiver based on modified architecture, 105
  complex networks, 126–30
    impedance matching tuners, 129–30
    RF power attenuators and splitters/couplers, 128–9
    single pole double throws and switching matrices, 127–8
  high performance, 106–26
    electromagnetic properties and mechanical actuation, 106–13
    electrostatically controlled RF MEMS device, 110
    inductors, 116–20
    lumped element network scheme, 109
    ohmic and capacitive switches, 120–6
    pull-in/pull-out characteristic of an RF MEMS, 112
    S-parameter behaviour of standard CPW, 108
    variable capacitors (varactors), 113–16
  RF MEMS for wireless applications, 100–31

passive levitation, 376
passive MEMS device, 493
passive wireless IOP sensors, 437–9
path loss, 60
Peltier coefficient, 389
Peltier effect, 389
PerMX, 259
PerMX 3050 polymer, 283
PerMX cap packaging, 282–5
phase-locked loop (PLL), 21
phase reversal keying (PRK), 45–6
phase shift keying (PSK), 521
phase shifters
   applications, 163–6
      design sample, 163–6
      insertion loss (S21) and return loss (S11), 165
      phase shift from 75 GHz up to 95 GHz., 166
      phased array, 163
      W-band switched-line phase shifter, 164
   distributed-line phase shifter, 150–5
   global manufacturing, 161–3
      implementation of the switched-line phase shifter and package side view, 163
      linearity and intermodulation studies, 161–2
      packaging issues, 162–3
      thermal study, 162
   loaded-line phase shifter, 142, 144–7
   mixed-architectures and exotic phase shifters, 155, 158–61
   overview, 136–9
      antenna array in a beamforming application, 137
      latest published comparison, 138
      reflection-type phase shifter, 148–50
      RF MEMS for wireless applications, 136–69
   switched-line phase shifter, 139–42
phased array antennas, 247
phased arrays, 163, 184–5
   MEMS-integrated phased array, 185
   X-band RF MEMS phased array and measured radiation patterns of three phase shifts, 164

photoresist, 248, 280
photovoltaic cells, 386–8
physical layer, 43–59
   modulation, 45–53
   orthogonal frequency division multiplexing (OFDM), 55–7
   software radio and cognitive radio, 59
   spread spectrum, 53–5
   system design, 63–4
   ultra-wideband (UWB), 57–9
PicoP, 579–80, 590
   microvision PicoP MEMS-based LBS projection engine, 579
piezoceramics, 348
piezoelectric energy harvesting, 346–50
   basics on transduction principle, 348–50
   output power measured on a piezoelectric generator, 349
   piezoelectric cantilever for energy harvesting applications, 349
   piezoelectric materials operation modes, 347
   properties and typologies, 346–8
   properties of piezoelectric materials for energy harvesters, 348
piezoelectric mechanism, 110
piezoelectricity, 346
PIN-diode, 209
Pixtronix Digital Micro Shutter, 574–5
   Pixtronix Perfect Light display device, 575
   schematic diagram of device, 574
Pixtronix PerfectLight, 574
planar inverted-F antenna (PIFA), 181
plasma enhanced chemical vapour deposition (PECVD), 13, 69
plastic deformation, temperature-induced, 294
plastic distortion, 359
pneumotonometry, 436
polarisation reconfiguration, 192–4
   multi-mode antenna with CPW patch structure, 194
   multi-mode antenna with microstrip patch structure, 194
   spiral antenna, 193
   techniques, 193

poly-methyl-meta-acrylate (PMMA), 467
polycrystalline ceramics, 348
polydimethylsiloxane (PDMS), 427, 467
polymer bonding, 259
polyvinylidene fluoride (PVDF), 348
Poole-Frenkel effect, 299
power spectral density (PSD), 57
power telemetry, 433–5, 449
predictive modelling, 554
printed circuit board (PCB), 468
prognostics approach, 554
pseudo-random chip sequence (PRCS), 53–4
pull-in voltage, 6, 14, 15, 111, 227
pull-out voltage, 112, 227
Pulse Doppler-radar, 521–2
pulse position modulation time-hopped ultra-wideband (PPM-TH-UWB), 58
Pyrex glass, 265

Q-factor, 117, 226
quadrature phase shift keying (QPSK), 50
Qualcomm IMOD display, 570–3
  biostability of device reflectance, 573
  colour pixel formed by RGB subpixels, 572
  device forming a wavelength-dependent switchable reflector, 571
  subdivision of RGB subpixels into subpixel elements, 572
quality factor, 363, 431–2

radiation pattern reconfiguration, 189–92
  MEMS-actuated pattern-reconfigurable vee antenna, 190
  MEMS patch array, 190
  pattern-reconfigurable antenna, 191
  pattern-reconfigurable lens-array for a pyramidal horn antenna, 192
  reconfigurable reflect-array antenna, 192
  techniques, 189
radiative powering, 496

radio-frequency identification (RFID), 477–8
radio frequency microelectromechanical systems (RF MEMS), 3–25
  antennas for wireless applications, 176–202
    design considerations, 197–201
    future trends, 201–2
    reconfigurable antennas, 185–97
    reconfigurable feeding networks, 179–85
  applications, 16–24
  automotive radar, 518–46
    components, 522–32
    examples of automotive radar front-end technology, 532–7
    unconventional MEMS radar beam-steering technologies, 537–46
  communication standards, 209–10
    mobile standard evolution, 209
  complex circuit fabrication, 244–9
    FBK RF MEMS fabrication process, 246
    pillars used as stoppers to avoid short circuits, 248
  conventional component technology, 213–15
  design challenges, 14–16
    high actuation voltage, 14–15
    packaging, 16
    reliability, 15–16
    yield and temperature stability, 16
  fabrication steps, 81–8
    bias circuitry with MIM or MAM capacitors, 87–8
    dielectric considerations in capacitive switches, 81–2
    movable membrane, 86–7
    sacrificial layer considerations, 82–6
  fabrication technologies, 67–96
  GSM system frequencies, 208
  high-performance devices, 250–3
    5 bit switchable phase shifter, 253
    building block for switching matrices, 252
    measured isolation parameters of SPDT switch, 251

SP4T switch, 252
integrated technology for microsystem implementation, 88–94
  hybrid integration, 90–1
  low frequency noise spectral densities, 90
  monolithic integration, 91–4
MEMS-based technology, 216–20
multi-input multi-output (MIMO) systems, 222–3
operation principle, 4–14
  components electromagnetic analysis, 9–13
  electromechanical analysis of electrostatic MEMS, 4–9
  fabrication, 13–14
  parallel-plate model, 5
passive components for wireless applications, 100–31
  applications, 102–5
  complex networks, 126–30
  high performance, 106–26
phase shifters for wireless applications, 136–69
  applications, 163–6
  comparison of W-band phase shifters, 167
  distributed-line phase shifter, 150–5
  global manufacturing, 161–3
  loaded-line phase shifter, 142, 144–7
  mixed-architectures and exotic phase shifters, 155, 158–61
  overview, 136–9
  reflection-type phase shifter, 148–50
  RF MEMS phase shifter summary, 168
  SP3T V-band switch, 169
  switched-line phase shifter, 139–42
possible system in a package using MEMS, 224
receivers, transmitters and transceivers, 210–13
  frequency spectrum received by antenna of a handset, 211
  receivers and transmitters diversity, 220–2

reliability, 291–338
  analytical modelling, 309–19
  charging, 297–309
  electrostatic discharge, 319–23
  failure mechanisms overview, 292
  issues of MEMS packages, 324–37
RF circuits, 68–78
smart technologies, 79–81
  switches, 79
  traditional movable process, 80–1
  traditional process flow devices, 80
  vertical and lateral displacement configurations, 80
systems-on-a-chip, 223
technology, 228–31
  cantilever-based series ohmic metal-to-metal contact switch, 229
  capacitive shunt switch, 230
technology for high performance passive components, 231–44
  capacitive contact switches, 237–40
  electrostatically actuated devices, 231
  inductors, 243–4
  movable structures, 233–4
  ohmic metal-to metal contact switches, 234–7
  RF signal lines and biasing lines, 232
  variable capacitors, 240–2
UMTS (3G) system frequencies, 208
wafer-level packaging technology, 258–88
  electrical effects of packaging material on packaged devices, 261–3
  packaging with hard cap materials, 263–74
  packaging with polymer cap, 274–85
  wafer-level zero-level packaging, 259–61
wireless application technologies, 94–6
  NEMS varactor with a CNT-based membrane, 95

radio frequency microelectromechanical
    systems (RF MEMS) (*cont.*)
  RF NEMS switch with a clamped-
    clamped CNT-based membrane,
    95
  wireless architectures and front-ends,
    207–24
radio link control (RLC), 41
rapid eye motion, 584
Rayleigh formulation, 366
receiver diversity, 220–2
  approaches, 221
reconfigurable antennas, 185–97
  compound reconfiguration, 194–7
  frequency reconfiguration, 186–9
  polarisation reconfiguration, 192–4
  radiation pattern reconfiguration,
    189–92
reconfigurable feeding networks, 179–85
  multi-antenna and multi-port
    switching, 181–4
  phased arrays, 184–5
  tunable feeding networks, 180
  tunable matching networks, 180–1
reflection-type phase shifter, 148–50
  comparison, 149–50
    3-bit reflection-type phase shifter,
      151
    schematic diagram, 150
  implementation
    tunable capacitor, tunable
      distributed loaded-line and
      switched reflection line, 149
  theory, 148–9
    implementation, 148
release time, 8–9
reliability, 291–338
  analytical modelling, 309–19
  charging, 297–309
    capacitive electrostatically driven
      RF MEMS switch, 298
    RF MEMs capacitive switch, 297–9
  definition, 291
  electrostatic discharge, 319–23
    damage caused by ESD to MEMS,
      322
    DC leakage measurements on
      unprotected MEMS, 323

  effect on MEMS, 321–7
  experimental charging evaluation,
    299–309
    accelerated testing, 304–7
    biasing scheme, 308
    C-V characteristic measurements,
      301
    capacitance measurements, C-V
      curve measurements and C-V
      curve evolution, 306
    component waveforms and
      resulting virtual voltage sources,
      308
    definition of C-V measurement
      main parameters, 302
    down-state and up-state
      capacitance of a switch, 304
    evolution of positive pull-in
      voltage of two different devices,
      307
    localisation of charging
      mechanisms, 307–9
    main difference between MIM and
      MEMS devices, 303
    motion measurement of MEMS
      beam, 300
    reliability testing techniques for
      charging assessment, 302–4
    results of an experiment where two
      sources of actuation waveforms
      were used, 309
    simplified MEMS structure, 303
    test structures, 302
    two charging mechanisms with two
      different time constant, 307
    voltage shift between two C-V
      curves, 305
  failure mechanisms in RF MEMS,
    292–6
    corrosion, 295
    creep, 294
    dielectric breakdown of the air gap,
      293
    dielectric breakdown of the
      dielectric, 293
    dielectric charging, 292
    electrical short, 296
    electromigration, 295

fatigue, 293
fracture, 295–6
friction, 295
fusing, 296
mechanical or acoustic coupling, 296
micro-welding and wear, 294–5
outgassing and adsorption, 296
self-biasing, 295
stiction, 293
temperature-induced elastic deformation, 294
temperature-induced plastic deformation, 294
hermeticity testing of packages, 328–37
cap deflection, 332–4
cap deflection in vacuum/air, 334–5
capped resonator, 329, 332
deflection measurements before and after He storage of sealed package, 336
deflection response to a change in pressure, 334
helium leak rate, 329–31
helium pressurisation, 335–7
measured Q factor of capped resonator during storage, 330
measured Q on a sealed resonator, 332
membrane deflection of two packages measured by inferometry, 335
MEMS switch packaged with Pyrex cap, 333
outgassing, 331–2
result of He fine leak test performed on Si package, 336
schematic cross-section of the test structure, 331
issues of MEMS packages, 324–37
closing time of RF MEMS switch as function of ambient pressure, 325
device parameters affected by ambient conditions, 324–8
measured pull-in and pull-out voltage of micromirror, 327
measured Q factor several MEMS resonators, 325
measured resistance of suspended beam, 326
measured response of RF MEMS switch at different pressures, 324
MEMS resonator in a wafer-level package, 328
non-uniform charge distribution in parallel-plate and generalised distributed plates approximations, 311–19, 320
charging induced asymmetry of C-V characteristic observed in case of cycling under bipolar actuation, 318
corresponding linear variations of air gap and equivalent charge distributions, 318
2D+ model description, 313–15
electrostatic force exerted on moving plate, 313
evolution of VPO and VPI vs σ^2, 317
model implications, 315–19
model of MEMS device with non-uniform trapped charge and air-gap distributions, 314
simulated narrowing of the d-V curve, 316
stable C-V characteristics, 319
stable C-V corresponding to the figure in case where $a0$ and $b0$ equal respectively to 1.5μm and 6μm, 320
stiction thought experiment, 312
thought experiment, 312–13
uniform charge in parallel-plate approximation, 309–11, 312
measured fast C-V characteristic, 312
schematic development of Wibbler's model, 310
simulated C-V curve with uniform charging, 311
reliability effect, 199–201
reliability models, 553
reliability research, 552

remote control, 401
resonance frequency, 10
resonance tuning, 371–2
restoring mechanical force, 114
retinal ganglion cells (RGC), 445
retinal prosthesis, 442
retinal scanned display (RSD) systems, 579
retinitis pigmentosa, 442–3
retransmission time-out (RTO), 34
RF circuits
  MEMS-based technologies, 68–78
    3-D broadside coupler, 78
    3-D integrated polymer technology with localised surface micromachining, 78
    attenuation and quality factors of bulk micromachined CPW, 70
    bulk micromachined antenna, 71
    bulk micromachined coplanar lines, 69
    bulk micromachined inductors, 72
    DRIE efficiency, 73
    inductors with and without micromachining, 73
    levels for bulk and surface-micromachined technologies, 76
    notching effect on large etched holes, 74
    surface-micromachined configurations, 75
    surface-micromachined CPW, 77
RF MEMS switches, 216–18, 522–4
  comparison of RF MEMS switches, 525
  electrostatically actuated MEMS switch types, 523
  in-line DC-contact MEMS series switch, 524
  layout of an early prototype MEMS antenna switch, 218
  quad-band antenna switch, 216
  SPDT and SPST switches, 217
RF power attenuators, 128–9
  schematic diagram, 128
RF signal lines, 232
rotating generators, 350
Rotman lens, 536
round trip time (RTT), 33–4

sacrificial layer, 82–6
  flat metallic MEM bridge, 86
  gold bridge anchorage, 84
  MEM planarisation process flow, 85
  non-flat metallic membrane due to bottom relief, 84
  shunt switch, 85
second-harmonic generation (SHG), 580
Second Sight, 451
Second Sight Medical Products, Inc., 446
Seebeck coefficient, 389
Seebeck effect, 388
self-actuation, 295
self-biasing, 295
self-inductance, 430
series switches, 12–13
  MEMS cantilever, 12
  MEMS switch circuit with metal-to-metal contact, 13
  RF MEMS cantilever, 12
short-range radar (SRR), 519–20, 522
  applications, 520
SHOWWX, 579
shunt bridge, 10
shunt capacitive switches, 9–11
  MEMS bridge to a coplanar line in up- and down-states, 10
  shunt capacitive MEMS switch circuit, 11
  shunt RF MEMS switch, 11
silicon controlled rectifier (SCR), 323
single-pole double-throw (SPDT) switch, 127–8, 182, 228
  schematic diagram, 127
single-pole four-throw (SP4T) switch, 228
single-pole single-throw (SPST) switch, 216
singlepole–quadruple-throw (SP4T) switch, 536
skip depth, 430
slide film damping, 361
slow-wave structure phase shifter, 160–1
  picture and measurement, 161
smart sensor nodes, 557
software radio, 59
specific absorption rate (SAR), 426, 503

spiral inductors, 243–4
splitters/couplers, 128–9
spread spectrum, 53–5
  basic DSSS, 54
spring force, 5
square loop inductor, 117
squeeze film damping, 361
static pull-in, 5–7
  electrostatic and spring forces
    magnitude acting on a
    suspended plate, 6
stiction, 293, 310
stochastic resonance, 375
stress concentration factor, 360
sub-carrier modulation, 501
subretinal prosthesis, 444
substrate-guide relay (SGR), 590
switchable capacitors, 9–11
  MEMS bridge to a coplanar line in
    up- and down-states, 10
  shunt capacitive MEMS switch
    circuit, 11
  shunt RF MEMS switch, 11
switched-line phase shifter, 139–42
  comparison, 142
    schematic diagrams, 143
  implementation for size reduction,
    140–2
    π-network, 142
    SP2T and SP4T architectures, 141
    transmission lines and semi-
      lumped architectures, 142
    two bit phase shifter based on
      SP2T and SP4T architectures,
      141
  rotary switches, 159–60
    microphotograph and performance,
      160
  standard implementation, 139–40
    shunt switch CPW 3-bit phase
      shifter implementation, 140
  theory
    3-bit switched-line phase shifter,
      139
switched-loaded-line phase shifter, 155,
  158
  schematic diagram, 158
  small UAV, 158
switching matrices, 127–8

switching time, 8, 15
Symbiq, 490
symbol error result (SER), 52
systems-on-a-chip, 223

tele-actuation, 401
tele-sensing, 401
telecommunications reliability
  monitoring
  issues, 551–4
    implications of electronics
      reliability, 552–3
    monitoring and construction of
      reliability models, 553
    prognostics solutions, 554
  multi-MEMS platform, 559–65
    case study results, 563–5
    corrosion sensors, 561–2
    gas flow sensors, 563
    gas sensors, 562–3
    humidity sensors, 561
    temperature sensors, 560–1
  using wireless MEMS, 550–66
    advantages of wireless MEMS,
      557–9
    current monitoring solutions, 555–6
    development of solutions using
      MEMS technology, 556–7
    scientific publications, 558
telemetry, 401
temperature sensors, 560–1
  typical temperature linear response,
    561
thermal/electro-thermal mechanism,
  110–11
thermal wafer-to-wafer bonding, 259
thermally stimulated depolarization
  current measurements (TSCD),
  299
thermoelectric generators, 388–91
thin-film deposition/growth bonding,
  259
Thomson coefficient, 389
Thomson effect, 389
time division multiple access (TDMA),
  210
tonometry, 436
Townsend arc, 293
transcutaneous powering, 496

transmission control protocol (TCP), 30, 31–3
transmission line junction, 139
transmission line pulsing (TLP), 320
transmitter diversity, 220–2
transmitter matching, 219–20
  impedance matching network, 220
transport layer, 31–5
  packet loss detected, 33
trap assisted tunnelling, 299
triboelectric charging, 320
Triggerfish, 484
true time delay (TTD), 138
tunable capacitor, 524–6
tunable filters, 24
tunable matching networks, 180–1
  input impedance of a GSM-900 PIFA antenna, 181
tunnel vision, 442
5-tuple, 36
2net hub, 502

ultra-wide band (UWB), 57–9, 519
  capacity vs. SNR and bandwidth, 58
  spectral masks, 57
Universal Mobile Telecommunication System (UMTS), 41
user datagram protocol (UDP), 31

variable capacitors (varactors), 113–16, 240–2
  RF MEMS fabricated in a surface micromachining process, 114
Vee-antennas, 546
  concept of micro-mechanically reconfigurable Vee-antenna, 545
  E-plane beam-steering patterns, 545
very large scale integrated circuits (VLSI), 416
virtual retinal display (VRD), 588
voltage-controlled oscillator (VCO), 103
  band-switchable 50/68 GHz, 19–22
    measured phase noise, 21
    micrograph, 20
    oscillation frequency, 21
    schematic diagram, 20
voltage standing wave ratios (VSWR), 22

wafer-level packaging technology, 258–88
  electrical effects of packaging material on packaged devices, 261–3
    CPW, Si cap-packaged CPW and PerMX cap-packaged CPW, 262
    Zc and εeff as function of cavity depth, 263
  example of zero-level packaging, 260
  packaging with hard cap materials, 263–74, 275
    concept of glass-cap packaging with BCB sealing ring, 266
    concept of Si cap packaging with AuSn sealing ring, 264
    concept of silicon-cap packaging with BCB sealing ring, 269
    fabricated glass cap and glass-cap packaged CPW, 268
    fabricated sealing ring before packaging, 265
    glass-cap packaging with BCB sealing ring, 265–8
    measured S-parameters before and after glass-cap packaging with BCB sealing ring, 268
    measured S-parameters before and after Si cap packaging with AuSn sealing ring, 265
    measured S-parameters before and after Si cap packaging with BCB sealing ring, 272
    measured S-parameters before and after Si cap packaging with PerMX sealing ring, 275
    packaged CPW line, 264
    packaging process flow, 267, 270
    PerMX 3050 process conditions, 273
    process flow of Si cap packaging using PerMX sealing ring, 273
    Si cap-packaged CPW with a PerMX ring, 274
    Si cap-packaged CPW with BCB ring, 271
    Si cap packaging with a AuSn sealing ring, 264–5

Si cap packaging with a PerMX sealing ring, 272
Si cap packaging with BCB sealing ring, 268
packaging with polymer cap, 274–85
  ANSYS modelling results on BCB cap deflection and chip deflection, 276
  BCB cap packaging, 275–80
  BCB cap-packaging results, 279
  BCB cap packaging with vertical interconnect, 280–2
  fabrication results, 282
  measured BCB cap profiles, 279
  measured PerMX cap profiles, 286
  measured S-parameter after PerMX cap packaging, 287
  measured S-parameter before PerMX cap packaging, 287
  measured S-parameters of BCB-capped CPW, 280
  measured S-parameters of RF test patterns, 284
  packaging process flow of flip-chip compatible BCB cap packaging, 281
  PerMX cap-packaged coplanar, 287
  PerMX cap packaging, 282–5
  PerMX packaging process, 285
  PerMX packaging results, 286
  process flow of BCB cap packaging, 278
  RF test patterns, 283

wafer-level zero-level packaging, 259–61
wafer-level zero-level packaging, 259–61
white light interferometry (WLI), 300
wireless data transfer requirements, 500–2
  bi-directional wireless data transfer circuit, 501
wireless epiretinal prostheses, 445–9
wireless intraocular pressure sensors, 437–42
wireless link budget, 59–63
wireless local area networks (WLAN), 35
wireless medical telemetry service (WMTS) spectrum, 502
wireless powering requirements, 496–500
    powering circuit with multiple (1–3) receiving coils, 500
    powering circuit with multiple (1–3) transmitting coils, 500
  wireless power circuit, 497
wireless retinal prosthetic systems, 442–9
wireless sensor networks (WSNs) technology, 551
  modules, 558, 559, 564
wireless subretinal prostheses, 444–5
Wisenet, 501
WLAN standard 802.11, 40

ZigBee, 501

Lightning Source UK Ltd.
Milton Keynes UK
UKOW03n2153180813

215569UK00002B/4/P